# Sexuality

**RAYMOND ROSEN**

*University of Medicine and Dentistry of New Jersey*
*Rutgers Medical School*

**ELIZABETH HALL**

RANDOM HOUSE
New York

# Sexuality

FIRST EDITION
9 8 7 6 5 4 3 2 1
Copyright © 1984 by Random House, Inc.

**Library of Congress Cataloging in Publication Data**

Rosen, Raymond, 1946–
    Sexuality.

    Bibliography: p.
    Includes index.
    1. Sex instruction.  2. Sex instruction for youth.
3. Sex.  4. Hygiene, Sexual.    I. Hall, Elizabeth, 1929–    II. Title.
HQ35.2.R67  1984      306.7      83-24726
ISBN 0-394-33248-2

Manufactured in the United States of America

Designed by Betty Binns Graphics

## *Permissions Acknowledgments*

From Athanasiou, R., P. Shaver, and C. A. Tavris, "Sex," *Psychology Today*. Reprinted from Psychology Today Magazine. Copyright © 1970 Ziff-Davis Publishing Company.

From Barbach, Lonnie, and Linda Levine, *Shared Intimacies: Women's Sexual Experiences.* Copyright © 1980 by Lonnie Barbach and Linda Levine. Reprinted by permission of Doubleday & Company, Inc.

From Barbach, Lonnie, *For Each Other: Sharing Sexual Intimacy.* Copyright © 1982 by Lonnie Barbach. Reprinted by permission of Doubleday & Company, Inc.

From Bell, A. P., M. S. Weinberg, and S. K. Hammersmith, *Sexual Preference,* Indiana University Press, 1981. Reprinted by permission of Indiana University Press.

From Bell, D. H., *Being a Man: The Paradox of Masculinity.* Copyright © 1982 by The Lewis Publishing Company. Published by The Lewis Publishing Company, Fessenden Road, Brattleboro, Vermont 05301.

From Bell, Ruth, et al., *Changing Bodies, Changing Lives.* Copyright © 1980 by Ruth Bell. Reprinted by permission of Random House, Inc.

From Berscheid E., E. Walster, and G. Bohrnstedt, "The Happy American Body, A Survey Report," *Psychology Today*. Reprinted from Psychology Today Magazine. Copyright © 1973 Ziff-Davis Publishing Company.

From Kolodny, R. C., "Evaluating Sex Therapy: Process and Outcome at the Masters and Johnson Institute," *Journal of Sex Research.* Copyright © 1981. Reprinted by permission of *The Journal of Sex Research,* a publication of The Society for the Scientific Study of Sex.

From Kriss, Regina, "Self-Image and Sexuality After Mastectomy." In David G. Bullard and Susan E. Knight (eds.), *Sexuality and Physical Disability,* St. Louis, 1981, The C. V. Mosby Co. Permission granted by C. V. Mosby Company and Regina Kriss, Ph.D.

From Lenz, R., and B. Chaves, "Becoming Active Partners." Quoted from the movie "Active Partners," by permission of the producer Marvin Silverman and authors R. Lenz and B. Chaves. Copyright © 1979.

From Masters, W., and Johnson, V. E., interviewed by M. H. Hall. "A Conversation with Masters and Johnson," *Psychology Today.* Reprinted from Psychology Today Magazine. Copyright © 1969 Ziff-Davis Publishing Company.

From Money, J., and C. Bohmer, "Prison Sexology: Two Personal Accounts of Masturbation, Homosexuality, and Rape," *Journal of Sex Research.* Copyright © 1980. Quoted by permission of *The Journal of Sex Research,* a publication of the Society for the Scientific Study of Sex.

From Moser, D. L., "Sex Guilt and Sex Myths in College Men and Women," *Journal of Sex Research.* Copyright 1979. Quoted by permission of *The Journal of Sex Research,* a publication of the Society for the Scientific Study of Sex.

From Perlmutter, L. H., T. Engel, and C. H. Sager. "The Incest Taboo: Loosening Sexual Boundaries in Remarried Families," *Journal of Sex and Marital Therapy.* © Copyright 1982 Brunner/Mazel, Inc.

From Rasmussen, P. K., and L. L. Kuhn, "The New Masseuse: Play for Pay," in C. Warren (ed.), *Sexuality: Encounters, Identities, and Relationships.* Copyright © 1977. Reprinted by permission of Sage Publications, Inc.

From Roberts, E. J., "Children's Sexual Learning: A Report on the Project on Human Sexual Development, 1974–1980." Television Audience Assessment, Inc., Cambridge, Massachusetts, 1982. © 1982 Elizabeth Jeanine Roberts. All Rights Reserved.

From Roth, Philip, *Portnoy's Complaint.* Copyright © 1967, 1968, 1969 by Philip Roth. Reprinted by permission of Random House, Inc.

From Rubin, Lillian, *Worlds of Pain.* Copyright © 1976 by Lillian Breslow Rubin. Reprinted by permission of Basic Books, Inc.

From Rubin Z., L. A. Peplau, and C. T. Hill, "Loving and Leaving: Sex Differences in Romantic Attachments," *Sex Roles.* Copyright © 1981. Reprinted by permission of Plenum Publishing Company.

From Sanford, L. T., *The Silent Children.* Copyright © 1980. Reprinted by permission of Doubleday & Company, Inc.

From Schulman, H., "Common Discomforts of Pregnancy," *Childbirth Educator.* Copyright © 1982 Harold Schulman. Reprinted by permission.

From Smith, D., "Spinal Cord Injury." In David G. Bullard and Susan E. Knight (eds.), *Sexuality and Physical Disability,* St. Louis, 1981, The C. V. Mosby Co. Reprinted by permission.

From Starr, Bernard D., and Marcella Bakur Weiner, *The Starr-Weiner Report on Sex and Sexuality in the Mature Years.* Copyright © 1981 by Bernard D. Starr, Ph.D., and Marcella Bakur Weiner, Ed.D. Reprinted with permission of Stein and Day Publishers.

From "A Survey of College Women's Experience with and Attitudes Toward Pelvic Examinations," *Women and Health,* Vol. 4, Copyright © 1979. Reprinted by permission of The Haworth Press, Inc.

From Sussman, L., and E. Bordwell, *The Rapist File.* Copyright © 1981. Reprinted courtesy of Chelsea House Publishers.

From Tanzer, D., "Natural Childbirth: Pain or Peak Experience?", *Psychology Today.* Reprinted from Psychology Today Magazine. Copyright © 1977 Ziff-Davis Publishing Company.

From Tavris, C. A., "Women in China: The Speak-Bitterness Revolution," *Psychology Today.* Reprinted from Psychology Today Magazine. Copyright © 1974 Ziff-Davis Publishing Company.

From *Teenage Pregnancy: The Problem That Hasn't Gone Away,* published by The Alan Guttmacher Institute, New York, 1981. Reprinted with permission.

From Tennov, Dorothy, *Love and Limerance.* Copyright © 1979 by Dorothy Tennov. Reprinted with permission of Stein and Day Publishers.

From Terkel, Studs, *Working: People Talk About What They Do All Day and How They Feel About What They Do.* Copyright © 1972 by Studs Terkel. Reprinted by permission of Pantheon Books, a Division of Random House, Inc.

From Thorton, V., "Growing Up with Cerebral Palsy." In David G. Bullard and Susan E. Knight (eds.), *Sexuality and Physical Disability,* St. Louis, 1981, The C. V. Mosby Co. Reprinted by permission.

From Tollison, C. D., and H. E. Adams, *Sexual Disorders: Treatment, Theory, and Research.* Copyright © 1979. Reprinted by permission of Gardner Press.

From Vance, E. B., and N. W. Wagner, "Written Descriptions of Orgasm: A Study of Sex Differences," *Archives of Sexual Behavior.* Copyright © 1976. Reprinted by permission of Plenum Publishing Corporation and the authors.

From Zilbergeld, Bernie, *Male Sexuality.* Copyright © 1978. Reprinted by permission of Little, Brown, and Company.

# To the Student

Sexuality is a far-reaching topic. It goes beyond basic facts about sexual activity and reproduction. The study of sexuality leads us to explore sexual identity and behavior from a variety of perspectives. It also addresses such questions as What makes us sexual beings? What forces shape and mold this central facet of our lives? What is the meaning of sexuality for each individual?

There is also a practical side to the study of sexuality. We need to know how to maintain sexual health and well-being, how sexual decisions are made, and how to deal with everyday concerns like contraception and sexually transmitted diseases. By such study, we should gain a greater understanding of our own behavior and the behavior of those around us.

If this were a textbook in chemistry or statistics, it would provide you with a set of facts and the skills to apply them. In a course on sexuality, however, facts become meaningful only in the context of beliefs, values, and emotions. Because we are convinced of the importance of this larger context, we have tried to write a textbook that places sexuality within a broad perspective that considers the "whole person"—the thinking person, the valuing person, the feeling person, and the behaving person. We have considered all these aspects when writing the book.

**Information** As a thinking person, you need to evaluate and assimilate large numbers of theories, facts, and research findings. Information about human sexuality has been expanding at a rapid pace. An understanding of the latest information about sexual biology and behavior is useful and important. This textbook contains the most recent research findings on sexuality; summarizes the historical developments that have brought us to our present understanding of sexuality; and provides comparisons with other cultures, which broaden our perspectives.

**Values** As a valuing person, you have notions of "good" and "bad," "right" and "wrong," that have grown out of your unique background and experience. Some of the information in this book may challenge your values, or at least provoke you to think seriously about your views of the sexual world.

There are no simple answers to questions about sexual values. We hope to give you the opportunity to examine your beliefs and to make them explicit. In the process, you may come to understand how and why such values have developed.

**Feelings** As a feeling person, the subject of sexuality may elicit emotions that reflect your perceptions about yourself and others. At the start of this course, you may feel anxious, fearful, or embarrassed. These feelings are normal and common reactions and should not be ignored or denied. Emotions are part of the learning experience. Like values and attitudes, our feelings need to be explored and understood.

**Behavior** As a behaving person, decisions about relationships, intimacy, love, sexuality, and friendship are an important part of your everyday life. This course will provide information that allows you to understand past decisions and to make better decisions in the future.

This is an ambitious task. We have tried to write a textbook that, through several techniques, will help you to get more out of the course. They are:

**Organization** The book approaches the topic of sexuality from several points of view. The first unit examines the sexual person, emphasizing the central concepts of gender identity, sex roles, and the sexual relationship. The second unit looks at the sexual body, describing sexual anatomy and sexual response. The third unit looks at sexual behavior, exploring sexual activities and interactions. The fourth unit examines sexual development over the life cycle, from infancy to old age, and describes sexuality in the context of our society. The fifth unit looks at sexual variations and complications, examining the clash between society and sexual freedom and investigating sexual coercion. The sixth and final unit examines sexual health and reproduction.

**Personal experience** Within each unit, the usual textbook information on theory and research findings has been enhanced by use of personal experience. Learning that there is a wide difference among people in their sexual reactions and expression is an abstraction. Hearing people describe their own experiences can give life to the abstract fact. So we have included quotations from our files and the files of other experts, as well as case histories that seem to make concepts easier to understand.

**Practical information** A subject as personal as sexuality has obvious application to our own lives. But transferring the conclusions of researchers into practical information can be tricky. To overcome this problem, we have included several chapters that provide concrete information on improving sexual awareness and body image (Chapter 6), sexual communication (Chapter 10), keeping sexual relationships alive (Chapter 13), solving sexual problems (14), and preventing or dealing with rape (Chapter 16), as well as practical information on sexually transmitted diseases and contraception.

**Focus features** Each chapter has at least one focus piece that often investigates a topic of current concern. The information in these features can help you to understand reports in the media and to evaluate them. For example, the features explore such issues as premenstrual syndrome, the value of circumcision, sex-change surgery, whether masturbation is harmful, and the existence of the G-Spot, and female ejaculation.

**Chapter outlines** Each chapter begins with a listing of the topics to be covered in that chapter. Reading the outline will give you advance information about the contents of that chapter. The outline can also be useful in reviewing for an exam. It emphasizes the topics you are likely to be tested on.

**Definitions** New terms are set in boldface type so that they stand out on the page and are defined clearly and simply. The bold type alerts you to the fact that you will be expected to know these terms.

**Glossaries** This book presents its glossary in two ways. Each of the boldface terms is defined in the margin of the page where you first encounter it. As you read the chapter, you can easily find the definition again if you need it. There is an additional glossary at the end of the book, so that you can refresh yourself on the meaning of a term when you come across it in later chapters.

**Chapter summaries** A brief summary at the end of each chapter repeats the central points made in the text. Reading the summaries as soon as you finish the chapter can help you to remember what you have just read, and when reviewing for an exam, the summaries will give you a quick overview of the chapter.

We hope you find this book both interesting and useful. It is meant to help you to think, to reassure you about some of your personal concerns, and to give you an understanding that should carry over into your own life. If it succeeds in these aims, we will have met our goals.

# To the Instructor

Teaching sexuality is very different today from what it was ten or fifteen years ago. At that time, courses in sexuality were a novelty on college campuses, and instructors were hard pressed to develop and justify an academically sound curriculum in what was viewed as a "soft" new area. The instructor's job was made more difficult because there was little in the way of a systematic research base, appropriate instructional resources, or available textbooks.

The education and interest levels of students have changed noticeably in recent years, and the curriculum has expanded into areas barely touched upon in the past. Perhaps most important of all, there has been a marked change in the educational objectives and philosophy that most instructors bring to the teaching of sexuality.

Today's sexuality course presents a unique set of challenges to the instructor. The teaching of basic facts about sexual biology and behavior, while necessary and important, is now seen as only one element of the task. In addition, instructors are expected to explore sexual attitudes and values, to discuss sexual options and decision making, and to provide practical information in many areas. At the same time, they must remain sensitive to the feelings, values, and concerns that students bring with them to class.

Students and instructors alike are aware that today's sexuality course presents the opportunity to consider some of the most interesting and personally meaningful topics in the college curriculum. The special nature of the subject matter makes the nature of a textbook in sexuality especially important.

*Sexuality* is intended to provide the reader with a balanced, contemporary perspective on all aspects of human sexuality. We have gone about the task in the following manner:

**General approach** This textbook defines human sexuality in its broadest terms. It provides students with the best available information on sexual anatomy and physiology, as well as the most recent findings and facts about contraception and sexually transmitted diseases. It recognizes the highly personal and individual nature of sexuality by drawing on the personal experience of individuals as well as on the norms and statistics of scientific research. It provides information in a way that can be applied to the student's life.

**Audience** Students need no background in psychology or physiology in order to use this text. The material is presented in such a way that students at two-year and four-year colleges and students who have had introductory courses in either psychology or physiology will also find it useful.

**A gender-based focus** Since society's concepts of masculinity and femininity have a powerful effect on the way sexuality is experienced, the book begins with a discussion of what it means to be male or female in the 1980s and continues this theme throughout the text. Sex roles are used as a lens through which to view the development and expression of sexuality.

**Emphasis on personal experience** Because of the differences in sexual perception, feelings, and behavior, knowing what "most people" do and feel tells us little about what the individual does and feels. To keep the student aware of these differences, we have included case histories, as well as many personal statements from our own files and the files of others in the field.

**Use of cross-cultural material** The temptation in writing a textbook in human sexuality is to place all the cross-cultural material in one chapter. While this may simplify organizational problems, it often leads students to think that contemporary middle-class American sexual attitudes and behavior are "normal" or "ideal" and that the attitudes and behavior of other groups are "strange" or "peculiar."

To dispel this notion, we have integrated findings from other cultures into the text. Special attention has also been given to the dominant subcultures within the United States. Black and Hispanic sexual attitudes and behavior are presented on their own terms.

**Inclusion of self-help information** Recognizing the need of many students to understand their own sexuality, we have included separate chapters on body image (Chapter 6), sexual communication (Chapter 10), and sexual problem solving (Chapter 14). This practical material, based on the experience and research of counselors and sex therapists, is aimed at making students more comfortable with their own bodies, removing barriers between partners, and aiding students in solving their own sexual problems.

**Organization** Text content has been organized in a manner that seems likely to result in a more balanced understanding of sexuality and its far-reaching effects on our lives:

**Part One—The Sexual Person** begins by examining gender identity and sex roles (Chapter 1), then goes on to explore the sexual relationship (Chapter 2). This unit provides a context in which the meaning of sexual development and behavior becomes clear.

**Part Two—The Sexual Body** covers basic sexual anatomy and physiology (Chapters 3 and 4), explores the nature of the sexual response (Chapter 5), and covers the topics of body image and body awareness (Chapter 6). It also presents up-to-date coverage of such topics as premenstrual syndrome, the Grafenberg spot, circumcision, and female ejaculation.

**Part Three—Sexual Behavior** builds on the material in Part Two, discussing solitary sexual activity (Chapter 7) and sexual interaction (Chapter 8). It includes in-depth treatment of sexual fantasy (Chapter 7), and homosexuality and bisexuality (Chapter 9). It closes with a chapter on sexual communication (Chapter 10).

**Part Four—The Human Life Cycle** further develops an understanding of sexuality by tracing its development throughout the life cycle. Separate chapters are devoted to sexuality in infancy and childhood (Chapter 11), in adolescence (Chapter 12), and in adulthood (Chapter 13), including sexuality among older adults. The unit concludes with a discussion of sexual problems and their solutions (Chapter 14).

**Part Five—Sexual Variations and Complications** explores aspects of sexuality that conflict with law or social norms, including all types of coercive sex. In addition to a chapter on common paraphilias (Chapter 15), a second chapter (Chapter 16) discusses coercive sex, explores rape, sexual harrassment, incest, prostitution, and the possible relationship of coercive sex and pornography.

**Part Six—Sexual Health and Reproduction** begins with a chapter on sexually transmitted diseases (Chapter 17), which presents the latest information on herpes and AIDS, as well as STDs generally covered in textbooks. An entire chapter (Chapter 18) is devoted to sexuality and health, exploring the effect of illness, disability, and drugs on the expression of sexuality. A chapter on contraception (Chapter 19) includes material on the new vaginal sponge as well as the latest findings on the long-term effects of birth-control pills. The text closes with a chapter on reproduction (Chapter 20) that includes material on home birth, artificial insemination, and test-tube fertilization.

In order to help the learning process, we have included a number of pedagogical aids for the student:

**Part introductions** Each of the six basic parts is briefly introduced in order to set the tone for the sort of material that will be covered.

**Chapter outlines** The major headings in each chapter are presented in outline form to give the student a preview of the content.

**Definitions** When each term is used for the first time, it is defined clearly in the text and printed in boldface type.

**Glossaries** As terms are introduced on a page, their definitions are also printed in the margin, thus providing a running glossary. This glossary places an additional definition in a prominent place. A second glossary, at the end of the book, gathers all the definitions in one place so students can easily refresh their memory while reading later chapters.

**Chapter summaries** The summary at the end of each chapter succinctly capsulizes the points made in the text, allowing students to review the material.

To assist both instructor and student, other aids are provided:

**References** A complete list of references is placed at the back of the book, for students who wish to explore a covered topic or for the instructor who wishes to expand text coverage at any point.

**Study guide** This guide, prepared by Dr. James Pitisci of Miami-Dade Community College, is keyed to the text. It reviews and enhances the text material. It includes practice quizzes and discussions of real life situations, which give students the ability to assess their own sexuality.

**Workbook** *Your Sexuality: A Personal Inventory* is a series of carefully designed questionnaires, exercises, and suggested readings that can help students assess and explore their sexual attitudes has been written by Robert Valois and Dr. Sandra Kammermann.

**Instructor's manual** This manual, designed by Beverly Palmer, a testing professional, provides class-tested teaching suggestions for both large and small classes, a list of learning objectives, and tests for each chapter.

## *Acknowledgments*

The writing of this book would not have been possible without the dedicated support and involvement of several key individuals. We are particularly grateful to Judy Rothman, senior psychology editor at Random House, for bringing together the team of Rosen and Hall, and for guiding the book from conception to delivery. Our developmental editor, Leslie Carr, also played a critical role in coordinating the project at every phase, and Anna Marie Muskelly, our project editor, applied meticulous care in shaping and refining the final manuscript. We are also grateful to Betty Binns Graphics for the talented and imaginative design of the book.

Several academic colleagues have also contributed in important ways. In particular, we appreciate the continuing support and guidance provided by our colleagues in the human sexuality program of Rutgers Medical School: Sandra Leiblum, Richard Cross, and Jeffrey Fracher. Special thanks are also owed to Joseph LoPiccolo of SUNY Stony Brook, for his painstaking critique of the entire manuscript, and to Gloria Bachman and Marjorie Nichols for many constructive suggestions on specific chapters. As always, we are indebted to our dearest friend and colleague, John Gagnon, for his invaluable insights and inspiration.

The ideas, comments, and suggestions of a good many academic reviewers improved the final manuscript. We are indebted to the following people:

Mary Kay Biaggio, University of Idaho; Rodney M. Cate, Oregon State University; Linda Carelli, The William Patterson College of New Jersey; Joseph Darden Jr., Kean College of New Jersey; Joan F. DiGiovanni, Western New England College; Andrea Parrot Eggleston, Cornell University; Beverly Fagot, University of Oregon; Shirley Feldman-Summers, University of Washington; Linda Joseph, Queensborough Community College; Sander M. Latts, University of Minnesota; Joseph LoPiccolo, SUNY Stony Brook; Dennis McClung, Saddleback Community College; Roger N. Moss, California State University Northridge; Wesley G. Morgan, University of Tennessee; Beverly B. Palmer, California State University Dominguez Hills; Bruce Palmer, Washington State University; Valerie Pinhas, Nassau Community College; James H. Pitisci, Miami Dade Community College; J. Randall Price, Richland Community College; Rae Silver, Barnard College;

And special thanks to Linda and Josh, and to Scott, who never ran out of patience or sympathy.

RAYMOND C. ROSEN

ELIZABETH HALL

# Contents

*Part One:* *The Sexual Person*                                             **1**

*Chapter 1*
*Sexual Roles*
*and Identities*

PAGE 4

*Part Five:* *Sexual Variations and Complications*      **383**

*Chapter 15*
*Unconventional*
*Sexual Behavior*

PAGE 386

*Chapter 16*
*Sexual Coercion*
*and Exploitation*

PAGE 412

*Part Six:* *Sexual Health and Reproduction*  447

# Part One

# The Sexual Person

Sexuality seems to be something we all participate in but few people feel easy talking about. We may swap jokes with friends or read sexy bestsellers, but a serious, open discussion of the topic makes many of us uncomfortable. Most of us learned as children that frank expressions of sexual feelings are taboo, and the lesson seems to have stuck. But because sexuality is such a basic part of our lives, it deserves to be looked at seriously and discussed honestly.

Sexuality is much more than a matter of biology. Each person's sexuality unfolds in the context of a particular time and a particular culture. Today, shifting standards and changing expectations may force us to face new challenges connected with sexuality, challenges our grandparents didn't have to face. Our understanding of sexuality will be made easier if we first consider what it means today to be a woman or a man. Society's concepts of masculinity and femininity influence the jobs men and women hold, their roles in the family, their social lives, their personalities, their attitudes, their relationships, and the way they dress. Hardly any aspect of life escapes this influence—including what men and women do in bed and how they feel about it.

So we start the examination of sexuality by looking at the sexual person. In the first of the two chapters in this unit, we explore the basis of sexual roles and identities; we see how both biology and culture shape the experience of being male or female. In Chapter 2 we look at the sexual relationship itself, focusing on emotions and the ways in which their expression is influenced by being male or female.

# 1 Sexual Roles and Identities

# Chapter 1

Imagine you have just had an encounter with a visitor from another planet. Was the creature male or female? How would you decide? And why does it matter?

Dividing the world in this way seems important to us. In the movie *E.T.,* the first question asked by the little sister of Elliott, the boy who discovered the extraterrestrial, is "Is it a girl or a boy?" Elliott, whose contact with the visitor has been extremely limited, confidently announces, "It's a boy." We are never told how he came by this information, and what we see of the alien does not tell us anything. As the film progresses, E.T. gives little indication of being male or female. But E.T.'s masculinity seems important to the boys, for when the little sister dresses E.T. like a girl they are outraged, and one exclaims: "You should give him his dignity. This is the most ridiculous thing I've ever seen."

It would seem that among human beings, the most enduring, consistent aspect of personal identity is that of being male or female. We use these concepts to identify ourselves, our friends, and the people we meet, hear, or read about. But although we use them easily, what they mean has changed a lot during the past two decades. What does it mean to be a woman? What does it mean to be a man? Once we were certain we knew the answers—or certain we could never know (Frieze et al., 1978). We accepted the standards of our culture as unchangeable aspects of life. Now, however, discoveries about culture, learning, chromosomes, and hormones have complicated our lives and our thinking. We are not nearly as certain about things as we once were. Masculinity and femininity are not as separate as we

# Sexual Roles and Identities

once thought, and we have found out that each is an intricate mix of biology and culture, hormones and learning.

In this chapter, we begin an attempt to answer the questions by describing some basic components and concepts: gender, gender identity, sex role, sexual orientation, and sexual scripts. Then we try to put sex differences in perspective by looking at their biological and environmental sources. In this context, transsexualism becomes a case of mistaken identity. Exploring the female and male experiences will give us a base from which we can examine the concept of androgyny. We close by looking at sexual identity as it develops and changes over the human life cycle.

Let's turn now to basic concepts, beginning with gender.

## ASPECTS OF GENDER: BASIC CONCEPTS

When a baby is born, people always want to know the infant's basic biological classification—whether it is a boy or a girl. But there is more to gender than the mechanics of the reproductive system.

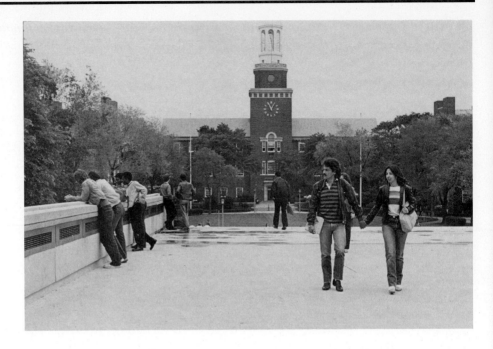

Concepts of masculinity and femininity change, affecting most aspects of life. The way we dress reflects our idea of what it means to be a man or a woman, and so does our sexual activity—and the way we feel about it. (© Hazel Hankin/Stock, Boston)

## *Biology and culture*

**gender** all differences between males and females, including biological, social, and psychological.

**imperative elements of gender** the physical differences that are necessary in order to carry out reproductive functions

**optional elements of gender** the social and psychological aspects of gender

**sex** the anatomical and physiological differences between males and females

The biological aspects of **gender** consist of the physical differences between men and women: woman's ability to menstruate, to carry a fetus until delivery, and to provide it with milk after birth, and man's ability to produce and transmit sperm are features of biological gender. But other aspects of gender, such as actions or personality characteristics, are influenced, shaped, and encouraged by culture. Some researchers distinguish between these elements of gender by calling the biological aspects **imperative** and the cultural aspects **optional** (Money and Ehrhardt, 1972). In this book, we refer to the biological aspects of gender as **sex** (Stoller, 1968).

Except for some rare genetic errors, biological sex is either-or. The vast majority of people have either male or female physiology, not both. Gender is more flexible. The shape of the genitals does not automatically lead a person to act in "masculine" or "feminine" ways.

The concepts of sex and gender are further complicated by the fact that when people meet for the first time, each assigns the other a "sex" label. That is, you decide—based on a person's appearance and actions—whether that person possesses male or female genitals. Some researchers now use the terms "male" or "female" only when referring to the reproductive aspects of gender and "masculinity" or "femininity" to refer to all the optional aspects (Freimuth and Hornstein, 1982). Among the optional aspects of gender are gender identity, sex roles, sexual orientation, and sexual scripts.

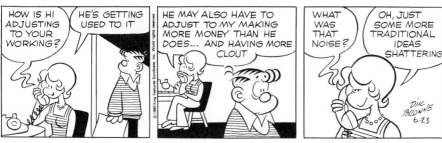

(© 1980 King Features Syndicate)

## Options: identity, role, orientation, script

**Gender identity** is invisible. It is the person's private sense of being male or female (Money and Ehrhardt, 1972). Gender identity develops during the preschool years. Because this identity is a way of feeling, it cannot be established from a person's appearance.

In traditional Western societies, aggression, independence, and logic have been considered masculine traits, and compassion, nurturance, and dependence have been considered feminine. These characteristics are part of **sex roles**, the patterns of attitudes, behavior, and beliefs dictated by society for members of each sex. A sex role includes some behaviors and prohibits others.

Most aspects of sex role have nothing to do with the biological differences between men and women. For example, although most cultures give women the responsibility for child care, men can just as well fill this role. Similarly, although men are generally expected to support the family, women can easily do so. Today, some members of each sex are exchanging traditional roles—by choice or by necessity. The imperative aspects of gender control physical reproduction; the optional aspects provide a social structure in which children can be reared.

Gender and sex, or the optional and imperative aspects of gender, do not always go together. For most people, there is a good fit between the two. Most people tend to act in ways that are expected of them on the basis of their anatomy. Boys generally behave in ways their culture labels "masculine"; girls learn to be "feminine." But there are individuals whose sexual anatomy does not match their gender. The most striking example is the **transsexual**, whose physical characteristics are at odds with both gender identity and sex role.

Yet another option is **sexual orientation**, which is sometimes called "sexual preference," the choice of sexual partner. A person's sexual orientation may be heterosexual (attracted to people of the other sex), homosexual (attracted to people of the same sex), or bisexual (attracted to members of both sexes). The definition relies on the sex—or the biological structure—of the preferred partner. These categories used to be viewed as fixed and distinct, like sex. Then, after Alfred Kinsey and his associates (Kinsey, Pomeroy, and Martin, 1948) interviewed thousands of American men about their sexual activities, it became clear that sexual preference may change during the course of a person's life and that sexual orientation is a mat-

**gender identity** a person's inner sense of being male or female

**sex role** the pattern of attitudes, behavior, and beliefs dictated by society for members of each sex

**transsexual** a person whose gender identity conflicts with his or her biological sex and prescribed sex role

**sexual orientation** a person's choice of sex partner, which may be heterosexual, homosexual, or bisexual; also called sexual preference

ter of degree. Many people do not fit neatly into any of the three categories. Kinsey's research may well have laid the basis for recent changes in society's attitude toward homosexuality. His discovery that many heterosexual men and women had had some sort of homosexual experience helped homosexuals to resist the 1950s' medical view that they suffered from some disorder, and it convinced many heterosexuals that their attitude toward homosexuality was unreasonable (Gagnon, 1975).

Kinsey's influence went far beyond matters of homosexuality. He probably did more than any other American to demystify human sexuality and make it an accepted part of life. His detailed interviews with nearly 12,000 men and women revealed to other Americans what their fellow citizens were doing in the bedroom and made public discussion of sexual behavior acceptable. The research of Kinsey and his associates is perhaps the most reliable source of information about American sexual behavior and this body of work remains the standard against which all other sex research is measured.

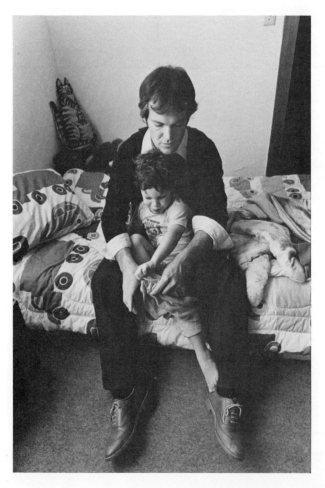

Although only a woman can bear a child and only a man can produce sperm, either can care for a child. Many men now share in child care and some are assuming complete responsibility in this traditionally feminine area. (© Hazel Hankin)

Alfred Kinsey probably did more than any other person to change American attitudes toward homosexuality, masturbation, and premarital sex. (Photograph by Dellenback. Courtesy, The Kinsey Institute for Research in Sex, Gender and Reproduction, Inc.)

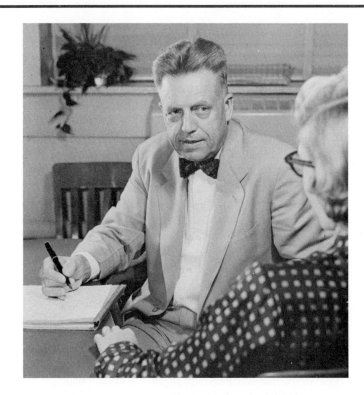

Today sexual orientation is generally seen as a continuum with heterosexuality at one end, homosexuality at the other, and bisexuality in between. A person's place depends on the similarity or difference between the person's biological gender and that of the partner and how often the person chooses a partner of that particular gender (Freimuth and Hornstein, 1982).

**Sexual script** is another optional aspect of gender; it refers to the often subconscious mental plan that guides a person's sexual activity (Gagnon and Simon, 1973). Scripts are so named because they direct and explain human action as surely as the script of a play guides the actor's interpretation of a role in the theater. Sexual scripts tell people whom they may have sex with; what sexual acts they can perform; when they can have sex—both time of day and time of life cycle; where they can enjoy these sexual acts; and why they have sex at all—whether for pleasure, lust, love, relaxation, exploitation, or duty. Scripts tend to steer behavior into paths the culture considers acceptable and to make us comfortable in social situations, for they help us to organize our behavior and to understand the behavior of others.

People develop sexual scripts just as they develop sex roles—by learning. Because each person has different experiences, individual scripts are somewhat different. However, the influence of the culture means that most scripts in a society are similar. The male script calls for a man to initiate sexual activity, and the traditional woman's script for her to respond and to set limits. Each person absorbs the script at an early age, as one woman recalled when interviewed about her sexual history:

**sexual script** the mental plan that guides a person's sexual activity

When I was in grade school, I got involved with a fast group. We used to go down in the basement with these guys and let them touch our breasts, even though at first all I had in there was tissue paper. It was mostly pressure to be accepted and to have a boyfriend. There were all kinds of rules on what to do and not to touch me down below. That was out because it was a slutty thing to do. The emphasis wasn't on "did it feel good"; the emphasis was on being part of the crowd and having the boyfriend. (Authors' files)

Sexual scripts become visible only when they are broken. Imagine a couple on their first date. As they sit on a couch, the woman slips her arm around the man's shoulders, kisses him lengthily, and begins fumbling with his clothing. Most men would be shocked, and most women would find it very difficult to act in this way, for such behavior is not part of the feminine script. Indeed, the constraints of sexual scripts can be so thoroughly absorbed that they interfere with sexuality. For example, sex therapists have discovered that the feminine script makes it difficult for many women to initiate sexual activities, even with their husbands (Gagnon, Rosen, and Leiblum, 1982).

## SEX DIFFERENCES IN PERSPECTIVE

According to popular ideas, men and women are opposites. Also according to these ideas, women have the negative characteristics and men the positive ones. Women talk too much; they cry a lot; they are indecisive, dependent, and timid. Men say little; they never get emotional; they are competitive, decisive, independent, and aggressive. These descriptions bear little resemblance to most men and women; they are **sex-role stereotypes**, exaggerated portrayals of the traits and behavior of each gender. We all know independent women and timid men, as well as indecisive women and aggressive men. Certainly there are differences between men and women, but the differences are not nearly so great nor so stable as stereotypes would have them. Only four kinds of sex differences have been solidly established: females excel in verbal ability; males excel in visual-spatial and mathematical ability and are more aggressive than females (Maccoby and Jacklin, 1974). But even these characteristics have been challenged as being shaped by culture. Girls are discouraged from studying math, and as we'll see, aggression is both expected and encouraged in boys, but regarded with alarm when it appears in girls.

The fact is that there is great overlap between the sexes. The average man is larger and stronger than the average woman—but some women are larger and stronger than the average man, and some men are smaller and weaker than the average woman. The same sort of overlap appears in attitudes, personality, and intellectual abilities. At one time the differences were seen as "natural"—they were the result of biology and impossible to overcome. Then research seemed to indicate that all differences could be explained as learned, stamped into children by cultural demands that they fit their prescribed sex roles. Although the degree of basic difference is still an issue, today's view is that some biological differences do exist, but that culture exaggerates them. What are small cracks become chasms.

**sex-role stereotype** exaggeraated concepts of the traits and behavior of each gender

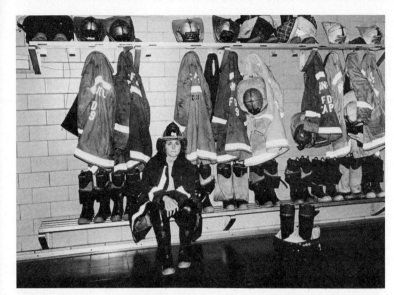

As more women and men take on nontraditional jobs, sex-role stereotypes begin to break down. We have discovered that the differences between the sexes are much smaller than we once thought and that to a great extent male and female abilities overlap. (© Abigail Heyman/Archive; © Mark Antman/Stock, Boston)

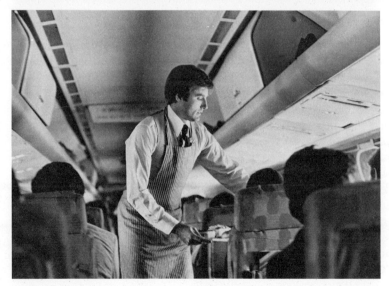

## The biological basis of differences

In lower animals, the biological basis for sex differences is clear. For example, male canaries sing and female canaries do not, and a corresponding sex difference has been found in the brain cells that control singing (Gelman et al., 1981). In human beings, however, establishing links between biology and behavior is extremely difficult. As we'll see in Chapter 3, male and female hormones, chemical substances secreted by the sex glands, determine which sex organs will appear and how they will function. But we do not know whether these hormones also affect behavior.

The clearest connection between hormones and behavior is that between male hormones and aggression. In one study (Reinisch, 1981), seventeen girls and eight boys whose mothers took male hormones during pregnancy showed a strong tendency to be physically aggressive. When asked how they would respond in sample situations involving conflict with other people, the children often chose hitting or kicking over yelling, running away, or settling the situation in some other nonaggressive way. The exposed boys were much more aggressive than their brothers, and the exposed girls were much more aggressive than their sisters. The children ranged from six to eighteen years of age, but neither age nor order of birth had any connection with a tendency to strike out. In line with other studies of sex differences in aggression, the boys who had not been exposed to extra prenatal hormones were much more aggressive than the unexposed girls.

Other studies have consistently indicated that exposure to hormones before birth causes male and female brains to develop differences in structure and function—a condition called **brain dimorphism**. Scientists agree that these differences affect cyclical functions, such as the menstrual cycle. Some investigators, however, believe that the brains of men and women differ in other ways, that the higher centers of the brain—which process and integrate information—also show dimorphism. An exaggerated version of this view was the nineteenth-century idea that young women were both physically and mentally weak and hence too frail for college life.

**brain dimorphism** sex differences in brain structure and function, believed to be caused by prenatal exposure to hormones

Assumptions about women's intellectual ability have changed, but the notion of brain dimorphism is still with us. In this view, separate brain mechanisms in males and females are responsible for differences in behavior. Although the display of masculine or feminine behavior may be influenced by the environment, it is supposed to be largely the result of programming in the brain before birth (Diamond, 1976). Researchers have also suggested that through their effect on the fetal brain, hormones may be responsible for some of the differences between men and women in sexual behavior, personality, and intelligence (Reinisch, Gandelman, and Spiegel, 1979).

This position is controversial because much of the evidence comes from animal research, in which hormones are removed or added and the animal's subsequent behavior observed. But the results of animal research cannot be applied directly to human beings, and similar studies could not be done with human subjects because of ethical problems. Perhaps a closer look at environmental influences will give us a better answer.

## The environmental basis of differences

Even though some sex differences appear to have a biological basis, the environment determines how they will be expressed. In the study of children with prenatal exposure to male hormones, for example, two girls and one boy showed a lower level of aggression than their unexposed siblings (Reinisch, 1981). These children may have lived in families that discouraged physical aggression. Biological predispositions may make certain kinds of behavior easy to learn—but if the conditions that encourage the learning never arise, the behavior may not appear.

Each culture shapes masculine and feminine behavior into the forms valued in that society. A review of anthropological studies shows that in most cultures women are expected to be nurturing, responsible, and obedient, and to tend the children. Men are expected to be self-reliant achievers and to fight wars (Tavris and Offir, 1977). Any other job or aspect of personality may differ widely from one culture to the next. Iranian women are cold and logical; Manu men love to play with children; Philippine men gossip. In Arab countries, a man is allowed to express his emotions and is expected to gossip at the market, while his wife farms and produces handicrafts (Yorburg, 1974). Because male and female traits, behavior, and social roles change from culture to culture, and because there is so much overlap in the behavior of men and women, it seems clear that many sex differences are the result of environmental influences (Frieze et al., 1978).

Males and females are treated differently from the moment of birth. In Chapter 11, we'll explore just how children come to behave according to the culture's rules for their own gender. The process begins in the family and is encouraged by playmates, teachers, other adults, and the media. As society has begun to relax its rules, this differential treatment has become plain. Even in areas that seemed obviously dictated by biology, there have been great changes.

Sports have always been considered a male domain—but now women have begun to close the gap in athletic performance. In 1964, the male Olympic record for swimming the 400-meter freestyle was 4 minutes, 12.2 seconds. In the 1980

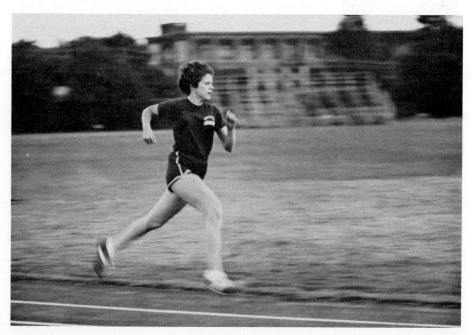

Although their body structure will always give men an advantage in most sports, women are now within 10 percent of the best male times in swimming and track. On races longer than 100 kilometers, women may one day equal the best male speed. (© Barbara Alper)

# Focus

## TRANSSEXUALISM—A CASE OF MISTAKEN IDENTITY

The existence of transsexuals raises basic questions about the meaning of gender and gender identity, because transsexuals' sex (biological structure) conflicts with their gender identity and sex role. To understand the transsexual's gender identity, imagine that you wake up one morning and find that during the night your body has changed to the other sex. If you're male, you discover that your penis and scrotum have vanished. You have breasts, a vagina, and a high voice. If you're female, your breasts have disappeared, and you've sprouted a penis. Your voice has deepened and as you rub your hand across your chin, you feel the beginnings of a beard. But inside you feel exactly as you had the day before. According to Deborah Feinbloom (1976), you'd be feeling just the way a transsexual feels every day of his or her life.

Most transsexuals say they sensed as children that things were "not right" and eventually came to feel that they were trapped in the body of the wrong sex. One transsexual wrote: "I really wanted to be like my sister and her girlfriends. It seemed like a very cruel joke that I wasn't" (Kessler and McKenna, 1978, p. 175).

Since gender identity is fundamental to personal, social, and occupational identity, this discrepancy between biological and

A sex change operation transformed Dr. Richard Raskind into Dr. Renee Richards. (Wide World Photos; Korody/Sygma)

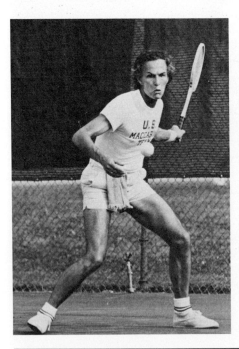 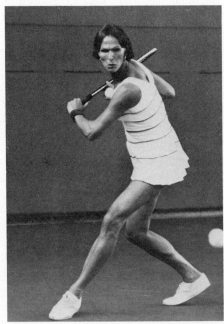

psychological role places the transsexual under continual stress. One biological male transsexual described the relief he felt when he tried living as a woman:

I almost can't express how happy and comfortable I feel in this role. It's almost as if it were meant to be. The inner peace I experience as Martha (my female self) is incredible—even though it's like being on a constant high . . . I really don't remember when I've felt so good or comfortable in my entire life. (Authors' files)

The strain of living in accordance with their biological sex is so great that many transsexuals request surgery to make their bodies correspond to their gender.

Many transsexuals feel they are "passing" when they are living in accordance with their biological sex. For example, "Jane," who was born "John," served as a sailor on an all-male ship. Although she had a penis, she felt she was a female passing as a male and deceiving her fellow sailors. Later she adopted a more comfortable female role (Kessler and McKenna, 1978).

To the world, however, transsexuals are passing when they live in accordance with their gender identity and sex role, so that observers would be likely to say that "Jane" was passing when she was living as a female. It's true that transsexuals must learn some aspects of the new sexual role when they begin living the role they feel is truly theirs. One female-to-male transsexual said he learned to behave like a man from reading *Playboy Advisor*.

Transsexuals first came to public attention in 1953 when Christine Jorgensen was operated on in Denmark and "her" sex was changed from male to female. Transsexuals remain relatively rare. There are probably about 10,000 in the United States, and about 2,000 of them have had sex reassignment by way of hormones and surgery (Feinbloom, 1976). Most transsexuals were born as biological males; it is estimated that there are from six to eight male transsexuals for every female (Levine and Lothstein, 1981).

Although the majority of transsexuals are sexually attracted to members of their own biological sex, they do not regard themselves as homosexuals. In fact, many male transsexuals would regard sexual activity with a woman as homosexuality, since their own gender identity is female. Transsexuals are different from homosexuals, because homosexuals have no wish to change their bodies, nor does their gender identity conflict with their genitals. In most cases, transsexuals find sexual experiences with either sex very unsatisfying because they are not in the "right" body.

Research is being conducted in the causes and effects of transsexualism at a number of universities. The primary goal is to find effective ways to help these individuals, many of whom are severely distressed. By solving the riddle of transsexualism, we may also learn more about the process of gender development in all human beings.

Moscow games, four women beat that mark (Gelman, 1981). Because of their larger proportion of muscle to fat, men will always have a biological advantage in certain sports, but the narrowing of the gap shows how far the environment had widened it.

Women and men are becoming alike in other ways as well. Today women feel less pressure to marry and rear children, and many have also become more assertive and independent, exposing an environmental influence on those "masculine" traits. Some now hold jobs once held only by men, such as construction worker or bank president. Men feel more freedom to show their emotions and to participate in child care; expressing emotions and nurturing are no longer exclusively feminine traits. Men can choose to become househusbands.

But despite these visible changes, some researchers claim that sex roles have not changed in any basic way. They hold that instead some of the punishments for violating cultural expectations have been lifted (Kessler and McKenna, 1978). Other rules, such as the prohibition of skirts on men, remain firmly in place.

The fact that the gap between male and female sex roles appears to be narrowing does not mean that men and women are necessarily alike. As biology and culture interact, the sexes have different experiences, develop different expectations, and see the world in different ways. They come to think of themselves as different, which maintains the gap (Tavris and Offir, 1977). This belief is probably responsible for a good part of the differences we see in sexual behavior.

## THE FEMALE EXPERIENCE

The experience of being a woman has probably changed more in the past century than at any time in the history of the human species. In every known society, women have always been subordinate to men. Their unlimited fertility resulted in a continual cycle of pregnancy, nursing, and pregnancy. In need of help while so tied down, women obeyed their male protectors and came to be regarded as inferior to men.

The situation that originally allowed men to dominate women no longer exists in technological societies. When women bear few children—or none at all—they no longer need continual protection. Theoretically, then, women should no longer be subordinate, and the experiences of men and women should become more similar.

In some aspects of life, this has happened. Recent changes in the role of women have reduced male dominance and increased female freedom. As a result of the changes, today women get conflicting messages about their "proper place," face new choices about education and careers, and encounter unrealistic messages from the media about the essence of being female. Many women who are old enough to have seen the great changes society has gone through in recent decades at times express anger or confusion:

> When I grew up the career choices were simple: schoolteacher, nurse,
> librarian, or secretary. None of them really appealed to me, but my parents

and high school advisers made it clear that those were the options. And they were only insurance, since I'd probably get married and not work at all. For a while I conformed, but I can still get angry at some of the smug assumptions I met—and accepted for a lot of years. (Authors' files)

Despite the new freedom of choice for women, custom, sex roles, and child-rearing practices keep alive much of the distance between the male and female experience. When in 1982 a male actor played a female role in the movie *Tootsie,* the gulf became apparent. His impersonation of a woman led Dustin Hoffman to examine his own life and changed his behavior and his attitudes. In an interview, he said: "If you are a woman for a month, the world is a different experience in ways you would never imagine" (Bennetts, 1982). A look at the separate experience of women and men may help to clarify Hoffman's reaction.

## Historical attitudes toward women

Tracing the history of attitudes toward women means discussing men's attitudes toward women, for until recently history was written by men. Although women were probably responsible for many of the technological improvements that made a stable society possible—basketry, weaving, pottery, domesticating grain and improving its yield—they were always considered to be the second sex (Bullough and Bullough, 1973). Some writers have suggested that human beings once lived in a matriarchy, a society in which women—aided by the power of religion—dominated men. However, most anthropologists now believe that women have never been truly dominant, although they have held important roles in some societies.

For whatever cause, women have been subordinate in all the cultures and traditions that influenced modern European and North American society—Judeo-Christian, Greek, and Roman. Old Testament Judaism was a male-oriented religion that regarded women as inferior. In addition to being inferior, women were also seen as aggressively sexual, so tempting to men that Eve had little trouble seducing Adam. There were only two possible roles for women in traditional Judaism—erotic lover and temptress or dutiful wife and loving mother. According to the ancient Greeks, woman was inferior. She was sensual and governed by the uterus, as opposed to the rational male, who was governed by reason. Most philosophers agreed that sexual intercourse was beastly and that the highest form of love was never expressed physically. Among the Romans, women had more privileges than they did among the Greeks, but they were still regarded as inferior, incompetent, and intensely interested in sexual pleasure. Christianity developed as a male-centered religion that regarded sex as evil and women as dangerous. Again, by arousing sexual desire and threatening their spiritual freedom, women tempted men from higher things. Women were not only legally inferior to men, as they always had been; in Christian societies, they were morally inferior as well (Bullough and Bullough, 1973).

The Judeo-Christian tradition was carried to the New World by European settlers. In the American colonies, the position of women varied somewhat by region. It was worst among the Puritans of New England, who regarded sexuality as interfering with spiritual life and woman as a dangerous temptress. Attitudes toward sexuality were more relaxed in the other colonies, but everywhere women were subordinate to men. Toward the end of the eighteenth century, as the middle class tried to shed its image as a frontier society, there was a conscious attempt to be "respectable." This led to the idea of the sexless woman, for "proper women" were supposed to be shocked by base, animal sexuality (Lewis, 1980).

Through all this period, American women were bearing as many children as possible. Families might have as many as fifteen or twenty children, a practice that only began to die out among middle- and upper-class families as Victorian ideas took hold in the nineteenth century. In the Victorian era men visited prostitutes to avoid forcing pure women, uninterested in sex, into degrading practices. At the time childbirth was so risky that many middle-class women may have owed their lives to their husbands' "consideration."

It was during the nineteenth century that safe and effective contraceptives were invented, reducing the fear that every act of sexual intercourse was likely to lead to a risky pregnancy. Malnutrition, pelvises deformed by childhood rickets, the possibility of hemorrhage, exhaustion from repeated pregnancies, miscarriages, and abortions, as well as the threat of deadly childbed fever, made childbirth dangerous, especially among the poor. In addition to lessening the risks of childbirth, contraceptives protected women from sexually transmitted diseases, which afflicted as many as 30 percent of nineteenth-century Americans (Lewis, 1980). Now able to rely on contraception, "respectable" women lost their fear of sex. By the 1880s, they were confident enough to wear alluring nightgowns for the first time (Tannahill, 1980).

The invention of the rubber feeding nipple and the pasteurization of milk

Until the nineteenth century, American women bore as many children as possible. Victorian ideas reduced family size by curtailing marital sexual activity, and it was not until effective contraceptives were available that most women lost their fear of sex. (Culver Pictures)

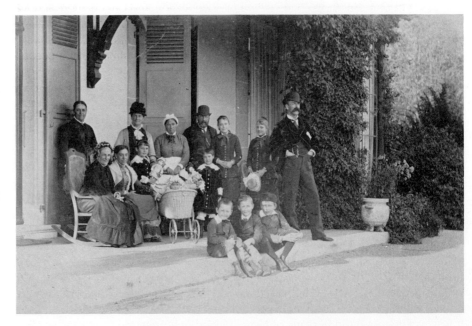

were also important in easing restrictions on women. The nipple made it possible to turn over infant feeding to others. The pasteurization of milk, among all scientific advances, was probably the most important in reducing infant mortality (McKoewn, 1977). And with more babies living, women were not obliged to produce so many.

Then, in the 1920s, the sanitary pad was marketed. For the first time, women had a simple, disposable way of handling menstruation. They no longer had to wear voluminous, long skirts to hide odor and bulky menstrual cloths (Bullough, 1980).

Despite the inroads made by the women's suffrage movement, it would be another forty years before women—taught from infancy that their place was in the home and that their job was bearing and rearing children—asserted their equality with enough strength to affect society's view of them. Perhaps it required the contraceptive pill, the availability of safe abortions, and a better understanding of female sexuality to make women realize that a redefinition of roles was possible.

## Growing up female

Our grandmothers grew up in a world in which women were expected to marry "till death do us part," become mothers, and stay home. Today, more people are staying single, nearly one marriage in two is destined for divorce, fewer people are having children, and more than half of all women with children are working outside the home. Many of the rules that governed women's lives for generations have been set aside, and women are learning to play by new ones.

**A woman's life** Women are taking their education and careers more seriously today than ever before. Most know they will be supporting themselves—and perhaps others as well—for part if not all of their lives. Discrimination in hiring, promotion, and salary still exists, but women now work in almost every occupation. Today the majority of insurance adjusters, bill collectors, real estate agents, photographic process workers, and production-line assemblers are women, and in some other traditional masculine areas women have made large gains (Prial, 1982).

But the fact that women should be prepared to assume an equal economic role may not be obvious in the schools. In a society that increasingly requires scientific and technological backgrounds for employment, women still seem reluctant to choose careers in those areas. Studies of high school students in the United States, Sweden, and England show that girls continue to fall behind boys in science courses. Most girls have less positive attitudes toward science than boys do, believe science is harder to learn, and take part in fewer elective science activities, even though as many girls as boys believe science is important. The differences researchers find in achievement and interest are apparently not biological, because girls in all-girl high schools in England tend to excel in chemistry and biology (Finn, 1980). Perhaps the presence of women as science instructors in all-girl schools and the absence of competing male students (who remind girls of the sex-role stereotypes) encourage girls in science classes.

### Table 1.1   College enrollment by sex (1960–1981)

PERCENTAGE ENROLLED IN COLLEGE

|  | 1960 | 1970 | 1980 | 1981 |
|---|---|---|---|---|
| **Males:** | | | | |
| 18–24 | 46.2 | 44.9 | 35.4 | 35.7 |
| 25–34 | 16.6 | 12.7 | 13.0 | 13.2 |
| TOTAL | 65.5 | 59.4 | 49.4 | 49.8 |
| **Females:** | | | | |
| 18–24 | 26.6 | 33.4 | 35.6 | 35.3 |
| 25–34 | 4.4 | 5.5 | 13.5 | 13.7 |
| TOTAL | 34.5 | 40.6 | 50.6 | 50.2 |

The ratio of males to females in college has reversed since 1960. Particularly in the over twenty-five group, the percentage of women entering college has increased dramatically in the past decade.

Source: Statistical Abstract of the United States, 1982–1983, U.S. Bureau of the Census (1982).

The goals of college students, however, certainly have changed in the past fifteen years (Table 1.1). When compared with women students in 1967, today's women no longer emphasize such reasons as making friends and developing social competence for attending college, but instead stress career goals. They are generally as interested in challenging careers as are college men, but they are less interested in earning money and becoming an economic success (Goldberg and Shiflett, 1981).

At one time, women decided whether they would have careers or marry and have children. If they chose marriage, they expected to work only until their first child was born. Today the decisions are more complicated. Women not only decide whether to marry, but *when* to do so (Frieze et al., 1978). Early or late marriage and early or late childbearing are additional alternatives their grandmothers did not have to evaluate.

**Attitudes and expectations**   Traditionally, women have been expected to define themselves in relation to men. The "proper" role has been that of "wife-companion," making home and husband the center of a woman's life (Rothman, 1978). A woman who follows the traditional path is primarily wife and mother, and if she works outside the home, her job is secondary. She derives her self-esteem from her relationships to loved ones. She is compassionate, nurturant, and dependent, and her attitudes and expectations hew closely to the traditional female sex role.

An increasing number of women have taken a nontraditional approach to their lives. Instead of defining themselves in relation to men, they focus on their own individual achievement. Whether or not they marry, they see their own success in an occupation as central to their identity and self-esteem. Nontraditional women tend to be independent and assertive.

The nontraditional picture of women has become more prevalent in recent years, and some young, well-educated adults have developed an image of the ideal woman that combines traditional and nontraditional qualities. Among *Psychology Today* readers, men and women agreed that the ideal woman was loving, warm, and gentle, as well as intelligent, self-confident, and able to stand up for her beliefs (Tavris, 1977).

Since both views of women have many adherents, girls and women receive conflicting messages about woman's role in the economic system, about family life, and about sexuality. Whether women decide to follow a liberated or traditional path, it is almost impossible for them to shut out the opposing messages.

The traditional message can be heard in many homes, schools, churches, and from the media. Nowhere does it come through so clearly as on television, and continued exposure to stereotypical images of weak and passive women and dominant men may still be shaping personalities and attitudes. Women in television programs tend to be submissive, illogical, incompetent, emotional, affectionate, and romantic. When they face problems, someone else solves them—less than 2 percent of the female characters solve their own difficulties (Roberts, 1980).

An analysis of more than 300 television commercials found that the difference between female and male sex roles is far greater than it is in society (Mamay and Simpson, 1981). Women are either mothers, housekeepers, creatures interested in beauty and cleanliness, or sensuous sex objects. Women's place is clearly in the home, and men continually explain household machinery or chemical products to women who say such things as, "I don't know why it works, it just does."

Tradition has also established a sexual role for women: to be sexually accessible—but not demanding (Slater, 1977). As we have seen, the female sexual script is primarily one of responding to male overtures and setting limits, and the absorption of this script shapes sexual attitudes and expectations. Today, however, popular magazines inform women that they may initiate sex, tell their partners what they like to do in bed, and explore new techniques in lovemaking. But as we'll see, receiving the message is easier than acting on it.

Nontraditional women appear to have carried their autonomy into the sexual area. Among a group of college women, they showed increased levels of intercourse and a greater insistence on contraception than did traditional college women (Scanzioni and Fox, 1980). It may be that women's wider participation in the world of work will cause further changes in their attitudes toward sex. The more committed a person is to a job, the less important sexual life often becomes. Among successful male executives and professionals, many value sex more as a release from tension than as a delightful pastime (Cuber and Harroff, 1965). If women begin to define themselves primarily in terms of their jobs, they may adopt this male approach to sex.

Women's primary expression of sexuality has traditionally been within the marriage relationship. Although matters that once were taken for granted by women and men are at least being discussed today—even in working-class families—it appears that beliefs about what is appropriate—whether the division of labor within the household or the care of children—are changing more radically than the behavior itself.

The traditional female position concerning such matters tends to place the family first and can be summed up as, "If the family does well, I do too." The traditional male position tends to place the family second and can be expressed as, "If I do well, the family does too." As men become less traditional, they tend to agree with their wives that decisions should be made jointly. But such men may not also accept the traditional male position as applying to both parties—a situation that can promote serious conflicts between sexual partners (Scanzioni and Fox, 1980). Whether continued shifts in sex roles will ease this tension remains to be seen. Although men continue to occupy most of the positions of authority and although they have historically provided the explanations and philosophies about "human nature" (which was always male nature), the experience of a man in contemporary society seems to be shifting in major ways.

## THE MALE EXPERIENCE

Today men are also receiving conflicting messages about their sex role, with the result that basic attitudes toward sex have undergone extensive change.

### Historical attitudes toward men

Until men's role in procreation was known, women may have been seen as a magical force. In primitive societies dominated by fear of the unknown, this view may have bolstered the power of women. Eventually, however, men learned of their role in procreation and used their greater physical strength to subjugate women. It was argued by Friedrich Engels (1884) that the transition to absolute male dominance was responsible for the development of private property and the rise of social and economic injustice.

Once men were firmly in control, they stayed there. A look at traditional attitudes toward men quickly shows that a history of men in the Western world is a history of Western thought and politics. Society seemed to be defined primarily in masculine terms. Men were seen as restrained, controlled, spiritual, and less susceptible to sexual impulses than women (Slater, 1977). The Greeks saw men as dominated by reason (the mind) and women by sexual urges (the uterus). It was not until the nineteenth century that men came to be seen as creatures driven by sexual urges and women as passively enduring the lust of men.

Because men were the dominant group, masculine values were rewarded by society and generally seen as superior to feminine values. It was better to be logical, to make decisions quickly, to strive for power, to engage in business or politics as ends in themselves rather than as means to an end, and to take a tough, aggressive approach to human problems. Traditional feminine values, such as compassion, were considered "nice but unrealistic" (Farrell, 1975). As late as the 1970s, a U.S. senator seeking the Democratic nomination for president was said to have destroyed his chances for the office by weeping in public.

## Growing up male

Our grandfathers grew up in a world in which men expected marriage to last forever and to provide the family's sole support. The recent social changes that have so radically altered women's lives have had a considerable impact on men, chipping away at their position as family provider and freeing them to experiment with roles that had been restricted to women.

As boys grow up, however, they still learn four things about being male: avoid doing anything "feminine," don't be dependent on anyone, become successful, and be aggressive (Brannon, 1976). The belief that boys must shun anything feminine has actually made the male sex role more confining than the female sex role. A girl can be a tomboy and no one objects. But when a boy plays with dolls or shows other feminine interests, parents generally become nervous, and most try to stamp out such "sissy" behavior (Green, 1974). Fathers become especially upset, apparently because they fear their sons may become homosexual. Few people seem to worry that tomboys will become lesbians.

**A man's life**  The rigidity continues into adulthood, with many men apparently confining themselves within the traditional male sex role because they are afraid they will be considered homosexual. In fact, among a group of young, college-educated men who were asked about their concepts of masculinity, some said that they felt masculine only in public when they were concerned about behaving "like a man" and not "like a homosexual" (Tavris, 1977). Numerous studies have shown that men seem more hostile toward homosexuals than women, and that the more strongly men believe in traditional definitions of sex roles, the more antihomosexual they are (Morin and Garfinkle, 1978).

As men have begun to share financial responsibilities and to question some of the stereotypical male values, their occupational and social goals may be shifting. When male college students today were compared with the students of 1967, most men had become more interested in the social reasons for attending college (Goldberg and Shiflett, 1981). They said that among their college goals were developing self-confidence and finding a wife. Although these students still wanted to make money and be successful, many had adopted social goals traditionally considered feminine.

Television has tended to perpetuate stereotypical male traits. Men are generally portrayed as ambitious, competitive, realistic, violent, independent, logical, intelligent, dominant, unemotional, and tall. They also solve women's problems (Roberts, 1980). Since many of these characteristics are perceived as superior to stereotypical female traits, men have a lot to live up to. If they are not more capable, more intelligent, and more successful in every way than their wives, sisters, or female acquaintances and co-workers, they may feel they are not truly masculine. If that happens, the burden shifts and men become defensive. They are driven to prove that they are not feminine, not dependent, not emotional, not passive, not afraid, not helpless. So the adult male stereotype can be as confining as its female counterpart (Goldberg, 1979).

Even when men want to break the stereotype, its power remains strong:

I still very much hold on to some of [my father's] ideas about being strong and potent, and these feelings used to scare me when I was younger, because I felt that I could never fill those images of masculinity. In some ways I still feel that I want to be king of my castle, just like him, and my wife and I joke about that a lot. It's also important to me to earn more money than she does, even though she's a professional, too, and I feel sometimes that I still want to hold on to the stereotypes about women that I got from my father, that basically women are emotional and are nincompoops. . . . You know, I try to filter out these attitudes or make light of them, but they're still buried deep inside. (D. Bell, 1982, p. 12)

**Attitudes and expectations** Curious as to what most adults actually believed about men, researchers examined a number of studies and discovered that popular beliefs about typical male characteristics broke down into three major categories: how a man handles his life, how he handles others, and how he handles his mind and emotions (Cicone and Ruble, 1978). In the first group are qualities such as adventurous, independent, ambitious, courageous, competitive, and active that describe a go-getting attitude toward life and promise success in the world. In the second group are qualities such as aggressive, powerful, dominant, and assertive that describe a person who dominates others. In the last group are qualities such as logical, realistic, stable, unemotional, and self-controlled that indicate a cool, self-contained person.

Other studies have found that many young middle-class people have a changed image of the ideal male (Figure 1.1). The macho male, who is tough, strong, and aggressive and has many sexual conquests, was rejected out of hand by 28,000 young, college-educated readers of *Psychology Today* magazine (Tavris, 1977). Only 5 percent of the men and 4 percent of the women admired him. Both sexes said that the ideal man combines self-confidence, success, and the willingness to fight for his family (traditional male qualities) with warmth, gentleness, and the willingness to lose (traditional female qualities). As one reader put it:

I'm tired of the American male stereotypes! I have a beard, two biceps, a penis AND I'm capable of showing warmth, sharing housework, and shedding a tear. Why are so many men threatened by that combination of characteristics? (Tavris, 1977, p. 35)

The male sex role is intimately involved with sexuality, for it shapes the way men think and feel about sex. For over a century, sex has generally been seen as more important and enjoyable for men than for women. The belief that men have a stronger biological sex drive persists despite the lack of evidence to support it (Gross, 1978). The idea that men are always ready and willing for sex and that their only problem is getting enough of it has become a cultural myth, as we'll see in Chapter 4 (Zilbergeld, 1978).

Perhaps as a result of this belief in the male need for sex, men tend to separate sex from other aspects of life. Many men find it difficult to establish—or even imagine—nonsexual friendships with women, even though most women easily separate sexual from nonsexual intimacy (Rytting, 1976). The masculine tendency to confuse a need for affection with sexual desire may be why in the past many men felt

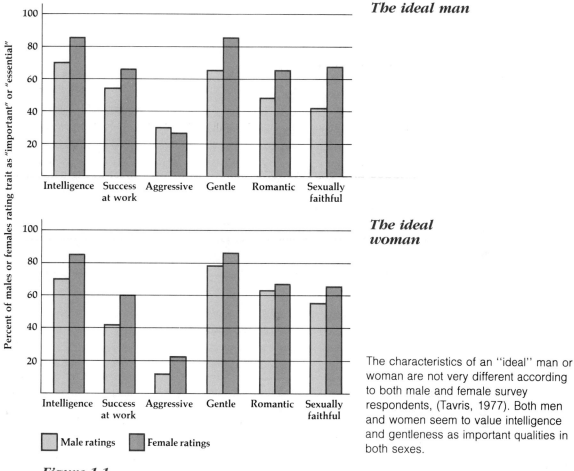

*The ideal man*

*The ideal woman*

Male ratings   Female ratings

*Figure 1.1*

The characteristics of an "ideal" man or woman are not very different according to both male and female survey respondents, (Tavris, 1977). Both men and women seem to value intelligence and gentleness as important qualities in both sexes.

no need to express their love after sexual intercourse—an omission that may make their sexual partners unhappy (Reik, 1960).

Traditional masculine characteristics may have had other influences on the expression of male sexuality (Gross, 1978). The ambitious, competitive achiever may transfer his preoccupation with success from business to bedroom; now he becomes preoccupied with orgasms, both his own and his partner's. A woman described how her husband's sense of manhood had come to depend upon her orgasms:

> It's really important for him that I reach a climax and I try to every time. He says it just doesn't make him feel good if I don't. But it's hard enough to do it once! What happens if he finds out about those women who have lots of climaxes? (Rubin, 1976, p. 92)

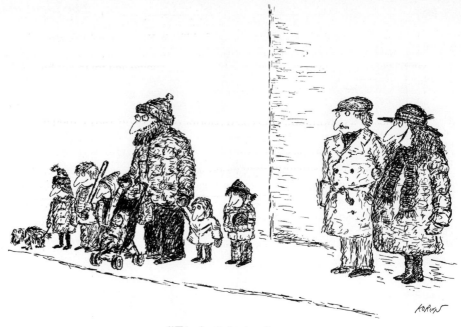

*"That's fathering."*

Similarly, a man who transfers the male characteristics of dominance and control to his sex life will insist on following the traditional male sexual script, initiating sexual interactions and directing each sexual encounter. He will also be unable to reveal any uncertainty or ignorance about sex.

The aggressive aspects of the male sex role are believed to be the basis of rape, a link we discuss in Chapter 16. Finally, the inability of many men to express their emotions stands in the way of communication and thus makes real intimacy between partners difficult.

Recent changes in men's sexual concerns may not be as radical as they seem. The transformation of the heterosexual male image from an insensitive sexual animal, interested only in self-gratification, to a competent lover who skillfully satisfies his partner may be a superficial shift (Gross, 1978). Whether the "typical" man will simply switch from counting sexual conquests to counting his partner's orgasms or come to enjoy a relationship between equal partners is uncertain. Perhaps an equal relationship requires us to rethink the concepts of masculinity and femininity.

## ANDROGYNY

Many people believe that the more masculine a person is, the less feminine, and vice versa. But when either men or women feel rigidly bound by sex roles, they may become as uncomfortable as this woman:

Sometimes I feel that the roles we play are so stifling and inhibiting. I sometimes enjoy being feminine and a bit helpless or submissive, but the problem is turning it on and off when you feel like it. How many times can somebody open a door for you before you start to wonder what's wrong with you? Ultimately, I would like to let go of being so feminine and try to just be more of myself. I wonder if it's really possible? (Authors' files)

If masculinity and femininity are thought of as two separate qualities, instead of as two ends of a continuum, suggested Sandra Bem (1974; 1981), then a person could be both highly masculine and highly feminine. She described such people as possessing **androgyny** and proposed that they would tend to be flexible, responding assertively when the situation demanded assertion and compassionately when the situation demanded compassion. Bem believes that androgynous people have an advantage over strongly **sex-typed** people; that is, women who possess only feminine characteristics and men who possess only masculine characteristics.

She designed a measure of androgyny, called the Bem Sex-Role Inventory, which allows people to rate themselves on qualities that are generally considered feminine (such as affectionate, cheerful, compassionate, warm), masculine (such as aggressive, ambitious, dominant, and self-reliant), or neutral (such as adaptable, friendly, sincere, and tactful). Scores on this measure indicate that a person is androgynous (high in both feminine and masculine traits), masculine (high in masculine and low in feminine traits), feminine (high in feminine and low in masculine traits), or undifferentiated (low in both masculine and feminine traits, although they may be high in neutral traits).

Androgyny, as measured by the Sex-Role Inventory, seems to be advantageous in a number of ways. For example, when placed in social situations, androgynous men and women were competent, effectively handling situations in which they had to show appreciation (such as complimenting a bank teller), as well as those in which they had to be assertive (such as returning an overcooked steak in a restaurant) (Kelly, O'Brien, and Hosford, 1981). Most of the sex-typed individuals were not as effective in the same situations, and undifferentiated people were the least competent of all.

Other sorts of social situations may also be affected by androgyny. In another study (Narus and Fisher, 1982), most androgynous men found it easy to share confidences and to communicate with either men or women. Sex-typed men tended to find such expressiveness easy with women but difficult with men, and undifferentiated men seemed to find it difficult to be expressive with anyone.

In attempting to explain such effects, Bem (1981) proposes that sex-typed people view themselves and the world primarily in terms of gender. Unlike androgynous people, they see most heterosexual interactions in sexual terms. If sex-typed people do place this interpretation on interactions with the other sex, it doesn't seem to make sexuality easier for them. Some studies (Walfish and Myerson, 1980) have found that sex-typed people tend to be less comfortable with their sexuality than androgynous women and men. Compared with androgynous people, sex-typed men and women seemed to feel more guilt about sex and found it difficult to express their sexuality freely or to talk about sex with others.

But the concept of androgyny is more complicated than it appears. Tests of

**androgyny** the presence of both traditional male and traditional female characteristics in the same person

**sex-typed** possessing only the characteristics of a single gender

androgyny tap only one aspect of sex roles: personality traits—primarily the personality traits society sees as desirable. American society demands that women have some masculine personality traits (a full-time homemaker and mother is expected to be independent and self-assertive in running her household) and that men have some feminine personality traits (a mechanic is expected to be considerate of others and able to love) (Spence and Helmreich, 1980). Although women generally have a preponderance of feminine traits and men of masculine traits, it is the situation in which a trait is expressed that makes it seem appropriately male or female.

Since the sex-role inventory rates traits in isolation, not in the context of life situations, androgyny may have no relation to other aspects of being male or female, such as gender identity, attitudes toward sex roles, and vocational and recreational preferences (Spence and Helmreich, 1981). An androgynous woman may be independent, self-reliant, assertive, and willing to take risks, as well as affectionate, gentle, tender, and warm. But she may choose a typically feminine role and find her greatest pleasure in rearing her children. An androgynous man may be compassionate, loyal, sympathetic, and understanding, as well as aggressive, competitive, independent, and willing to take risks. But he may be a truck driver and an avid fisherman and football fan.

It may be that androgyny gives people an advantage in aspects of life that have little to do with gender because such individuals have, in effect, many talents (Spence, 1979). They are able to adapt to a wider variety of roles and situations than either the sex-typed individual (who is talented in only one direction) or the undifferentiated person (who displays few of these socially desirable talents).

Sexual identity continues to develop and change throughout life. Biological events, such as sexual maturation, pregnancy, menopause, and aging, affect sexual identity as do social events such as marriage, divorce, getting or losing a job, the departure of children from the home, and retirement.

## SEXUAL IDENTITY THROUGH THE LIFE CYCLE

The concept of the life cycle is based on the notion that every human being follows a common path from conception to death. Although the path varies in different cultures, it nevertheless passes some of the same landmarks and reaches them in the same basic order. For instance, everyone undergoes the physical changes associated with sexual maturation. In some cultures, these changes are celebrated with elaborate rituals that mark the passage to adulthood; in others, they are virtually ignored.

A second concept that is basic to the notion of the life cycle is that each life consists of predictable stages, such as infancy, childhood, adolescence, young adulthood, middle age, and old age. Development through these stages is not smooth and continuous; it proceeds in fits and starts, stimulated by biological and social events. Each event, such as puberty or retirement, brings with it the need to adjust, to learn, and to grow. The way in which changes are experienced depends on both the nature of the event—say, childbearing—and the person's view of it. The woman who has always expected and wanted to bear children will probably respond to birth in an entirely different way from the woman whose goals and life style are disrupted by the event.

Sex roles themselves seem to change during the life cycle, alternately tightening and loosening (Schell and Hall, 1983). They are usually rigid in early childhood, when children first establish gender identity. They tend to loosen during middle childhood, then tighten again during early adolescence when conformity to sex roles may be more important than at any other time of life. In late adolescence sex roles again relax, only to become strong again with parenthood. Beginning with late middle age, roles tend to lose their rigid quality. No longer concerned with childbearing, women feel free to express their masculine qualities and men to express the feminine side of their nature (Guttman, 1975).

As people meet the developmental tasks of life, they often modify their concepts of masculinity and femininity. For example, the adolescent boy may see traditional masculinity as important and desirable. As he enters young adulthood and leaves the family, he finds that establishing new personal relationships requires a different sort of masculinity from that of the adolescent male, for whom expressions of vulnerability or of positive feelings toward other men are forbidden. He must also establish a new kind of relationship with women that requires intimacy and emotional expressiveness. As concepts of masculinity and femininity are modified, the old standards are not discarded; instead, the young man may incorporate new dimensions. By late middle age, men too take on androgynous qualities (Moreland, 1980).

Little is known about the process of development over the life cycle among homosexual men and women. Since most homosexuals are alike only in their sexu-

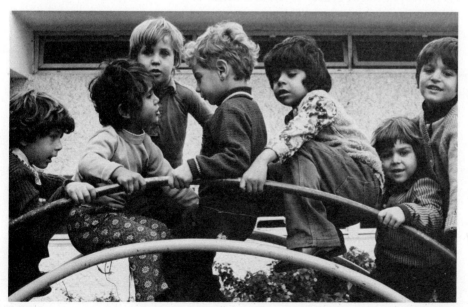

In early childhood, sex roles are much more rigid than they are a few years later. With the development of a firm gender identity, children do not feel quite as bound by the requirements of sex-role stereotypes. (©Marvin E. Newman 1981/ Woodfin Camp & Assoc.)

al orientation, their lives can take many paths. Individuals who are not exclusively homosexual may marry and have children and confront the same developmental tasks as heterosexual men and women who marry. But most homosexuals face a special task in late adolescence or early adulthood. They may experience a profound conflict between their identity in a heterosexual world and their attraction toward members of their own sex. This conflict may be accompanied by guilt, anxiety, and family disruption, and it can even result in alienation from the family:

> When I told my folks that I was a lesbian they totally freaked out. It was so against their religion, their life style and friends, that they just couldn't deal with it. I'm not living at home anymore and I hardly ever talk with them. I hope after a while they'll mellow out about it." (Bell, 1980, p. 120)

The resolution of this conflict may leave the homosexual woman or man better equipped to meet other life tasks, or it may leave a deep sense of anger or vulnerability (Kimmel, 1978).

Looking at human sexuality across the life cycle draws our attention to the individual while stressing the universality of certain life changes. In addition, it emphasizes the internal, or subjective, aspects of sexuality—not only what happens to each person, but how it seems to the individual involved. The subjective aspects of sexuality are a large part of the human experience. Most of us spend far more time thinking about sexuality than actually engaging in sexual acts. For that reason, studies of sexuality that simply count the frequency of intercourse or masturbation and ask about sexual techniques may overlook the important role of subjective experience.

Another value of the life cycle perspective is its recognition of the interaction between biology and experience. At each phase of life, the body has different sexual capacities. In turn, these biological changes influence the nature of the sexual experience, although not necessarily in a single direction. Although slowed sexual response might at first distress an older man or woman, this same slowing down often leads to more relaxed and caring interaction.

Each person moves through a predictable sequence of developmental stages, but the transition from one stage to another is relatively easy for some and not for others. Cultural patterns have a powerful influence on the relative ease of these transitions. In tribal cultures, for example, children are generally allowed to masturbate, to observe adult sexual activity, and to engage in sex play with one another (Ford and Beach, 1951). For these children, the transition to adult sexuality is not an abrupt break with the past. In contrast, Americans generally restrict the expression of childhood sexuality. Children are usually discouraged from sex play and guarded from exposure to sexual information. For American children, adulthood brings a new set of sexual questions and responsibilities for which most have had little preparation.

Stresses may also occur when a person enters a particular stage much earlier or later than peers. Society generally sets a "right time" for various transitions, but not all individuals are punctual. If puberty, or sexual maturation, takes place at age sixteen or seventeen instead of in the early teens, the late maturer may suffer several years of embarrassment or discomfort at being out of step. One woman whose puberty was delayed recalled her own unhappiness:

I remember waiting and waiting for my first period to come. I was about two years later than my friends. Everyone, including my mother, was really panicked about it. She took me to three or four different doctors before it finally came. (Authors' files)

Similarly, people who never pass such sexual milestones as the loss of virginity, marriage, or childbirth may also feel out of step. Pressures to adhere to a rigid timetable are less severe than they once were. In the past decade or so, American society has become more "age-irrelevant," so these milestones may be early or late without evoking much comment (Neugarten and Hall, 1980). However, people who miss one of the milestones—the person who decides to remain celibate or the couple who decide not to have children—often feel compelled to justify their choices.

In addition to its emphasis on predictable patterns, the life cycle perspective also brings into focus the experience of the individual. Although there are many universal sexual experiences, each person has unique feelings, thoughts, and actions. All snowflakes follow the same physical laws, yet each snowflake has a unique shape. In the same way, the physical and social laws that govern sexuality interact with but do not obscure each individual's unique identity.

# Summary

**1** **Gender** includes all the biological (or **imperative**) and cultural (or **optional**) aspects of being male or female. The biological aspects are also referred to as **sex**. **Gender identity**, which develops during the preschool years, is a person's private sense of being male or female. **Sex roles** are the attitudes, behavior, and beliefs dictated by society for members of each sex. Sex roles are exaggerated consequences of the physical differences between the sexes, and most aspects of each sex role can be performed by either men or women.

**2** The sex (biological structure) of a **transsexual** conflicts with his or her gender identity, so that transsexuals feel as if they are trapped in a body of the opposite sex. This discrepancy places the transsexual under considerable stress, and many transsexuals request surgery to make their bodies correspond to their gender identity. Although most transsexuals are sexually attracted to members of their own biological sex, they are different from homosexuals. Homosexuals have no wish to change their bodies and their gender identity corresponds to their biological sex.

**3** **Sexual orientation**, which refers to a person's preference regarding the sex of the sexual partner, falls along a continuum. Sexual orientation may be heterosexual, homosexual, or bisexual. Sexual activity is generally guided by a **sexual script**, a learned mental plan. Each person's sexual script is unique, although it is heavily influenced by the general sexual script for his or her gender in a particular culture.

**4** Sex roles become translated into **sex-role stereotypes**, exaggerated concepts of the traits and behavior of each gender. Although the biological basis for sex differences in lower animals is clear, establishing such a link in human beings is difficult. Sex hormones do influence brain structure and function before birth, but the proposal that they are responsible for differences in the way male and female brains process information is controversial. Male hormones appear to be linked with a tendency toward aggression. However, males and females are treated differently from the moment of birth and many sex differences are the result of environmental influence. In recent years, the gap between male and female sex roles seems to have become smaller.

**5** Women have been subordinate to men in all the cultures and traditions that influenced modern European and North American society. Such inventions as reliable contraceptives, rubber feeding nipples, pasteurization of milk, and sanitary pads probably played a major role in enabling women to assert equality with men and push for a redefinition of sex roles. As sex roles change, women are taking education and careers more seriously than ever before, and are deciding when and whether to marry, whether to have children, and how to combine occupational and domestic roles. Beliefs about sex roles, sexuality, and the marriage relationships appear to be changing faster than actual behavior, and it is very difficult for some women and men to break out of the traditional scripts. Traditional women are primarily wives and mothers, but to nontraditional women, occupation is central. Despite changes in sex roles, the media— especially television—continue to portray men and women in terms of sex-role stereotypes.

**6** The rigid male stereotype teaches men to avoid "feminine" activities, to be aggressive, independent, and successful. Younger, highly educated men appear to be moving away from stereotypical attitudes. In the male stereotype men have strong sex drives, a belief that apparently leads them to separate sex from other aspects of life and to transfer their preoccupation with success from business to the bedroom.

**7 Androgyny,** or the combination of male and female personality traits in a single person, may lead to flexible behavior, whereas **sex-typed** people, or those who possess only the qualities attributed to a single sex, may be more rigid. Androgyny appears to affect comfort with sexuality and behavior in social situations. However, androgyny may bear no relation to any other aspect of gender except personality traits.

**8** Sexuality changes and develops across the life cycle, with every human being following a common path of development through predictable stages. Sex roles seem to tighten and loosen at predictable points during the life cycle. Homosexuals face an additional task, the conflict between their identity in a predominantly heterosexual world and their sexual orientation. Seeing sexuality across the life cycle makes both individual and universal aspects of sexuality clear; it also highlights the interaction between biology and experience. Transitions through the life cycle are heavily influenced by culture, and stresses in sexual development may occur if a person enters a stage too quickly or too slowly, or if the person misses some sexual milestone.

## a woman's view

The most important factors in a good sexual relationship are emotional closeness, mutual caring, sensuality, and tenderness. Of all of these I think emotional closeness is the most important, because if there are feelings lacking or if there is anger brewing in the background, I can't experience a very close relationship. The true essence of love making is a real emotional closeness. (Barbach and Levine, 1981, p. 34)

## a man's view

My relationships with women have changed so dramatically since my college days. When I think back to how I was always on the make, and how important it was to "score" with every date, I realize just how far I've come. Now I can be really close to a woman and open myself up to her, and it doesn't have to lead to sex. On the other hand, it's a long time since I've been to bed with someone I wasn't emotionally involved with. (Authors' files)

# 2 The Sexual Relationship

# Chapter 2

---

Sex is different from food or air or water; any of us could survive without it, although most of us wouldn't want to. Sexual activity serves three basic human needs. First, it is procreational: sex can lead to reproduction and the survival of the species. Next, it is recreational: sex can be a form of play. Finally, it is relational: sex gives us a way of expressing our feelings toward another person.

For thousands of years, these last two aspects of sexuality were difficult to separate from procreation, although procreation was always easy to separate from sex's other functions. A person can engage in sex dutifully, without delight or affection, for the purpose of providing an heir—and many people have. But until reliable methods of birth control were developed, the possibility of producing a child accompanied each episode of hetereosexual activity, no matter what its purpose.

American society has emphasized the relational aspect of sexual behavior in the belief that sexual activity is at its best within the context of an intimate relationshp. The contemporary American ideal is two people who have formed a pair bond, developed intimacy, and are deeply in love. Since people are not always ready or willing to take on the responsibility of an intimate relationship, the nature of sexual relationships varies widely and expresses a variety of human needs.

In this chapter, we'll explore the sexual relationship, and even attempt to discover just what love is. We'll take up the question of men and women in love, and try to find out whether the experience is different for the two sexes and—if so—how a man in love differs

# The Sexual Relationship

from a woman in love. After investigating the Judeo-Christian view of the sexual relationship, we'll look at love and sexuality in two quite different cultures. By contrasting black, Hispanic, and white views of the sexual relationship, we can explore the influence of ethnic background on love. The chapter will close with a brief review of the study of human sexuality.

## THE SEXUAL RELATIONSHIP

Most of us want our sexual encounters to occur within the context of a sexual relationship. Ideally, that relationship is marked by intimacy, love, and pair bonding, but it may not include all three. The possibilities of sex are not limited by the bounds of an intimate relationship. For some people, some of the time, sex is just fun.

### Sex as play

Sex can be an extremely pleasurable form of adult play, as many people have discovered. According to one woman:

> With my present sexual partner, lovemaking is mostly lighthearted and playful. The best part of it is that we can tease each other and fool around a lot—he really makes me laugh! I think most of us need some way to let our hair down once in a while—life is too serious otherwise. (Authors' files)

Recreational sex can be more than fun; it can also serve an important function. Playful sex without intimacy has a place in our lives at times when we do not want an ongoing relationship, but also do not want to give up sex. Just after a divorce or the breakup of a love affair, for example, recreational sex may be extremely helpful. At such times, there is a need to attain emotional freedom from the former lover or spouse, as well as a desire to avoid a premature emotional commitment or marriage on the rebound (May, 1981). If the end of the relationship has been painful, recreational sex can reassure a person that he or she is still an appealing sex partner, or it can help to wipe away the memories of the unhappy relationship.

In some instances, divorced people who steer clear of recreational sex may find that their need to prove successful in an intimate relationship may spoil sex for them. One man recalled how his need to prove himself hampered his ability to see that sex is also play:

> When my marriage broke up, it seemed reasonable that I would get right into a relationship with Emily, a woman I had known as a friend for a long time. I felt this tremendous pressure building up to prove myself as a good family man who could maintain a steady connection with a woman despite the fact that my marriage had ended. . . . We both felt a lot of anxiety over whether we could be intimate and whether we could make a relationship together. What was on the line, we felt, was potential success in cementing a *Commitment*. So we were always off balance, and things were completely different from the way we had been as friends. (D. Bell, 1982, p. 90)

Recreational sex becomes a problem when people reject the idea of emotional intimacy and treat all their sexual encounters as "nothing but" recreation. This can lead to the development of too many relationships that lack any kind of emotional intimacy. Some therapists see this behavior pattern as trivializing sex, draining it of meaning and making it no more important than a handshake (Bach and Torbet, 1982). In the view of psychologist Rollo May (1981), the habitual practice of sex without intimacy can turn the sexual act into sensation without emotion, so that there is little difference between intercourse and masturbation.

Our concern that sex be playful may lead us to overlook the fact that recreational and intimate sex are not always separate. Laughter and play are important features of many intimate relationships. In fact, intimate relationships that include playful sexual encounters are probably the most durable kind.

## Intimacy

**intimacy** an emotional state marked by acceptance, self-disclosure, and feelings of trust and closeness

Whether a sexual relationship lasts only a few weeks or a lifetime, it has little lasting meaning for either partner unless it includes intimacy. **Intimacy**, which is an emotional state marked by acceptance, self-disclosure, and feelings of trust and closeness, is not restricted to sexual partners. Intimacy can develop between family members, friends, or colleagues at work.

Within the sexual relationship, intimacy has many dimensions. The way it is expressed depends on the partners' needs and expectations and on the kind of relationship. The same person may express intimacy in different ways in different relationships. But if a relationship is to be intimate and not exploitative, each partner will care for the other (Bach and Torbet, 1982). A twenty-one-year-old woman told why intimacy was important to her:

> I need to have a person who's very aware of my feelings, who's going to be in tune with me emotionally and physically, somebody who, first and foremost, I want to wake up in bed with the next morning. If it's not an ongoing kind of sharing, then I don't feel that secure. If it's just going to be a one-night stand, I don't want to be part of that. I've been in enough of them to know there's a feeling of dissatisfaction that's too overwhelming and just not worth it for me. (Barbach and Levine, 1981, pp. 33–34)

An intimate relationship requires some degree of spontaneity, but it can range from what seems like totally spontaneous "love at first sight" to a long, considered building of intimacy from a neutral first impression. Even partners who tumble head over heels are unlikely to develop any lasting intimacy unless they also have common interests, backgrounds, and goals (Wong, 1981).

Psychologists who have analyzed intimate relationships see them as composed of two kinds of attachment: liking and loving (Walster and Walster, 1978). Some relationships are high on passionate love but low on companionate love (liking); others are high on companionate love but have little spark or passion. Rarely is a relationship high on both factors. In a highly passionate relationship, lovers feel

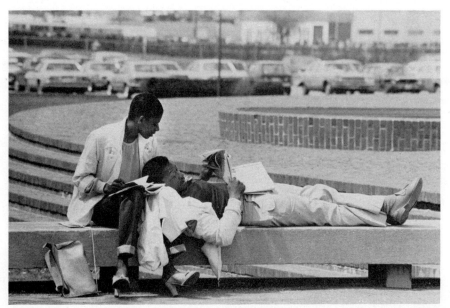

This couple exemplify the ideal sexual relationship in today's United States. They have formed a pair bond, developed intimacy, and are deeply in love. (© Ellis Herwig/Stock, Boston)

they can confide in the partner, and the thought of never being with the partner plunges them into misery. In a highly companionate relationship, lovers believe the partner is unusually well-adjusted, have great confidence in the partner's good judgment, and think the partner is one of the most likable people they know.

If an intimate relationship is to be satisfying, it needs to be honest. In an honest relationship, the partners agree on the level of the relationship's intensity (liking or loving), on whether the relationship is limited (as with the lovers in the film *Same Time, Next Year,* who spent one weekend each year in an intimate, loving, sexual relationship and never saw each other between their annual meetings) or extended to all areas of life, and on its duration (for the summer, till graduation, for a lifetime) (Wong, 1981). When agreement is lacking, one partner is likely to be hurt.

## Love

There are probably as many definitions of love as there are people in the world, for love is a uniquely personal experience. Our attempts to define love run into the roadblock of the English language, which uses one word to describe feelings that other languages have three words to express. In Greek, love is either *eros, philia,* or *agape* (ah-gah-pay); in Latin, it is *amor, delictio,* or *caritas. Agape* and *caritas* describe unselfish love—the love of God or the altruistic love of others. In the Bible when St. Paul speaks of love as being patient and kind, never envious, selfish, or conceited, he used the word *agape. Philia* and *delictio* describe the love of one friend for another. This sort of love is sometimes called sisterly or brotherly love. *Eros* and *amor* describe erotic or sexual love, the sort of love that is at the basis of intimate sexual relationships.

But it's possible to feel different kinds of love for the same person—and for the mixture to change over time. Erotic lovers can be moved by unselfish love to nurse one another in illness, to comfort one another in sorrow. Friendly love can be at the basis of shared delight in a conversation, a walk in the woods, a sail on a summer's day. In fact, partners can feel more than one kind of love for each other at the same time.

In contrast with the idealized version of love at its highest level—gentle and unselfish, timeless and enduring—is the more down-to-earth love most of us know. Love may be unselfish, but it can also be the basis of possessiveness and jealousy. Love may be extremely pleasurable, but it can also be intensely painful. Love may last a lifetime, but it can also be fickle and short-lived. Love expands options for some people, but inhibits or stifles others. Hate, loneliness, or selfishness seem to be the opposites of love, yet for some people these qualities are bound up in the love relationship.

Such great individual differences in the experience of love might lead us to Voltaire's conclusion: "There are so many sorts of love that one does not know where to seek a definition of it." To some, love is an expression of our basic humanity and goodness; to others, love means sex or security or possessions or "never having to say you're sorry." Any definition can be valid for a certain person at a specific time and place. But despite the lack of a universal definition, none of us has any difficulty in identifying our love relationships.

**The origins of love** There have been two basic approaches to untangling the nature of love. One sees love as an instinctive force that shapes human behavior from within, and the other sees it as learned, shaped by culture and personal experience.

Sigmund Freud, the Viennese physician who developed an instinctive approach to love, viewed it as a transformation of the basic sexual instinct, or life force, which he called the libido.

**libido** the basic sexual instinct, or life force

In 1905, Freud published *Three Essays on Sexuality,* which shocked the scientific community by proposing an elaborate theory of infantile sexuality. Freud attempted to trace the origins of adult emotional disorders to disturbances in childhood sexuality and to show the significance of childhood sexuality for all aspects of personality development. He maintained that it was society's suppression and redirection of the sexual instinct that led to the development of culture. In large part through his influence, sexuality came to be seen as central to the formation of character and the development of culture (Gagnon, 1975). To modern psychoanalysts, love is a manifestation of instinctive urges that must be expressed in one form or another. And since all forms of love originate from the libido, even the care-giving mother-child relationship is based on sublimated sexuality.

In the learning approach, love is a learned reaction that varies from culture to culture and at different times in the same culture. The United States is a love-oriented culture—love between parent and child and between adults is highly valued. Americans seem unable to conceive of a normal life that does not contain love relationships. Novels, films, and popular music are filled with love themes, and children grow up believing love and marriage are a necessary part of adult experience.

Our culture reinforces us for being in love, and most of us feel deprived and incomplete without it. But in other cultures there is no such emphasis on love. Marriage is far more likely to be based on financial or family considerations than on personal feelings. Among Australian aborigines and in some African societies, for example, when a girl reaches puberty she may be married to a man who is old enough to be her grandfather. Far from being tragedies, such marriages are generally successful (Montagu, 1962).

In one version of the learning approach, passionate love is seen as having two components: a physiological state of arousal and a process of mental labeling (Walster and Walster, 1978). In the arousal portion of any strong emotion, the palms sweat, the face is flushed, and the heart pounds. A person standing at the edge of a precipice might label these sensations "fear." A person who is arguing with an enemy might label them "anger." And a person who is in the presence of an arousing sexual partner might label them "love." Although the labeling process is more complicated than this, the point is that we ourselves decide the label. Even in the presence of an appealing partner, we might call the emotion "love," "lust," "infatuation," or "annoyance."

Many of our ideas about love come from novels, popular music, and movies. The films of Spencer Tracy and Katherine Hepburn taught a generation of Americans that love relationships were essential and that they always led to marriage. (The Museum of Modern Art–Film Stills Archive)

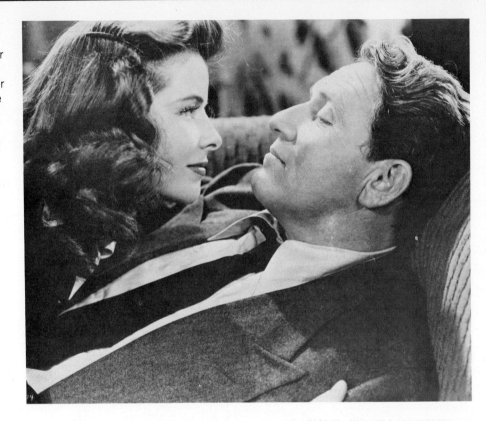

### The course of passionate love

The way we feel when we are passionately in love has been studied by Dorothy Tennov (1979), who wondered just how the feelings connected with companionate love differed from those of passionate love, which she called **limerence**. She found that many people's experiences with sex and love showed no trace of desperate passion, but that when the passion was strong, the relationship eclipsed all others.

**limerence** passionate love

People who were passionately in love were in a wildly emotional state, on a seesaw between bliss and jealousy. They were obsessed with thoughts of their loved one; their mood depended on the loved one's actions; they longed for a response, and when it came, they felt they were walking on air. They could be so passionately involved with only one person at a time. One person described these feelings in a diary:

> This obsession has infected my brain. I cannot shake those constantly intruding thoughts of you. Every thought winds back to you no matter how hard I try to direct its course in other directions. (Tennov, 1979, p. 34)

Why does passionate love strike? It may be that each of us carries around an idealized, individual image of a perfect mate. If for some reason we project this image onto another person, bells ring, lights flash—it's love. The loved person is seen as a dream come true. But this impassioned love is not for the real person; it is for the idealized image (Money, 1980). Obviously, such an intense feeling can't last forever. The delirium may last for days, for weeks, or for six months, but its natural lifetime seems to be about two or three years—long enough to court, mate, and produce a child.

If the partners are unlucky and share nothing but passion, when the passion burns out the relationship goes dead. For the fortunate, it turns into a companionate love, a more tranquil erotic affection sparked by brief episodes of passion (Walster and Walster, 1978). One man described such a transformation:

> There are two kinds of love, crazy love when you are just zapped when you first meet someone and then the deep love that may develop after you get to know a person. They are not the same. The first kind sends you into the clouds, you feel as if you are walking on air. . . . The second kind comes of knowing someone very closely, of becoming super-familiar with her, of trusting her implicitly and always feeling at ease with her. It is a relaxed and comfortable feeling, not as exciting and heady as the first kind but far more rewarding and secure. (Hite, 1981, p. 126)

Women have had similar experiences:

> I do love him tremendously. My whole life is built around him, and I'm sure that if you'd asked me that question ["Do you feel that you are 'in love' with Jim?"] during our most unsettled, if not actually stormy, second year, I'd have said yes without hesitation. But my feelings for Jim are not the kind of thing you read about in romantic stories. I don't know how I'd feel if I suspected he was having an affair with his secretary, or losing interest in me, but as things stand, I say I am not "in love" with Jim, but rather feel a very deep, very solid love and affection for my husband and the father of my precious babies. (Tennov, 1979, pp. 10–11)

Given the wildly emotional nature of limerence, it's probably best for all of us that the intensity doesn't last.

## Pair bonding

Whether love is passionate or companionate, the partners often form a **pair bond,** an intimate, committed relationship. To get a better understanding of such relationships in human beings, researchers have studied animal mating systems.

The members of many species form pair bonds, typically between an adult male and female, and generally involving a sexual element. Among human beings, pair bonds are usually distinguished by intimacy and long-term commitment—the promise that the intimacy will be permanent. Another feature of many pair bonds is exclusivity, based on the belief that intimacy can exist only when it is not shared outside the primary relationship.

Biological approaches to pair bonding divide the process into three phases: **proception,** the attraction of the partner, which corresponds to courtship; **acception,** or genital sexual activity, including vaginal, anal, and oral sex; and conception, including gestation and parenthood. During parenthood, the pair bond

**pair bond** an intimate committed relationship, generally involving a sexual element

**proception** the courtship phase of pair bonding, which includes the solicitation and attraction of the partner

**acception** the phase of pair bonding that consists of genital sexual activity, including vaginal, oral, and anal sex

**conception** the phase of pair bonding that consists of conception, pregnancy, and parenthood

expands to form a nonsexual bond with the child. With the development of birth control, the **conception** phase has been eliminated from many human pair bonds, as more and more couples are childless by choice (Schwartz, Money, and Robinson, 1981).

The nature of adult sexual relationships in any species appears to be partly determined by patterns of child care. If the male participates in the care and rearing of the young, pair bonding is common (Beach, 1976). Among the northern wolf, where child care is shared by the parents, the adult pair bond is so strong that the partners remain faithful until one or the other dies. Lengthy courtships and pair bonding do not develop if the male contributes nothing to childrearing. Members of such species are likely to have many sexual partners, with competition or sexual advertising common among males. The female chooses the most desirable male for each successive mating.

**monogamy** pair bond made up of one male and one female

**polygyny** pair bond made up of one male and several females

**polyandry** pair bond made up of one female and several males

**sociobiologist** scientist who attempts to explain social behavior by looking at biological processes

In many species, child care is neither equally divided nor exclusively the responsibility of the female. Various types of pair bonds have developed to cover these situations. Species in which the female alone cannot provide sufficient food for her young live in **monogamy** (one male and one female). In those species in which the male contributes little to the nourishment or rearing of offspring, such as cattle or deer, **polygyny** (one male and several females) is the general rule. A natural example of **polyandry** (one female and several males) occurs among some birds. The male incubates the eggs, freeing the female to find another mate, who may then take on the role of incubating a second batch of eggs.

**Sociobiologists**, who attempt to explain social behavior by looking at biological processes, believe the same basis underlies human pair bonding. Since human infants are born totally helpless, offspring need both parents to survive. As a result,

The nature of sexual relationships varies from one species to another. Pair bonding is strongest when the male helps care for the young. (Animals, Animals)

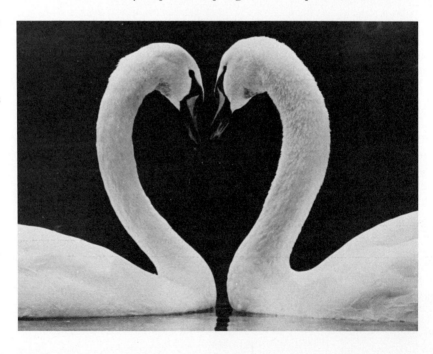

a strong, exclusive, and relatively permanent pair bond develops (Barash, 1977). Human societies may be monogamous, polygynous, or polyandrous. Pair bonding may be altered or weakened in societies where a father is not crucial to the rearing of his children.

Pair bonding in American society appears to be a mixture of Mediterranean and Nordic traditions (Money, 1977). Mediterranean pair bonding developed thousands of years ago around the eastern end of the Mediterranean. It grew out of urban culture and the system of slavery, and featured the ownership and control of women by men. It was marked by arranged marriages, virgin brides, and a double standard of morality for men and women. The Nordic tradition developed in the prehistory of northern Europe. It grew out of a family-centered fishing and farming culture in which men and women were more nearly equal, and it featured marriage based on romantic love, premarital sex between engaged couples, and a single sexual standard. The two traditions merged, and the dominant American pattern became romantic love, virgin brides, and the double standard. Now that the conception phase of pair bonding no longer dominates human sexuality, pair bonds can develop for nonbiological reasons—to avoid alienation and loneliness, to enhance emotional security, to express and receive love, to share physical intimacy. Human beings are social beings, and they will always tend to seek out others of their kind with whom they can be intimate.

Some authorities believe that when human beings never develop emotional bonds with adults in infancy, they may be unable to form stable pair bonds when they grow up (Schwartz, Money, and Robinson, 1981). They may find themselves falling in and out of love with great rapidity. They may develop "anxious" bonds, in which they are pulled toward a partner, only to draw away when the relationship promises to become intimate. Or they may become so centered on themselves that they cannot develop a bond. They may never be able to trust a partner, to commit themselves to a relationship, or to find pleasure in intimacy or physical contact. In Chapter 11, we'll see how important infancy and childhood are in the development of sexuality. Now we turn to the different experiences of men and women in love. Emotional intimacy and love may be expressed differently by men and women, in good part because men's and women's sex roles are so dissimilar.

## MEN IN LOVE

From early childhood, men learn to suppress emotional display and generally to appear tough, confident, and self-reliant no matter how they feel inside.

In the stereotypical view, men need sex more and love less, so men are seen as using love to get sex while women are seen as using sex to get love. It appears, however, that love and intimacy are often as important for men as for women, although men express these needs differently. One man testified to the importance of love in his life:

Love is the ultimate in heartfelt affection between a man and a woman. Being loved and knowing I am loved by my wife is the very foundation of my existence. Take it away and I would surely perish. (Hite, 1981, p. 123)

Studies of passionate love have found no universal sex differences in the way men and women experience this passion. However, fewer men than women say they often daydream about the loved one or lie awake at night thinking about their beloved. And when asked about the unhappy aspects of limerence, men say they fear rejection or heartbreak less than women do (Tennov, 1979). But in studies that followed the course of more than 200 college relationships, men tended to fall in love more easily than women and to be slower in falling out of love (Rubin, Peplau, and Hill, 1981). Men were more likely to say that the desire to fall in love was an important reason for beginning a love relationship and to be strongly attracted to the partner at the first meeting. Like men in earlier studies (Knox and Sporakowski, 1968), these men believed in love at first sight and were certain that love could overcome any obstacle—racial, religious, or economic. Among couples who broke up over the two-year period, the men were more often depressed, lonelier, and unhappier than the women.

In their nonsexual relationships, men seem to find intimacy more difficult to achieve, especially when their friend is another man (Fischer and Narus, 1981). This reluctance to establish intimacy with other men is apparently influenced by sex roles and early learning. Many American men grow up without male models who demonstrate physical intimacy among men. When television news programs show Arab men in emotional embraces of greeting or leave-taking, American male

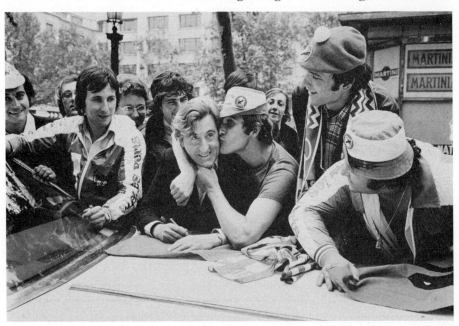

Most American men feel uncomfortable about any physical intimacy with another man. Among some ethnic groups, however, male sex roles allow men to embrace one another. (© Bernard Pierre Wolff/Magnum)

viewers may react with snickers or snide comments. The fear of being regarded as homosexual leads men to avoid touching other men except in contact sports. And since men are supposed to be competitive and never show weakness, they are unlikely to disclose their weaknesses or problems to other men (Lewis, 1978). One man expressed exactly this attitude, saying:

> I haven't had a friend since I was in college. The business world taught me that friendships are a luxury one cannot afford. They leave one vulnerable, with great chinks in one's armor. (Hite, 1981, p. 89)

Yet in another study of a group of young, educated, single adults, this generally accepted male characteristic failed to appear. Men were as willing to disclose their strengths and weaknesses to their male friends as women were to reveal themselves to their female friends. What's more, men were not more likely to confide in women than in men (Hacker, 1981). Although the inhibitions and restrictions of the male sex role do make intimacy difficult for men, its power is probably diminishing. Men today are learning to be more flexible as a wider range of behavior becomes available.

## WOMEN IN LOVE

Changing sex roles have also had an impact on the way many women act and feel in love relationships. Traditionally, women's identities have been closely linked to their love relationships. Although love relationships are still important today, many women no longer expect them to fill their lives to the exclusion of other roles in the larger society.

Love has public significance for most women in American culture because it is the accepted reason for marriage and because a woman's social role has been defined by her husband's position. It may be this increased vulnerability that makes women more likely to say they have been depressed over a love affair, or to be "terribly afraid" that their beloved will stop loving them (Tennov, 1979). But if this is so, why do women seem to fall in love less easily and break off relationships faster than men? A young woman who had ended a relationship reported:

> I don't think I ever felt romantic [about her partner]—I felt practical. I had the feeling that I'd better make the most of it because it won't last that long. (Rubin, Peplau, and Hill, 1981, p. 829)

Perhaps women tend to take a practical approach because the social consequences of marriage make them cautious about investing their love in the first place. For many young women today, the sexual revolution has meant premarital sex with a man they love deeply and intend to marry. They are "serious" about love because they are more likely than men to make the practical connection between love and life choices (Laws and Schwartz, 1977).

The still-prevalent female attitude shows in the words of a twenty-six-year-old woman:

I was a virgin until this year. I spent my life believing that sex should be reserved for a marital or other strongly committed relationship. So I waited until I found the right person. This year I found him. Interestingly, my lover held the same views I did, and he too was a virgin. I decided I was ready for intercourse with this man, because I was fairly certain the relationship will lead to marriage and I am fairly certain we can make the marriage work. (Wolfe, 1981, pp. 314–315)

Although some women have severed the connection between love, intimacy, and sex, most women have not. Such factors as love for their partner and the comfort, familiarity, and security of an intimate relationship are very important to them (Barbach and Levine, 1981). An emotional bond generally requires time to develop, but women report that on rare occasions, it is apparent almost as soon as they meet a man. It seems to be primarily divorced or widowed women who go through a period of sex without caring before they decide some kind of emotional commitment is necessary. One woman's experience is typical of this group:

After I got divorced, it was like every sexual experience that I went through was new and each time I got something new out of it. It was exciting and satisfying at first, but what I've learned about myself during the past four years is that caring about somebody and loving somebody is more important. That's when I can really enjoy sex. (Barbach and Levine, 1981, p. 31)

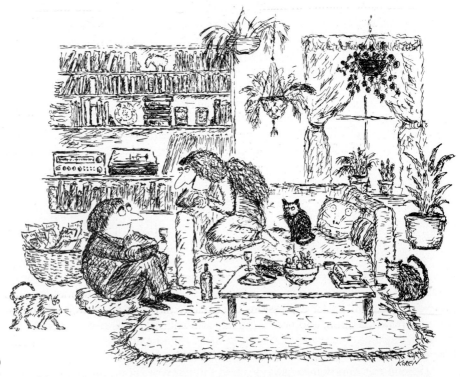

*"I'm very, very fussy when it comes to men."*

Women appear to link sex and love. However, when men and women were asked about their love experiences, women were much more likely to say that they had been in love without feeling the need for sex, and half the women but only a fifth of the men said they thought about sex a lot more when they were in love (Tennov, 1979). Among the 200 college couples, women who had had intercourse with their boyfriends were more likely to be in love with them than those who had not had sexual relations. However, there was no relationship at all between a man's love for his girlfriend and whether they had had sex (Peplau, Rubin, and Hill, 1977).

All these studies of men and women in love have been conducted in American society, and most have been limited to white, middle-class individuals. In other societies, other social classes, and among other ethnic groups, love and sexual relationships may be approached in a different manner.

# CULTURAL AND ETHNIC ASPECTS OF THE SEXUAL RELATIONSHIP

Certain aspects of sexuality are common to all cultures. Sexual customs vary from one society to the next, from one segment of a culture to another, and at different times in the same culture. In many cultures, religious traditions are the basis for sexual customs. The American view of the sexual relationship, for example, has been shaped by the Judeo-Christian tradition.

## *The Judeo-Christian influence*

Just as cultural standards change, so the sexual values proposed by any religion often evolve over time or are interpreted differently. Many of the Judeo-Christian values that are taken for granted today come not from the Bible, but from the later pronouncements of religious authorities.

Despite the changes, it is possible to generalize about the influence of the Judeo-Christian tradition on current sexual practices. Overall, this tradition can be described as the most sexually restrictive of all the major religions (Bullough, 1976). In some respects, Jewish and Christian approaches to sexuality differ sharply. In traditional Judaism, sexual intercourse was a sacred activity—but only within marriage (Gordis, 1977). Marriage had two goals: procreation and companionship. Marital sex was seen as cementing the marital relationship as well as producing offspring. Celibacy, or abstinence, had no place in Judaism for either priests or the general population. Other expressions of sexuality did not fare so well. Masturbation was frowned upon, and homosexuality and adultery were condemned. In the book of Leviticus, homosexual activity by men called for the death penalty, and when the woman was married, both partners in adultery were killed.

**celibacy** abstinence from sexual intercourse

Despite the importance placed on marital sex, the subordinate position of women and the double standard were always clear. When a married man had intercourse with an unmarried woman, the act was considered not adultery, but fornication. And as the book of Deuteronomy makes clear, women who were not virgins at marriage were to be stoned to death. (A woman "proved" her virginity by bleeding on the nuptial bedclothes.)

Judaism's stress on the positive aspects of marital sexuality did not carry over into Christianity. Jesus said little about sex except for his admonishments against divorce, in which he attempted to hold men to the same standards that bound women (Bullough and Bullough, 1973). The early Christians adopted the Greek attitude that sex was low and unworthy, and celibacy exalted (Hiltner, 1977). Primarily as a result of the writings of St. Paul, all forms of sensual pleasure were prohibited—even pleasure within marriage. St. Paul believed that profound spiritual enlightenment could be achieved only through abstinence. He advised those who were unable to maintain this state to marry, for it was better to marry than to suffer the torments of unsatisfied desire or to risk the sin of nonmarital sex.

Over the centuries, the position of the Catholic Church on sexual matters continued to harden. The writings of St. Augustine (A.D. 354–430) had a great impact on the increasingly antisexual position of the Church. With his conversion, Augustine became celibate and renounced all forms of physical and sexual pleasure. Due largely to his influence, Christianity in the Middle Ages developed into a religion of sexual asceticism.

The leaders of the Protestant Reformation rejected the Roman Catholic position on celibacy and took a more positive attitude toward sex within marriage. Martin Luther (1483–1546) agreed with St. Augustine that sexual desire was sinful, but urged marriage for procreation and to prevent sexual immorality. He believed

In traditional Judaism, marriage was meant to provide companionship as well as children. Sexual intercourse was sacred, but only within the bounds of marriage. (© Abigail Heyman/Archive)

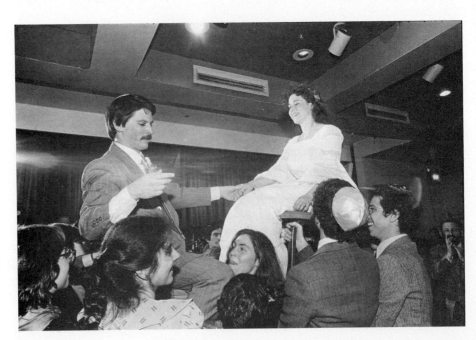

that—for men—sexual gratification was as necessary as eating and drinking. John Calvin (1509–1564), the father of Puritanism, believed that woman's primary role was that of a companion, not a producer of children (Phipps, 1973). But neither Luther nor Calvin recognized the sexual rights of the individual, and both regarded masturbation and homosexuality with revulsion.

The overall effect of Western religious tradition has been the classification of most sexual conduct as sin. This set of sexual standards has been honored more in the breach than in the observance, but certainly, there have been personal costs for those who have failed to live up to the sexual demands of their religious beliefs.

Religious values have also been used to justify the oppression of sexual minorities and women. For example, the use of contraceptives continues to be a major issue within the Roman Catholic Church, as does the status of homosexuals. In contrast, the Church has begun to take a more positive attitude toward the pleasures of sexuality within marriage (Hiltner, 1977). And signs of change have appeared within Christian churches in general. Certain groups, such as the Unitarians and the United Methodists, have begun sex education programs for young people. Clergy have been taking an active role in counseling adults with sexual problems. Shifting sexual values have also caused changes within the Roman Catholic Church, as an increasing number of the American clergy have followed their consciences on such matters as homosexuality, divorce, and contraception. Such signs indicate that the traditional attitude of the churches toward sexual conduct is changing. But the influence of tradition is still strong.

## Cultural variations

Human beings respond to their history and environment, and almost every aspect of their sexuality can be developed, shaped, and altered by the social context in which it takes place. Because so much of human sexual activity is learned, questions of "normality" and "morality" can be answered only within a specific cultural context. What seems "normal" to Americans may hold little appeal for people in Europe, Asia, or Africa. Indeed, American sexual standards and practices have themselves changed radically in this century. Not many decades ago, Americans believed that masturbation was dangerous to body and soul, that women never enjoyed sex, and that too many orgasms depleted a man's strength. Given the sweeping changes that have taken place, what was "normal" sexual expression for a married couple in 1900 would be considered unusual, if not unhealthy, in the 1980s.

One of the first researchers to make a serious study of the sexual customs of other cultures and to describe differing customs was Havelock Ellis, a nineteenth-century Englishman. Ellis was influential in popularizing the concept of individual and cultural relativism in sex and in persuading people that the value of any sexual custom had to be considered in relation to the culture in which it was found (Bullough, 1976). He made extensive use of the case-history method, documenting with individual histories the wide range of sexual variation that can be found in all

# Focus

SEXUAL
CUSTOMS
IN TWO
CULTURES

A look at Mangaia and the People's Republic of China, two very different cultures, may help to put American sexual practices in perspective.

The people who live on the small island of Mangaia in the South Pacific have a relaxed attitude toward sexuality. Children are free to watch the "private" sexual activities of parents and siblings within the one-room Mangaian home. Their masturbation and sex play are accepted as long as they are conducted "in private." Circumcision in Mangaia is a rite of passage, during which a youth is instructed in sexual technique by a male expert. After two weeks of instruction, the boy has intercourse with a mature and experienced woman, who teaches him about the timing and positions that bring a woman to orgasm. Since a woman who cannot reach orgasm is virtually unknown in Mangaia, a man who

fails to provide his partner with several orgasms gets a reputation as a poor lover.

Mangaians are especially concerned with frequent and lengthy intercourse and show little interest in foreplay, sexual position, or demonstrations of affection. Affection or intimacy is not required for intercourse. Young men and women have many partners before deciding to marry. As might be expected, many Mangaian women become pregnant or bear children before marriage. These children are not considered illegitimate, and pregnancy does not necessarily lead to marriage.

The rate of intercourse in Mangaia is far higher than in most Western cultures. However, love as Americans know it—warm and affectionate feelings between sexual partners— does not seem to play a major role in Mangaia. Mangaians select their

sexual partners on the basis of physical attractiveness or prowess in sexual techniques, but with little regard for long-term emotional attachment or love (Marshall, 1971).

In contrast to the permissive society of Mangaia is the restrictive society of the People's Republic of China. Sexual attitudes and behavior in China reflect the country's political needs. Since society's requirements are considered to be far more important than those of any individual, love and sex are considered counterrevolutionary activities. Personal gratification is supposed to come from work and participation in the Communist system, and not from fulfilling selfish desires for romance and sexual pleasure. Sexuality gets little scientific attention, and the Chinese receive almost no sex education, prefer not to talk about sex, and have few sources of help for sexual problems. A Chi-

*Ellis,*
*no judgements*

societies. Instead of making judgments, Ellis simply observed and collected information. On the basis of the case histories, Ellis wrote *Studies in the Psychology of Sex,* which was published in six volumes between 1897 and 1910. Although Ellis covered a wide range of subjects, his opinions on masturbation, homosexuality, and female sexuality were particularly influential. He argued that masturbation was an essentially harmless activity, that homosexuality was a genetically determined but nonpathological sexual variation, and that women had a sexual response equal to that of men. During the twentieth century, the understanding of varying customs was broadened by studies conducted around the world by anthropologists.

nese woman told an American psychologist who was visiting China that her mother waited until her daughter's wedding day to explain the "true purpose of marriage" (Tavris, 1974).

This seemingly Victorian approach toward sexuality is fairly recent. In pre-Communist times, the Chinese had a relatively matter-of-fact attitude toward sex, considering it a natural urge that, like eating or sleeping, should be satisfied at the right time and in the right place. An-

cient Chinese writings contained explicit descriptions of sexual activity, and prostitution was tolerated. However, love and romance were unimportant; marriages were based on economic and social considerations.

In today's China, romantic love continues to play only a small role in most marriages. Since China is a sexually segregated society, a go-between is often used to introduce eligible men and women. Courtship and dating are not common. Women

rarely marry until they reach their mid-twenties, and men are older than that. Couples may not marry without the approval of the Communist Party secretary at their place of work. After marriage, there are strong incentives for having only one child, and birth control is easily available.

Within this social system, sexual satisfaction is rarely seen as an important goal, and the Chinese seem mildly amused at the interest in sex shown by American visitors.

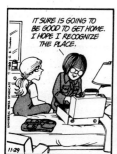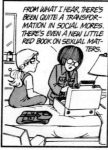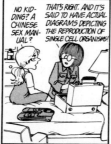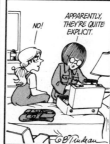

Young people in China receive very little sex education at home or in school. Chinese sex manuals are extremely conservative by western standards. (© 1980 G. B. Trudeau. Reprinted with permission of Universal Press Syndicate. All rights reserved.)

## *Ethnic variation*

The United States is a pluralistic society, with many ethnic groups. So attitudes and approaches to sexual relationships vary widely, both among regions and among particular subcultures. One historic difference has been that between the white and black cultures. Although these differences appear to have narrowed sharply in the past decade, there are still variations in the way many blacks and whites approach the sexual relationship.

Traditional attitudes toward sexual relationships among American blacks originated in African cultures and evolved within the institution of slavery. In African societies, sexuality was under family and community control, and in many societies women had a strong role in the family and in the culture, although they were not dominant (Ladner, 1971; Staples, 1972). Transported to American slaveholding states, blacks were not allowed to marry and families were frequently separated. Slaves were often bred like animals, and black women were considered the sexual property of their owners (Staples, 1972).

After the Civil War and emancipation, economic and social pressures continued to shape black sexual and family patterns. Many black women had to take partial or full responsibility for supporting the family, so women continued in strong roles. Because blacks had not been allowed to marry under slavery, a system of common-law marriage grew up that resulted in a deemphasis on legal marriage. And because blacks viewed sexuality as a natural human function, premarital sex was not heavily censured (Ladner, 1971). Concern over premarital sex tended to be not with the act itself, but with any possible pregnancy that might result (Staples, 1972). This tolerance of sexuality included an acceptance of illegitimate birth and made it common for grandparents to rear a teenage daughter's baby.

With the development of the black middle class and the elimination of discriminatory laws, many blacks began to adopt the traditional white American patterns described earlier in the section on pair bonding. Among male college students, for example, the rate of premarital intercourse is virtually the same for blacks and whites (Staples, 1971). Only a single vestige of traditional black patterns seems to linger among black college students, both men and women: Their admiration of strong and independent women is deeper than that of white students (Crovitz and Steinmann, 1980).

As blacks have been moving away from their traditional pattern, middle-class whites seem to be adopting many of its elements. Women are taking partial or full responsibility for the family's economic support, sexuality is increasingly seen as a natural function, premarital intercourse is accepted, couples live together without marriage, and illegitimate births are less stigmatized.

Among the most rapidly growing ethnic group in the United States, the Hispanic-Americans, sexual patterns have strong roots in the Mediterranean tradition of pair bonding. Within the Hispanic tradition are several subgroups, including Mexican-Americans and Puerto Ricans.

Mexican-American family and sexual patterns are heavily influenced by Spanish traditions, absorbed during the 300 years of Spanish rule that resulted in a fusion of Spanish and Indian cultures. The traditional patterns are strongest among families in rural areas, in the working class, and in low-income groups.

Mexican-American relationships are pervaded by the idea of *machismo*—the aggressive, sexually experienced, courageous male who protects the family women (wife, sisters, mother) and children. Family honor is linked to the daughter's virtue, so that virginity is jealously guarded. The ideal woman is humble, submissive, and virtuous, although she may wield a good deal of power as the self-sacrificing mother. In fact, the love of a mother for her children is regarded as stronger and more important than the tie between woman and man. The marital relationship is almost

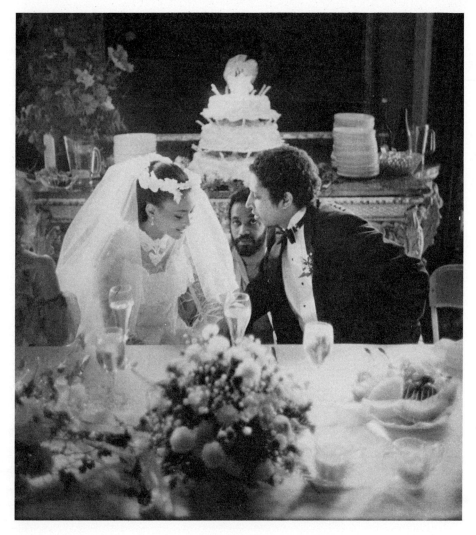

In traditional Christianity, sexual intercourse was confined to marriage and permitted only for procreation. Although views of sexuality have changed, the bride in a traditional wedding still wears the white that symbolizes virginity. (© George W. Gardner)

formal, characterized by respect and consideration. There is little hostility between husband and wife, but neither is there any deep intimacy (Falicov, 1982).

While Mexican-American traditions are influenced by Spanish and Indian cultures, Puerto Rican traditions have been shaped by Spanish, Indian, African, and Corsican cultures. As with Mexican-Americans, the traditional patterns are strongest among rural, working-class, and low-income families. Among the middle class, women are becoming more independent and men less dominant: some of the same shifts in sex roles described in the dominant U.S. culture are occurring in this group as well.

*Machismo* also dominates Puerto Rican sexual patterns, and men are expected always to be ready for sex and to behave seductively around women. Women learn to repress their sexuality and to look upon sex as an obligation to their husbands. As with Mexican-Americans, female virginity is important and is protected by family men. The double standard prevails before and after marriage, with men expected to stray and women to be faithful (Garcia-Preto, 1982).

Puerto Rican marriage is a uniting of two families, not two individuals, and the extended family can be relied on for emotional and tangible assistance. The husband controls the family and provides for it, and he demands respect. One Puerto Rican husband told his wife:

> Respect between husband and wife means that as a wife you must be loving, considerate, and never have negative thoughts about me. (Garcia-Preto, 1982, p. 171)

Despite these demands, wives often exert power behind the scenes while paying public respect to their husbands.

What we have learned about sexual attitudes and practices in various ethnic groups has come from research on human sexuality. These studies have given us much information, but they also have certain limitations.

## STUDYING SEXUALITY

For centuries, social codes and religious prohibitions have kept sexuality hidden. Each of us has had access to only one sexual history—our own. Given the private nature of sexual experience, at some time or another most of us probably wonder if our responses are "normal." In the search for information, most sources turn out to be inadequate or questionable. Because few people speak openly or honestly about their own sexual experiences, information from friends may not be accurate. Besides, how do we know our friends are "normal"?

Books, movies, TV, and magazines provide some information, but again there are limitations. The media report on what is new and different, rather than on what is average and ordinary. A flood of articles on "swinging" is interesting reading, but may not necessarily reflect the sexual customs of most people. Nor do X-rated movies provide information about what "most" people do.

**sexology** the science of human sexual behavior

Only within the last century have fairly reliable answers begun to come from **sexology,** the science of human sexual behavior. Research with animals has provided one perspective on sexual behavior, although the picture it gives us lacks the profound influence of language and culture that are so important in human behavior. Research on other cultures has provided another perspective and made us aware of the many variations in human practices.

Perhaps the most revealing information has come from surveys of large numbers of people by interviews or questionnaires. Such research gives us access to many more sexual histories than we could reach on our own. When using survey data, however, we need to be aware of its limitations. One major limitation on survey data is the possibility that those who responded to the questions do not reflect the population as a whole. For example, people who are sexually liberal may be

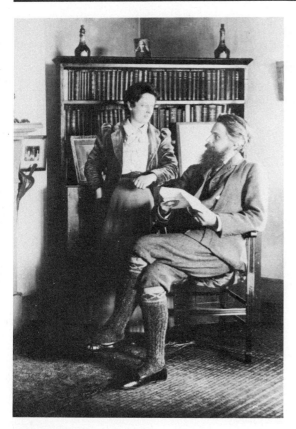

Havelock Ellis, shown with his wife, Edith Lees Ellis, was a pioneer of sexology. He argued that sexual customs were relative to each society, that sexual response was as strong in women as in men, that homosexuality was not pathological, and that masturbation was harmless. (Courtesy, Lafitte Collection)

more likely to answer questions about sex than those who are sexual conservatives. People who are extremely satisfied with their sex lives may see no value in sex research and so decline to participate, whereas those who have sexual problems may either be eager to participate in the hope of finding solutions or refuse to take part because they find the topic of sex distasteful (Tavris and Sadd, 1977). Even the research done by Kinsey and his associates (Kinsey, Pomeroy, and Martin, 1948; Kinsey et al., 1953), discussed in Chapter 1, has been criticized for underrepresenting blacks, the poor, and the uneducated, as well as for the problem of possible bias caused by the differences between people who volunteer to answer questions about their sex lives and those who do not.

Another source of sexual information comes from laboratory observations of human sexuality, which have given us information about the physiology of sex and in the process have dispelled a number of myths about what actually happens during intercourse. This observational research has been indispensable to our knowledge of human sexual response. A landmark study was carried out by William Masters and Virginia Johnson (1966), who observed more than 14,000 sexual acts in nearly 700 men and women between the ages of eighteen and eighty-nine. Most subjects were paid volunteers who agreed to masturbate or perform intercourse

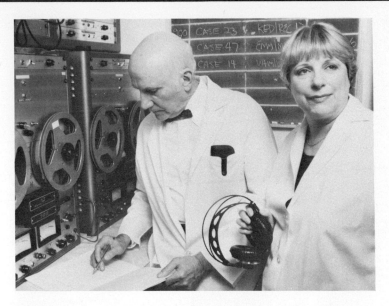

William Masters and Virginia Johnson have done the most extensive laboratory research on the psychophysiology of sexual arousal and orgasm. Their findings have dispelled many sexual myths and demonstrated the value of sex research. (© Dirck Halstead/Liaison)

with their partners while being filmed or recorded by physiological measurement devices. This research dispelled several sexual myths and led to a change in public attitudes toward sex research. Because Masters and Johnson were able to demonstrate the practical value of laboratory research in dealing with sexual problems, research on human sexuality is now seen as a valuable contribution to the health and behavioral sciences.

But even this landmark research is not perfect. Masters and Johnson have been criticized for using prostitutes as subjects. In addition, their use of volunteer subjects and their concentration on people older than twenty, as well as the higher than average educational level of their subjects, may mean that their data are not applicable to some groups.

Finally, laboratory experiments, in which a researcher makes systematic changes in some factor that affects sexual attitudes or behavior and then observes the result, can also confirm or disprove popular beliefs and the ideas of early sexologists. The limitation of such research is that the artificial laboratory situation, in which, for example, a person responds to fantasy or explicit sexual tapes, may be too far from the context of daily life to be applied to other situations.

Although all these types of research are flawed, they do give us an idea of the wide range of sexual activities and responses among human beings. We cannot use this research to generalize about what is "normal" sexual behavior, but by putting together information from all these sources, we can now talk about human sexuality with a good deal more confidence than before. Throughout this book, we will draw on all these sources as we explore human sexuality in modern life.

# Summary

**1** Sexuality serves three basic human needs: procreation, recreation, and closeness. Until reliable methods of birth control were developed, it was virtually impossible to separate sex as play or an expression of feeling from its reproductive function.

**2** Recreational sex is a form of adult play. It can be important when people do not want an ongoing relationship but also do not want to give up sex. Recreational sex can become a problem when people restrict their sexual activity solely to play. **Intimacy** is important in relational sexuality, and the way intimacy is expressed depends on the partners and the character of the relationship. Intimate relationships may be primarily passionate (loving) or primarily companionate (liking), or a combination of the two.

**3** Love can be seen as an instinctive force or as learned behavior, shaped by culture and experience. Sigmund Freud saw love as instinctual, a transformation of the **libido**, or life force. Some learning theorists see it as a combination of physiological arousal and a mental label attached to the arousal. **Limerence**, or passionate love, may last for days, weeks, or months, but usually has a fairly short time span. When it fades, the relationship goes dead or companionate love develops. Whether love is passionate or companionate, the partners tend to form a **pair bond**—an intimate, committed relationship. Pair bonding goes through three phases: **proception**, or courtship; **acception**, or genital sexual activity; and **conception**, or gestation and parenthood. The type of pair bond that develops in a culture seems to be based on its child-care patterns. In human societies the pattern may be **monogamous** (one male and one female), **polygynous** (one male and several females), or **polyandrous** (one female and several males). Pair bonding in the United States appears to be a combination of Mediterranean (arranged marriages, virgin brides, the double standard) and Nordic (romantic love, premarital sex between engaged couples, a single standard) traditions.

**4** No universal sex differences have been found in the way men and women experience passionate love. However, men tend to fall in love more easily than women and to be slower to fall out of love. Men seem to find nonsexual intimacy more difficult to achieve than women do.

**5** Love is the accepted reason for marriage in the United States, and women's social roles have customarily been defined by the husbands' position. Women tend to take a practical approach to love, perhaps because of the social consequences of marriage. For them, the sexual revolution has often meant premarital sex with a loved partner whom they intend to marry. Women appear to link love and sex closely. In their nonsexual relationships, women generally focus on personal liking and feelings, as opposed to the male focus on shared activities.

**6** The Judeo-Christian tradition seems to be the most restrictive of all major religions in attitudes toward sex. Traditional Judaism, while seeing the woman as inferior, viewed sexual intercourse as a sacred activity within marriage. Early Christians accepted the Greek attitude that sex was low and unworthy, and that **celibacy** was the highest human state. Through the centuries, the Catholic Church became increasingly restrictive in sexual matters. The Protestant churches formed after the Reformation were only slightly less rigid in their teachings on sex.

**7** Because almost every aspect of sexuality can be so heavily influenced by society, it is virtually impossible to say that any one kind of sexual activity is "normal." Different groups within a society often develop their own sexual ethic. In American society, blacks developed their own tradition that in recent years has primarily characterized low-income blacks. Hispanic-American traditions are heavily influenced by Mediterranean pair bonding.

**8** **Sexology,** the science of human sexual behavior, has developed only within the last century. Our present information on sexual activity has come from studies with animals, interviews and surveys, laboratory observations of human sexuality, and laboratory studies. All these types of research are limited, but they do give us an idea of the wide range of sexual activities and responses among human beings.

# Part Two

# The Sexual Body

Ask most any five-year-old how you can tell a girl from a boy, and the answer is likely to be correct. But there's more to being male or female than the possession of a penis or a vagina. In addition to the obvious physical differences, there are major internal differences in the sex organs, in the balance of hormones that course through the bloodstream, and in the makeup of each cell in the body. It's no wonder, then, that despite many similarities in male and female sexuality, there are also major differences.

Until recently, information about the structure and function of the sexual systems was primarily the property of scientists and physicians. Most people thought it was "not quite nice" for the average person to know too much about the reproductive organs and how they work. But without a knowledge of its anatomy, sex remains a mystery. Although people have had adequate sex lives without ever knowing much about sexual anatomy, except "what" to put "where," a basic knowledge of our reproductive organs and how they work can allay worries and increase sexual satisfaction. Many of us have questions about our own anatomy and these doubts can interfere with a positive sexual self-image.

Since the genitals are usually kept hidden, few people have ever really compared their own genitals with those of others. The study of sexual anatomy can fill this informational gap and help to dispel the negative attitudes we may have grown up with. When a sense of the intricate and wonderful ways in which these organs function is allowed to develop, feelings of discomfort may change to appreciation or even awe. In the four chapters that make up this unit, we will examine the female and male sexual systems, discover how each responds to sexual stimulation, and see how knowledge about the systems relates to our feelings about sex and our self-awareness.

## a woman's view

Being a woman certainly has some advantages. I don't have to worry about hiding an erect penis if I'm aroused at an inopportune moment. And I don't have to worry about 'getting it up' when I want to have sex. (Authors' files)

A few times when I've been feeling good about myself I got really high just before my periods. It was like a drug high, even though I didn't take anything. It came and went, totally unexpected. (Boston Women's Health Book Collective, p. 35)

# 3 The Female Sexual System

# Chapter 3

Although most of our sexual activity is either for fun or to express intimate feelings, investigations of sexual anatomy generally take a reproductive point of view. The sexual anatomy of a male is seen as a sperm delivery system and that of the female as a system for conception, pregnancy, and childbirth. Such obviously different roles require anatomy that differ in important ways. Yet there are many similarities in the architecture of the male and female sexual systems. And there should be, because both sexes start out very much alike.

Because of the similarities, we'll begin with prenatal development. A discussion of the way male and female sexual organs are formed will give us a basis for understanding the structure and function of the female sexual system. A look at how menstruation works will increase our understanding of an aspect of female function that is currently the focus of debate, the premenstrual syndrome. Finally, we'll examine the evidence for any connection between female sexual interest and changes in hormone levels.

## SEXUAL ORGANS AND HOW THEY FORM

The Bible tells us that Adam was created first and that Eve was an afterthought, created from Adam's rib to be his mate and companion. From this creation myth came the conventional wisdom of the West: man is the primary and natural sex and woman a derivation. Research

# The Female Sexual System

does not support the biblical view of sexual development. In fact, a careful look at the development of the fertilized egg reveals that if there is a primary sex, it is female.

A child's sex is determined at the moment of conception, when the father's sperm unites with the mother's **ovum**, or egg cell. Until research established just how that determination took place, people were free to speculate. Some believed the father was responsible, others that it was the mother. Some said that the right testicle produced boys and the left, girls. One group maintained that the direction of the penis at the time of insemination was crucial: a right-facing penis could produce males; a left-facing one, females. And some believed that the decision was made by the mother's ovaries, with eggs from one ovary producing girls and eggs from the other producing boys.

There is no longer any doubt. The sex of a child is determined by the nature of the sperm that impregnates the egg. Each sperm, like each ovum, contains twenty-three single **chromosomes**, beadlike structures made up of many genes carrying the information required to turn a single cell into a human being. When sperm and ovum unite, the fertilized cell contains twenty-three *pairs* of chromosomes, and every cell in the new individual's body will contain those same twenty-three pairs.

Only one pair of chromosomes is involved in the determination of sex. Normal eggs carry an X chromosome, and normal sperm carry either an X or Y chromosome. If an X-carrying sperm penetrates the egg, a girl (XX) is produced. If a Y-carrying sperm penetrates the egg, a boy (XY) is produced. The same pair of sex chromosomes will appear in every cell of the new individual's body.

**ovum** the egg cell produced by the female ovary

**chromosomes** beadlike structures made up of many genes carrying the information required to turn a single cell into a human being

Despite this chromosomal difference, at conception and for the first six weeks of development, male and female embryos appear identical and proceed along a common path. The original XX or XY cell multiplies millions of times, with each new cell carrying the same genetic message.

The rudiments of male and female internal organs exist in both sexes. Each embryo has a pair of **gonads,** or sex glands, that will become either ovaries or testes, and two sets of internal sexual structures that can develop into either female or male internal organs.

The external genitals develop from a common structural base, a small swelling of external tissue that may become a **clitoris,** the female erectile organ, or a **penis,** the male erectile organ.

Since female anatomy and male anatomy develop from a common set of primitive structures, there are many homologues in adult sexual anatomy. **Homologues** are organs or structures that have the same origin. For example, the female clitoris and the male penis are homologous (Figure 3.1). They do not, however, play the same role in adult sexual function. The penis is involved in reproduction, urination, and sexual response. The clitoris is involved only in sexual response. But homologous structures can play similar roles. For example, the testes and ovaries, which develop from the same primitive tissue, are both involved in the production of sex cells (sperm and ova) and the secretion of sex hormones.

The event that shifts development in the masculine direction suggests that the species begins as essentially feminine, because a male can develop only if something is added to the embryo about six weeks after conception. The crucial ingredients are **androgens,** or male hormones. Around this time, the Y chromosome in the male embryo sends a message to the undifferentiated gonads that causes them to develop as male testes and to secrete a mixture of predominantly male hormones.

The new testes also secrete a substance that inhibits the **Mullerian ducts,** the primitive sexual structures that would develop into female internal reproductive organs. Under the influence of this substance, the Mullerian ducts begin to disintegrate, although remnants never disappear, even in the adult male. At the same time, the hormone mixture secreted by the testes causes the **Wolffian ducts,** the primitive sexual structures that will become the male internal reproductive organs, to develop.

In the absence of a Y chromosome—that is, when it does not receive instructions to the contrary—the embryo develops along a female path. It continues in an undifferentiated state for another six weeks, when the gonads begin to develop into ovaries. This female development does not require any ovarian production of **estrogens,** or female hormones, and although the ovaries do not secrete a hormone mixture at this time, they do develop a supply of immature egg cells that will last until menopause, when the supply of eggs is exhausted. When no male hormones affect the embryo, the Wolffian ducts atrophy and disappear, indicating that the natural baseline of sexual tissue in the embryo is female.

The final stage of sexual differentiation is the molding of the external genitals. If no male hormones are added, the external genitals take on a female appearance. The original swelling of external tissue shrinks and becomes the clitoris. The genital folds become the **labia minora,** or "inner lips," and the clitoral hood. The geni-

---

**gonads** sex organs, called testes in the male and ovaries in the female

**clitoris** the female erectile organ, which is highly responsive to sexual stimulation; part of the vulva

**penis** the male erectile organ, which is highly responsive to sexual stimulation

**homologues** organs or structures with the same embryonic origin, such as the clitoris and the penis

**androgens** male hormones

**Mullerian ducts** primitive sexual structures that develop into female internal reproductive organs

**Wolffian ducts** primitive sexual structures that develop into male internal reproductive organs

**estrogens** female hormones

**labia minora** inner lips surrounding the vaginal opening; part of the vulva

**(1) UNDIFFERENTIATED**

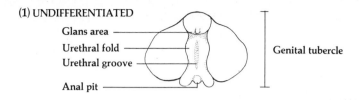

Glans area

Urethral fold

Urethral groove

Anal pit

Genital tubercle

**(2) PARTIALLY DEVELOPED** (45–50 mm)

Male

Female

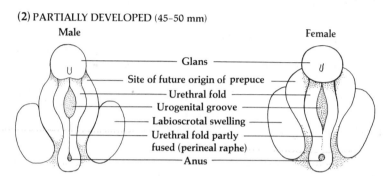

Glans

Site of future origin of prepuce

Urethral fold

Urogenital groove

Labioscrotal swelling

Urethral fold partly
fused (perineal raphe)

Anus

**(3) FULLY DEVELOPED**

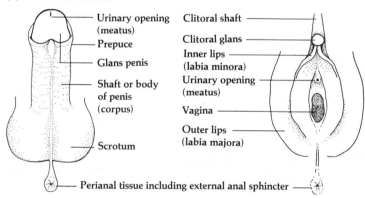

Urinary opening
(meatus)

Prepuce

Glans penis

Shaft or body
of penis
(corpus)

Scrotum

Clitoral shaft

Clitoral glans

Inner lips
(labia minora)

Urinary opening
(meatus)

Vagina

Outer lips
(labia majora)

Perianal tissue including external anal sphincter

*Figure 3.1  The stages in the differentiation of male and female external genitalia.*

(1) Undifferentiated stage—appears during the second month of pregnancy. (2) Differentiated stage—about the third month of pregnancy. (3) Fully developed stage—at the time of birth.

tal swelling turns into the **labia majora**, or "outer lips," and the single opening is divided in two, separating the vaginal opening from the urethral entrance that will allow the passage of urine.

When male hormones are present, the original swelling grows to become the penis. The two folds of skin fuse around the penis, and the two swellings also fuse together to form the **scrotal sac**, a pouch behind the penis. When the fetus is about seven months old, the testes usually descend into this sac. The single opening, which is enclosed in the penis, will become the urethral tube, connecting both the internal sexual organs and the bladder and allowing the passage of both semen and urine.

**labia majora** outer lips surrounding the vaginal opening; part of the vulva

**scrotal sac** the pouch behind the penis that holds the testes

By the time of birth, male and female sexual organs can usually be identified with a single glance. With sexual maturity, the difference in genitals makes it seem wildly improbable that they could have had a common origin. But our examination of the male and female systems will turn up many homologous structures.

## EXTERNAL ANATOMY

**vulva** the external female genitals

The common origin of the male and female sexual systems will become apparent as we look at external female anatomy. Until the twentieth century, the external genitals, or **vulva**, received scant scientific attention, perhaps because they are primarily associated with sexual response. What may have been the first major study of female external anatomy was carried out at the turn of the century by Robert Latou Dickinson (1933), an American gynecologist. His careful, detailed drawings, sketched from life, reveal wide individual differences in normal sexual anatomy. Within broad anatomical limits, a woman's external genitals show distinct and individual characteristics in their size, shape, coloring, skin texture, hair distribution, and positioning.

*Figure 3.2   Front view of the vulva (external genitalia) of a mature woman.*

Below: enlarged view of the clitoris showing the clitoral hood (prepuce) adjoining the inner lips (labia minora). Stimulation of the inner lips is generally transmitted to the nerve endings in the clitoris.

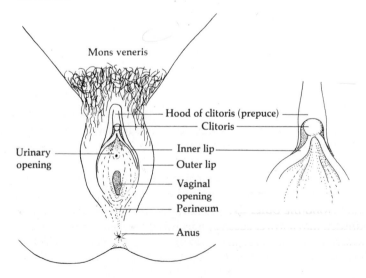

Mons veneris

Urinary opening

Hood of clitoris (prepuce)
Clitoris
Inner lip
Outer lip
Vaginal opening
Perineum

Anus

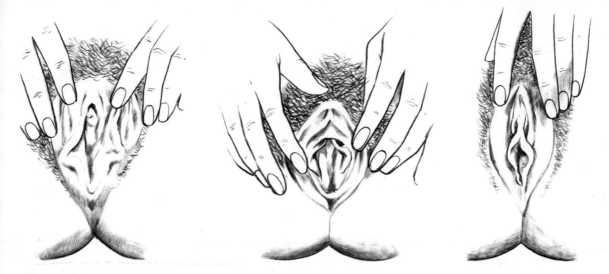

## Figure 3.3

There are many variations in the shape and appearance of the vulva from one woman to the next.

## The labia majora

The soft, fatty tissue at the base of the abdomen that is covered with pubic hair is known as the *mons veneris,* called the "mount of Venus" in deference to the Roman goddess of love (Figure 3.2). Extending from the bottom of the mons are two folds of skin called the labia majora. The outer surfaces of these lips are also covered with pubic hair, but the inner surfaces are smooth and thicken toward the front of the body. They contain numerous sebaceous (oil-producing) glands, sweat glands, and fat cells, and have a rich blood supply. In the sexually unstimulated woman, they normally meet to enclose and protect the organs located between them.

## The labia minora

Enclosed within the outer lips are a smaller, thinner set of deeply pigmented skin folds called the labia minora. These inner lips have been compared to the petals of a flower (Figure 3.3). They have neither sweat glands, fat cells, nor hair, but many small sebaceous glands are located close to the surface. The labia minora also have a rich network of blood vessels and nerve cells, which makes them extremely sensitive to touch. In some women, these lips remain tucked between the labia majora; in others, they extend beyond the outer lips. One side is often longer than the other. Each lip can be divided into a lower section, which surrounds the vestibule, and an upper section, which meets the other lip above the clitoris to form the fold of skin that is the **clitoral hood.**

**clitoral hood** upper part of the labia minora which meet, partially covering the clitoris

## *The vestibular area*

**vestibule** area between the labia minora containing small mucous glands

**vestibular bulbs** two masses of tissue on either side of the vaginal opening that swell when sexually stimulated

Between the labia minora is an area known as the **vestibule**, which contains small mucous glands that secrete fluid. Both the urethra and the vagina open into the vestibule, with the vaginal orifice located below the urethral orifice. On either side of the vaginal opening, beneath the labia minora, are the **vestibular bulbs**, two masses of tissue that swell and fill with blood when stimulated. The bulbs are surrounded by the pubococcygeus (PC) muscles, which contract involuntarily during orgasm, and which some therapists believe can be strengthened by exercise, as we'll see in Chapter 6.

## *Bartholin's glands*

**Bartholin's glands** glands on either side of the vaginal opening that secrete fluid

Behind the vestibular bulbs on either side of the vaginal opening are **Bartholin's glands**, also called the vestibular glands. These small, rounded bodies are homologous to Cowper's glands in the male, which will be discussed in Chapter 4. Each gland secretes fluid into the vestibule through a small duct that opens beside the hymen.

Bartholin's glands were once thought to be the source of the vaginal lubricant secreted during sexual arousal. Then research by William Masters and Virginia Johnson (1966) showed that the glands secrete no more than a few drops of mucus, which do not appear until long after a woman is sexually aroused. Masters and Johnson concluded that any secretion from Bartholin's glands during sexual activity was minute compared with secretions coming from the vaginal walls.

## *The hymen*

**hymen** a thin membrane that separates the vagina from the external genitals

At the entrance to the vagina is the **hymen**, tissue with no known physical function. For centuries, however, it has been assigned a cultural function: to determine whether a woman was still a virgin. Although examination of the hymen provides no clear evidence about a woman's sexual activity, the intact hymen remains a symbol of virginity in many cultures and its condition has affected the course of many women's lives.

Typically, the hymen is a thin membrane that separates the vagina from the external genitals. Both its inner and outer surfaces are covered by a layer of mucous membrane. Hymens come in many sizes, shapes, and thicknesses. Despite their role as guardian of virginity, most hymens have an opening large enough to allow the passage of menstrual fluid and the insertion of a tampon. Only in rare cases does the hymen form such an impenetrable barrier that menstrual fluid collects behind it—a condition known as imperforate hymen.

The hymen may stretch in a variety of ways, and sexual intercourse is only one method of widening the vaginal opening. It may also be stretched by finger pressure or by masturbation within the vagina. In some women, the opening is so large that little discomfort accompanies first intercourse:

> My first sexual experience was not at all like what I expected. On the one
> hand, I was very relieved that it was much less painful than I had expected.
> On the other hand, I was surprised—and I think even a little disappointed—
> that there was no blood on the sheets afterwards. (Authors' files)

Not all women find their first intercourse this easy; some may feel pain unless the
membrane is gradually stretched in advance. Even among sexually active women,
however, remnants of the hymen are often visible around the vaginal opening.

## The clitoris

Western scientists ignored the clitoris for many centuries, probably because the organ is not necessary for reproduction. Its only purpose seemed to be the enhancement of female sexual pleasure, and since many cultures have been unconcerned
with female sexual pleasure—or even doubted its existence—it is not surprising to
find that only in recent years has the clitoris been considered a suitable topic for
scientific study.

Although our culture has ignored the existence of the clitoris, other cultures
have not. When attention is paid to this small organ, it tends to be either extremely
negative or extremely positive (Huelsman, 1976). Among tribal societies that take a
negative approach, such as certain Arab and African groups, the clitoris is surgically
removed as part of the ritual passage into adulthood. There is evidence that clitoral
removal was performed in ancient Egypt; it has also been found among people as
diverse in geographic location as the aborigines of Australia and some South American Indians. Among certain Muslim groups, the removal of the clitoral hood—
which amounts to female circumcision—is performed to this day.

The most drastic forms of surgery have been performed in areas where males
and females are socially isolated from each other, where the male role is extremely
dominant, and where female sexual pleasure is ignored (Huelsman, 1976). According to Mary Jane Sherfey (1973), some societies believe the female sexual drive is
so strong that order can be maintained only if males use drastic measures to curb it.
Genital surgery would accomplish this purpose.

Not all peoples have regarded the clitoris negatively. Many Polynesian and Mi-
cronesian cultures believe that a large clitoris is a sign of sexual power, in much the
same way that a large penis is thought to indicate male potency. In some of these
cultures, attempts are made to enlarge the clitoris and the labia through manual
and oral stimulation. Societies with this positive approach to the clitoris tend to accept and even encourage female sexual pleasure.

Western medical science has traditionally dealt with the clitoris in a negative
manner. In the eighteenth century, surgical removal of the clitoris (**clitoridectomy**)
was common. A woman who suffered from epilepsy, nymphomania ("excessive"
sexual desire), "excessive" masturbation, or who simply had a large clitoris was often treated by the removal of her clitoris. Removal of the clitoral hood (**clitoridotomy**) was also recommended by many Victorian physicians as an effective guard
against what they regarded as the dangers of masturbation.

**clitoridectomy** sur-
gical removal of the cli-
toris

**clitoridotomy** surgi-
cal removal of the clito-
ral hood

The clitoris is not found only in the human species. The females of all mammals, various species of reptiles, and some birds have a clitoris (McFarland, 1976). In many mammalian species, its anatomy is quite similar to the human clitoris. Whether nonhuman females experience orgasm is uncertain, although the clitoris may serve several functions. In some species, manipulation of the clitoris is necessary to induce ovulation; in others, females will not accept male sexual advances unless the clitoris has been stimulated.

**crura** leglike structures that join to form the clitoral body

**clitoral glans** the small rounded portion of the clitoris, which is visible on the body surface

**corpora cavernosa** hollow, spongelike cylinders found in both the clitoris and the penis

**Clitoral anatomy** The clitoris consists of a pair of **crura** (legs) that join to form the clitoral body, which ends in a small, rounded **clitoral glans**. Only the glans is visible on the surface of the body, although it is usually covered by the clitoral hood. The crura lie beneath the surface of the skin, where they are attached to the pelvic bone structure and covered with two small muscles. The clitoral body is suspended from the pubic bones by a ligament. Like the penis, the clitoris consists of erectile tissue; within the clitoral body are two hollow, spongelike cylinders, or **corpora cavernosa**. In addition to a rich network of blood vessels, the clitoris has a large number of nerve endings that make it sensitive to touch.

The average size of the clitoral glans is about .18 in. (4 to 5 mm) in diameter. In their research, however, Masters and Johnson (1966) saw clitoral glans measuring from .08 in. (2 mm) up to .39 in. (1 cm), a range considered normal. The length of the clitoral body and the crura also vary greatly. The crura may be long and thin or short and thick; and their size bears little relationship to the size of the clitoral glans.

**Sexual responsiveness and the clitoris** In attempting to explain variations in female responsiveness, many people have turned to clitoral anatomy. As a result, myths regarding clitoral size and placement have become widely accepted.

According to one myth, the intensity of a woman's sexual response is related to the size of her clitoris—a myth also prevalent in Pacific cultures that have a high opinion of the clitoris. Research has shown that there is absolutely no relationship between clitoral size and either the speed or the intensity of sexual response (Masters and Johnson, 1966).

The second myth is that female sexual response is related to the distance between the clitoral glans and the vaginal opening. Supposedly, the farther the glans is placed from the vaginal orifice, the more difficult it will be for a woman to reach orgasm. With close placement, the clitoris gets direct stimulation during intercourse and a woman will reach orgasm quickly. This myth was exploded nearly half a century ago by Dickinson (1933), the same gynecologist who first studied female sexual anatomy. Dickinson found that women whose clitoris and vaginal orifice were close together were no more likely to be orgasmic than women in whom they were widely separated. More recently, Masters and Johnson (1966) reported that even when the two organs are quite close, the penis rarely makes direct contact with the clitoris. In addition, penile stimulation of the clitoris during intercourse is usually indirect, because the clitoris automatically retracts as a woman nears orgasm. In fact, as we'll see, portions of the internal female sexual system have been linked with intense sexual responsiveness and orgasm.

# THE INTERNAL ORGANS

Because the internal sexual organs are directly involved in reproduction, quite a bit is known about their structure and function. These organs are located within the pelvic bone structure, which encloses them in a protective ring. The muscles of the pelvic diaphragm form a hammock that holds the organs in place and helps to maintain the position of the uterus. The female pelvis is lighter, more rounded, shallower, and wider than the male pelvis, because it must accommodate the growing fetus during pregnancy and allow the passage of the baby's head at delivery.

The internal organs fill both reproductive and sexual roles (see Figure 3.4). The major sexual organs within the female pelvic basin are the vagina, the cervix, the uterus, the ovaries, and the Fallopian tubes.

## *The vagina*

> There is a space, a special place, inside me. It's warm and wet, and feels so good. (Authors' files)

As this woman's words indicate, the **vagina**, a canal leading from the vulva to the cervix, plays an important role in sexual arousal. It is also important in reproduction, and these roles often overlap. For instance, the vaginal lubricant secreted

**vagina** the canal extending from the vulva to the cervix

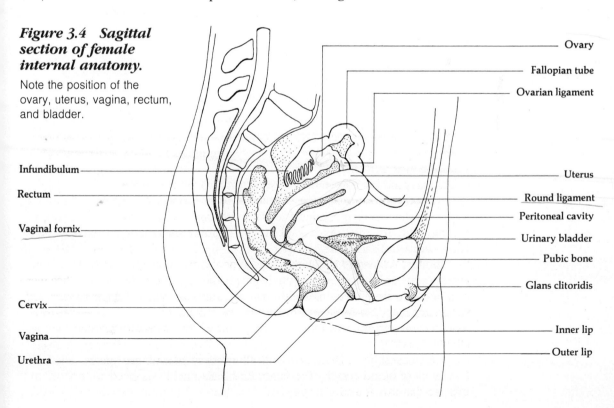

**Figure 3.4  Sagittal section of female internal anatomy.**

Note the position of the ovary, uterus, vagina, rectum, and bladder.

Infundibulum

Rectum

Vaginal fornix

Cervix

Vagina

Urethra

Ovary

Fallopian tube

Ovarian ligament

Uterus

Round ligament

Peritoneal cavity

Urinary bladder

Pubic bone

Glans clitoridis

Inner lip

Outer lip

## Focus

### THE GRAFENBERG SPOT— A NEW EROGENOUS ZONE?

**Grafenberg spot (G spot)** a small area within the vagina that supposedly is highly responsive to sexual stimulation

Recently, some researchers have suggested that the clitoris is not the only focus of sexual sensation in women. It has been proposed that an area deep within the front vaginal wall responds to stimulation much as the clitoris does and that continued stimulation of this **Grafenberg spot,** or **G spot,** can produce orgasm (Ladas, Whipple, and Perry, 1982). The G spot is said to be located about halfway into the vagina and just beneath the urethra. If you imagine a clock inside the vagina with 6 o'clock at the vaginal opening, the G spot would be found somewhere between 11 o'clock and 1 o'clock, with the precise spot—and its size—varying from woman to woman.

The spot is about the size of a small bean, but when stimulated it supposedly swells until it is as large as a dime, or even a half dollar in some women. Some women seem to have discovered the G spot on their own:

I have always had orgasms, but I have never had much stimulation when the penis was completely inside my vagina. In fact, sometimes my excitement and arousal would end abruptly when the penis entered me completely. I have always been most excitable when the penis was only one-half or one-third its way into my vagina. Now I know why—at that point it hit my "magic spot." (Ladas, Whipple, and Perry, 1982, p. 40)

Some women claim that when orgasm follows stimulation of the G spot, they release fluid as if they were ejaculating. In Chapter 5, we'll discuss the topic of female ejaculation.

At present, however, the existence of the G spot as an actual anatomical structure has not been established. In laboratory studies gynecologists have been able to find the spot in fewer than half the women they examined (Zilbergeld, 1982). So it's not clear that all women have a G spot or just where the spot is located. In addition, the G spot's overall importance in sexual response seems to vary greatly from one woman to the next.

---

when a woman is sexually aroused eases the entrance of the penis during intercourse and may also help the sperm to survive in the first part of the journey toward the egg. Similarly, the muscular contractions that take place during sexual orgasm may aid the movement of the sperm through the cervix.

The vagina is normally a small organ, with little internal space. In the resting state its walls touch. But vaginal muscles are capable of considerable expansion. During childbirth, the vaginal walls expand enormously to allow the passage of the baby's head and shoulders.

In most women, the vagina is placed at about a 45-degree angle, slanting up and back toward the spinal column. In shape, the vagina resembles an elongated S, changing direction three times, although the angles are slight. Typically, the vagina is between 3.2 and 4 in. (8 and 10 cm) in length. It is shorter in the prepubertal girl and tends to shrink in women who have passed the **menopause,** when the menstrual cycle ends.

**menopause** the time of the last menstrual cycle, which usually comes at about age fifty-one

Like most other sexual organs, the connective tissue of the vagina is filled with a network of blood vessels. The outer third is also richly supplied with nerve endings, so that it is sensitive to physical stimulation. The inner two-thirds, however, has relatively few sensory nerve endings, and is usually insensitive to physical stimuli except pressure.

Before puberty, the vaginal membranes are thin and fragile. After the first menstrual period, these membranes thicken in response to rising hormone levels. Unlike the uterus, the vagina shows only minor changes during the phases of the menstrual cycle. After menopause, lowered hormone levels cause the vaginal walls to thin so that their supply of blood is reduced. At this time, lubrication in response to sexual stimulation may be so scanty that sexual intercourse is uncomfortable unless an artificial lubricant is used.

## *The cervix*

Extending into the vagina is the **cervix**, which is the passageway between the vagina and the uterus. The cervix is actually the bottom, or neck, of the uterus, and at its center is a small opening. Glands within the cervix secrete different types of mucus at successive stages of the menstrual cycle, and their consistency varies. During ovulation, when an egg has been released by an ovary, the mucus is thin and clear and easily penetrated by sperm; at other times the mucus is thick and pasty, forming an impenetrable plug that acts as a barrier.

**cervix** the neck of the uterus, which is the passageway between the uterus and the vagina

## *The uterus*

The **uterus**, or womb, is involved in both reproduction and sexual function. During pregnancy, it provides a hospitable and protective environment for the growing fetus; during childbirth, contractions of its muscles propel the fetus through the birth canal. The muscles of the uterus also contract during orgasm.

**uterus** the womb

Although the uterus is held in place by a series of ligaments its position is not fixed, and it shifts when the bladder or rectum is full. When a woman is standing and her bladder and rectum are empty, the uterus tends to lie in an almost horizontal position, with the top toward the front of the body.

The uterus is made up of three layers: an outer covering, a layer of muscle, and a mucous layer called the **endometrium**. The bulk of the uterus is muscular tissue; these muscles are dense, firm, and interlaced in all directions. During pregnancy, the fibers expand greatly in size and new ones are added. When changing hormonal levels trigger childbirth, the uterine muscles contract in powerful spasms that move the fetus toward the cervix. The cervical opening expands so that the fetus may pass into the vagina.

**endometrium** the inner lining of the uterus

Two patterns of change can be seen in the uterus, a lifelong pattern and a cyclical pattern. The lifelong pattern commences before birth, when in response to increased estrogen levels in the mother, the uterus begins to grow rapidly during the seventh month of fetal life. This growth lasts until a few days after birth. During infancy, cut off from the maternal estrogen, the uterus shrinks and remains small until a few years before the first menstrual period. Then, in response to increased hormone levels, the uterus grows to its adult size. In women who have not had children, it is a pear-shaped organ about 3 in. (6 to 8 cm) long. After childbirth the uterus tends to be larger in size (9–10 cm), although its shape remains the same. Finally, after the menopause the uterus again shrinks in size and may become as small as it was before puberty.

The second pattern of uterine change and development coincides with the menstrual cycle. Each month, the endometrium develops a thick, glandular coating. The purpose of this change is to provide a nourishing environment should pregnancy occur. If the woman fails to conceive, the endometrial lining is shed during menstruation. Although the major uterine changes take place in the endometrium, the outer layers of the uterus and its muscles may also change in shape and appearance.

## The ovaries

**ovary** female sex organ, which secretes sex hormones and produces ova

The **ovaries** serve two functions: they secrete sex hormones, and during the childbearing years they mature and release an ovum at each menstrual cycle. At birth, the ovaries contain about 400,000 immature cells that will develop into mature ova. Since the average woman releases only about 400 mature ova during her menstrual years, the vast majority of these cells degenerate without reaching maturity.

In the infant the ovary is a pale, smooth structure, shaped like a tiny sausage. Gradually it increases in size and weight, with most of this growth occurring after the first menstrual cycle. In the adult woman, the ovary is about the size and shape of an unshelled almond. During the menstrual years, the ovary turns a grayish color and the surface becomes increasingly pitted and irregular. This change comes about because each egg released during ovulation breaks through the ovarian wall. Although this rupture is rapidly repaired, it may be accompanied by a small amount of bleeding and may leave a scar. Finally, in the woman who has passed menopause and no longer releases ova, the ovary shrinks and becomes puckered.

The two ovaries are located on either side of the uterus (Figure 3.5). They are held in place by ligaments that run between the pelvic walls, the ovaries, and the uterus, but the exact position of the ovaries varies from one woman to another. After childbirth, their position may be slightly altered.

**follicle** one of many compartments within the ovary where ova mature

Each ovary contains a number of compartments, called **follicles**, at various stages of development (Figure 3.6), and within each follicle is an ovum. As a follicle develops it moves toward the center of the ovary, where there is a plentiful supply of blood. This development, which is stimulated by changes in hormone levels, continues for about twelve days, when the follicle moves back toward the outer surface of the ovary. Then, in a process we do not yet understand, one of the follicles continues to grow while the other maturing follicles begin to degenerate. Generally, only one follicle matures during each cycle.

**corpus luteum** "yellow body"; the ovarian follicle after the eruption of the ovum

As this follicle matures, it locates itself next to the ovarian wall. Ovulation occurs about fourteen days before menstruation, when the expanding follicle wall opens and the egg, together with some surrounding cells, is released through the wall of the ovary and into the body cavity. After the egg erupts, the follicle—still within the ovary—becomes the **corpus luteum**, or "yellow body." Its role now be-

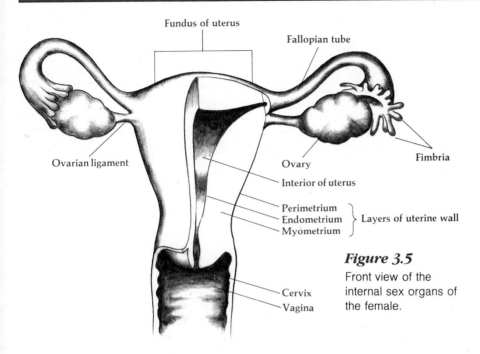

Fundus of uterus

Fallopian tube

Ovarian ligament

Ovary

Fimbria

Interior of uterus

Perimetrium
Endometrium
Myometrium
} Layers of uterine wall

Cervix
Vagina

**Figure 3.5**
Front view of the internal sex organs of the female.

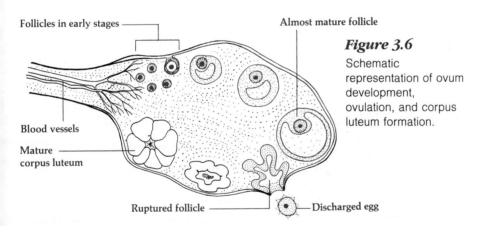

Follicles in early stages

Almost mature follicle

Blood vessels

Mature corpus luteum

Ruptured follicle

Discharged egg

**Figure 3.6**
Schematic representation of ovum development, ovulation, and corpus luteum formation.

comes to secrete hormones that prepare the uterus for the egg and help maintain a pregnancy. If conception does not take place, the corpus luteum shrinks and degenerates, the menstrual period occurs, and the process begins again.

Usually, the ovaries alternate in the maturation and release of egg cells, with each ovary releasing an egg every second month. It is possible, however, for a woman to ovulate and become pregnant with only one functioning ovary. Further, the ovaries may sometimes release more than one egg during the menstrual cycle. When both eggs are fertilized, fraternal, or nonidentical, twins may develop.

## The Fallopian tubes

**Fallopian tubes** the
tubes that transport ova
from the ovaries to the
uterus

The two **Fallopian tubes,** or oviducts, which guide the egg cell toward the uterus, also facilitate the movement of sperm toward the egg. The tubes provide a hospitable environment and nutrition for survival.

Each Fallopian tube is about 4 in. (10.16 cm) long, and extends from the top of the uterus to one of the ovaries. The wall of the tube has three layers: an outer layer, a double layer of muscle, and a mucous lining. The muscular layer produces a wavelike motion that moves the ovum toward the uterus, while within the tube, cells with tiny hairlike appendages sweep the egg along. Other cells secrete nutrients for the ovum.

There is no direct connection between the Fallopian tubes and the ovaries. When the ovum erupts from the ovarian wall, it must travel a short distance to enter the fringed end of the tube. It is not clear just how this transfer of egg from ovary to tube is accomplished. Perhaps the egg is swept into the tube by the action of fingerlike projections that surround the opening of the tube. Or perhaps some type of chemical attraction exists between the egg cell and the Fallopian tube.

The journey from ovary to uterus usually takes about seven days. However, the ovum can be fertilized only at the beginning of its journey—for less than twenty-four hours after it bursts through the ovarian wall. Fertilization generally takes place in the third of the tube closest to the ovary. By the time the egg has passed through this section of the tube, it can no longer be fertilized. If fertilization has occurred, the fertilized egg continues to travel along the tube, which narrows as it approaches the uterus. At the place where the tube enters the uterine wall, its opening is smaller than the head of a pin. Once the fertilized egg passes through, it implants itself in the uterine wall. (In rare instances the egg may implant itself in the wall of the tube, resulting in an ectopic pregnancy. If this should occur, the fetus usually does not survive.)

The egg that is fertilized is an exception. Most ova degenerate and are expelled from the body in the menstrual flow, a process we'll discuss later in the chapter.

## THE BREASTS

Although the breasts are not part of the genital system, they are certainly considered sex organs in American culture. Just as a large penis symbolizes male potency, large breasts symbolize female eroticism. The ideal woman, as portrayed by such male-oriented magazines as *Playboy,* is generally large-breasted. In contrast, the ideal woman of such fashion-oriented magazines as *Vogue* is usually small-breasted, so that the clothes she is modeling will hang better.

Breasts are such a powerful cultural symbol that women often worry about the size and shape of their breasts. In response to these fears, surgical procedures have been developed to reduce breasts that are "too large" and medical procedures have been used to augment breasts that are "too small." Such procedures may have dramatic effects on the way a woman feels about herself:

Most people find it hard to understand why I had silicone injections to develop my breasts. But to me it was really important to feel good about my body and the way it looks. Getting bigger breasts definitely improved my self-image a lot. (Authors' files)

In addition to their symbolic function, the female breasts play a very real role in two aspects of female sexuality. First, some women respond sexually to breast stimulation, and their breasts show a variety of changes during the sexual response cycle. The response can be so strong that the woman experiences orgasm through breast stimulation alone. Second, breasts provide nourishment for the young; all mammals have mammary, or milk-producing, glands.

During the life cycle, the breasts undergo a variety of changes. In the newborn—both male and female—small but distinct mammary glands are present. Some infants even secrete a small amount of a milklike fluid in the first few weeks after birth. This secretion is stimulated by the extremely high level of hormones that cross the placenta while the fetus is in the uterus. Several weeks after birth, when these hormones have disappeared from the infant's body, the breasts go into a period of quiescence that lasts through childhood. At the onset of puberty, rising hormone levels stimulate breast development in the female.

## The structure of the breast

The female breast consists of fat cells, glandular tissue, and fibrous tissue. The number of fat cells, which seems to be determined in part by heredity, is the main factor in breast size—the more fat cells, the larger the breast. Yet the size of the breast has almost no effect on a woman's ability to breastfeed or on the sexual sensitivity of the breast.

Each breast contains about fifteen to twenty milk glands, or **mammary lobes,** which are held in place by connective tissue. A series of ducts, rather like a system of pipelines, connects these milk-producing lobes to the nipple (see Figure 3.7)

**mammary lobes** milk glands within the breast

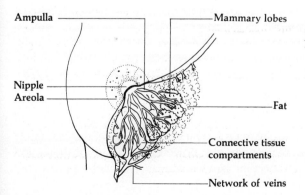

Ampulla

Mammary lobes

Nipple
Areola

Fat

Connective tissue compartments

Network of veins

### Figure 3.7

Internal anatomy of the breast in a mature woman.

and small collecting chambers between each duct and the nipple can store milk. The size of the mammary glands varies with a woman's age and childbearing status; they grow throughout pregnancy and are most highly developed just after childbirth.

During the course of a normal pregnancy, high levels of hormones cause a series of changes that prepare the breasts to produce milk, a process we'll examine in Chapter 20. Finally, after menopause, when hormone levels have fallen, the size and structure of the breast shift once again. In addition to these long-term changes, the breasts regularly alter in size and structure as hormone levels fluctuate during the menstrual cycle. Despite these changes, women of the same age and childbearing status all have about the same number of mammary lobes, so that a woman with small breasts is likely to have a generous supply of milk after childbirth.

**nipple** the conical structure in the center of each breast containing the outlet of the milk ducts

**areola** the dark circular area surrounding the nipple

Each of the fifteen or twenty ducts from the mammary lobes terminates in a very small hole on the surface of the **nipple**, the breast's most obvious feature. Nipple erection is caused by the contraction of small involuntary muscles in the **areola**, the dark circular area surrounding the nipple. When the breast is stimulated—whether by sexual stimuli, by cold, or by the pressure of tight clothing—these muscles contract and the nipple becomes erect. The surface of the areola is slightly bumpy because of the sebaceous glands that lie near the surface. These glands create a lubricant that protects the nipple from irritation by the infant's saliva during nursing. Hair sometimes grows sparsely around the outside of the areola. This hair growth is most often related to hormonal changes and tends to increase with age.

## Common breast problems

**fibroadenoma** a multiplication of cells enclosed within a fibrous capsule that forms a harmless lump in the breast

**mastodynia** tender, swollen, lumpy condition of the breasts that is common just before menstruation

Since the breasts are functioning glands that respond to a variety of hormonal changes, they are prone to a number of physical problems. Certain of these problems are extremely common, but almost never serious. For example, sometimes cells multiply to form a harmless lump, called a **fibroadenoma**, which is enclosed in a fibrous capsule so that it cannot invade the breast. At other times, the lump is a cyst, or a membrane filled with fluid. In an especially common condition known as **mastodynia**, women find that their breasts become lumpy, tender, and swollen just before menstruation. The lumps are typically round and movable, and are due to the buildup of fluids and tissues throughout the body during this phase of the menstrual cycle. The condition usually disappears as menstruation begins, and often disappears altogether or becomes less noticeable after pregnancy (Cope, 1978). Once women reach their forties, the lumpiness and swelling may increase and fail to disappear completely during menstruation. After menopause, the condition vanishes unless women take estrogen.

Although the lumps may cause women a great deal of concern, they are rarely related to any form of cancer. Women should, however, be aware of them, and learn to examine their breasts and become familiar with any changes—a procedure explained in Chapter 6.

# FEMALE SEXUAL FUNCTION

The features of a woman's sexual anatomy change in predictable ways when she is sexually stimulated, just as they do during the menstrual cycle. In response to sexual stimulation, her organs change in size, color, and texture. The changes typical of the menstrual cycle come in response to shifts in hormone levels.

## *Arousal*

When a woman becomes sexually aroused, blood flows into the pelvic area, filling the labia majora and causing them to swell and separate slightly. The labia minora may increase two or three times in diameter and their color may change, varying from deep pink to purplish-red. The vestibular bulbs also fill with blood and become firm. The clitoris increases slightly in length and width, and the hood thickens and expands.

Within the vagina, blood fills the network of blood vessels, and as the pressure of the pooled blood increases, the internal mucous layer of the vagina "sweats" drops of fluid. This fluid, which appears within twenty seconds after stimulation begins, lubricates the vagina for the insertion of the penis (Masters and Johnson, 1966). If a young woman is not aware of this response, the first time it occurs she may be worried or embarrassed:

> When I was about fifteen, I was making out with my boyfriend in the back
> seat of his car, and my pants started to feel very wet. I didn't really know what
> was happening, and I remember trying to keep him from seeing what was
> going on. I was so embarrassed about it. (Authors' files)

The uterus undergoes marked changes during sexual arousal and orgasm (Masters and Johnson, 1966). During arousal, it becomes increasingly elevated, changing the position of the cervix. After orgasm, the uterus returns to its unstimulated position. Contrary to long-held opinion, the cervix secretes no mucus during sexual stimulation. After orgasm, the cervical opening widens in some women, a response that may aid the sperm's journey to the uterus.

At orgasm, the muscles of the uterus contract in a series of waves from top to bottom, a pattern that resembles the early stages of childbirth. The direction of these contractions led Masters and Johnson (1966) to conclude there is no truth to the belief that the uterus "sucks up" seminal fluid, since the pattern moves in the wrong direction to create suction. In fact, these contractions may be responsible for the increased bleeding immediately after intercourse reported by many menstruating women. The powerful contractions of the uterine muscles during orgasm expel menstrual fluid into the vagina.

## *Menstruation*

The menstrual cycle has long been surrounded by myth, misunderstanding, and confusion. Although it is a natural event that is experienced by half the population between the ages of twelve and fifty, it has generally been treated as an illness and regarded as a "curse." In many tribal societies, the menstruating woman is considered taboo. Among the Arapesh of New Guinea she must withdraw to an isolated mountain hut; among the Eskimo she is thought to bring bad luck to the hunter; and among some groups in India she is forbidden to prepare food.

Although we now understand the physiological basis of the menstrual cycle, many myths persist. In industrialized countries, restrictions on the menstruating woman have been replaced by "protective" limitations and concerns. The menstrual cycle has been used to rationalize restrictions on women's activities and responsibilities at work. It has been proposed that women are unsuitable for important positions because of the "menstrual handicap." By suggesting that women require special consideration and treatment, some opponents of the Equal Rights Amendment perpetuated the myth that menstruation is a handicap.

In most societies the menstruating woman is considered "unclean" and hence an unsuitable sexual partner (Ford and Beach, 1951). Concern for the woman is not the basis for these restrictions; most of the prohibitions are meant to protect the health of the man. There is no evidence that intercourse during menstruation is harmful to either partner, so there is no health reason to restrict sexual activity. But many modern societies have replaced the myth of danger with esthetic prohibitions. For example, American culture reinforces the notion that menstruation is messy and embarrassing. Advertisements suggest that the menstruating woman has a secret that can be concealed only by using the proper tampons and deodorants. Yet even the esthetic argument against menstrual sex seems unnecessary. A woman can easily use a diaphragm (a contraceptive device, described in Chapter 19) to catch her flow during intercourse, demolishing any esthetic objectives.

Although we have a good understanding of the way the menstrual cycle works, we are only beginning to understand the causes of painful menstruation and the premenstrual syndrome. And the effect of the menstrual cycle on a woman's desire for sexual activity has not yet been solidly established.

**How the menstrual cycle works**  Early explanations of the menstrual cycle were often distorted by male prejudice and medical ignorance. Many theories began with the notion that women have too much blood. The menstrual cycle was meant to eliminate this excess, which collected either because of some internal defect in women or because women were not as physically active as men. The extra blood left the body through the uterus because this was the weakest part of the body (Delaney et al., 1976). These exploded theories have left a legacy that persists in the face of medical knowledge; many people still see menstruation as an unnatural process or some sort of illness.

**menarche** the first
menstruation

In our society, **menarche,** or the first menstruation, generally occurs at the age of twelve or thirteen. For about two years before this time, hormone levels rise steadily. With menarche, they begin to rise and fall in a regular monthly pattern that continues until menopause—unless interrupted by pregnancy, stress, or illness. The length of the cycle varies widely among individuals, but its average length is about twenty-eight days. Illness, drug use, or physical deprivation can affect the length of the cycle, as can such psychological factors as stress.

In each woman the duration of menstrual flow is predictable, but there are

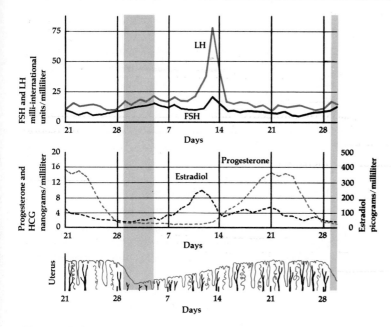

### Figure 3.8

(above) Hormone levels during the menstrual cycle. (below) Changes in the uterine lining during a typical cycle. The rise in FSH level early in the cycle causes the ovaries to secrete estrogen. The LH peak brings on ovulation and the development of the corpus luteum. The latter secretes estrogen and progesterone in the second part of the cycle. If conception does not occur, the corpus luteum disintegrates, causing the endometrium to be shed. (Data from Christopher A. Adejuwon of the Population Council)

wide individual differences. Although the period lasts about five days in most women, its length may vary from three to seven days. During each menstruation, approximately two to three ounces (just over a quarter of a cup, or 57 to 85 g) of menstrual fluid is released. This substance is made up of the discarded uterine lining and blood.

The menstrual cycle is controlled by hormones and regulated by a complex interaction of the ovaries, the pituitary gland, and the hypothalamus—a structure that lies deep within the brain. Each of these organs is sensitive to levels of hormones within the bloodstream and at the correct time signals other glands to secrete appropriate hormones. These hormones cause the maturation and release of an egg, the buildup of the lining of the uterus, and—if there is no pregnancy—the shedding of this lining.

The menstrual cycle consists of three overlapping phases: the proliferative phase, the secretory phase, and the menstrual phase. During the *proliferative phase*, the pituitary secretes the hormone FSH (follicle-stimulating hormone), which travels through the bloodstream to the ovaries and stimulates the growth of an egg follicle (Figure 3.8). In turn, cells in this follicle, called the **Graafian follicle,**

**Graafian follicle** the ovarian follicle that is in the process of maturing an egg

secrete increasing amounts of estrogen, causing a buildup of the endometrium that lines the uterus.

Just before midcycle, the pituitary releases a sudden burst of LH (lutenizing hormone). About thirty-six hours after this burst, ovulation takes place. On average, ovulation occurs about fourteen days after the start of the last menstrual period and about fourteen days before the start of the next period.

After ovulation, the *secretory* phase begins. Now LH transforms the ruptured Graafian follicle into the corpus luteum, which secretes two hormones: estrogen and progesterone. These hormones cause the endometrium to produce substances that can nourish a fertilized egg.

If fertilization takes place, the corpus luteum expands and continues to secrete estrogen and progesterone to maintain the pregnancy. If the egg is not fertilized, however, the corpus luteum will begin to disintegrate, producing decreasing amounts of these hormones. When this happens the endometrium can no longer be maintained; it is shed, marking the menstrual phase of the cycle. At this time, low levels of estrogen again trigger the pituitary to secrete FSH, beginning the cycle anew (Figure 3.9).

**Dysmenorrhea**   Some women breeze through their menstrual periods with little discomfort:

> I never know I'm menstruating until the flow appears. So my period is simply a nuisance. The big problem is when I forget that I'm menstruating and don't change a tampon soon enough. (Authors' files)

**dysmenorrhea** painful menstruation

Such women are probably in the minority. Most women have some sort of mild discomfort, and many suffer from **dysmenorrhea**, severe abdominal cramps that may be accompanied by nausea, vomiting, headaches, backache, diarrhea, dizziness, weakness, or insomnia. At one time a woman who complained of such symptoms was simply patted on the shoulder and told she'd have to live with her monthly disorder. It was often suggested that her pains were all in her mind and that perhaps she was rejecting the "feminine role" (Gannon, 1981).

Today we've begun to understand the causes of dysmenorrhea. Although it's probably true that cultural attitudes toward menstruation can increase the severity of pain and discomfort, researchers seem to have established a real physical basis for dysmenorrhea.

The culprit appears to be *prostaglandin,* a common chemical found in both men and women. Prostaglandins are produced in many body tissues, including the uterus, and they can stimulate muscle contractions. Toward the end of the menstrual cycle prostaglandin levels rise, apparently peaking at menstruation, and it's suspected that progesterone regulates their production. In some women, an oversupply of prostaglandins seems to make the uterus contract, shutting off the flow of blood and causing a pain that researchers have compared to the sharp pains of angina suffered by cardiac patients (Dingfelder, 1982).

This constriction of blood flow probably was at the basis of the cure for dysmenorrhea traditionally suggested by gynecologists: have a baby. At one time it

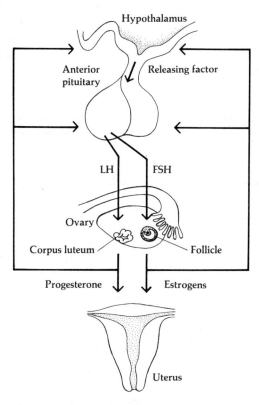

*Figure 3.9    Feedback
mechanisms controlling the
female reproductive cycle.*

Note that the hypothalamic secretions stimulate
the pituitary gland to secrete FSH and LH. FSH
causes one or more follicles in the ovary to
develop and produce estrogen. The LH triggers
ovulation and the formation of the corpus
luteum. In turn, hormones secreted by the
corpus luteum cause the hypothalamus and
pituitary to inhibit or stimulate further secretions.

was thought that the cervical enlargement which followed pregnancy was responsible for the frequent disappearance of dysmenorrhea after a woman gave birth.
Now, however, physicians believe that structural changes in the uterus, particularly
the permanent increase in blood vessels that accompanies pregnancy, is responsible (Dingfelder, 1982).

Today, most physicians prescribe prostaglandin inhibitors for women with
clear-cut cases of dysmenorrhea. A number of these drugs are on the market and
they have been effective in eliminating or reducing symptoms in most women (Bu-

# *Focus*

## THE PREMENSTRUAL SYNDROME

**premenstrual syndrome (PMS)** an uncomfortable condition, with both physiological and emotional symptoms, that can develop just before menstruation

The notion that women's moods fluctuate with phases of the menstrual cycle has long been an accepted part of our folklore. The most distressing changes, believed to take place in the week before menstruation begins, have achieved the status of a syndrome—the **premenstrual syndrome (PMS).** The status of PMS varies: it has been treated as an illness requiring medication and ignored as the dramatizing of neurotic women. Arguments about PMS center on whether it exists, and if so, what causes it and how many women experience it.

Although the scientific status of PMS is uncertain, women accused of murder and child abuse have attempted to use it as a defense. Two British women received lighter sentences for crimes committed under PMS stress, but an American woman who claimed that PMS caused her to beat her four-year-old daughter dropped her defense and pleaded guilty to child abuse (Bird, 1982).

Some research has found that premenstrual women are more prone to accidents and injuries, more likely to enter a mental hospital, and more likely to call in sick at their place of employment than

women in other phases of the cycle (Dalton, 1964). But this relationship between the premenstrual phase and such behavior is not necessarily caused by hormone levels. Since psychological stress can alter the menstrual cycle, it is just as likely that the cause runs in the other direction (Parlee, 1976).

In severe cases of PMS, a woman says that her breasts are swollen and tender, her abdomen bloated, and her hands and feet swollen. She may complain of headaches, constipation, fatigue, depression, irritability, or tension. Her skin may develop acnelike blemishes, and she may be extremely thirsty or crave sweet or salty foods. When menstruation begins, the symptoms quickly disappear (Reid and Yen, 1981).

Although many women spontaneously report symptoms of PMS, Mary Brown Parlee (1976) maintains that no one has yet shown that the syndrome exists. For example, when asked to describe any premenstrual symptoms, many women provide evidence for PMS. Yet these data appear to be influenced by cultural beliefs and attitudes toward menstruation, for when women are simply

asked to record their daily mood changes, evidence for PMS dwindles.

What's more, few studies of PMS compare findings from the premenstrual phase, gathered from women who complain of PMS, with the same women's behavior in other parts of the cycle. And researchers rarely check these findings against women who do not complain of PMS. Our angle of vision may be tilted. Instead of viewing the premenstrual phase as a time when such moods as irritability increase, we might view the midcycle as a time when women experience a mood upswing.

Some researchers claim that PMS exists, but that women learn to experience it. According to Karen Paige (1976), mood and behavior changes are not caused solely by fluctuating hormones, but instead are social and cultural responses to menstruation. Her research with fifty-two women who were using a pill that minimized hormonal fluctuations supports this view. A frequent side effect of the pill is reduced menstrual flow. If PMS is not linked to hormone levels, but is instead a response to menstrual bleeding, then women whose flow is reduced would be less likely to complain of the "premenstrual blues." This was the case. Women with a reduced menstrual flow showed less anxiety than women whose flow remained normally heavy. In addition, Catholic and Jewish women in the study, whose religions tend to view the menstruating woman as "unclean," showed more premenstrual anxiety than did Protestant women. Despite this evidence of a psychological influence on PMS, researchers have been unable to find any common personality factors or emotional problems among women who complain of the syndrome (Blank, Goldstein, and Chatterjee, 1980).

Although many studies have reported cyclical mood changes, few of them suggest that all women experience these changes. For example, among nearly a thousand wives of graduate students at a large university, only about 20 percent complained of moderate to severe irritability, mood swings, or tension in the premenstrual phase (Moos, 1969). Estimates of the syndrome's occurrence vary: researchers have found that as few as 15 percent or as many as 90 percent of women

show signs of PMS.

Arguments about whether PMS has a physical or a psychological origin are not likely to fade away. Some of those who favor a physical cause suppose that shifting levels of estrogen and progesterone lead to water retention, a symptom that might be related to other types of premenstrual discomfort. Others blame vitamin deficiencies, low blood sugar, or a woman's allergy to her own hormones. Most recently, researchers have suggested that PMS develops when the brain releases certain chemicals erratically. These chemicals, known as peptides, can affect hormone balance, thirst, appetite, water retention, mood, and behavior (Reid and Yen, 1981). Since there's no agreement on the cause of PMS, treatment varies widely; physicians prescribe progesterone injections, changes in diet, vitamin supplements, antidepressants, and diuretics to reduce water retention.

However, none of the proposed causes of PMS explains why women's symptoms differ or why social factors influence its occurrence. Perhaps hormones or peptides set the stage for PMS, but psychological and social factors shape women's

attitudes toward menstruation. American culture expresses negative attitudes and expects the premenstrual phase to be distressful. Growing up in this atmosphere may lead some women to feel distress or increase the intensity of distress in others.

The status of PMS has been the center of heated debate because it is related to the status of women in American culture. Because PMS is often used as a rationale for denying women positions of authority, many feminists prefer to deny its existence. Others agree that it exists, but react to it in different ways. Some suggest that during the premenstrual phase a woman is behaving in the same way that a man, with his relatively constant hormone levels, behaves all the time. Others claim that PMS is taught to women by a sexist society. Yet others, angered that PMS is viewed by some as being "all in a woman's head," claim that premenstrual symptoms have real physical causes. On the basis of the information we now have, none of these views can be accepted or rejected.

doff, 1982). For years, women with dysmenorrhea took aspirin, and the discovery of the prostaglandins' role in the disorder supports that practice. Aspirin is a weak prostaglandin inhibitor; however, its effect seems to be too weak to bring relief to many women (Heinrichs and Adamson, 1980).

Prostaglandin inhibitors do not help all women, but there are other treatments that can provide relief. Birth control pills that prevent ovulation also prevent prostaglandin buildup, so that for some women, taking a contraceptive pill may end menstrual pain. Sexual intercourse sometimes reduces cramps, but only if the woman has an orgasm (Lanson, 1975). So sexual activity—either masturbation or with a partner—may be helpful.

An old but effective method of decreasing menstrual pain is heat. Spending a half-hour soaking in a hot bath or with a hot water bottle on the abdomen often relieves cramps. Regular exercise is also helpful. Swimming, running, walking, or bicycling—any exercise that strengthens lower abdominal and upper leg muscles—can reduce menstrual pain. Among several hundred young women with dysmenorrhea who followed a prescribed exercise routine, about 70 percent found that within four months their menstrual discomfort was sharply reduced (Lanson, 1975).

**amenorrhea** absence of menstruation

**Menstruation and exercise**   Although moderate exercise can relieve menstrual problems, intense exercise has been implicated in cases of **amenorrhea**, or the absence of menstruation. This effect has been found only among girls and women who exercise strenuously and regularly, at the level common among ballet dancers and competitive swimmers or runners. In young girls, menarche may be delayed; in women, menstrual periods may cease or become extremely irregular.

Swimmers and runners who begin training before menarche generally begin to menstruate at about fifteen, and each year of strenuous training seems to postpone menarche about five months. It's been suggested that this delay is due to the low proportion of fat in the bodies of women who exercise strenuously. When body fat drops much below 17 percent, estrogen levels may be so low that ovulation does not begin.

Among women runners, from 7 to 10 percent seem to develop amenorrhea. These women tend to weigh less, run longer distances and faster, lose more weight when running, eat less protein, and find running more stressful than do runners whose periods are regular. Researchers have suggested that a woman whose amenorrhea is due to strenuous exercise may be able to reestablish her menstrual cycle by increasing the quality of her diet, upping her cholesterol intake to the maximum recommended level, gaining weight, and slowing her running speed (Brody, 1982).

**toxic shock syndrome** a violent pathological reaction to the growth of a bacterium, Staphylococcus aureus, which has been connected with tampon use

**Toxic shock syndrome**   In the past few years, many women have become concerned about **toxic shock syndrome**, in which a sudden onset of high fever, vomiting, and diarrhea is rapidly followed by extremely low blood pressure and shock (U.S. Public Health Service, 1980). Sometimes toxic shock syndrome is fatal. Toxic shock victims are generally women younger than twenty-four, and the disease is most likely to develop during the menstrual period.

Toxic shock is caused by a bacterium, Staphlyococcus aureus, which finds a hospitable home in tampons soaked with menstrual fluid. The highly absorbent tampons seem most closely linked with toxic shock, either because women change them less frequently or because they absorb more of the menstrual fluid, leaving the vaginal walls drier and open to irritation.

Since women who have had toxic shock once are highly susceptible to a second attack, it's been suggested that they discontinue using tampons. Using regular tampons is apparently riskier for all young women than using sanitary pads; however, the chances of developing toxic shock are slight, even for tampon wearers. The disease is extremely rare. Not all menstrual disorders occur during menstruation; a relatively common problem precedes the onset of the monthly flow.

**Sex and the menstrual cycle**  It would seem logical that regular changes in hormone levels would affect women's sexual activity. In lower animals, the female is receptive to males only during ovulation. Of course, lower animals do not have true menstrual cycles, in which the uterine lining is shed. Among chimpanzees, who do have menstrual cycles, females show a period of strong sexual desire during the high-estrogen phase of the cycle. Ovulation occurs, the female is fertile, and she generally accepts the sexual advances of any male. But social factors also affect her sexual behavior; during nonfertile periods, a female chimpanzee will accept a favorite male and reject others (Ford and Beach, 1951).

Although social factors have an enormous influence on human sexuality, we would expect hormones to have some effect on sexual behavior. If sexual receptivity is tied to hormones in a way that ensures the survival of the species, women would show a sexual peak at midcycle, when ovulation occurs. But social factors appear to overpower any such effect.

In some cultures, women's sexual desire is indeed expected to be strongest at specific times in the menstrual cycle, but rarely is midcycle (the fertile period) seen as the height of receptiveness. For example, members of the Masai society believe that a woman's receptiveness rises sharply just after her menstrual period, and Hopi Indians believe that a woman is most ardent just before and just after menstruation.

These expectations are in line with sexual behavior that is dominated by social factors. Living in a society that frowns on sexual contact during her menstrual period, a woman may well show heightened desire just before and after her period as a way of compensating for her socially dictated abstinence. Social factors could influence sexual behavior in other ways as well. For example, since many women know that pregnancy is most likely to occur at midcycle, they may abstain at that time, causing intercourse rates to drop.

Research on sexual response across the menstrual cycle has produced inconsistent results. Some studies indicate that sexual activity peaks just before and just after menstruation (McCauley and Ehrhardt, 1976). This finding suggests that desire is strongest at times when a woman is least likely to conceive. Apparently, hormones either do not heighten desire at ovulation, or if they have this effect, it is almost obliterated by social influences. In the light of such research, hormonal contributions appear minor when compared with the effect of attitudes and emotions.

No trace of shifts in sexual responsiveness during the menstrual cycle appeared when women listened to tapes of a man and woman enacting a sexual encounter. In this study (Hoon, Bruce, and Kinchloe, 1982), the date of ovulation was established for each woman, and her physiological responses to the erotic material were recorded. As measured both by their physiological responses and their own judgment of their arousal, these women responded similarly to erotic material in every stage of the menstrual cycle.

Although hormone levels do not seem to have a direct effect on a woman's sexual response, they may influence her general mood and feelings of well-being. Such an influence could lead to variations in sexual interest in the course of a cycle. In another study (Adams et al., 1978), hormone levels seemed to have some effect on women's sexual interest. At midcycle, when estrogen levels are highest, there was an increase in sexual activity initiated by women—but only among women who did not take a contraceptive pill. Since the pill prevents ovulation by keeping estrogen and progesterone levels fairly steady, the failure of women on the pill to show a peak at midcycle strengthens the possibility of a link between hormones and sexual interest.

Generalizing about hormone levels and sexual activity is difficult because there are striking individual differences in both the amount and timing of hormonal secretions (Whalen, 1975). Two women who have cycles of equal length may have very different patterns of hormone release.

The probability of sexual intercourse depends on many factors that have nothing to do with hormones. The availability of an attractive partner, general health and well-being, available time and appropriate place, and the opinions of others are just of a few of the influences that contribute to sexual activity. If all these factors remained constant, hormonal influences on sexuality might become clear. But since the factors vary considerably, they probably mask whatever hormonal influences there are.

# Summary

**1** The sex of a child is determined at conception by the type of sperm that unites with the **ovum**, or egg. Sperm that carry X chromosomes produce girls; sperm that carry Y chromosomes produce boys. At first male and female embryos are identical, and it is six weeks before male and female development diverges. In male embryos, the **gonads**, or sex glands, develop into testes, and in female embryos, the gonads develop into ovaries. Because of this common beginning, some of the sex organs in males and females are **homologous**; that is, they have the same origin.

**2** The **vulva**, or external female sex organs, show wide individual differences. The major external sex organs in the female are the **labia majora**, or outer lips; the **labia minora**, or inner lips; the vestibular area; Bartholin's glands; the **hymen**; and the clitoris. The **clitoris**, which is highly responsive to sexual stimulation, contains hollow, spongelike cylinders, or **corpora cavernosa**, so that the clitoris, like the penis, is an erectile organ. There is no relationship between the size of a woman's clitoris and the intensity of her sexual response, just as there is no relationship between sexual responsiveness and the distance between the clitoral glans and the vaginal opening.

**3** The major internal sexual organs in the female are the vagina, cervix, uterus, ovaries, and Fallopian tubes. It has been proposed that deep within the vagina is a small area called the **Grafenberg spot**, which—like the clitoris—is extremely responsive to sexual stimulation. As yet the existence of the G spot has not been scientifically confirmed. There are two patterns of change in the **uterus,** or womb. The lifelong pattern consists of prenatal growth, shrinkage immediately after birth, regrowth with sexual puberty, and shrinkage at **menopause,** when menstruation ceases. The cyclical pattern follows the menstrual cycle. The **endometrium,** or inner uterine layer, develops and, if pregnancy does not occur, is shed at each menstruation. The ovaries secrete **estrogens,** or female hormones, and mature and release an ovum during each menstrual cycle. Each ovary contains a number of **follicles,** or compartments for maturing ova. The **Fallopian tubes** guide the ova from the ovary to the uterus.

**4** Female breasts are a powerful cultural symbol; they play a role in sexual response and in providing nourishment for the young. The breast consists of fat cells, glandular tissue, and fibrous tissue. Its milk glands, **or mammary lobes,** produce milk that passes along milk ducts to the nipple. Breast stimulation causes small muscles in the **areola,** the dark, circular area surrounding the nipple, to contract and the nipple to become erect. Because the breasts' size and shape vary in response to hormonal changes, many women find that their breasts become tender and swollen just before menstruation, a condition known as **mastodynia.**

**5** When a woman becomes aroused, blood flows into the pelvic area, causing her sexual anatomy to change in predictable ways. Although the menstrual cycle is a natural event, it has been surrounded by myths and often treated as an illness. The menstrual cycle is controlled by hormones and regulated by interaction of the ovaries, the pituitary gland, and the hypothalamus. In the proliferative phase of the menstrual cycle, the hormone FSH stimulates the growth of an egg follicle, called the **Graafian follicle,** which secretes estrogen and causes the endometrium to build up. Just before midcycle, the hormone LH causes ovulation—the release of the ovum through the ovarian wall. Now the secretory phase begins: The follicle becomes the **corpus luteum** and is set to help prepare for pregnancy and to maintain it. If conception does not occur, the corpus luteum degenerates and the menstrual phase of the cycle begins. The endometrium is shed and new secretion of FSH begins the cycle once more.

**6** Some women are troubled by **dysmenorrhea,** or painful menstruation, a condition now believed to be the result of excessive prostaglandin production. Prostaglandin inhibitors relieve dysmenorrhea in most women; other women are relieved by oral contraceptives, orgasm, heat, or regular exercise that increases muscle tone. Intense exercise has been implicated in **amenorrhea,** or the absence of menstruation. **Toxic shock syndrome,** in which bacteria cause a severe pathological reaction, has been linked to wearing highly absorbent tampons.

**7** Some women report physiological symptoms and mood changes just before menstruation that are known as **premenstrual syndrome (PMS).** The precise cause of PMS is unknown, although it may be due to fluctuating hormones, water retention, vitamin deficiencies, low blood sugar, a woman's allergy to her own hormones, or the erratic release of brain chemicals. Although no common personality traits have been found in women who report PMS, some investigators believe that cultural attitudes toward menstruation play an important role, and other investigators believe that its incidence is exaggerated and its existence not established.

**8** The effect of hormones on women's sexual behavior has not been established. Some studies have shown that sexual activity peaks just before and just after menstruation, when a woman is unlikely to be fertile. Some studies have found no difference in sexual responsiveness at any time during the menstrual cycle; however, other studies have found an increase in the initiation of sexual activity at midcycle among women who do not take contraceptive pills. But so many social and psychological factors affect sexual activity that any hormonal influence is probably masked.

*a man's view*

I'm glad to be a man. It's usually easy to reach orgasm, I can have sex just by opening my zipper, and I get to initiate the action. Best of all, I can't get pregnant. (Authors' files)

Let us consider the penis, probably the laziest part of a man. Your heart, lungs, and brain are working all the time.... In contrast, most of the time your penis does exactly nothing. While it serves as a tube through which urine passes, it has no active part in the process. And a penis is not necessary for your survival. Even if you didn't have one, or had one that never became erect, you could live a long, healthy, and perhaps happy life. So, despite fashionable ideas of penises being necessary and always active, hopping about with lots of throbbing and crashing, the real penis is much given to rest and relaxation. (Zilbergeld, 1978, p. 92)

# 4 The Male Sexual System

# Chapter 4

Men grow up surrounded by the male mystique, a set of myths about male sexuality that leaves many men uncertain about their own sexual capacity. The mystique builds from the first whisperings between small boys, who repeat gossip, exaggerated jokes, and misinformation. Among the most common myths, for example, is the belief that boys and men are informed, experienced, and eager about sex. Because much of a woman's sexual apparatus is hidden while a man's organs are in plain sight, there is another myth that sex is mysterious and complicated for women, but simple and straightforward for men. According to this myth, women reach orgasm only with a patient and skillful lover, whereas men can climax any time, any place, and with a minimum of effort. Women supposedly require tenderness and affection, but men simply want a place to insert their penis.

Part of this mystique indicates that the mythical man is supposed to have sex frequently and to have no doubts or questions about how, when, or where to do it. This being the case, a man who asks a question about sex or expresses some concern is mistakenly perceived as not a "real man." The problem is that few men are as experienced or skillful or unconcerned as the male mystique would have it, but most men hide their doubts and questions. They pretend they know more than they do, have sex more often than they do, and have no questions, even while many of them are worrying about themselves and their masculinity. They worry about what other men do, about their own thoughts, about why sex is not as wonderful as the myth implies, and about whether they're fulfilling their sexual "duty" to their wives or lovers (Zilbergeld, 1978). It appears that the carefree, never-ending sex of male-oriented magazines and locker room stories is outside of most men's experience.

# The Male Sexual System

In this chapter, we begin with a description of male sexual anatomy, which may well dispel some of the concerns generated by the male mystique. After we investigate the practice of circumcision, we'll turn to the male sexual function and the effect of male hormones on sexuality. We'll end by investigating the variable—and sometimes surprising—effects of castration on sexual activity.

## EXTERNAL ANATOMY

The external organs of the male sexual system—the penis, scrotum, and testes—are highly visible, and their prominence may help to explain why complete female nudity is more acceptable in Western cultures than complete male nudity. The male sexual system, like the female system, is designed to fulfill both sexual and reproductive roles.

### The penis

No other part of male anatomy carries the emotional significance of the penis. The phallus, or penis, has been regarded as a primary symbol of power in almost all cultures. The importance a culture places on the penis often shows up in art. The ancient Roman god of fertility, Priapus, was an exceedingly ugly child with enormous genitals. Many Romans kept statues of Priapus in their gardens and wore charms in the shape of a penis, his symbol, to ward off the evil eye and bring good luck. Similarly, the erotic art of Japan abounds with huge penises, some of them larger than their "fortunate" owners.

The power of the penis has been so profound in European culture that Sigmund Freud (1974), the founder of psychoanalysis, based his theory of masculinity and femininity on the male's possession of a penis and the female's lack of one. Girls, he proposed, are born "castrated," and as soon as a little girl discovers the splendid organ that is attached to each boy's lower abdomen, she is consumed with **penis envy**. Freud believed that girls never overcome this feeling, and that it casts a shadow over their lives. Through a peculiar chain of reasoning, Freud decided that penis envy made women morally and culturally inferior to men. As might be expected, this aspect of Freudian theory has been criticized more than any other. These symbolic meanings may have little to do with an individual's personal experiences, but they are bound to influence the way a man views his own sexuality.

From a reproductive view, the simple but important function of the penis is to convey semen containing sperm into the vagina. In accomplishing this task, the size and appearance of the penis are of little importance. But the penis has other important functions: it is the primary organ of male sensory pleasure, and it passes urine from the bladder out of the body.

**Penile anatomy** The penis has two major parts: the head and the shaft. The head is also called the **glans** (see Figure 4.1), from the Latin word for acorn. The urethra passes through both the shaft and the glans and ends in a slit-shaped opening called the **meatus**. Some boys are born with the opening of the urethra on the underside of the penis instead of at the tip, a condition called **hypospadia**. If the opening is on the underside of the glans no treatment is needed, but if it occurs too far back on the underside of the shaft, the condition can be corrected surgically (Brooks and Brooks, 1981).

Dickinson (1933), who pioneered in observations of the female sexual system, noted that the tissue of the glans is especially soft and yielding. He suggested that it had adapted through evolution to avoid injury to a woman's internal organs during intercourse. The surface of the glans is generally smooth or wrinkled in appearance. Although the area of greatest sensitivity varies from one man to another, the shaft of the penis and the **corona**—a ridge of tissue separating head from shaft—are generally most responsive to stimulation by touch. A third sensitive area is the **frenulum**, a thin strip of skin attached to the glans on the underside of the penis. The undersurface of both glans and shaft are usually more sensitive than the upper surface.

Within the shaft of the penis are arteries, veins, small blood vessels, and erectile tissue. Unlike the organ in some other mammals, the human penis contains no bones. Inside the shaft are three hollow, spongelike cylinders that run the length of the penis. Like the cylinders in the homologous clitoris, the two upper cylinders are called the corpora cavernosa; the lower cylinder, through which the urethra runs, is

**penis envy** the Freudian belief that envy of the male penis overshadows the life of girls and women

**glans** the head of the penis

**meatus** the slit-shaped opening in the head of the penis

**hypospadia** a condition in which the urethra opens on the underside of the penis instead of at the tip

**corona** the ridge of tissue separating the head of the penis from the shaft

**frenulum** a thin strip of skin attached to the glans on the underside of the penis

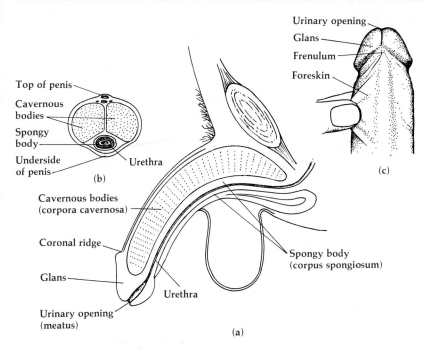

Urinary opening

Glans

Frenulum

Foreskin

(c)

Top of penis

Cavernous bodies

Spongy body

Underside of penis

Urethra

(b)

Cavernous bodies (corpora cavernosa)

Coronal ridge

Glans

Urethra

Urinary opening (meatus)

Spongy body (corpus spongiosum)

(a)

*Figure 4.1  Internal and external anatomy of the penis.*
Three different views show: (a) a side view of the internal anatomy; (b) a cross-section of the internal structures; and (c) the underside of the penis and the location of the frenulum.

known as the **corpus spongiosum**. When an erect penis is forcibly bent, one of the cylinders can tear. This is called a penile fracture, and it can be corrected by surgery (Brooks and Brooks, 1981).

At the base of the penis, the cylinders form *crura* (legs) that anchor the penis to the pubic bone. The lower, spongy body does not attach directly to the pubic bone; instead, it enlarges into the *bulb* of the penis, which is located within the groin. Two sets of muscles enclose the root of the penis; one set fastens around the crura of the cylinders, and the other is wrapped around the bulb. Contractions of these muscles aid in expelling semen or urine through the urethra.

**corpus spongiosum** the hollow cylinder within the penis through which the urethra runs

**Penile size and sexual satisfaction**  The intense cultural focus on the penis has led many men to worry about the size of their penis. Many believe their penis is the wrong size—and the wrong size is always too small. The penis that runs through most male fantasies comes in three sizes: large, gigantic, and too big to get through the door (Zilbergeld, 1978). Once a man becomes convinced his penis is "too small," he may become preoccupied with the notion:

> I can remember when one of the guys on my team made a comment about what a "tiny dick" I had. Even though I knew that he was just trying to put me down, I couldn't help worrying about it for years afterwards. (Authors' files)

# *Focus*

## IS CIRCUMCISION NECESSARY?

**foreskin** the fold of skin that covers the glans

**circumcision** an operation in which the foreskin is pulled forward over the penis and cut away, leaving the glans permanently exposed

**smegma** secretion that accumulates beneath the foreskin

At birth, a boy's penis is covered with a layer of thin, loose skin. Part of this skin folds over on itself and covers the glans; the fold is called the *prepuce,* or **foreskin.** In many national and religious groups, the foreskin is pulled forward over the penis and cut away, leaving the glans exposed. This process is called **circumcision.**

The practice of circumcision originated in ancient times and is often associated with religions, including Islam and Judaism. The ancient Egyptians may have been the first culture to practice widespread circumcision of males and females. Pictures of circumcised males appear on the walls of Egyptian tombs, and writings indicate that it was a religious rite, performed by priests. Among ancient Jews, circumcision was an act of religious faith, and God's instructions to Abraham, ordering circumcision as a sign of the covenant, can be found in the book of Gen-

esis. Although the Koran does not order ritual circumcision, it is an act of religious faith among Muslims. Perhaps Mohammed simply adopted a common Arab custom (Bullough, 1976).

Circumcision is also practiced in many tribal cultures as part of an initiation rite that signifies a young boy's passage into adult status and privileges. In many African societies, young men were not allowed to have sexual intercourse until they had gone through these rites (Ford and Beach, 1951).

Among developed nations, including the United States, circumcision is far more likely to be performed for "hygienic" reasons than as an act of religious or social faith. The medical arguments for circumcision include cleanliness and the prevention of cancer. The uncircumcised penis, the argument goes, may accumulate dirt and secretions, called **smegma,** which can lead to infection. Supposedly, circumcised men

have a lower rate of penile cancer than do uncircumcised men. What is more, their female partners are reputed to have a lower rate of cervical cancer than other women.

Both reasons have been attacked. The relationship between cancer and circumcision is not at all clear. Penile cancer is as rare in France, Sweden, Norway, Finland, and Denmark, where circumcision is not a routine practice, as it is in the United States, where more than 80 percent of newborn boys are circumcised (Kesselman, 1982). What is more, there's no evidence that circumcision in her male partners reduces a woman's chances of developing cervical cancer (Wallerstein, 1980). As far as cleanliness goes, an uncircumcised boy can easily learn to clean beneath the foreskin—a simple procedure—and eliminate the chances of infection. One of the few situations in which circumcision is clearly called for is a rare condition known

Some men worry that their penis is too small to satisfy a woman. This concern was also evident in ancient India. The *Kama Sutra,* the Hindu guide to sexual techniques, classified men as belonging to one of three groups—Hare, Bull, or Horse—depending on the size of the penis. Women were classified as Deer, Mare, or Elephant, according to the depth of the vagina. The *Kama Sutra* advises men to select a female partner from the corresponding group. For men and women from differ-as **phimosis,** in which the foreskin is so tight it cannot be pulled back for cleaning.

The effect of circumcision on sexual functioning was long a topic of controversy. Depending on which group you listened to, it either heightened or reduced sexual stimulation.

One group believed that constant exposure of the sensitive glans in circumcised men would make intercourse so stimulating that men would begin to ejaculate too soon. They also maintained that uncircumcised men, whose glans is generally covered, were not as sensitive to erotic stimulation. Thus, circumcision intensified sexual stimulation, making life sexier but perhaps leading to sexual problems.

The other group took a contrary position. They said that it is the foreskin that is especially sensitive, because it contains many nerve endings. Removing the foreskin would reduce stimulation. As a matter of fact, circumcision became popular in the United States during the nineteenth century because it was supposed to make masturbation less pleasurable. The twentieth-century argument focused on intercourse. Since a circumcised man's glans is constantly exposed, it would become tough and less sensitive, enabling him to prolong intercourse. This group recommended circumcision as a treatment for premature ejaculation (Kesselman, 1982).

Both groups appear to be wrong. Laboratory research has found little difference in ejaculatory control between circumcised and uncircumcised men (Masters and Johnson, 1966). And the two groups show similar sensitivity to light touch. In addition, the foreskin retracts during sexual intercourse, leaving the glans of an uncircumcised man as exposed to stimulation as it is in a circumcised man.

When men are asked about circumcision, both circumcised and uncircumcised men seem satisfied. Most circumcised men seem to give little thought to their condition, but appear to be glad to be rid of a foreskin:

I was rather surprised and disbelieving when I first found out about circumcision, as I thought I had been born the way I was. I still did not want to be uncircumcised; it seemed natural. (Hite, 1981, pp. 397–398)

Yet the uncircumcised men seem just as happy to have escaped the operation, although some American men admit to having felt "different" as boys:

When I was younger, I thought everyone else was circumcised and felt strange that I wasn't, and never wanted to expose my penis to other boys. But now I think that having a foreskin has made the head of my penis more sensitive and enhanced sexual pleasure for me. (Hite, 1981, pp. 398–399)

**phimosis** a condition in which the penile foreskin is so tight that it cannot be pulled back

ent groups who wanted to have intercourse, the manual described positions that minimized the disparity and increased the pair's pleasure.

Scientific measurement of the penis indicates that most masculine concern is misplaced. Dickinson (1933), again one of the first researchers to measure penile size, reported that the average erect penis was 6.2 in. (15.5 cm) long. Dickinson's findings were confirmed by Masters and Johnson (1966), whose research de-

*Figure 4.2*

The external genitals
of the male vary
widely in
appearance.

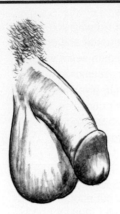 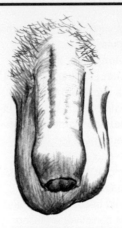 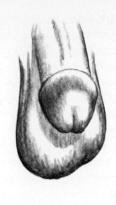

stroyed the myth that the larger the flaccid, or limp, penis, the larger the organ would be when erect. They found that smaller penises generally increased more in size than did larger penises. Among the men they studied, the flaccid penis ranged in size from 3.4 in. (8.5 cm) to 4.2 in. (10.5 cm), with the average being about 3.8 in. (9.5 cm). (See Figure 4.2.) Yet with full erection, the difference usually disappeared. For example one man, whose penis measured 3 in. (7.5 cm) when flaccid, had an erection that measured 6.6 in. (16.5 cm); a second man, whose flaccid measurement was 4.4 in. (11 cm), also had an erection that measured 6.6 in.

A second myth about the penis is that skeletal and penile size are related; that is, that a very tall man will have a long penis. Research has demolished this belief. The largest penis measured by Masters and Johnson (1966), which was 5.6 in. (14 cm) when flaccid, belonged to a man who was only 5 feet 7 inches tall and weighed 152 pounds. The smallest flaccid penis they observed measured 2.4 in. (6 cm) and belonged to a man who was 5 feet 11 inches tall and weighed 178 pounds.

Finally, the relationship between penile size and sexual satisfaction is often highly exaggerated. As sexual advice columns repeatedly stress, penile size is far less important than sexual technique. Among one group of four hundred women, not one mentioned penis size as an important factor in sexual satisfaction (Zilbergeld, 1978). This doesn't mean that women are unaware of differences in penis size. Like men, women are susceptible to cultural fantasies. But few of them let these fantasies affect their choice of sexual partner.

### The testes

What would you think of a man who placed his hands over his genitals when making a promise? Strange as it may sound today, this custom was prevalent among ancient Romans, and the words "testis" and "testicle" are derived from the same Latin word as "witness." In fact, other English words, such as "testify" and "testimonial," come from the same source. In ancient Rome, a man's word was literally as good as his testes.

Such examples show that culture may endow the testes as well as the penis with symbolic meanings. The slang expression for showing such "masculine" qualities as courage, boldness, or assertiveness is "having the *balls* to do it." As a result, just as some men confuse the size of the penis with masculinity, others express concern over the size or shape of the testes. Most of these concerns are largely unfounded, although testes do show a wide range of normal variation.

As we saw in Chapter 3, the testes and the ovaries are homologous organs: both develop from the same primitive structures and both perform the same basic functions. The ovaries mature egg cells and release primarily female hormones; the testes produce sperm cells and release primarily male hormones.

**Anatomy** The testes differ from the ovaries in their location. The ovaries are located deep within the body. The testes are highly visible on the exterior of the body within a pouch of skin called the **scrotum**. Before birth, the testes move from the abdominal cavity into the scrotum in most boys. In a few babies, however, this descent does not take place before birth; between 1 and 7 percent of male babies are born with undescended testes, a condition called **cryptorchidism**. In most cases the testes descend by themselves within a few months. No one is sure just what triggers the descent, but it has been suggested that the mother's hormones are involved in the process.

Inside the testes of a young boy, tightly coiled tubes gradually expand into **seminiferous tubules**. It is within these tubes that sperm develop. (See Figure 4.3.)

**scrotum** scrotal sac; pouch of skin that holds the testes

**cryptorchidism** a condition in which the testes do not descend from the abdomen into the scrotum

**seminiferous tubules** the tightly coiled tubes within the testes where sperm develop

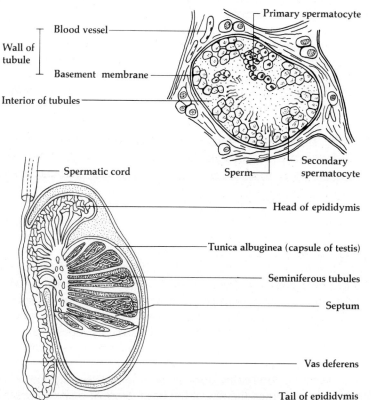

*Figure 4.3*

(left) Cross section of an adult male testis. (right) The inside of a seminiferous tubule, with the sperm cells in various stages of spermatogenesis.

**spermatogene-sis** the process of sperm development

The process, called **spermatogenesis**, begins before puberty and is functioning efficiently by the time a boy is about sixteen years old. Spermatogenesis continues throughout life, although as men become older the process slows markedly. It has been estimated that a healthy man produces several billion sperm each year. Despite this continual production, some men believe the supply is limited:

> Every time I masturbated, I used to feel bad that I was using up all my sperm. Someone once told me that your testicles could dry up if you did it too often. A lot of the men I know have the same idea. (Authors' files)

Hormones are intimately involved in sperm production. The interaction among gonads, the pituitary gland, and the hypothalamus is much like that found in women, although men do not have a well-defined hormonal cycle comparable to the menstrual cycle. The hypothalamus releases the hormones ICSH and FSH from the pituitary. ICSH is chemically identical to the LH released by the female hypothalamus, but gets the name ICSH (interstitial cell-stimulating hormone) because it stimulates the production of **testosterone** (a male hormone also found in women) in the interstitial cells of the testes. FSH, which stimulates ovulation in women, stimulates sperm production in men.

**testosterone** male hormone

Sperm cells take from sixty to seventy days to mature, and in the course of their development they pass through several stages. A mature sperm cell, or spermatozoon, consists of three parts: an oval-shaped head, a neck, and a tail that tapers off at the end. The chromosomes are located in the head and, as noted in Chapter 3, whether one of the chromosomes is an X or a Y determines the sex of the new individual. Under a microscope, X-bearing (female) sperm appear slightly shorter than Y-bearing (male) sperm and have larger, more oval-shaped heads. Sperm cells are much smaller than human eggs; whereas sperm measure only about .005 in. (.06 mm), an ovum can be seen with the naked eye and is about the size of a period on this page.

In the adult male, the testes are oval-shaped organs about 1.5 in. (38 mm) in length. They are suspended in the scrotum by the spermatic cord. The left testis usually hangs a little lower in the scrotum than the right. The skin on the outside of the scrotum is wrinkled, sparsely covered with hair, and contains many sweat glands.

Inside the scrotum, each testis is covered by a thick capsule that protects the seminiferous tubules. These tiny tubes are coiled into about 250 chambers; if uncoiled, they would stretch almost a mile. Between the tubes are a number of large cells that secrete male hormones.

**epididymis** a system of ducts within the testes where sperm mature

**vas deferens** a long duct that transports sperm from the epididymis to the urethra

Sperm move from the seminiferous tubules into another series of ducts, then into a third convoluted duct system called the **epididymis**. Although this system is no longer than 1.5 in. (3.8 cm), if it were unrolled, it would stretch another twenty feet. Sperm remain in the epididymis for about two weeks. Once they are mature, they pass into the **vas deferens**, a long duct that transports them to the urethra. During ejaculation, sperm leave the body through this route.

**Keeping the testes cool**   If sperm are to generate and grow, the testes must be kept cooler than the rest of the body. Normal body temperature is 98.6°F., but sperm production drops, sperm become sluggish, and sperm may even undergo spontaneous mutation if scrotal temperature rises above 93.2°F (34°C.). Sperm are so sensitive to heat that tight underwear or a long, hot bath can temporarily reduce a man's fertility.

Through evolution, several mechanisms have developed to keep the scrotum at an optimum temperature. The sweat glands on the surface of the scrotum help to speed heat loss through evaporation. A network of tiny blood vessels speeds cooling by conduction. Finally, muscular action moves the testes toward or away from the body's heat. When the surrounding temperature rises muscles relax, moving the testes away from the groin so that they may cool. During emotional stress or sexual excitement, these muscles contract, elevating the testes close to the body. It seems possible that, by keeping the testes against the body, chronic emotional stress could reduce fertility by interfering with the processes that regulate the temperature of the testes.

## THE INTERNAL ORGANS

A man's internal organs are set to deliver sperm. As they move from the testes to the urethra, sperm mix with fluids from three glands: the prostate, the seminal vesicles, and Cowper's glands (Figure 4.4). These internal organs play an important role in balancing the chemical composition of the seminal fluid, or **semen**. In fact,

**semen** the fluid produced by the prostate, seminal vesicles, and Cowper's glands in which sperm are carried from the body

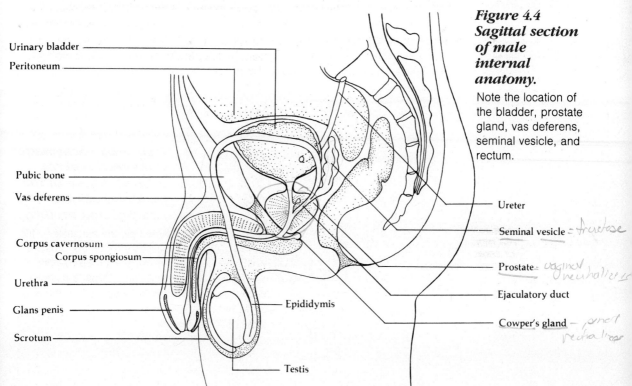

*Figure 4.4 Sagittal section of male internal anatomy.*

Note the location of the bladder, prostate gland, vas deferens, seminal vesicle, and rectum.

Urinary bladder

Peritoneum

Pubic bone

Vas deferens

Corpus cavernosum

Corpus spongiosum

Urethra

Glans penis

Scrotum

Epididymis

Testis

Ureter

Seminal vesicle

Prostate

Ejaculatory duct

Cowper's gland

the teaspoonful of semen ejaculated is mostly fluid from these glands. Little of its bulk consists of sperm. Although impregnation can take place without these fluids, a properly balanced seminal fluid helps sperm to live longer within the acid environment of the uterus. In addition, prostaglandins in the fluid cause the uterus to contract and may aid in fertilization. So the chemicals produced by internal organs enhance male fertility.

## The seminal vesicles

**seminal vesicle** a coiled and bulging tube that secretes part of the seminal fluid

**ejaculatory duct** the continuation of the vas deferens through the prostate to the urethra

Just off each epididymis, in a spot between the bladder and the rectum, is the **seminal vesicle**—a single coiled and bulging tube. These tubes secrete a fluid that is high in fructose, a natural sugar that increases the movement of sperm. As the vas deferens enters the **ejaculatory duct** the seminal vesicle joins it, and it is here that secretions from the seminal vesicle mix with sperm. On its way to the urethra, the ejaculatory duct passes through the prostate.

## The prostate

**prostate** a gland that secretes the portion of the seminal fluid that gives semen its characteristic color and odor

**fibrinogenase** a substance in the prostatic secretion that causes semen to coagulate temporarily when deposited in the vagina

The **prostate**, located below the bladder (Figure 4.5), is usually smaller than a golf ball and weighs about an ounce (28.3 g). Within this gland is an intricate series of ducts that secrete prostatic fluid, which gives semen its milky, white appearance and characteristic odor. Besides prostaglandins, the fluid contains a number of other important biochemical substances. One of them, **fibrinogenase**, causes semen to coagulate temporarily once it is within the vagina. This sudden thickening of the fluid increases the chances of conception by keeping the semen from dripping out of the vagina. Since prostatic fluid is alkaline, it neutralizes the acidity of the vagina, keeping sperm alive.

Before a boy reaches puberty, the prostate is inactive. Then, as hormone levels

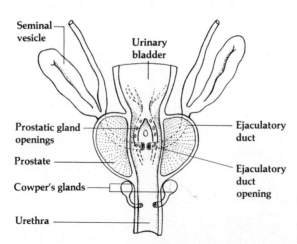

Seminal vesicle

Urinary bladder

Prostatic gland openings

Prostate

Cowper's glands

Urethra

Ejaculatory duct

Ejaculatory duct opening

***Figure 4.5 Schematic cross-sectional representation of the prostate, seminal vesicles, and urethra.***

Note how the ejaculatory duct passes through the prostate and where the ejaculatory duct and Cowper's gland openings join the urethra.

rise, the prostate increases in size and begins to secrete fluid. In the sexually mature male, the gland continually secretes its fluid, which is either discharged during ejaculation or mixed with urine from the bladder.

If the prostate becomes inflamed—a condition called **prostatitis**—it may cause considerable discomfort or pain. Among the symptoms of prostatitis are a swollen sensation in the penis (although the penis looks perfectly normal) and a continual, intense desire to urinate. Although this inflammation is common and not dangerous, it often has an emotional impact far out of proportion to its severity (Silber, 1981). For example after a bout of prostatitis, some men develop erectile difficulties.

The prostate can be felt or stimulated directly through the rectum. This placement may make the prostate quite sensitive to stimulation, especially during anal intercourse. Homosexual men often report such prostatic stimulation triggers ejaculation. During a medical examination, a physican can assess the size of the prostate through the rectum.

> **prostatitis** inflammation of the prostate

## Cowper's glands

Each **Cowper's gland** is about the size of a pea, and one is located on each side of the urethra just below the prostate. These glands also produce an alkaline secretion, but its function is to neutralize the acidity of the urethra, not the vagina. Since the urethra is the outlet for urine and urine is an acid fluid, it is important to neutralize this acidity before the alkaline ejaculatory fluid passes through the tract. Cowper's glands produce only a few drops of fluid, and it is released before ejaculation. The precise amount of fluid released varies from one man to another and from one sexual encounter to the next.

Although sperm is neither produced nor stored in Cowper's glands, sperm can be secreted into the urethra from the ejaculatory duct before ejaculation, only to be carried along with the alkaline fluid produced by Cowper's glands. For this reason, it may be possible for a man to impregnate a woman even if he withdraws before he ejaculates.

> **Cowper's gland** a gland located on either side of the urethra whose alkaline secretion neutralizes the normally acid urethra

## BREASTS

In the 1980s, few people regard male breasts as part of the male sexual anatomy, even though many men find stimulation of the breasts sexually exciting:

> Does a man like to have his nipples touched? I don't know how other men feel about this, but I recently found out that I can get very turned on by having my nipples sucked or lightly pinched by my partner. I always thought that this was something only women enjoyed. (Authors' files)

In the Victorian era, men's breasts carried sexual meaning. A man who exposed his nipples was regarded as indecent, and men's bathing suits always covered the torso. Today, bathing suits cover only the penis and scrotum, and even on the street a "topless" man hardly draws a second glance.

Anatomically, there are some similarities between male and female breasts. The areola and nipples are similar in form, although in the male they are generally smaller. Like their female counterparts, male nipples contain sensitive nerve endings and may become erect in response to tactile stimulation or a drop in temperature. As we've seen, some men enjoy breast stimulation. Men also have rudimentary mammary glands, and at birth baby boys sometimes secrete a small amount of breast milk when these glands are stimulated by hormones from the mother's body. Unlike female breasts, the male breast has little underlying glandular tissue or fatty padding.

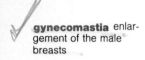

**gynecomastia** enlargement of the male breasts

However, male breasts can become swollen or enlarged, a condition known as **gynecomastia**. Such swelling is especially common during adolescence, and approximately half of all adolescent boys show some degree of gynecomastia. Boys' breasts may swell because some estrogen production accompanies the rising androgen levels of puberty. One boy with this condition reported:

> When I was in the eighth grade my nipples felt so sore that it hurt to wear any shirt at all. (Bell, 1980)

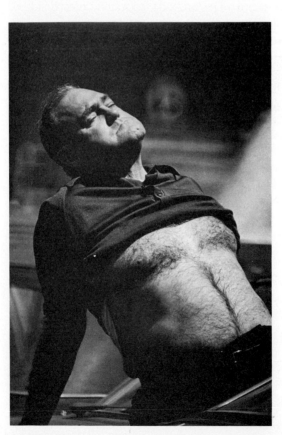

As men age, their breasts sometimes become noticeable—a condition that is not a true gynecomastia. (© Ellis Herwig/Stock, Boston)

Although boys find their enlarged breasts embarrassing, the condition is temporary and usually lasts no more than a year or two.

Gynecomastia sometimes afflicts adult males, with about 7 percent of men showing some degree of breast enlargement (Kolodny, Masters, and Johnson, 1979). The swelling is often a side effect of various prescription drugs, and the enlargement disappears when treatment is stopped. In some cases, however, there may be a hereditary tendency toward gynecomastia. For example, President John F. Kennedy once complained about a photograph that showed him shirtless at the helm of a sailboat, saying that it showed the "Kennedy breasts."

## MALE SEXUAL FUNCTION

When a man is sexually stimulated, his sexual anatomy undergoes predictable changes, some of them resembling the changes in women's sexual organs described in Chapter 3. For example, the scrotum responds to sexual arousal in much the same way as the labia majora, with increased flow of blood accompanied by muscular tension (Masters and Johnson, 1966).

Just before or during ejaculation, this increased muscular tension suddenly pulls the testes close to the groin. After orgasm, the muscle relaxes and the scrotum returns to its normal position. If arousal extends over a lengthy period the muscle goes through cycles of tension and relaxation, producing an up-and-down movement of the testes. Since this is an involuntary movement, most men are unaware of it. The muscular tension may be related to reproductive function, because men whose testes fail to elevate during orgasm ejaculate with diminished force (Masters and Johnson, 1966).

The most obvious and important aspects of male sexual arousal are erection and ejaculation. The influence of male hormones, like that of female hormones, is uncertain.

### *Erection*

The penis becomes *erect* when the flow of blood into the three penile cylinders sharply increases. These cylinders are like a compressed sponge. During sexual arousal, the spaces within the sponge fill with blood, thickening and lengthening the penis. At one time it was believed that erection was caused by the narrowing of veins in the penis, but it now appears that the change is primarily the result of the active opening of arteries and small blood vessels (Masters and Johnson, 1966).

The arteries that supply blood to the penis are controlled by nerves from the bottom part of the spinal cord. When these nerves are stimulated, nerve impulses cause blood vessels in the penis to expand, permitting blood to fill the three cylinders (Figure 4.6). Since the spongy, erectile tissue is enclosed in a tough membrane, increasing pressure causes the erect penis to become firm, making it easy to penetrate the vagina. It is a paradox that the firmness of an erection is related to the

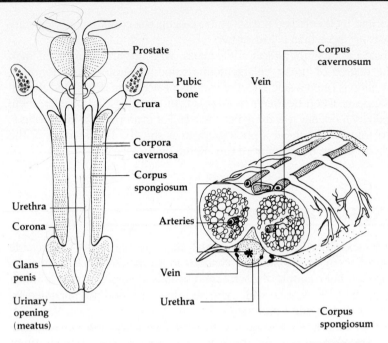

*Figure 4.6*   *Two schematic cross sections of the penis.*

(left) Longitudinal section: Note how the corpora cavernosa (upper bodies) form the crura, which attach to the pubic bone. (right) Cross section through the shaft indicating the major blood vessels of the penis. Erection is caused when the spongy bodies (corpora), which are composed of erectile tissue, fill with blood.

relaxation of blood vessels within the penis (Dickinson, 1933). If emotional or physical stress interferes with this relaxation response, a man may find it difficult to get or keep a full erection.

The mechanims of **detumescence**, or loss of erection, are less well understood. Detumescence seems to take place when small arteries and blood vessels constrict, partially shutting off the flow of blood into the penis. There may also be a slight increase in blood flow through the veins and out of the penis during detumescence, but this has not been clearly demonstrated. When detumescence fails to occur, a condition known as **priapism** develops. In this condition, the erection may persist for lengthy periods even though the man no longer feels sexually aroused.

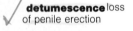

**detumescence** loss of penile erection

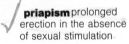

**priapism** prolonged erection in the absence of sexual stimulation

### *Ejaculation*

**ejaculation** expulsion of semen during orgasm

Ejaculation, the expulsion of semen during orgasm, takes place in two stages: emission and expulsion. During the *emission* phase, sperm and seminal fluids move through the ejaculatory duct to the urethra. A sphincter muscle located between the urethra and the urinary bladder contracts to prevent these fluids from traveling into the bladder. During the *expulsion* phase, semen is ejaculated from the urethra. This expulsion is caused by a strong contraction of muscles located at the base of the penis. The force of the expulsion is affected by age, degree of sexual arousal, and time elapsed since the last ejaculation.

Under certain circumstances, instead of coming out through the urethra, the ejaculate may be forced back up into the bladder, a condition known as **retrograde ejaculation.** This "backward ejaculation" usually occurs when the bladder sphincter fails to remain closed during emission. When this happens, the seminal fluid mixes with urine in the bladder and then passes from the body during urination. Retrograde ejaculation can be caused by surgery in the prostate area, by drugs, or by certain conditions present at birth (Avellan, 1980).

**retrograde ejaculation** "backward" ejaculation into the bladder instead of out through the urethra

For most men, orgasm and ejaculation take place at the same time. Under some circumstances, however, a man can ejaculate without having an orgasm, or have an orgasm without ejaculating. For example, men with spinal cord injuries sometimes reach orgasm without ejaculating:

> When I first got out of the hospital after the accident, sex was very frustrating for me because I couldn't ejaculate. Even though I could still get a good hard-on, I was very hung up on not coming. One day I discovered that I could have a certain kind of orgasm, and this was the big breakthrough for me. (Authors' files)

Some men report having several orgasms before a final orgasm accompanied by ejaculation, a process we discuss in Chapter 5.

## Sex and hormones

Although most people believe that the male sexual drive is fueled by hormones, the relationship between sexual interest and hormone levels is extremely complex. Low levels of testosterone do not necessarily indicate low sexual interest, nor do high testosterone levels always ensure high sexual interest. As with women, hormones affect sexuality within a larger context that includes individual differences in experience, expectations, and physiology.

**Patterns of hormone release** Although men have no well-defined hormone cycle, they do show rhythmic as well as sudden patterns of hormone release. Levels of testosterone in the blood are not stable, but show irregular, abrupt increases, suggesting that hormones are released in spurts (Schiavi and White, 1976).

These cycles may be as short as thirty minutes or as long as a year. For example, there is a daily rhythm in blood testosterone levels. Testosterone, ICSH, and FSH levels all fluctuate during sleep, but only testosterone shows a general pattern (Schiavi et al., 1982). As a man sleeps, each fluctuation of testosterone tends to peak at a higher level, reaching its highest peak early in the morning. Levels decrease during the day and reach their lowest point late in the evening. Yet late evening, when the testosterone level is lowest, is when sexual intercourse is most likely to take place.

# Focus

## CASTRATION

**castration** removal or destruction of the testes or their function

Much of what we know about the role of hormones in male development and sexual functioning comes from research on the effects of **castration:** the removal or destruction of the testes or their function. Centuries before any research was done, castration was widely used. Farmers knew it kept livestock docile, and they castrated pigs, bulls, lambs, and colts shortly after birth, a practice that is still routine. Some religious sects, such as the Skoptsky of Russia, demanded castration as a condition of membership. In eighteenth-century Europe, women's roles in opera and soprano parts in church choirs were sung by *castrati,* men who had been castrated as boys to keep their voices from changing. In the Middle East, servants in harems were always **eunuchs,**

**eunuch** a man who was castrated before puberty

men who had been castrated as boys in order to eliminate sexual desire and fertility—although the procedure did not interfere with erection.

Since castrati and eunuchs have their testes removed before puberty, they have no beards, sparse body hair, and thinly muscled, spindly arms and legs. But they never become bald. They do have pubic and axillary (armpit) hair, for these characteristics are under the control of hormones secreted by the adrenal glands. Little information exists about the sex lives of such men. Men who are castrated before puberty will probably be apathetic about sexual activity unless they receive hormone replacements. However, exceptions to this general rule exist. Some prepubertal castrates are capable of erection, although they cannot ejacu-

late (Money and Ehrhardt, 1972). This makes sense, because erection is common in young boys, and some of them are capable of orgasm. It seems possible that little or no male hormones are necessary for orgasm.

Sometimes castration is performed after puberty. It may be used to halt the spread of cancer, and in several European countries castration is used as treatment or punishment for male sex offenders. Obviously, castration of sex offenders is meant to reduce sexual activity. But does it?

A man who is castrated after puberty keeps his beard, his muscle mass, his deep voice, his larger penis. The major effect of castration is a drastic reduction in testosterone levels.

The effects of castration after puberty vary widely. In some men, sexual drive

---

There are, however, large individual variations in these daily patterns. One man's testosterone level may peak at 5 A.M., while another man's may not peak until 8 A.M. Short-term swings in testosterone release may widen these variations. It's been suggested that men also have annual cycles, with peaks in the summer and early autumn, and valleys in the winter and early spring, as well as additional regular cycles ranging from eight days to more than a month.

Testosterone levels may also be influenced by changes in the external environment. Physical or emotional stress can lower testosterone levels in the blood. When a man is under stress, the hypothalamus sends chemical messages to the pituitary, telling it to stop stimulating the testes. This relationship has shown up in several studies. For example, combat troops in Vietnam had lower testosterone lev-

and capacity may diminish and disappear within weeks. In others, sexual interest may persist in spite of lessened ability to have erections and orgasm. Some men maintain both sexual interest and ability for years. In such cases, the amount of ejaculate during orgasm diminishes and finally disappears. Among 157 Norwegian men ranging in age from twenty-five to fifty-four who had been castrated for medical or legal reasons, more than two-thirds ceased sexual activity and lost all interest in sex within a year of the operation. In the remaining third, interest and activity persisted, sometimes for as long as ten years (Bremer, 1959). Among thirty-nine German sex offenders who had been castrated, most reported a diminished interest in sexual thoughts and a decrease in intercourse and masturbation. Yet nearly a third of this group were still able to engage in intercourse, with convicted rapists being the most sexually active. The effects of castration were connected with age: virtually all the men who were more than forty-five years old when castrated gave up sexual activity, but nearly three-fifths of the younger castrates were still sexually active (Heim, 1981).

Testosterone appears to be only one factor in sexual activity. Psychological factors play a major role in sexual arousal, and they also appear to be deeply involved in the aftereffects of castration. The adult male castrate may have had considerable sexual experience before the operation, and the memory of past sexual contact may prolong sexual capacity. The availability of a supportive sexual partner is also likely to be important. In addition, psychological and physical health are probably related to the outcome. A man who is castrated to curtail criminal sexual behavior may react differently from a man castrated to halt the spread of cancer. Finally, a man's attitude is likely to have a great effect on his reaction. If he is convinced that the procedure will leave him unable to engage in sexual activity, his conviction may prove to be a self-fulfilling prophecy. But if he expects to function normally afterward, he may well be able to do so.

Such complex interactions make it plain that the male sexual system is every bit as complicated as that of the female. In Chapter 6, we'll see how body awareness and sexual feelings are intertwined.

---

els than soldiers in basic training or on noncombat duty. And men in officer candidate school had low testosterone levels at the beginning of the course, when pressure was greatest. As pressure decreased, testosterone levels went up.

There seems to be a strong relationship between testosterone secretion and psychological state. Increased testosterone levels are generally associated with the presence of a sexually attractive and possibly available partner, sexual stimulation, and sexual activity. Decreases are associated with depression, defeat and humiliation, and chronic stress (Kaplan, 1974). In Chapter 1 we noted the effects of exposure to male hormones before birth on the development of aggression in children. Evidence of the effects of testosterone levels after birth on male aggression is inconclusive, although some researchers have found an association under certain conditions. For example, prisoners with long histories of violent and aggressive crimes have been found to have much higher testosterone levels than other prisoners (Rubin, Reinisch, and Haskett, 1981).

Female hormone levels have been suspected of affecting a woman's mood, as we saw in Chapter 3. The same sort of connection has been found among men. When male hormone levels and mood were compared over a ten-week period, the higher the men's testosterone level, the more hostile and anxious they felt. However, the closeness of the relationship varied considerably from one man to the next. There is no way to predict how hormones will influence the mood of any one individual (Houser, 1979).

**The effect of hormone levels** A certain amount of male hormones is necessary for normal sexual function, but most men seem to have far more than they need. Exactly how much testosterone is required is unknown, and the minimum amount may vary from one man to another (Bancroft, 1981). When testosterone drops below a certain level, sexual desire may disappear. For example, men who are born with an abnormal chromosome condition that results in extremely low testosterone production are sterile and lack any interest in sex. When they are given testosterone they often begin to have sexual fantasies, to show sexual interest, and to become sexually active (Rubin, Reinisch, and Haskett, 1981).

It would seem only reasonable, then, that hormone levels determine sexual desire. But some evidence indicates that it works in the opposite direction: sexual desire and activity increase hormone levels. In several species of animals, including monkeys, bulls, rabbits, and rats, levels of testosterone increase after mating. When male rhesus monkeys were put with receptive females, their testosterone levels increased following mating and fell to former levels within a week after they were separated from the females (Rose, 1972).

Sexual activity also appears to alter hormone levels in men. Over a two-month period, testosterone levels among a group of young men in their twenties showed wide differences from one man to another and in the same man on different occasions. These men also kept diaries of their sexual activity, but there was no relationship between a man's average testosterone level over the two months and frequency of intercourse. However, there was a striking relationship between each incident of sexual activity and temporary hormone levels. A majority of the men had significant rises in testosterone level on the morning *after* intercourse. In other words, increases in testosterone were not the cause but the result of sexual activity. It may be that when testosterone falls below a critical level, a man's body attempts to raise it by increasing the probability of sexual activity (Kraemer et al., 1976). Similar effects have been found in connection with masturbation. Levels of several androgens, including testosterone, climbed among one group of men after masturbation (Purvis et al., 1976).

The relationship between sexual activity and hormone levels is not clearly understood (Schiavi and White, 1976). Not all researchers have found elevated hormone levels after sexual activity. It may be that sexual arousal, rather than sexual activity, elevates hormone levels. Among men who were shown a sexually arousing film but had no opportunity for sexual activity, testosterone levels increased, peaking after sixty to ninety minutes (Pirke et al., 1974).

Sometimes the effect of testosterone can be dramatic. In the case of a man who had been born without testes, sexual interest and activity were totally dependent on injections of testosterone. At eighteen, this man had gone through an artificial puberty with the aid of hormone injections. After each injection he had an intense desire for sex, but by the time ten days had passed and his hormone levels had dropped, his sexual desire vanished, only to be reinstated by the next injection. His sexual interest and activity became steady only after he received the transplant of a testis from his twin brother and his testosterone level ceased its wild fluctuations (Silber, 1981). In Chapter 14, we'll look at possible connections between hormones and some sexual problems.

# Summary

**1** The external organs of the male sexual system include the penis, **scrotum,** and testes. The profound symbolic significance attached to the penis by most cultures influences most men's view of their sexuality. The functions of the penis are to convey sperm into the vagina, to provide sensory pleasure, and to pass urine out of the body. Three hollow cylinders run the length of the penis: the two corpora cavernosa and the **corpus spongiosum,** which carries the urethra. Although many men are concerned that their penis is too small, most of the penile size differences seen in the flaccid state disappear when the penis is erect. There is no relationship between skeletal size and penis length, and the connection between penile size and sexual satisfaction is highly exaggerated.

**2** **Circumcision,** or the cutting away of the **foreskin** that covers the **glans,** is practiced in many cultures. In the United States circumcision has been practiced for hygienic reasons, although research has found little support for the practice. Circumcision has been reputed to increase or reduce sexual stimulation, but there appears to be little difference in sexual response between circumcised and uncircumcised men.

**3** When the testes do not descend from the abdominal cavity into the scrotum before birth, a boy is born with **cryptorchidism,** a condition that usually corrects itself. Within the testes are the **seminiferous tubules,** where sperm develop in a lifelong process known as **spermatogenesis.** The hormone ICSH stimulates the production of the hormone **testosterone** in the testes, and the hormone FSH stimulates sperm production. Sperm mature in about sixty days, and each sperm has an oval-shaped head, a neck, and a tapering tail. Sperm move from the seminiferous tubules through a series of ducts into the **epididymus,** where they mature before passing into the **vas deferens.**

**4** The internal sexual organs of the male include the seminal vesicle, the **prostate,** and **Cowper's glands.** The secretions of these three glands combine to form the seminal fluid that transports sperm from the body. Secretions of the seminal vesicle increase the movement of sperm; secretions of the prostate neutralize the acidity of the vagina, coagulate semen within the vagina, and cause the uterus to contract; secretions of Cowper's glands neutralize the acidity of the urethra. The prostate may become inflamed, a common, uncomfortable, but not serious condition known as **prostatitis**.

**5** There are some similarities between male and female breasts, and some men find breast stimulation sexually exciting. **Gynecomastia**, or enlarged breasts, is common in adolescent boys and appears in about 7 percent of all men.

**6** In response to sexual stimulation, a man's sexual anatomy undergoes predictable changes. When blood flows into the penile cylinders, the penis becomes erect—a change that appears to be the result of the active opening of arteries and small blood vessels. Since relaxation of the blood vessels is required for erection, emotional or physical stress may interfere with the response. **Detumescence** may be the result of a constriction of small arteries and blood vessels. When the penis remains erect despite the lack of sexual stimulation, the condition is known as **priapism**. **Ejaculation** is the expulsion of **semen** during orgasm. In **retrograde ejaculation**, the semen is forced back into the bladder instead of out through the urethra. Although orgasm and ejaculation usually take place at the same time, either can occur without the other.

**7** Men have rhythmic as well as stable patterns of hormone release. There is a daily rhythm to blood testosterone levels, with the peak coming very early in the morning and the lowest level late in the evening. However, there are large individual variations. Either physical or emotional stress can lower testosterone levels, while the presence of a sexually attractive partner, and sexual stimulation and activity can raise the levels. Although there is no way to predict the way testosterone will affect an individual's mood, high levels may be linked to hostility, anxiety, and, in some cases, aggression. A minimum amount of testosterone is required for sexual function, and most men have far more than they need. There appears to be some relationship between testosterone levels and sexual activity, but most studies have found that the hormone rises *after* activity.

**8** **Castration**, or the removal or destruction of the testes, has provided information on the role of hormones, since the major effect of castration is a drastic reduction in testosterone levels. **Eunuchs**, who are castrated before puberty, do not ejaculate and may be apathetic about sexual activity. However, some are capable of erection and perhaps orgasm. Castration after puberty sometimes leads to a lessening or disappearance of sexual interest and activity, although some castrated younger men remain sexually active. Attitudes toward castration, sexual experience, availability of a partner, and physical health can affect the response to castration.

# 5 Sexual Response in Men and Women

# Chapter 5

A certain look, caress, or physical setting may be immensely stimulating to you but completely unarousing to someone else. Some people must have direct physical stimulation to become aroused; others are quickly aroused by mental imagery and fantasy. Such enormous differences in individual response to sexual stimuli develop because the human brain is intimately involved with the sex organs. For most people, sex is primarily psychological (Beach, 1969).

Because sexual response involves learning, memory, emotion, and imagination, your past experiences play an important role in determining which sights, sounds, tastes, smells, and touches arouse you and which have little erotic value or destroy any chance of arousal. These learned sexual stimuli are called **psychogenic** because they are processed by higher brain centers. When a sexual stimulus consists only of touching or caressing the sex organs, it is called **reflexogenic** because the sensation is processed in the spinal cord and arousal is reflexive, in the same way as your knee automatically jerks if someone hits you just below the kneecap (Weiss, 1972).

In this chapter, we'll begin by considering how psychogenic stimuli develop and how they combine with reflexogenic stimuli. Then we'll discover just what happens in a typical experiment on human sexuality. This information will give us some background for an exploration of the role of the nervous system in sexuality and the sexual response cycle. We'll look at the controversy over female ejaculation. Next, we'll investigate orgasm in women and men as well as the debate over multiple orgasms. We conclude with a brief look at what happens after orgasm.

**psychogenic** arising from the mind; processed by higher brain centers

**reflexogenic** involuntary physiological response; processed in the spinal cord

# Sexual Response in Men and Women

## INDIVIDUAL DIFFERENCES IN SEXUAL RESPONSE

Sexual arousal and orgasm are profound emotional responses, and human emotions have both a psychological and a physiological dimension. A person who is afraid, for example, experiences a feeling of fear and also shows measurable physiological change (the heart pounds, sweat breaks out). The same is true of sexual arousal and orgasm. They involve changes in bodily function and in emotion.

The interaction between higher mental processes and the responses of muscles and body organs is known as **psychophysiology**. One of the fundamental principles of psychophysiology is that our past experiences influence our physiological response to any stimulus.

**psycho-physiology**
study of the connection between mental processes and bodily responses

### How individual differences develop

The process of learning about sexual stimulation often begins in childhood, when a young girl or boy feels pleasure when touching the genitals. These pleasurable sensations lead to more touching. Any particular sights, smells, or sounds in the environment while this fondling is going on may become associated with erotic pleasure and later serve as psychogenic stimuli. For instance, while taking a bath a girl may discover that as she cleans her genitals, she feels pleasure. During subsequent baths she repeats this action, and before long the sound of water or the smell of soap may become associated with pleasure, until simply running the bath water may evoke feelings of sexual pleasure.

This process continues during adulthood, as an individual's sexual experience widens and as he or she enters successive phases of the life cycle. The association isn't always with stimuli that evoke pleasure, however; sometimes the learning process involves associating stimuli with unpleasant sexual consequences. Suppose a man has trouble attaining an erection while with a woman who wears a certain brand of perfume. After several such experiences with this woman, he may be unable to respond to any woman who wears the same perfume. Or suppose a woman and her partner are interrupted by her parents; the anxiety or guilt generated by this episode may become associated for that woman with future sexual interactions.

Most psychologists believe that psychogenic stimuli are created by a process known as *conditioning,* in which the repeated association of two events eventually makes one event call forth any response that was originally connected with the other event. Many sex researchers believe that conditioning is more powerful than anatomy or physiology in creating variations in adult sexual behavior (Kinsey et al., 1953). For this reason, it may be necessary to look into that person's past experience to understand why a person finds a certain stimulus sexually arousing.

One way experience affects learning is through cultural standards. Stimuli considered highly arousing by the culture generally become arousing to its members, so that some psychogenic stimuli will be exciting to most people. But people have unique histories, and the repeated pairing of certain sounds, sights, or other sensations with particular sexual consequences often condition a man or woman to a special set of stimuli. Often we don't know why a particular stimulus has become arousing. For example, one woman discovered that she responded to an odd sound:

> Once I worked in a fast-food place, and every time the refrigerator turned on,
> I'd get a sexual rush. It was the sound that did it. (Wolfe, 1981, p. 76)

Information and imagination also affect sexual response. Thoughts, images, fantasies, and memories can create sexual arousal with no direct, physical stimulation of the genitals. One adolescent boy found this out:

> I was in class the other day thinking about feeling and screwing the girl across
> from me. Then the bell rang. Here I am sitting, afraid to get up 'cause I've got
> this gigantic hard-on and it wouldn't go away. (Shanor, 1978, pp. 151–152)

In the case of reflexogenic stimuli, direct stimulation causes automatic sexual arousal. Stroking the penis or the clitoris sends a signal to the spinal cord, which relays the signal back to the sexual organ. That the higher brain centers have no part in this reflexive arousal is shown by the fact that some men with spinal cord injuries can have reflexive erections although they have no sensation in the pelvic area.

In many instances, reflexogenic and psychogenic stimulation combine to cause sexual arousal. During masturbation, people commonly use direct tactile stimulation accompanied by psychogenic stimulation in the form of fantasy or erotic literature. During sexual intercourse, most couples are aroused by a combination of body contact (reflexogenic) and the sight and sound of the partner (psychogenic). This sort of interaction between the physical and the psychological is called **synergism**. For example, a man who sees an erotic photograph will probably need less physical stimulation to produce an erection than a man who lacks such psychic stimulation. In the same way, anxiety or guilt may inhibit the response to physical stimulation (Weiss, 1972).

**synergism** interaction of psychogenic and re-flexogenic stimuli to achieve a single goal or response

## *Mood and sexual response*

If you're "in the mood" for sex, you're likely to initiate sexual advances or to respond quickly to a partner's signals. This mental state is affected by thoughts, feelings, beliefs, attitudes, and fantasies. At times you may know perfectly well why you are in the mood; at other times you may not. Feelings are sometimes spontaneous and uncomplicated, but they can also be hindered by conflicts and hesitation. Because human emotions and thoughts are so complex, the sexual experience can vary greatly from one occasion to another.

When placed in a potentially arousing situation, an individual's response is affected by information, emotion, and imagination. The information includes beliefs, labels, and expectations concerning sexuality. For example, a person who believes that fellatio (oral stimulation of the penis) is a perversion or a sign of mental disorder is likely to be turned off by the idea of performing fellatio. But a person who thinks fellatio is a healthy and desirable activity would be turned on by the prospect.

Any emotion that can accompany a sexual experience, such as joy, guilt, or anxiety, can either heighten or diminish a person's sexual reaction. For example, a loved partner is probably a more arousing sexual stimulus than a disliked person.

Imagination, in the form of mental images and fantasies evoked by a stimulus, also affects sexual response. Memories of past sexual experiences, for example, may heighten a person's response to an immediate stimulus. Indeed, most people can quickly learn to turn themselves on and off by using arousing fantasies and images (Rosen, 1973; Rosen et al., 1975).

These three mental components—information, emotion, and imagination—interact, as shown in Figure 5.1. For instance, the belief that fellatio is unhealthy influences feelings about the act and imagery concerning it. Or a disagreement between fantasies about fellatio and beliefs about it, as when a person fantasizes about it but believes it is an unhealthy practice, can lead to conflicting emotions. This type of conflict is common when people contemplate extramarital sexual activity. A man or woman may fantasize that an affair would be pleasurable, but at the same time be put off by the belief that such behavior is wrong or destructive. Finally, there is an interaction between physiological response and the erotic stimulus—as indicated by the arrows on the outside of the diagram. As an awareness of physical arousal to a particular stimulus increases, the stimulus is perceived as increasingly arousing.

A final factor that plays a crucial part in determining sexual response is wheth-

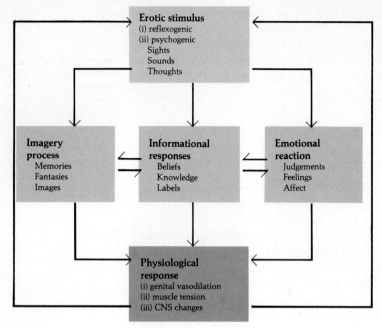

**Figure 5.1   How erotic stimuli are processed: This diagram shows the major psychological components that mediate a sexual response.**

Psychological factors affect physiological responses and vice versa. This model of sexual arousal shows the way in which sexual responses are mediated by cognitive and affective processes. (Adapted from Byrne and Byrne, 1977, p. 502)

er the individual is paying attention to the stimulus. If a potentially arousing stimulus escapes notice, or if some distraction is present, there may be no response at all. For example, men who listened to erotic tape recordings through one side of a set of earphones while arithmetic problems were played through the other side had smaller erections than men who listened only to the erotic tape (Geer and Fuhr, 1976). In daily life, a person may be distracted from a sexual stimulus by the sound of a television in the next room, by the aroma of freshly cooked food, or by thoughts of tomorrow's exam.

As the complexity and variety of psychogenic stimuli indicate, a delicate interaction between physiology and psychology appears to determine when and where sexual responses will occur. Researchers have explored this interaction in laboratory studies.

## MAPPING THE EROGENOUS ZONES

When sexual arousal is reflexogenic, stimulation usually takes the form of touch: caresses, strokes, pats, rubs, tickles, licks, sucks, nibbles, or light scratches. Nerve endings pick up this stimulation and transmit it to the spinal cord. Since these nerve endings are concentrated in some areas and sparse in others, the body responds unevenly to tactile stimulation.

Those areas that are especially responsive to touch and are heavily involved in sexual arousal are known as **erogenous zones.** In addition to the sex organs themselves—the clitoris, labia minora, vestibule, and vaginal canal in women and the penis (especially the corona and underside of the glans and shaft) in men—the breasts (especially the nipples), the mouth, the anus, and the skin between genitals and anus are all extremely sensitive. Stimulating other areas can also produce or heighten sexual arousal. Stimulation of the buttocks, thighs, neck, abdomen, earlobes, small of the back, palms of the hands, and soles of the feet is highly arousing to many people.

**erogenous zone** a body area that is especially responsive to touch and involved in sexual arousal

This variation in sensitivity to physical stimulation is nearly as great as the variation in psychogenic stimuli. Some people find having their earlobe sucked or nibbled highly arousing; others respond not at all. Women have even reported orgasm from caresses applied to the eyebrow or the crook of the arm (Kinsey et al., 1953). The required intensity of touch also varies. Some people respond to a featherlight caress and find a heavy touch unpleasant; others must have vigorous stimulation to respond at all. Since each person's response is so different, it takes some experimentation to map a sex partner's erogenous zones.

Apparently we are not born with these extended erogenous zones. Instead, experience and expectations can create them nearly anywhere on the skin. We even learn to endow certain touches with a sexual meaning, so that a touch occurring in a sexual context is arousing, but the same touch in a situation we interpret as nonsexual is not. For example, most women feel no arousal at all during a gynecological examination. It would seem that despite the reflexogenic nature of most physical stimulation, learning plays an enormous part in extending responsiveness from primarily sexual areas to other parts of the body. We should not expect a new partner to enjoy the same sort of caress in the same places that the last partner found so exciting.

## SEXUAL RESPONSE AND THE NERVOUS SYSTEM

All sexual stimuli, whether psychogenic or reflexogenic, are processed by the nervous system, which is the communications network of the body and can be compared with the telephone system of a modern city. The nerve fibers function like telephone cables, transmitting electrical signals to all parts of the body. The brain and spinal cord contain the relays and switchboard. The messages received and transmitted through the nervous system determine thoughts, feelings, and behavior. For example, if a man sees a nude woman, the nerve cells of his eyes code the stimulus, which is transmitted as a message to the brain. If the brain processes the message as "sexy," the nervous system sends out the word, triggering responses of glands, muscles, and sexual organs.

Anatomically, the nervous system is divided into the **central nervous system**

**central nervous system (CNS)** the brain and spinal cord

# *Focus*

## EXPERIMENT IN HUMAN SEXUALITY

**penile plethysmograph** a device that measures penile arousal through changes in the flow of electrical current

The penile plethysmograph is used to study male erection in the laboratory. The thin rubber ring slips over the penis; as the penis expands, even tiny changes in size are recorded on the connected polygraph.

Although much of what we know about the effects of various stimuli on sexual response has come from laboratory experiments, few people know what it means to participate in this work. Many of these research projects take place on college campuses. By following Ken, an undergraduate who has volunteered to act as a subject, through one of these investigations, we can discover just how these experiments are done.

At the scheduled hour, Ken is met at the lab by a male graduate student wearing a white lab coat. On the far side of the room stands a polygraph—a device that will transform the electrical signals produced by Ken's body into a pen-and-ink record. The polygraph has several dials for adjusting the signals, and a set of pens that record the signals on a moving sheet of paper.

The researcher explains to Ken that the purpose of the experiment is to find out how much voluntary control a person can exert over sexual response. Ken will be asked to increase and decrease his sexual arousal using only mental imagery. In the course of the experiment, he will also watch an erotic movie.

Before the experiment begins, Ken fills out a short questionnaire in which he describes the state of his physical health, whether he uses any legal or illegal drugs, and the extent of his sexual experience. He also signs a notice of "informed consent," in which he states that he understands the purpose of the experiment and agrees to participate.

After completing the paperwork, Ken and the researcher walk to an adjoining soundproof room containing a projector and screen. In the center of the room is a comfortable reclining chair. Next to the chair is a table covered with bottles, cotton swabs, and various types of equipment. Wires from the equipment pass through a small hole in the wall to the polygraph in the next room.

Ken sits in the chair while the researcher hooks him up to the devices. A belt is strapped around his chest to measure his breathing. Several small flat metal disks, called electrodes, are taped to his chest to measure his heart rate. A second set of electrodes is taped to his arm to measure muscle tension.

Finally, Ken is asked to unzip his pants and place the **penile plethysmograph** around his penis. The plethysmograph looks something like a thin rubber band with an attached wire (see photo), and it measures sexual arousal. It is actually a thin rubber tube that is filled with a strand of mercury. A very weak electrical current comes through the attached wire and flows through the mercury. As Ken's penis becomes erect the tube will stretch, making the strand of mercury thinner and changing the flow of electrical current. These changes in

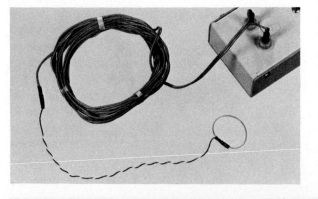

electrical flow will be recorded by the polygraph. With this technique, even tiny changes in the diameter of the penis can be measured. The device is so sensitive that every pulse of blood into the penis can be measured.

If Ken had been Karen, her arousal would have been measured by a **vaginal photocell plethysmograph** (see photo). This instrument, shaped rather like a tampon, measures the amount of light reflected from the walls of the vagina. When a woman is sexually aroused, the vaginal walls fill with blood. The resulting lubrication reduces the light that is reflected to the photocell, so the polygraph records increases in blood flow (Sintchak and Geer, 1975). Because both penile erection and vaginal lubrication are caused by the same basic physiological process—the pooling of blood in the pelvic area—the results of research with the vaginal plethysmograph are basically comparable to results obtained with the penile plethysmograph.

After all the measuring devices are in place, the researcher turns down the lights and leaves the room. Over the intercom, a voice tells Ken to relax for the next few minutes.

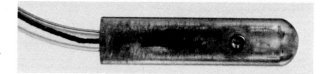

The vaginal plethysmograph is used to study female sexual arousal in the laboratory. The device is inserted into the vagina, where it uses changes in reflected light to measure increases in vaginal blood flow that accompany arousal.

Then, after what seems like a long time, the voice tells Ken to try, using only mental imagery, to produce an erection. Ken concentrates on his last sexual experience with his girlfriend. Just as he is beginning to enjoy himself, the voice instructs him to try to return to the unaroused state. This time, Ken concentrates on unpleasant imagery—he imagines his last exam, and when that does not work, he recalls a film he has seen about sexually transmitted disease.

Now Ken hears the sound of a projector, and the movie screen in front of him lights up. As he watches the erotic film, he knows he is again becoming aroused. But just as his sexual response becomes intense, the voice instructs him to remain unaroused while he watches the film. This time the task is even more difficult, and Ken finds that he is tensing his body as he tries to think

about unpleasant things. Finally, the screen goes dark and the researcher returns to remove the recording equipment.

The researcher shows Ken his polygraph record. As the researcher explains what each of the lines means, Ken can see that the line recording his sexual arousal shows a clear rise and fall as he produced and then lost his erection. He also notices that both his breathing and his heart rate increased when he became excited.

From experiments like this one, scientists have explored the role of sexual fantasy in arousing men and women, the effects of drugs on sexual arousal, and the mental processes that control sexual response (Rosen, 1981). In the course of the proceedings they have learned a great deal about the ways in which the nervous system processes sexual signals.

**vaginal photocell plethysmograph** a device that measures vaginal arousal through changes in the reflection of light

**peripheral nervous system (PNS)** nerve fibers that link muscles, glands, and sense organs with the central nervous system

**somatic nervous system** that part of the PNS connecting the CNS with muscles used in motor activity

**autonomic nervous system** that part of the PNS connecting the CNS with organs involved in functions that operate without conscious control

**sympathetic system** the division of the autonomic nervous system that dominates during periods of stress

**parasympathetic system** the division of the autonomic nervous system that dominates during periods of relaxation

(CNS), which consists of the brain and spinal cord, and the **peripheral nervous system (PNS)**, which consists of nerve fibers that link the muscles, glands, and sense organs with the CNS. Input for the system consists of messages from the sense organs and other parts of the body. Output consists of messages that travel from the brain or spinal cord through the peripheral nervous system to various muscles and glands.

These outgoing messages use either the **somatic** or the **autonomic** branch of the peripheral nervous system. In broad terms, the somatic nerve fibers connect the CNS with muscles that are necessary for motor activity, such as walking or talking. Muscle tension during sexual arousal is caused by stimulation of the somatic nervous system. But other signs of sexual arousal, such as vaginal lubrication or penile erection, are stimulated by the autonomic nervous system. In general the autonomic nervous system is in charge of functions that are mostly outside conscious control. It is much harder deliberately to change the rate of the heartbeat, for example, than it is to raise an arm or a leg.

The autonomic nervous system is further divided into the sympathetic and parasympathetic branches. The **sympathetic system** generally responds during periods of stress, when there is a need for vigorous activity. The **parasympathetic system** is dominant during periods of relaxation. Their functions are sometimes described as antagonistic, since more of one tends to mean less of the other. The two systems have different pathways within the body and use different chemical substances to activate the muscles and glands that are their targets. For example, the parasympathetic system uses acetylcholine to transmit its messages; the sympathetic system uses adrenalin and noradrenalin.

The sexual organs receive messages from both autonomic systems. An erect penis or a lubricated vagina results from the action of the parasympathetic system, which has expanded arterial blood vessels. As arousal becomes intense, the sympathetic nervous system increases its activity, raising blood pressure and speeding up the heart. At orgasm, the sympathetic nervous system takes over. Ejaculation is set off by a sudden discharge in the sympathetic system. This sudden release of adrenalin creates a temporary imbalance, which is quickly compensated for by a release of acetylcholine from the parasympathetic nervous system. It is this release of acetylcholine that helps to create the feeling of warmth and relaxation that often follows orgasm.

## THE SEXUAL RESPONSE CYCLE

**sexual response cycle** the orderly sequence of physiological responses identified with sexual arousal

The physiological responses identified with sexual arousal can be organized into a **sexual response cycle**. Although researchers agree that the cycle has an orderly sequence of stages, they do not agree on how many stages it contains or just where one stage ends and the next begins. As we'll see, there are two-, three-, and four-stage models, and each takes a somewhat different view of sexual response.

## Two-stage model

Before Masters and Johnson changed the way most people viewed the sexual response cycle, writers generally described it as having two important stages: **tumescence**, which corresponds to the flow of blood into the pelvic area; and detumescence, which corresponds to the flow of blood out of the area. The stages were given these names by sexologist Havelock Ellis (1906), who saw the terms as signifying the process of building up and discharging sexual energy. He referred to tumescence as the "piling on of fuel" and to detumescence as "the leaping out of the devouring flame" (p. 142). Energy accumulated during tumescence, only to be freed during detumescence, which began with orgasm.

This sexual energy was a fundamental part of human life for Ellis, but the process was not totally automatic. He believed that sexual arousal (tumescence) included a conscious and voluntary "courtship," in which a sexual partner was approached and sexual energy accumulated. Even among couples who had been sexual partners for years, Ellis believed, an abbreviated courtship period that consisted primarily of physical stimulation was included in every sexual act.

**tumescence** the condition arising when blood flows into the pelvic area during sexual arousal

## Three-stage model

The model of the sexual response cycle developed by sex therapist Helen Kaplan (1979) contains three stages: desire, excitement, and orgasm (Figure 5.2). Kaplan based this model on her work as a therapist, for she found that sexual problems tend to fall into one of these categories and that a person can function normally in any two of the categories while being inhibited in the third.

Desire, Kaplan's first stage, is unique to her model of the sexual response cycle. Desire does not involve the genitals, but consists of sensations that motivate a person to seek out sexual experience or to become responsive to it. Excitement consists of sexual arousal and lasts until orgasm begins. Kaplan believes that the three stages are physiologically related, but that each is governed by a separate neurophysiological system. A person who lacks desire, if pressured to participate in a

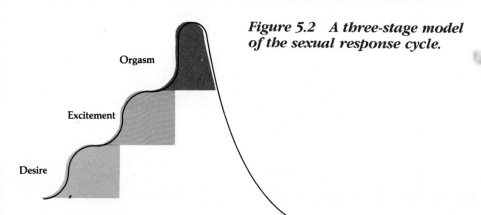

**Figure 5.2  A three-stage model of the sexual response cycle.**

Orgasm

Excitement

Desire

sexual encounter, might become as aroused and orgasmic as a person who is highly motivated to seek out sex.

## Four-stage model

Many members of the scientific community as well as the general public have accepted Masters and Johnson's (1966) four-stage model of the sexual response cycle. The model has had a profound effect on the way people think about human sexual response. It was born in the physiological laboratory, where it was derived from experiments much like the one described earlier. The data upon which the model was built came from hundreds of men and women who volunteered to have their responses recorded during masturbation or intercourse. Since desire is basically a subjective experience that cannot be measured in a laboratory, it is not part of Masters and Johnson's objective, physiological model.

The four stages of their model are excitement, plateau, orgasm, and resolution (Figure 5.3). **Excitement** involves gradually increasing levels of sexual arousal. In males, the most common sign of excitement is erection; in females, it is vaginal lubrication. During the **plateau stage**, the maximum level of arousal is reached. The term "plateau" may be misleading, since it implies that the level of arousal is continuously high. In fact, most people's arousal increases and decreases before they reach orgasm. During **orgasm**, muscle tension and blood flow into the genitals are at a maximum. Muscles contract rhythmically. In men, these contractions are usually accompanied by ejaculation. After a man ejaculates, he experiences a **refractory**

**excitement stage**
first stage of the Masters and Johnson model of the sexual response cycle

**plateau stage** second stage of the Masters and Johnson model of the sexual response cycle

**orgasm stage** third stage of the Masters and Johnson model of the sexual response cycle

### Figure 5.3    *A four-stage model of the sexual response cycle.*

(left) The typical male pattern, with the refractory period immediately after orgasm. The dotted line suggests that after the refractory period, additional arousal and orgasm may be possible. (right) Three variations of the typical female pattern. In (A) the pattern most closely resembling the male cycle, the woman is shown as able to have additional orgasms; there is no refractory period. In (B) the pattern shows a woman who reaches plateau but not orgasm. In (C) the response shown is that of a woman who rises rapidly to orgasm, without a plateau phase, and then returns quickly to the unaroused state. According to Masters and Johnson, there is more variability in the female response cycle than in that of the male. (Masters and Johnson)

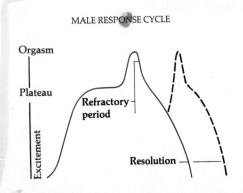

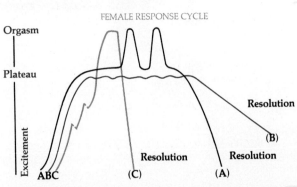

period, when the penis will not respond to further stimulation. There is no necessary female refractory period, however, and some women are capable of having several orgasms during the same period of stimulation. In the final stage, **resolution,** the body returns to its unstimulated state.

Despite the general acceptance of this model, neither a subjective nor a physiological justification for distinguishing between the stages of excitement and plateau has ever been established. Subjectively, a sexually aroused person does not seem to be able to distinguish between the two stages. Physiologically, the changes that begin during excitement generally continue into the plateau stage. In fact, one critic (Robinson, 1976) has argued that the four-stage model is entirely irrelevant to the male sexual experience and creates the impression of scientific precision where none exists.

Like all models, the Masters and Johnson four-stage model is an abstraction of human sexual response. Such models are helpful in organizing the response cycle into an orderly sequence of stages, but are not absolute standards. Further, since they are derived from studies of large groups of people, the models do not necessarily show how any one individual will behave during a sexual experience.

Yet all the models described can be helpful, for each draws our attention to a different aspect of sexual response (Table 5.1). Scientists need to develop models of behavior in order to direct their research, and different models are developed for different purposes. As our understanding of human sexuality continues to grow, new models of sexual response will undoubtedly be developed.

**refractory period** a period after ejaculation when a man's penis will not respond to stimulation

**resolution stage** fourth stage of the Masters and Johnson model of the sexual response cycle

## HOW THE BODY RESPONDS IN SEXUAL AROUSAL

Although learning, memory, and imagination are often responsible for sexual excitement, it is the body that responds in ways that can be observed and measured. Some of the physical changes that accompany arousal and orgasm take place in

### Table 5.1   The sexual response cycle

| TWO-STAGE MODEL | THREE-STAGE MODEL | FOUR-STAGE MODEL |
|---|---|---|
|  | Desire |  |
| Tumescence | Excitement | Excitement |
|  |  | Plateau |
|  | Orgasm | Orgasm |
| Detumescence |  | Resolution |

Each model of the sexual response cycle divides the cycle in different ways, calling attention to different aspects of sexual response.

**sex flush** a measlelike rash that spreads over the skin of some people as orgasm approaches

**vasocongestion** increased blood flow due to the dilation of small blood vessels

**myotonia** increase in muscle tension

almost everyone. For example, virtually all men and women have muscular contractions during orgasm. Individual differences are also the rule. Some changes, such as the **sex flush,** a measlelike rash that spreads over the skin as orgasm approaches, appear in some people, but not in others. And even when two people show the same physiological changes, their own perceptions of these changes probably differ.

During arousal and orgasm, the body responds with two basic physiological processes: vasocongestion and myotonia. **Vasocongestion** refers to the widening, or dilation, of the small blood vessels in the pelvic area. When the flow of blood into the area exceeds the amount of blood being drained out, the tissues become engorged, or congested with blood.

This pooling of blood leads to some of the sensations commonly associated with sexual arousal. Some people experience this engorgement as a feeling of warmth or heaviness. Others have a tingling or itching sensation in the genitals. In fact, the word "prurient," which means obsessively interested in sexual matters, comes from the Latin word *prurire,* meaning, to itch. With full engorgement of the blood vessels, a woman or man may also experience a pulsing or throbbing sensation.

**Myotonia** refers to increases in muscle tension. During sexual arousal, tension increases in both involuntary and voluntary muscles. Some people deliberately increase muscle tension by contracting the muscles of their thighs, abdomens, or buttocks. This increase in the level of muscle tension can produce a more powerful orgasm. Although patterns of myotonia differ greatly among individuals, some degree of muscle tension is a reliable part of the sexual response cycle. Perhaps the easiest way to understand these body responses is to look at women and men separately.

## The sexually stimulated woman

The first and most obvious physiological sign of sexual arousal in women is vaginal lubrication. The lubricant is secreted by the vaginal walls as blood fills the small vessels and the resulting pressure causes small drops of liquid to form.

Although the amount of lubricant varies greatly from one woman to another, vaginal lubrication appears to be a universal sign of sexual arousal. Some women are aware of a moist, sometimes sticky, feeling in the vagina soon after sexual stimulation begins. The quantity of liquid produced may be so great as to be mistaken for a female ejaculation or so scanty as to produce only a thin film over the tissues.

Vasocongestion changes the color and shape of the vagina and surrounding tissue. Increased blood flow turns the vaginal walls a deep red or purple. As excitement builds, myotonia raises the uterus and causes the inner two-thirds of the vagina to lengthen and expand. During what is referred to as the plateau stage in the four-stage model, marked vasocongestion spreads to the outer third of the vagina, sharply narrowing the diameter of the canal and creating what Masters and Johnson (1966) called the **orgasmic platform.**

**orgasmic platform** narrowing of the vagina during the plateau stage of the sexual response cycle

With vasocongestion, the labia minora enlarge and thicken. They may show

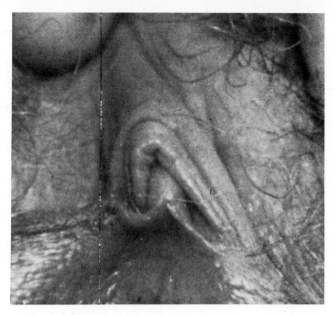

As blood flows into the pelvic area during sexual arousal, the clitoral glans becomes engorged, increasing in length and width. The process is similar to penile erection in men and is caused by the same process. (Courtesy, Gorm Wagner, M.D., and Focus International, Inc.)

striking color changes, deepening to dark shades of red or purple. In women who have given birth, the labia majora also fill with blood, changing in size and color. Before a woman has given birth, the outer lips tend to separate and are somewhat flattened during sexual arousal.

The most sexually sensitive female organ, the clitoris, also changes during excitement. Both length and width increase, although these changes may not be noticed by the woman or her partner. The clitoral hood thickens and expands as its tissues fill with blood.

Other parts of the body also change in response to vasocongestion. For example, when blood fills the small vessels close to the skin surface, a skin flush is produced that resembles a rash. Most women show some degree of this sex flush, although there are wide individual differences in the extent to which it spreads over the chest, throat, neck, and stomach (Masters and Johnson, 1966).

The breasts also enlarge from vasocongestion. Although the actual increase varies among women, a woman's breasts may expand as much as one quarter in size. In addition, the size and color of the areolae often change.

As sexual excitement builds, tension increases in all muscles. For example, one of the earliest signs of a woman's arousal is nipple erection, a response caused by the contraction of involuntary muscles. With the approach of orgasm, some women also have voluntary, spasmodic contractions of muscles in the buttocks, thighs, and abdomen. Facial tension is also common, and a woman may scowl, grimace, or frown as the muscles contract.

As excitement builds, additional changes occur in the cardiovascular and respiratory systems. Blood pressure rises, and the heart beats rapidly. As orgasm approaches, breathing may become faster and deeper. Whether ejaculation sometimes accompanies orgasm in women has recently become a topic of controversy.

*Focus*

DO WOMEN
EJACULATE?

"Then Alice spent frantically, plentifully bedewing my finger with her virginal distillation!" (Anon., 1968). This line from Victorian pornography illustrates the centuries-old belief that women as well as men ejaculate at sexual orgasm, emitting some kind of reproductive fluid. Modern sex researchers, including Kinsey and Masters and Johnson, rejected the notion and assumed that female ejaculation was simply a male fantasy, based on the assumption that since men ejaculate during orgasm, women react in the same way.

If ejaculation is limited to the emission of a fluid that contains sperm, clearly women cannot ejaculate. But if the term is defined as emitting a fluid during orgasm, the possibility of female ejaculation exists.

Some women say they emit a jet of fluid at orgasm, but sex researchers

have denied that it is ejaculation. Some explained that what seemed like an ejaculation was simply the expulsion of vaginal lubricant by powerful muscular contractions during orgasm. Since the fluid was secreted earlier in response to sexual stimulation, it could not be considered an ejaculate. Other researchers said that women who believed they were ejaculating were simply confusing ejaculation with the escape of urine at orgasm.

These explanations have been challenged by researchers who have observed orgasm in women who claim to ejaculate. In one case (Addiego et al., 1981), a woman said she ejaculated in reponse to vaginal stimulation but not when her orgasm was the result of clitoral stimulation. It appeared that the source of the stimulation was the Grafenberg spot. When she experienced or-

gasm in response to stimulation of the Grafenberg spot, a translucent, whitish liquid was expelled from the urethra. Laboratory analysis of the liquid showed that its chemical content was similar to fluid from the male prostate gland, which is emitted during ejaculation by men and which transports the sperm.

Other studies have failed to confirm this similarity. For example, some analyses have found no chemical difference between female "ejaculate" and urine (Zilbergeld, 1982). Further, direct stimulation of the G spot doesn't seem to be required for ejaculation. Some women say they ejaculate in response to clitoral stimulation:

I use a vibrator regularly. During a clitoral orgasm, I noticed a sudden discharge of fluid. I thought it to be urine, but on closer examination, I found this

## *The sexually stimulated man*

Sexual arousal in the male is usually identified with penile erection, which was described in Chapter 4. Vasocongestion causes the cylinders to fill with blood and become firm. At the same time, the escape of blood through the veins is decreased by the closing of tiny valves. If the process continues, pressure builds until the penile sheath reaches the limits of its expansion. At this point, the penis is firm and fully erect.

Erection, like vaginal lubrication, is controlled by the autonomic nervous system. It is this control that explains why men are unable to "will" an erection in the

fluid to be similar to, if not the same as, the fluid ejaculated during a vaginal orgasm.
(Ladas, Whipple, and Perry, 1982, p. 68)

Yet the comparison of female ejaculate to prostatic fluid makes biological sense, for women do have a homologous structure to the male prostate. The primitive tissue that in men develops into the prostate in women becomes a system of very small glands located around the urethra. Both the source and the chemical content of the female fluid suggest that if women do ejaculate, the process has a similar origin in both sexes.

Anatomists have found a wide variability in the amount and location of prostatic tissue in women. Perhaps women with large amounts of prostatic tissue or women whose prostatic ducts are anatomically exposed are more likely to ejaculate than other women. Or perhaps muscle tone has something to do with it.

In an attempt to explain why the expulsion of fluid is limited to only a few women, John Perry and Beverly Whipple (1981) studied forty-seven women. About half of them said they sometimes exuded a large amount of fluid at orgasm, the other half said they did not. Suspecting that muscle tone might be involved in female ejaculation, the researchers placed over each woman's cervix a small plastic device that measures muscle contractions. Then they asked the women to contract their internal pelvic muscles. Sure enough, the women who said they ejaculated produced much stronger contractions than women who did not ejaculate.

Perry and Whipple speculate that learning may also be responsible for the lack of female ejaculation. Men are expected to ejaculate and are rewarded for it, both by impregnating women and by social prestige. But since female ejaculation does not make conception more likely and since women often are told that such escaping fluid is urine (a social disaster) or perhaps some "pathological" condition, they are punished for ejaculating. As a result, they learn to restrain the response.

Meanwhile, the debate continues. Some women do seem to expel liquid during orgasm, but its source and chemical content, as well as whether the tendency is confined to a small group of women or is a reponse that can be learned, are unlikely to be determined without careful laboratory research.

same way that they can move a finger. Further, since the parasympathetic branch has the major role in causing an erection, a man who enters a sexual experience with a high degree of anxiety or fear—which would call the antagonistic sympathetic branch into action—might find himself unable to have an erection.

Once erection is present, it is usually maintained until the man ejaculates or the stimulation is lost. A man who is temporarily distracted during intercourse may lose some of his erection. But if stimulation is resumed, in most cases he will quickly recover the erection.

Men show many of the same signs of arousal as women. About 30 percent of men show the sex flush on some part of their body. Most men also show some

## Table 5.2  Four-stage sexual response cycle

| STAGE | WOMEN | MEN | BOTH SEXES |
|---|---|---|---|
| Excitement | Vagina becomes lubricated<br>Inner two-thirds of vagina lengthens and expands<br>Clitoris increases slightly in length and width<br>Uterus elevates<br>Labia majora separate and flatten<br>Labia minora enlarge<br>Sex flush often spreads over torso<br>Nipples erect; breasts enlarge | Penis erects<br>Scrotal sac elevates<br>Testes enlarge and begin to elevate<br>Nipples may erect | Myotonia increases<br>Vasocongestion occurs<br>Blood pressure and heart rate increase |
| Plateau | Orgasmic platform develops<br>Clitoris retracts<br>Uterine contractions may begin<br>Labia minora change color<br>Areolae may swell and change color<br>Bartholin's glands secrete fluid | Penile corona increases in size<br>Testes press against groin<br>Nipples may erect<br>Cowper's glands secrete fluid | Myotonia increases<br>Sex flush may appear<br>Heart rate and blood pressure increase further<br>Respiration increases |
| Orgasm | Orgasmic platform contracts rhythmically<br>Uterus contracts | Seminal fluid forced into urethral bulb<br>Semen ejaculated | Muscles spasms occur<br>Anus contracts<br>Brain waves change<br>Blood pressure, heart rate, respiration peak |
| Resolution | Film of sweat may cover body | Palms and soles may sweat<br>Refractory period occurs | Muscle tension disappears<br>Sex flush fades<br>Organs return to normal size and color<br>Blood pressure, heart rate, respiration become normal |

nipple erection. As sexual excitement builds, the pulse rate generally quickens, and breathing becomes faster and deeper. At this point, blood pressure may rise sharply, and signs of muscle tension similar to those seen in women become noticeable.

During the early stages of sexual arousal, the scrotal sac thickens and elevates, as noted in Chapter 4. Muscles shorten, pulling the testes upward toward the body. With further sexual arousal, the testes may increase as much as 50 percent in size. Just before ejaculation, the testes are drawn up close to the groin. This testicular elevation is generally a reliable sign that a man is on the verge of ejaculation (Masters and Johnson, 1966).

In both sexes, the tension that builds during arousal is discharged through orgasm. Table 5.2 compares the responses of men and women during the four stages of sexual response.

## THE SEXUAL ORGASM

What is orgasm? To say, as the *Random House Dictionary* does, that an orgasm is "the physical and emotional sensation experienced at the culmination of a sexual act," has meaning only for someone who is already familiar with the sensation. The essence of orgasm is a feeling, and it cannot be described without taking into account what goes on in the head as well as the physiological reactions of the body. A polygraph record of two orgasms may be identical, yet they may be experienced in vastly different ways.

Scientists have investigated orgasms in the laboratory, recording the body's reactions on a polygraph, and have found little physiological difference among orgasms, regardless of the type and source of stimulation or whether it is experienced by a man or a woman. Yet some women insist that they experience two distinct kinds of orgasm, one from clitoral stimulation during masturbation and an entirely different sort from vaginal stimulation during intercourse. Long ago, Freud claimed that the clitoral orgasm was "immature" and that what he called the "vaginal orgasm" was a sign of emotional maturity. Women were urged to strive for vaginal orgasms, and for decades many women who enjoyed clitoral orgasms believed that they were somehow sexually maladjusted.

Now that research has demonstrated that the orgasms are physiologically equivalent, however, there is no reason to believe that one kind is "better" than another (Masters and Johnson, 1966). Indeed, if we are to classify orgasms by source of stimulation, there would be "eyebrow orgasms," "breast orgasms," "anal orgasms," and "crook of the arm orgasms," since some people have had orgasms from such stimulation. Because each orgasm combines responses of mind and body, the subjective experience may differ from person to person and from one occasion to another in the same person. As one man put it:

> An orgasm can range from BLAH to a bang-bang, shoot-'em-up delirious
> almost high feeling. Depends on who you're with. (Shanor, 1978, p. 19)

Whatever its source, orgasm is experienced as an intense, immensely satisfying sensation that lasts only a few seconds by the clock but often seems to go on and on. Orgasm is difficult to describe. It eluded even so fine a writer as D. H. Lawrence (1928), who depicted Lady Chatterley's orgasm as "pure deepening whirlpools of sensation swirling deeper and deeper through her tissue and consciousness, till she was one perfect concentric fluid of feeling" (p. 158). Perhaps portraying the feelings that course through the body at orgasm is beyond the power of language. Our vocabulary for orgasm is limited, and most descriptions focus on such words as "tension," "buildup," and "release."

The similarities between male and female orgasm seem to outweigh any differences. The buildup and discharge of sexual tension are physiologically the same in both sexes. There are also clear similarities in the subjective experience. Consider the following descriptions:

> A sudden feeling of lightheadedness followed by an intense feeling of relief and elation. A rush. Intense muscular spasms of the whole body. Sense of euphoria followed by deep peace and relaxation.

> Basically, it's an enormous buildup of tension, anxiety, strain followed by a period of total oblivion to sensation, then a tremendous explosion of the buildup with a feeling of wonderfulness and relief.

> Intense excitement of entire body. Vibrations in stomach—mind can consider only your own desires at the moment of climax. After, you feel like you're floating—a sense of joyful tiredness.

> I really think it defies description by words. Combination of waves of very pleasurable sensations and mountings of tension culminating in a fantastic sensation and release of tension.
> (Vance and Wagner, 1976, pp. 93–94)

Given these, along with forty-four other descriptions—some written by men, others by women—neither gynecologists nor psychologists could detect the sex of the writer (Vance and Wagner, 1976).

## Physiological responses in orgasm

**orgasm** an intense physiological reflex that releases sexual tension

In both sexes, sexual **orgasm** is a physiological reflex that is brought about by a specific stimulus. Because of its sudden, explosive discharge of tension, orgasm has been likened to a sneeze that involves the entire body (Kinsey et al., 1953).

The typical stimulus for orgasm is stimulation of the nerve endings in the genitals, but this is not always true. Some people—more women than men—claim to be able to reach orgasm purely through fantasy (Kinsey et al., 1953). Some women report reaching orgasm through breast or anal stimulation, and male homosexuals sometimes reach orgasm through stimulation of the prostate gland during anal intercourse. Despite these exceptions, genital stimulation is the commonest trigger of the orgasm reflex.

As noted earlier, vasocongestion and myotonia build markedly just prior to orgasm. There may be involuntary spasms and jerkings of muscle groups. Although the pattern of myotonia varies from one individual to another, muscle tension is a critical component of the orgasmic experience. In fact, the buildup of muscle tension during arousal is a major factor in stimulating the orgasmic response.

Cardiovascular changes become most pronounced during orgasm. Heart rate, which climbs from its normal resting rate of about seventy beats per minute, may jump to more than 150 beats per minute during orgasm. Blood pressure also peaks during orgasm. Respiratory changes are common. The average resting respiration rate is about twelve breaths per minute, but rates as high as forty-one breaths per minute have been recorded during orgasm (Fox and Fox, 1969). Rapid breathing is not always the case; some men and women stop breathing just before orgasm. The physiological effects of these different breathing patterns are not yet understood.

During orgasm itself, there may be muscle spasms throughout the body. The toes may curl or spread. At the same time, there are regular, rhythmic contractions of the muscles surrounding the genital organs at intervals of about .6 to .8 second. In women, these contractions involve the vagina, uterus, and anal sphincter, the circular muscle that controls the anal opening.

In men, similar contractions occur in the muscles located at the base of the penis, the seminal vesicles, the prostate, and the anal sphincter. When men's orgasms were monitored by inserting an anal probe, wide individual differences appeared in the duration, intensity, and number of anal contractions. The average orgasm lasted almost twenty-six seconds and consisted of seventeen contractions, but orgasmic length varied from six to fifty-six seconds and the number of contractions from eight to thirty-three. However, each man's pattern of contractions remained stable from one orgasm to the next (Bohlen, Held, and Sanderson, 1980).

## Brain changes in orgasm

Since orgasm is both a mental and physical experience, it is to be expected that changes throughout the body will be paralled by striking changes in brain function. Orgasm is accompanied by a unique pattern of brain waves, and this pattern is found in both men and women (Cohen et al., 1976).

Early studies (Muscovich, quoted in Kinsey et al., 1953) showed that during orgasm the brain produced extremely large, slow waves that were compared with the activity during mild epileptic seizures. Since that time, researchers (Galin and Ornstein, 1972) have tried to connect brain activity with different states of consciousness. Such studies have found what appears to be a division of labor in the brain. Among most right-handed people, the left hemisphere seems to be connected with verbal or logical thought processes and the right hemisphere with spatial or intuitive thought.

Brain waves recorded during masturbation show similar differences in the ac-

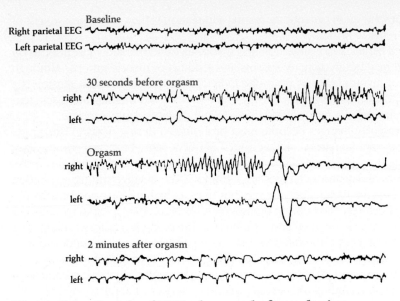

Baseline
Right parietal EEG
Left parietal EEG

30 seconds before orgasm
right
left

Orgasm
right
left

2 minutes after orgasm
right
left

### *Figure 5.4   Graph of EEG changes before, during, and after orgasm.*

EEG recordings from the right and left sides of the brain during sexual response. During orgasm the brain waves are much larger on the right (non-dominant) side.

tivity of the right and left hemispheres just before and at the moment of orgasm (Cohen et al., 1976). With right-handed men and women, brain waves in the right hemisphere became larger and slower, while brain waves in the left hemisphere showed much less change (Figure 5.4). It made no difference which hand a person used to masturbate; the pattern of brain activity was the same.

These brain wave patterns are quite unlike those observed under any other laboratory circumstances. Perhaps this unique brain activity explains why people find it so difficult to describe orgasm in words: the experience simply cannot be compared with any other state of consciousness.

### *Multiple orgasm*

**multiple orgasm** a succession of orgasms in which the person drops back to the plateau phase, then—with further stimulation—has a second, third, or more orgasms; also called sequential orgasms

In 1953, Kinsey reported that about 15 percent of the women interviewed in his study sometimes had several orgasms during the same sexual encounter. This finding was greeted with some skepticism. After all, it was only fifty years since Havelock Ellis had struggled to convince his contemporaries that women do experience sexual arousal and orgasm—and in much the same ways as men.

The skepticism faded when Masters and Johnson (1966) presented evidence of **multiple orgasm** from their laboratory studies of sexual response. They showed that after she has an orgasm, a woman can drop back to the plateau phase and after further stimulation may experience orgasm a second, third, or even more times. In none of these women does muscle tension drop below the plateau phase after orgasm. The orgasms are sometimes so close together that they appear to merge into one long, continuous orgasm.

After surveying many women, journalist Shere Hite (1976) argued that only the continuous orgasm should be called a multiple orgasm and that orgasms separated by several minutes and resulting from restimulation should be called *sequential orgasms*. Many women, she claimed, were capable of sequential orgasms, but multiple orgasms were much rarer. Some women in her survey wanted no more than one orgasm because the clitoris had become too sensitive for further stimulation. Other women said that multiple orgasms were more intense and more satisfying.

The number of orgasms women prefer is largely determined by individual history, learning, and the partner's cooperativeness. A woman may be satisfied with one orgasm during intercourse but prefer to have more than one when masturbating. Another woman may be emotionally satisfied by intercourse without orgasm. A third may find she has multiple orgasms with one partner and cannot reach orgasm with another.

Kinsey (1948) had also attributed multiple orgasms to men. He reported that some men had several orgasms, each with ejaculation, during a single sexual encounter. The capacity declined with age, from a peak of 15 to 20 percent of men in their teens and twenties to about 3 percent of men past the age of 60.

Research from Masters and Johnson's laboratory indicated that these multiorgasmic men apparently were men with very short refractory periods—the time after ejaculation when further sexual stimulation is ineffective and sometimes even unpleasant. In young men the refractory period often lasts only a few minutes; in older men it could last for hours.

Yet some men continued to report multiple orgasms. Further laboratory studies (Robbins and Jensen, 1978) suggest that these men have a series of "preejaculatory" orgasms culminating in a final orgasm with ejaculation. Physiological measures of heart rate, respiration, and muscle tension indicate that preejaculatory orgasms are real orgasms. Perhaps men who learn to reach orgasm without ejaculating may experience multiple orgasm in much the same way as women do. Apparently, the orgasm and ejaculation responses can be separated—at least for some men. This finding coincides with a report that a woman who said she sometimes ejaculated seemed to go through a refractory period after ejaculation. Although at times she had two or three orgasms during a sexual encounter, after ejaculation she found further sexual stimulation unrewarding (Belzer, 1981).

It seems that multiple and sequential orgasms are a physiological reality. Most men in our culture have learned to expect only a single orgasm, but this pattern does not necessarily reflect any limit on male capacity. Similarly, some women are content with one orgasm, although they may be able to have several. The limits on orgasm may be more a reflection of cultural conditioning than of physiological potential. The wide individual differences in orgasm preference once more indicate that there is no "ideal" pattern of sexual orgasm.

## AFTER ORGASM

During the resolution phase, the physiological processes involved in sexual arousal are reversed. Blood begins to flow out of the tissues and muscles in the pelvic area. Detumescence takes place and genital swelling decreases. A thin film of sweat sometimes covers much of the body. As muscle tension relaxes, a person often feels calm and relaxed. Laughter or tears are also common. Because of the warmth that sometimes suffuses the body following a sudden release of acetylcholine, this period after orgasm has also been called "afterglow" (Van de Velde, 1926).

As with arousal and orgasm, there are wide individual differences in subjective experience after orgasm. Some people feel a sense of blissful peace. Some are filled with a sense of exhaustion and often sleep. Others feel refreshed and invigorated. Reactions vary from letdown or even mild depression to elation or euphoria. Gender seems to have no effect on such responses; men and women show similar wide variation in their feelings.

After orgasm, both women and men often feel particularly close to their partners. When this feeling is present, the period is generally characterized by touching, caressing, or intimate conversation. One woman described the importance of such closeness to her:

> My orgasm subsides into a warm glow of well-being. This afterglow is short if
> I am not emotionally close to my partner, otherwise, it is long and rich and
> almost the best part. (Hite, 1976, p. 166)

What happens after orgasm can make a considerable difference in the way the whole sexual experience is perceived.

# *Summary*

**1** Sexual response involves learning, memory, emotion, and imagination as well as direct physical stimulation. Learned sexual stimuli, which are processed by higher brain centers, are called **psychogenic**; direct physical stimuli, which are processed by the spinal cord, are called **reflexogenic**.

**2** Individual differences in sexual response to various stimuli appear to develop through conditioning, in which the repeated association of a stimulus in a sexual context gives that stimulus sexual meaning. Psychogenic and reflexogenic stimuli often interact to create sexual arousal in a process called **synergism**. Mental states can increase or decrease sexual responsiveness because a person's response is affected by information, emotion, and imagination. Finally, sexual response also depends on whether a person is paying attention to a stimulus.

**3** Much of what we know about the effects of stimuli on sexual response has come from laboratory experiments, in which individual sexual response is monitored and measured. Breathing and heart rate are measured for both men and women. Men's sexual arousal is measured by the **penile plethysmograph**, a device that records blood flow into the penis by measuring changes in electric current. Women's sexual arousal is measured by the **vaginal photocell plethysmograph,** a device that monitors blood flow into the vaginal area by measuring changes in light reflection.

**4** Areas that are especially responsive to touch and heavily involved in sexual arousal are known as **erogenous zones.** Genital and breast areas are primary erogenous zones, but any part of the body can become an erogenous zone through learning. In addition, some touches are arousing in a sexual context but not in a nonsexual context.

**5** All sexual stimuli are processed by the nervous system. The **peripheral nervous system** (**PNS**) consists of nerve fibers that link muscles, glands, and sense organs with the **central nervous system** (**CNS**)—the brain and spinal cord. The **autonomic nervous system** (the division of the PNS that governs functions outside conscious control) is divided into branches that are intimately involved in sexual response. The **sympathetic** branch releases adrenalin and nonadrenalin; this system increases blood pressure and heart rate in response to sexual stimulation and controls orgasm. The **parasympathetic** branch responds to orgasm by releasing acetylcholine, which creates a feeling of warmth and relaxation.

**6** The **sexual response cycle,** an orderly sequence of physiological response, has been viewed in several ways. In the two-stage model proposed by Havelock Ellis, there are **tumescence** (corresponding with the flow of blood into the pelvic area) and detumescence (corresponding to the flow of blood away from the pelvic area). In the three-stage model proposed by Helen Kaplan, there are desire (the sensations that make people responsive to sexual experience), excitement (sexual arousal), and orgasm. In the four-stage model proposed by Masters and Johnson, there are **excitement** (gradual increase in sexual arousal), **plateau** (the maximum level of arousal), **orgasm,** and **resolution** (a return to the unstimulated state). Each model draws attention to different aspects of sexual response.

**7** The basic physiological processes involved in arousal and orgasm are **vasocongestion,** or congestion of blood in the pelvic area, and **myotonia,** or increased muscle tension. In women, sexual response is characterized by vaginal lubrication, changes in the color and shape of the vagina and surrounding tissue, a sharp narrowing of the vagina that creates the **orgasmic platform,** a lengthening and thickening of the clitoris, nipple erection, increased blood pressure and heart rate, and often a **sex flush** and rapid breathing. It has been proposed that some women ejaculate at orgasm, especially in response to stimulation of the Grafenberg spot, but the proposal is controversial. In men, vasocongestion makes the penis erect; increases blood pressure, heart rate, rate of breathing, and muscle tension; and draws the testes up toward the body. In addition, some men show nipple erection and a sex flush.

**8** Orgasm is an intensely satisfying physiological reflex that discharges sexual tension. No matter what part of the body is the focus of stimulation, the physiological responses are the same in both women and men. Genital stimulation is the commonest trigger of orgasm. During orgasm there are regular, rhythmic contractions of muscles surrounding the genital organs and the anal opening; there may also be muscle spasms throughout the body. Orgasm is accompanied by a unique pattern of brain waves. Some women have **multiple orgasms**, dropping back to the plateau stage before each new orgasm. Some men may have a series of orgasms without ejaculation, then enter a refractory period after ejaculation.

**9** The resolution phase of the sexual cycle is also known as "afterglow" and is accompanied by wide individual differences in subjective experience. The character of interaction between sexual partners during this period can have a strong effect on the way the entire sexual experience is perceived.

# 6 Sexual Feelings and Body Awareness

# Chapter 6

How many words does the English language have for penis? For vagina? For intercourse? You could probably rattle off at least a dozen in each category without pausing for breath. In addition to all the common terms, there is a scientific vocabulary as well as a private vocabulary we invent to express personal feelings. D. H. Lawrence (1928) called Lady Chatterley's vagina "Lady Jane" and her lover's penis "John Thomas."

Writers sometimes become lyrical about sexuality, as when Eric Berne (1970) described the journey of the ovum to the uterus as ovaries dropping "their ripened eggs like apples near the openings of the Fallopian tubes, whose gentle petals waft them down the tunnel toward the womb" (p. 41). But most of the words we use for anything to do with sexuality betray a profound uneasiness, as do our reactions to nudity. Working on the assumption that this uneasiness may come in part from an unfamiliarity and discomfort with the body, we'll begin with the language of sexuality and cultural attitudes toward nudity. We'll then consider male and female differences in awareness of the sexual response. Following a brief examination of the role of physical attractiveness, we'll explore various ways of developing body awareness.

## THE LANGUAGE OF SEXUALITY

It's generally agreed that when a society regards something as extremely important, it develops many verbal expressions for it. So one way to look at the abundance of sexual terms in our culture is to see it as an indication of the importance of sex.

# Sexual Feelings and Body Awareness

Yet that explanation does not fully account for the many expressions available. Few in this wealth of words are considered appropriate in "polite" conversation. Most are considered slang at best, and often regarded as "dirty." To call a penis a "weenie" sounds juvenile; to call it a "cock" sounds harsh. Many of us feel uncomfortable using these expressions, but feel prudish or pretentious using scientific terms. Speaking of a sexual act as "coitus" seems as pompous as referring to a kiss as an "osculation." To avoid sounding like a snob, some of us choose to use the sexual slang.

Until quite recently, sexual slang appeared to be used primarily by men. Perhaps because the stereotypical little girl was seen as "nice" and not interested in sex, women grew up without using much sexual slang. Since the stereotypical little boy was seen as "naughty" and curious about sex, men grew up hearing a lot of sexual talk and most learned to use earthy terms with ease. Outside the home, men and women tended to live separate lives, with most working women concentrated in only a few occupations. As society and sex roles have become less rigid, and as men and women interact in the same work force, the language of the sexes has come to sound more alike.

One problem with most of the common words for body parts and intercourse is their bluntness—they strip sex of any connection with either liking or loving and make it sound cynical and mechanical (Table 6.1). The forceful, vivid vocabulary of sexual slang is often biased, narrow, and simple-minded, and using these sometimes funny words may hinder our attempts to understand sexuality.

There's another problem with using sexual slang. Our underlying discomfort with sex is reflected in the way we apply sexual terms in other areas of life, almost always with a

## Table 6.1 Genital slang

| STANDARD TERM | SLANG TERM |
|---|---|
| anus | asshole, bung hole, butt hole |
| breasts | boobs, headlights, jugs, knockers, tits |
| buttocks | ass, behind, buns, butt, fanny, rear |
| clitoris | button, clit, joy button |
| gonorrhea | the clap, a dose, the drip, gleet, morning drop, a strain, the whites |
| hymen | cherry, maidenhead |
| menstruation | the curse, wearing the rag |
| penis | cock, dick, dong, joy stick, meat, organ, pecker, peter, poker, prick, rod, tool, wang, weenie |
| rectum | ass, cornhole |
| scrotum | bag, sack |
| semen | come, cream, cum, jism, load, love juice |
| sexually transmitted disease | social disease, VD |
| syphilis | bad blood, haircut, Old Joe, pox, siff, syph |
| testicles | balls, family jewels, gonads, gones, nuts, rocks |
| vagina (or vulva) | bearded clam, bearded lady, beaver, box, cunt, honey pot, manhole, muff, poontang, pussy, quim, snatch, toolbox, twat |

Adapted from E. J. Haeberle, *The Sex Atlas.* Seabury Press, 1978, p. 491.

negative connotation. To call a man a "prick" says that he's foolish, smug, or contemptible. To call a woman a "cunt" says that she's contemptible. And to say that someone has been "screwed" or "fucked over" means they have been cheated or deceived. Our standard curses are "fuck you" or "screw you" (Wentworth and Flexner, 1975).

Words that are regarded as offensive in one culture may be considered quite proper in another. In the United States, words like "fuck," "cock," and "cunt" are considered vulgar. In Nigeria, these same words, brought into the language by sailors and traders, are considered appropriate for conversation and used freely on television (Money, 1980).

When we use sexual slang, then, the negative overtones that accompany our words may impart an unwarranted tone to discussions of sexual activity. To avoid these connotations, we'll use standard scientific terms throughout the book. As we'll see, however, words are not the only way a culture passes along its sexual attitudes.

## ATTITUDES TOWARD NUDITY

People also convey the way they feel toward sex and the body through laws and customs surrounding the exposure of the body. Just how much nudity the public will accept varies from one culture to another and from time to time in the same culture. It also depends on gender.

### *Nudity isn't always shameful*

Some cultures thrive on partial or total nudity; in such societies, a bare body is not considered a sexual display. People in other cultures cover most of the body, and the parts that must be kept covered are the ones considered sexually arousing. In Samoa, it is the navel; in the Celebes, the knee; in some Muslim societies, it is the lower half of a woman's face (Gebhard, 1982). Occasionally, a society finds the display of almost any body part offensive. In the Irish island community of Innis Beag, a man may not allow another man's wife to see his bare feet (Messenger, 1971).

Among the ancient Greeks, nudity was common. All sporting events took place in the nude. A well-proportioned body was admired. Body hair was thought to detract from this beauty, so both men and woman plucked or singed body hair,

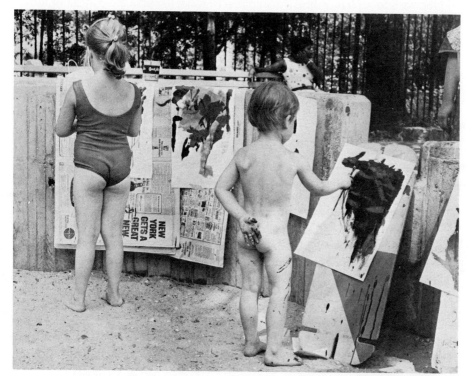

Young children are not self-conscious about their bodies and feel no instinctive shame in public nudity. A concern over genital display is taught by the culture.
(© Bettye Lane)

and hairy masculine legs were considered especially offensive. In one ancient Greek town, every bit of body hair was removed, and people went about in sheer robes (Sussman, 1976). In Sparta, young women were expected to dance naked in public ceremonies. This nudity was encouraged because it was thought the display of their bodies would encourage women to care properly for them.

Unlike the Greeks, who separated sex and esthetics, the Romans invariably connected nudity with sexuality. They stressed the well-proportioned, well-groomed body, but regarded public nudity as indecent. Not until public baths became common was any nudity tolerated.

In later centuries, Western ideas about nudity varied. The medieval Church regarded the body as shameful. Public nudity must have been uncommon; if it had been generally accepted, there would be no meaning to the exploits of the legendary Lady Godiva, who rode naked through the town of Coventry, England, in order to persuade her husband to lower local taxes (Bullough, 1976). Despite the Church's attitude, men, women, boys, girls, monks, and nuns shared the public baths in many cities. Nightgowns were unknown and beds were few, so several nude people commonly slept in one bed. Since a clothed sleeper was suspected of being diseased or disfigured, naked strangers of both sexes customarily shared beds in inns (Sussman, 1976).

This situation lasted until the sixteenth and seventeenth centuries, when syphilis spread through Europe, and an urban middle class developed. Fear of contagion and the wish to appear "refined" combined to make the intimate contact of former centuries seem unhealthy or disgusting. As a concern with privacy grew, the wealthy began to wear nightgowns (Haeberle, 1978).

The most prudish period was during the nineteenth century, when sexual temptation was taboo and almost everything seemed to be sexually stimulating. Breasts were tightly bound to the chest and referred to as "bosoms." The legs were so sexually charged that they could only be called "limbs," and piano legs were draped to keep the thoughts of Victorian males from straying to sex. This prudery was not confined to women; male nipples were always kept covered as well.

## Body attitudes and the double standard

Victorian attitudes may seem odd, but a double standard still exists in our supposedly "modern" society. We have different customs and assumptions regarding male and female nudity, and our prohibitions generally seem aimed at protecting men from being aroused by women's bodies.

These ideas are not peculiar to the United States. In cultures where nudity is customary, women are taught to keep their legs closed to avoid exposing the genitals. But in some of these same cultures, the penis is not covered (Gebhard, 1982). Scientists have supposed that this double standard may be based on differences in male and female arousal—that men need no more than the sight of a bare woman to be aroused, but that women do not respond unless the man's personality is also involved (Symons, 1979).

Whether women are indeed less responsive to nudity than men, most erotic

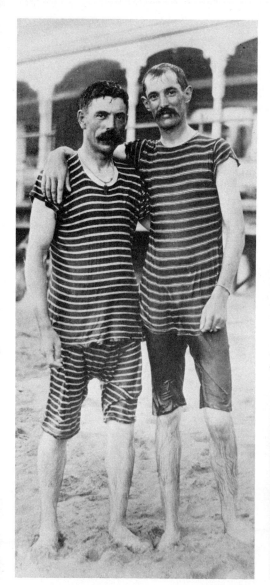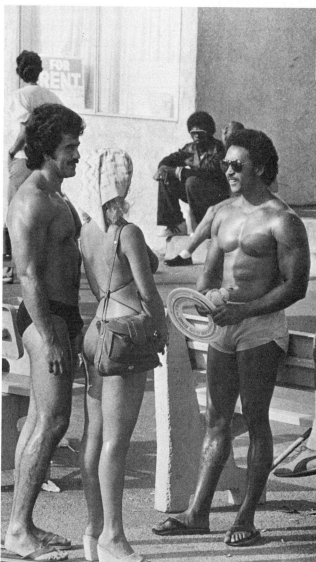

In the Victorian era, bathers covered most of their bodies. As public attitudes toward nudity changed, bathing suits shrank. (left: Brown Brothers/right: Ellis Herwig, The Picture Cube)

magazines and films are aimed exclusively at men. They feature female nudity—unless they are meant for homosexual men. Despite the appearance of such magazines as *Playgirl,* male nudity is still much less common in the media than female nudity.

And the overwhelming preponderance of female nudity in the media does not contradict a cultural concern over arousing males. Erotic media consciously break social standards, for their intent is to arouse. For example, in American society a woman's nipples are generally hidden, even in a bikini, so their exposure in a magazine or movie is regarded as titillating. Male nipples are not regarded as arousing and men often go shirtless—although the obligatory chest-baring scene in many films indicates that moviemakers may not believe women are unresponsive. A middle-aged woman recalled her own adolescent response:

> When I was a teenager, I went to see *West of the Pecos*—a mediocre western—eight times just to watch Robert Mitchum take off his shirt. His bare chest really turned me on. (Authors' files)

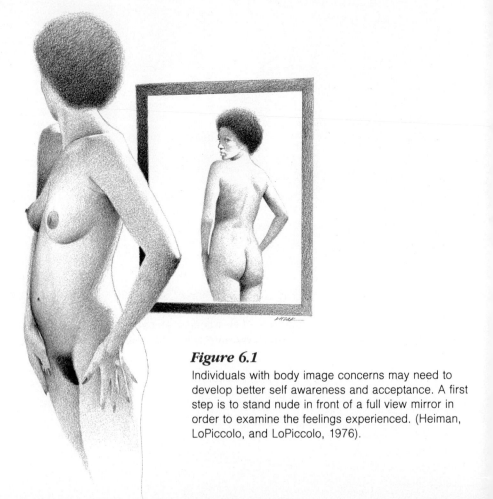

### Figure 6.1

Individuals with body image concerns may need to develop better self awareness and acceptance. A first step is to stand nude in front of a full view mirror in order to examine the feelings experienced. (Heiman, LoPiccolo, and LoPiccolo, 1976).

Other aspects of the double standard indicate an assumption that women are less comfortable with their bodies than men are. When a woman has a pelvic exam, some gynecologists drape her with a sheet so that only her vulva is exposed. But when a man goes to a urologist, he simply drops his pants. He would be astounded if the urologist draped his stomach and thighs.

Part of the difference between male and female attitudes may be due to anatomy. Male genitals are exposed and accessible. A man sees his own genitals several times each day and handles his penis each time he urinates. The placement of the penis almost ensures its stimulation.

Female genitals are internal. Many women never see their own genitals—indeed, without a mirror they cannot see them. A woman may never touch her genitals except for brief washing or to insert a tampon. The clitoris is partially covered by the genital lips and is much less likely than the penis to be inadvertently stimulated.

All this means that men may naturally become more familiar with their genitals—and perhaps more comfortable with them. But anatomy is not enough to account for the difference in attitudes. Society expects men to know what their genitals are, where they are, and what to do with them. Although society's attitude toward women is changing, many people still believe that women are better off if they don't find out too much about their bodies too soon. This disparity in standards of sexual modesty may play some part in the development of differences in men's and women's awareness of their own bodies and sexual response (Figure 6.1).

## AWARENESS OF AROUSAL: HOW MEN AND WOMEN DIFFER

Women and men respond to sexual stimulation in similar ways, as we saw in Chapter 5. Yet men seem to be more keenly aware of their arousal—or at least they are said to describe their feelings more accurately.

Does this mean that women are less in touch with their own genital responses than men are? Perhaps. The greater accessibility of male genitals and men's generally greater experience and possible comfort with them may cause men to be more conscious of their sexual arousal. But the difference in awareness may be more complicated than it seems. Folklore and the media agree that men generally have sex on their minds, and society approves when men report sexual interest. But women—who aren't supposed to know too much too soon—get no approval for saying that they're turned on. They may even be seen as not quite "nice" (Steinman et al., 1981).

There is no reason to believe that women are incapable of the same sexual awareness found in men. When women are told to pay attention to their genital sensations, their verbal reports of arousal are much closer to their physiological measures (Geer, in press). It may be that women simply need to be prompted. Because the culture is not geared to evoking female sexual response, women may have learned to deny or ignore their physiological reactions unless they are in an appropriate situation. As one woman said:

> For years I did my best to hold back my sexual feelings. Now that things have changed, I'm finding it hard to let go, even though there's no reason not to. (Authors' files)

It's even possible that the culture dampens women's sexual awareness through the heavy emphasis placed on physical beauty. A woman's feeling that she is not an attractive sexual partner could lead to such discomfort about sex that she might deny her sexual responses.

The discrepancy became clear when hetereosexual men and women watched a series of films portraying explicit sexual activity. Each movie was different: sex between a woman and a man, between two men, between two women, and among a group of men and women. Men's reports of their feelings agreed with their physiological arousal, which was recorded as in the experiment described in Chapter 5. The women's did not. Men accurately said that they were most aroused by group sex, but women—whose physiological recordings also showed the highest arousal during the group sex film—said that both the heterosexual film and the lesbian film were more exciting than the film portraying group sex (Steinman et al., 1981).

## BODY TYPES AND PHYSICAL ATTRACTIVENESS

Many people believe that their bodies are unattractive, and such a feeling is likely to increase discomfort about sex. Worries about breasts, penis, thighs, a spare tire, or some other physical imperfection can cast a shadow over the prospect of undressing in front of a partner. Since in the United States most people are mostly clothed most of the time, the standard of comparison tends to be the media image of the ideal body. Television, movies, or the carefully posed body looming large on the billboards can make men and women feel that their own bodies are unattractive and that no one could ever be interested in them.

After years of exposure to such images, people may develop a distorted body image and see themselves as less attractive than they are. When male college students were asked to pick the photograph that most resembled them from a group of ten pictures, men who were more than fifteen pounds overweight generally selected a photograph of a man who was fatter than they were (Schonbuch and Schell, 1967).

Despite the attention paid by the media to the ideal body, there's been little scientific research to find out what sorts of bodies people actually find attractive. In some times and some places, fat women have been considered beautiful. The idealized models painted by Peter Paul Rubens in the seventeenth century and American beauties of the late nineteenth century would feel out of place in the United States today. Today's fashion models would be regarded as emaciated and unattractive in those societies.

Americans are especially weight-conscious. In a large study of young, middle-

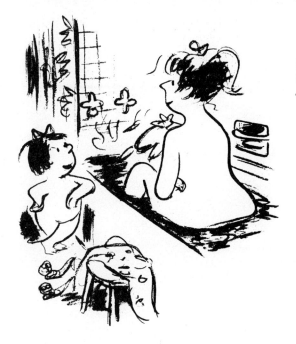

*"Hey, Ma. How come I'm so plain and you're so fancy?"*

class women and men (Berscheid, Walster, and Bohrnstedt, 1973), about half of the women worried about the size of their hips—more than were concerned with breast size—and twice as many men worried about a spare tire as fretted over the size of the penis. These women and men may be closer to the general public attitude than media attention to the importance of breast and penis size would indicate. In one of the few scientific studies (Horvath, 1981) of what people find attractive in bodies, a bulge around a man's waist was regarded as unattractive by both men and women, and broad shoulders were seen as attractive. Neither men nor women liked too many billowing curves on a woman. Nor were they attracted by large breasts. Women didn't like them at all, and men regarded breast size as immaterial—although they did notice it. Yet believing the common wisdom about breast size can lead to unhappiness, as one woman recalled:

> In my 22 years, I'd never met a man who wasn't foaming at the mouth over big boobs. Not until I met my husband did I realize that even a girl with small breasts can be considered sexy and attractive. (Berscheid, Walster, and Bohrnstedt, 1973, p. 121)

Since feelings about the body can add to discomfort about sex, it might be comforting to know that in a group of 28,000 men and women, less than a third of the women required their ideal man to be physically attractive and less than half of

By today's standards, these slender, active, and athletic women are attractive, but a hundred years ago the ideal woman was plump, passive, and rather helpless. (© Jerry Berndt 1982/Stock, Boston)

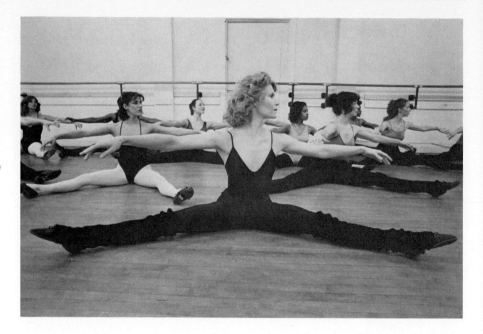

the men demanded physical attractiveness in their ideal woman (Tavris, 1977). Although our culture seems to place great emphasis on body shape as a source of sexual attraction, some researchers have wondered if we shouldn't investigate the role of odors.

## BODY ODORS AND SEXUAL ATTRACTIVENESS

If we can believe the commercials, perfumes, colognes, and after-shave lotions are surefire sexual attractants. A look at the enormous sales of these products indicates that many of us accept the claims. But what if substances normally secreted by the body also attract sexual partners? Such substances are known as **pheromones**, a term applied to any chemical messenger produced by one individual that influences the behavior of another.

**pheromone** any chemical messenger produced by one individual that influences the behavior of another individual of the same species

We know that insects, rodents, foxes, cats, dogs, coyotes, pigs, deer, cattle, horses, and some monkeys respond sexually to chemicals secreted by members of their own species (Keverne, 1977), and from time to time the possibility of human pheromones has been discussed. Two substances, copulins and androstenol, have received a good deal of attention.

Copulins, which appear to stimulate sexual interest in rhesus monkeys, have been found in human vaginal secretions. In an attempt to test their effectiveness on human sexual activity, researchers (Morris and Udry, 1978) had women rub perfume on their chests each night before they went to bed. The women used four perfumes, only one of which contained copulins, and tried a different scent each night. Every morning the women and their partners filled out separate questionnaires about the previous night's sexual urges and activity. None of the perfumes appeared to affect either desire or sexual activity.

Androstenol is found in armpit sweat of men, as well as in the urine of men and women. Since the same substance is produced by boars and appears to make sows sexually receptive, some perfume manufacturers have been adding androstenol to their products, claiming that it can "increase beyond normal fragrances, a person's attractant powers" (White, 1981). However, tests of androstenol, in which male and female researchers applied the chemical to their wrists and behind their ears before interacting briefly with a member of the opposite sex, indicated that the substance has no sexual effect on human beings. Whether the researchers used androstenol, a musklike fragrance, or no scent at all, they were perceived as equally attractive by members of the other sex (Black and Biron, 1982).

Do human sexual pheromones exist? We still don't know, but it appears that pheromones are unlikely to play a role in the initial attraction of sexual partners. It's possible, however, that during sexual activity the secretions of either partner might have an odor that heightens sexual arousal. Some men say they find vaginal odors exciting, and some women say they are aroused by the odor of semen. Since these responses may be learned, such testimony doesn't get us very far. If odors do play a role in human sexual attraction, it's probably not a large one. At any rate, our culture's widespread use of deodorants and perfume may keep us unaware of natural body odors, just as many of us are unaware of our bodies.

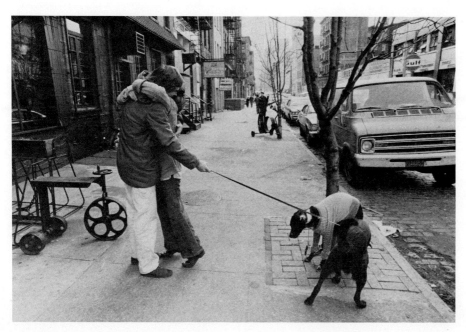

Among dogs, genital scents act as chemical messengers that directly affect sexual behavior. Although human sexual pheromones may exist, they are unlikely to play a major role in sexual activity. (© Leonard Speier 1983)

# Focus

BETTY DODSON
BODYSEX
WORKSHOP
PROGRAM

If you were shown a thousand photographs of human faces, you would have no difficulty in selecting your own picture. You are so familiar with your facial features—their unique shape, coloring, size—that you recognize yourself instantly. But if you were given only two or three photographs of genitals, the chances are that you'd be unable to recognize your own.

Most women learn about genital anatomy by studying diagrams and charts like those in Chapter 3. Such illustrations generally focus on structure— which tube is connected to which—and ignore the appearance of the external genitals. When external genitals are shown, it is usually in the form of a diagram that gives no hint of the enormous variability among women. A woman who compares these anatomical diagrams with her own genitals often finds differences that may lead her to question her own normality.

Just such an assumption of deformity led Betty Dodson, a New York erotic artist and feminist lecturer, to develop a program of workshops that teach women self-exploration and body awareness. When she was about ten years old, Dodson inspected her genitals in a mirror. She was horrified:

I had the same funny looking things that dangled from a chicken's neck. I was obviously deformed and I knew it was because I played with myself. At that awful moment of discovery, I swore off "doing it" on the spot, and made a deal with God. If he got rid of those things that hung down, I promised to stop swearing, keep my room clean, and to love my little brothers. (Dodson, 1983, p. 33)

Thinking that other women would benefit from more information about female anatomy, as she had, Dodson organized workshops for women interested in learning more about their own sexuality. As she had expected, Dodson found that many other women were concerned about their bodies.

Dodson's workshops consist of four sessions, and they are conducted in the nude. Women undress as they arrive, and begin by sitting in a circle. One by one, each woman tells how she feels about her own body. Next come lessons in breathing and posture. Each woman examines her posture in the mirror and notes the change in her body as she stands correctly, as well as the way altering her posture changes her feelings about her body.

One session begins with photographic slides of female genitals, a way of demonstrating that genital features vary as widely as facial features. During this session, each woman examines her own vulva and vagina, using a gynecologist's speculum and a mirror so that she can see her internal organs. Women are also taught to locate and tighten vaginal muscles, using exercises similar to those discussed below. In the final workshop session, women learn to massage their bodies and to enjoy the sensation.

These workshops teach women to become familiar with and to accept their own genitals. Women who have trouble experiencing orgasm may find such a genital self-examination an important step in learning about sexual response (Barbach, 1976).

# DEVELOPING BODY AWARENESS

Most of us have been taught to ignore our bodies, but observations of youngsters indicate that we didn't always behave that way. Small children often inspect themselves, exploring their crevices and protrusions, poking at nipples and navels, and probably enjoying the sensations. But all too often, as the small hand wanders to the genitals, an adult voice issues a stern warning or a large hand firmly pulls away the questing fingers. It takes few such experiences to teach children that it's not nice to handle the genitals, that it's dirty "down there."

It's no wonder, then, that so many of us are out of touch with our bodies. Sex therapists often find that this lack of body awareness contributes a great deal to sexual problems. Most programs of sex therapy begin with exercises to increase self-awareness and improve body image. But even people without specific problems may find it valuable to become more aware of their bodies and to learn to be comfortable with them.

The benefits of body awareness go beyond any possible increase in sexual satisfaction. A reluctance to inspect the genitals can lead to health problems. If you don't know how your genitals look when they're healthy, you're not likely to notice early signs of disorders. One positive result of the new interest in health has been an emphasis on regular self-examination by both women and men.

## Self-exploration for women

Self-exploration can be valuable for women of all ages. Successful self-exploration has four major goals: to become familiar with important parts of the body; to identify the feelings associated with different parts of the body; to overcome any inhibitions about looking at the genitals or touching them; and to develop a positive body image.

That's a big order for a simple series of exercises, but many women have learned their cultural lessons well and are so inhibited about touching their bodies that they have inadvertently dampened their sexual feelings. The prohibitions of childhood are worse for girls than for boys. Boys are praised for handling the penis when they urinate, but most girls are taught to keep their hands away. Later, the adolescent girl finds that the burden of deciding "how far to go" has been placed upon *her* by society. Steady practice in keeping sexual feelings under control for fear of "letting" a boyfriend do something that would "make him lose respect for me" can easily result in a woman who has simply turned off these feelings (Barbach, 1976).

**Getting in touch with your body**   Give yourself forty-five minutes to an hour to get acquainted with your body. The following self-exploration exercise has been distilled from the work of a number of therapists (Barbach, 1976; Gochros and Fisher, 1980; Heiman, LoPiccolo, and LoPiccolo, 1976).

Begin with a bath in which you soap yourself with your hands while concentrating on the sensations as your fingers move slowly over your body. After closing your eyes and visualizing your body, look at yourself in the water and react to what you see.

A full-length mirror is essential to every exercise. Standing nude in front of the mirror, look once again at your body. Examine your entire body with your eyes and fingers, feeling skin texture, muscles, bones, and fat. Look closely at each part of your body. Stand, kneel, and sit; open your legs and close them. Now think about your body, and decide what parts you like or dislike. Then try to figure out where you got the idea that parts of your body are ugly. Reflect on the fact that those slim, young women pictured in the media with large, firm breasts, perfect teeth, shining hair, flawless skin, and not an ounce of extra body fat are not typical women and that it probably took hours of preparation to get them ready for the camera—not to mention years of expensive dental work, exercise, and rigid diet. Consider that tastes in breast size vary and that breasts that are too large or too small this year are soon likely to be fashionable again. Remember that a little superfluous hair is normal and that it can be removed if it bothers you. Remember that most women have stretch marks, even if they have not borne children. One woman found she could come to terms with her "imperfections":

> My body has changed tremendously since I had children. I like some of the changes, like the fact that my breasts seem fuller and more round. But there are some other changes that I am not happy with—I've got some stretch marks, and my stomach is not as firm. I was self-conscious about this for a while, but my husband reassured me that I was still attractive, and now I've learned to see these changes as part of my growth and maturity. (Authors' files)

Now you are ready to touch your body again, concentrating on the feeling in the areas you caress as well as the feeling in your caressing fingertips. Finally, you accept the idea that it's all right to look the way you do. As the focus feature suggests, becoming familiar with your genitals is an important part of accepting your body.

**Examining your vagina**   Regular examination of their own internal organs can do more than make women comfortable with their bodies and with sexuality. It can lead to the early detection of medical problems and radically change a woman's approach to pelvic examinations. As most women know, the internal pelvic examination conducted by a gynecologist is staged so an observer would think a complicated medical procedure is taking place, even though the process itself is simple and safe.

The woman slides down to the end of an examining table, spreads her knees, and inserts her feet into metal stirrups. The gynecologist first inserts a speculum, a plastic instrument that holds apart the vaginal walls so that the vagina and cervix can be inspected. The gynecologist looks inside to check their condition. If the woman is scheduled for her annual Pap smear (a test for abnormal cell development), the gynecologist painlessly takes a few cells to be examined under microscope from the cervix with a cotton swab. The speculum is then removed, and the gynecologist conducts a "bimanual vaginal examination." (See Figure 6.2.) One

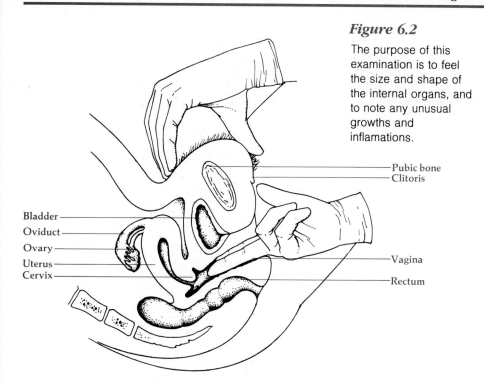

### Figure 6.2

The purpose of this examination is to feel the size and shape of the internal organs, and to note any unusual growths and inflamations.

Pubic bone
Clitoris

Bladder
Oviduct
Ovary
Uterus
Cervix

Vagina

Rectum

hand is placed on the woman's abdomen and a finger or two of the other hand, encased in a lubricated rubber glove, is inserted in the vagina. Now the gynecologist feels for the size, shape, or position of the internal sexual organs, checking for swelling, growths, or any tenderness. The procedure should not be painful.

Members of the women's health movement have been critical of the way these examinations are conducted, on the grounds that they debase and humiliate women, that they are disease-oriented, and that the gynecologist's approach—intentionally or not—deprives women of knowledge about the normal functioning of their bodies (Sloane, 1980). As one young woman put it:

> I think that position is really undignified. There's something about lying there on my back with my legs up and spread open that I just think is gross. (Bell, 1980, p. 157)

It is not certain whether women generally agree with these criticisms, although just under a half of the women in one study (Tiefer, 1979) said such gynecological exams embarrassed them, and nearly three-fifths said they disliked the experience. However, most women wanted to be draped with a sheet, less than half wanted a mirror placed so they could watch the examination, and nearly all recoiled at the idea of having a friend or lover present. What virtually all women said they would like is more information from the gynecologist—before, during, and after the examination. One of the women in this study said:

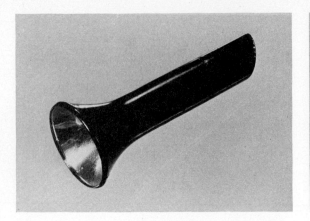

Speculums were first used for female gynecological examinations during the 19th century. This glass speculum, introduced about 1840, was wrapped with tinfoil and coated with hard rubber. (Courtesy, R. Rosen)

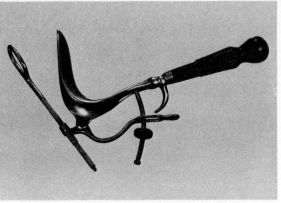

James Marion Sims, regarded as the "founder of gynecology," devised the duck-billed vaginal speculum. This adjustable model was introduced about 1875. (Courtesy, R. Rosen)

I still don't really know what the exam is or what they checked for or what I ought to be on the lookout for. (Tiefer, 1979, p. 393)

One way for women to get this kind of information is to examine their own bodies periodically. For this, you need a speculum (available at many drugstores or from hospital supply companies), a long-handled mirror, a flashlight, and K-Y Jelly. Begin by lying on a firm surface with your back supported—perhaps on a rug with your back against the side of a couch. Lubricate the speculum with K-Y Jelly, insert it into the vagina, and lock it open. Now shine the flashlight into the mirror, which you should hold so to direct the light toward the back of the vagina. You will be able to see the walls of the vagina, which are about the same color as the inside of the mouth, and if the speculum is inserted properly, a smooth, pink ring of muscle that is the cervix. Using a speculum properly takes some practice, but instructions can be found in self-health publications and pamphlets (Berry, 1977/1978).

Once you are accustomed to the sight of your healthy vaginal tissues, you can note such signs of disorder as changes in color or condition, a sharp increase in the normal vaginal discharge, or any change in its texture, color, or odor. (Some of these conditions will be discussed in Chapter 18.) It's also possible to check the placement of birth-control devices, to note changes in cervical mucus that denote a fertile period, or to spot early signs of pregnancy (Berry, 1977/1978).

**Examining your breasts** Vaginal self-examination is urged by the self-health movement and regarded dimly by the medical establishment. With breast self-examination the scales tip in the opposite direction; the medical establishment pushes monthly breast examination, but some members of the self-health movement take the position that they are of little value on the grounds that a focus on the search for disease in healthy women is itself unhealthy (Napoli, 1980). There is no argument, however, that self-examination detects breast cancer and other disorders earlier than they would ordinarily be found. In addition, the familiarity with your breasts that comes with monthly examination can help make you more comfortable with your body.

About a week after the menstrual period is a good time to examine your breasts, because any premenstrual tenderness or swelling will have subsided. The examination as recommended by the American Cancer Society has three parts. (See Figure 6.3.) The first part takes place in a shower or bath, since fingers glide easily over wet skin. Place your left hand behind your head and move the flat part of the fingers on your right hand over every area of the left breast, checking for lumps, knots, tender spots, or any change in the size and consistency of the breast tissue. There is a normal ridge of firm tissue in the lower crescent of each breast that should not be confused with lumps. Now, place your right hand behind your head, and use your left hand to examine the right breast in the same manner.

For the second part of the examination, stand naked in front of a mirror with your arms at your sides. Raise your arms over your head and check for any swelling, puckering, or dimpling in the breasts. Look for any depression or swelling, any redness or skin irritation. Then look for a whitish scale on the nipples, a distortion of the areola's circular shape, or a nipple that points to one side. Now place your palms on your hips and press down firmly, contracting chest muscles in order to outline the breast structure. Repeat the visual inspection.

For the final part of the examination, lie down with a pillow or folded towel beneath your right shoulder and place your right hand behind your head. Press down on the outer edge of the breast with the fingers of the left hand, moving them around the outside of the breast in a circle. Then move the fingers about an inch toward the nipple and repeat the process. This is done with increasingly smaller circles until the entire breast, including the nipple, has been examined. Next, squeeze the nipple and check for any discharge or bleeding. Moving the pillow to

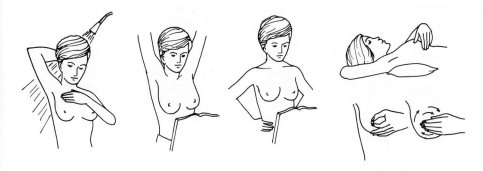

*Figure 6.3*
Breast self-examination can be performed in the shower, while standing in front of a mirror, or lying down.

your left shoulder, repeat the process for the left breast. Again, you are checking for lumps, dimples, or discharges.

Finding a lump should not send you into a panic. Because most self-examination campaigns focus on breast cancer, many women are unnecessarily upset when they discover a lump. As one woman recalled:

> The first time I found a lump in one of my breasts I nearly panicked. All the news media stuff on breast cancer is enough to scare anyone, and I was convinced I had it. It wasn't anything important, but I had a bad week. There must be a better way of preparing women to take care of their health. (Authors' files)

Most lumps are harmless. The majority are due to mastodynia. Some lumps are simple cysts, fluid-filled sacs that can be treated in the physician's office by withdrawing the fluid through a hollow needle. Other lumps are wartlike growths in the lining of a mammary duct or noncancerous tumors, which account for a quarter of all breast tumors (Kradjian, 1980). Few breast lumps are cancerous. But since one woman in eleven develops breast cancer at some time during her life, any lump should be reported to a physician.

## Self-exploration for men

The male anatomy is accessible; men are accustomed to handling their penises several times a day; and most men have had more experience with masturbation than most women. But many men still have a lot to learn about their own anatomy.

American attitudes toward sex hinder men's awareness of their own bodies, too. Since the man has traditionally been expected to court the woman—making love to her instead of having her make love to him—men do most of the stroking and caressing. As a result, some men's sexual awareness is limited to the penis; they lack awareness of the sensual potential of other parts of the body (Nowinski, 1980). As with the exercises for women, the major goals of male exercises in self-exploration are to increase awareness of the body, to get in touch with feelings about different body parts, to improve body image, and to learn about self-examination as part of taking responsibility for personal health care.

**Getting in touch with your body** There are many similarities between exploration exercises for men and for women. Like women's exercises, those developed for men are best done at a leisurely pace. The exercise that follows combines one developed by Joseph Nowinski (1980) with one by Bernie Zilbergeld (1978).

This exercise, too, begins in the shower. After soaping and rinsing, stand beneath the running water and focus on your sensations as the water hits your face, neck, arms, shoulders, chest, genitals, buttocks, thighs, legs, and feet. Move around, changing your position so that the water hits you from different angles. Now change the temperature, trying both warmer and cooler water on various parts of your body. Change the intensity of the spray and go through the same rou-

tine. When you step out of the shower, dry yourself slowly and notice the sensations as the towel strokes your body.

The full-length mirror is essential to male self-exploration. Inspect your body
from head to toe in the mirror, looking closely at each body part in turn. Take a
deep breath and notice how the line in your chest and stomach changes. Do you
fell differently about your body when your chest is inflated and your stomach is
drawn in? Now inspect your genitals. Turn sideways and inspect them again. If you
believe that your penis is too small, note that every man who has visited the Men's
Reproductive Health Clinic in San Francisco with bitter complaints of miniature
genitals has been found to have genitals of normal size (Castleman, 1978).

Lie down in bed and once more look at each part of your body. Take your
time. Inspect your fingers, hands, wrists, arms, chest, and stomach. Look at your
toes, feet, ankles, and legs. With a hand mirror, look closely at your genitals from
various angles. See how all the parts fit together. Look at the area between the scrotum and the anus. What do you like about your genitals? What do you dislike?

The next step is to explore your body with your hands, concentrating on the
sensations. Using a soft, stroking movement, explore your head, face, and neck.
Move to your hands, arms, and chest. Lightly caress your stomach, then your
thighs. Now turn on your stomach and stroke your back and your buttocks. Turn
over and caress your toes, feet, and legs.

It's now time to explore your genitals. Press the skin above your penis and
note your pubic bone. Gently prod the area between your scrotum and anus to
find the bulb of your penis. Now place one finger in front and another behind the
scrotum and gently squeeze above your testes. The cord you feel is the vas deferens.

Feel the texture of your pubic hair. Stroke your penis lightly and focus on the
sensation. Touch its various parts with caresses of differing intensity and notice
which parts are more sensitive. Move to your scrotum and do the same thing.
When you have finished, relax for ten minutes.

**Examining your body** Although men's genitals are more easily visible and
simpler to examine than women's, few men regularly examine their testes. This is
an important examination for younger men, because testicular cancer, although
rare, is one of the commonest cancers among men under thirty-five. If the cancer is
detected early, the survival rate is high. So examining the testes should be part of a
regular health routine.

The time to examine your testes is after a hot bath. As noted in Chapter 4,
sperm require a relatively cool environment, so the heat of a bath causes the testes
to move away from the body, making them easier to examine. Using both hands,
examine the left testis with the left hand and the right testis with the right. Place the
thumb on top of the testis and the index and middle finger beneath, probing the
flesh. The testes should feel firm, rather like an earlobe. With your fingertips, check
for small, hard lumps (Castleman, 1978). An early testicular cancer is usually painless and about the size of a pea, although later symptoms include a heavy feeling in
the testis, an enlarged testis, or a sudden accumulation of fluid in the scrotum.

Regular self-examination can detect testicular cancer, a form of the disease that, although rare, is one of the commonest cancers among men younger than thirty-five. (© Teri Leigh Stratford 1981)

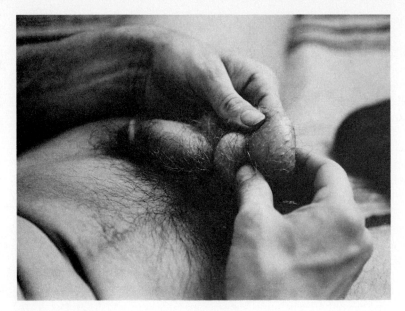

Diagnosing ailments of the prostate is the responsibility of a physician, but men can examine their own prostate glands by lying on the side in a fetal position with the knees drawn up to the chin. Now insert a thoroughly lubricated finger slowly and gently into the anus. A healthy prostate gland feels rather like the palm of your hand (Castleman, 1978).

Much is said about breast cancer in women, but few men know that it is occasionally found in men. However, it's so uncommon that for every hundred women who develop breast cancer, less than one man develops it. As a precaution, simply make a habit of examining your breasts regularly while in the shower. Following the method described in the section on women's breast examination, move your fingers in a circular pattern over every area of each breast, checking for lumps. The discovery of a painless lump should send you to a physician.

Developing body awareness and examining the body regularly can go a long way toward making men and women comfortable in sexual situations. Another technique that may increase sexual pleasure is to strengthen muscle tone in the pelvic area through exercise.

## TONING UP SEXUAL MUSCLES

Exercises originally developed by Arnold Kegel (1952) to help women strengthen their pubococcygeal (P/C) muscles after childbirth are said to increase sexual enjoyment in both men and women. Some women have reported heightened sensation during intercourse or stronger orgasms, and men have reported increased feeling, stronger erections, and more pleasurable orgasms (Zilbergeld, 1978). As a result, many sex therapists recommend the exercises to their patients, despite the fact that laboratory tests have not established any connection between the strength of these muscles and the frequency or intensity of orgasm (Chambless et al, 1982).

The first step is to locate the muscles involved. When urinating, try to cut off the flow. These muscles are the ones involved in the Kegel exercises.

Once you've located your P/C muscles and identified the sensation, you can try contracting them. Tighten the muscles, then release them. In order to make certain the right muscles are being exercised, women can insert a finger into the vagina and men can place a finger on each side of the penile base between the scrotum and the anus. As the muscles contract and release, you can feel them move.

There are three exercises in the series; the first two are for both men and women, the third for women only:

**1** Squeeze the muscles for three seconds, then relax. Wait three seconds and squeeze again. Do this "long Kegel" ten times.

**2** Contract the muscles again but release them immediately. Do this "flutter Kegel," a squeeze and release, ten times.

**3** Women can imagine trying to suck a tampon into the vagina by using these muscles, then holding it for three seconds. Do this ten times. Now bear down as if you were having a bowel movement, but concentrate on the vaginal area. Do this ten times.

As you get used to the exercises, gradually increase the number until you are doing each exercise twenty times. The entire series should be repeated three times a day—oftener if possible (Barbach, 1976; Gochros and Fisher, 1980). Since the exercises are invisible, they can be done almost anywhere—while watching television or riding in a car. Kegel exercises improve muscle tone and increase blood flow into the pelvic area. It takes about six weeks of regular exercise for the improved muscle tone to become noticeable.

Now that we've looked at the sexual architecture of women and men and their sexual responses and attitudes toward their bodies, we can begin to see why there are such wide individual differences in response to sexual situations. In Part Three we'll use this information as a basis for our examination of specific sexual activities.

# *Summary*

**1** Americans have many terms for genitals and sexual activity, but most of the common words sound harsh, cynical, and mechanical. The negative applications of these terms to other areas of life reveal an underlying discomfort with sexuality.

**2** Nudity is common in some cultures and strictly regulated in others. Different customs and assumptions govern male and female nudity, and most prohibitions seem aimed at protecting men from being aroused by women's bodies. The double standard for nudity may indicate the belief that men are aroused by the sight of a nude woman, but that women do not respond simply to the male body. Another basis for this double standard may be that cultural pressures have made women less comfortable with their bodies than men are.

**3** Men are believed to be more keenly aware of their arousal than are women, probably because men's genitals are more accessible and because men are rewarded for being so aware. Women may be capable of the same degree of sexual awareness men display, but they have been carefully taught to deny or ignore their sexual arousal except in certain situations.

**4** Many people believe their bodies are unattractive, a belief that is probably encouraged by the media image of the ideal body. Although such feelings can increase discomfort concerning sex, one study has shown that more than two-thirds of women and more than half of men do not require physical attractiveness in their ideal sexual partner.

**5** **Pheromones**, chemical messengers that affect the behavior of others, play a role in the sexual response of many animals. Some of these same chemicals have been found in human beings, but none of them have yet been shown to act as sexual pheromones.

**6** Most people have learned to ignore their bodies, and this lack of body awareness may contribute to sexual problems. Developing body awareness can increase sexual satisfaction and help people detect health problems. Women can learn to examine their breasts and vagina regularly, and men can learn to examine their testes, prostate, and breasts. Exercises developed to strengthen the pubococcygeal (P/C) muscles may increase sexual enjoyment for both men and women.

# Part Three

# Sexual Behavior

What makes any act sexual? From a reproductive view, any activity that can lead to pregnancy is sexual. But reproduction is only one of the many motives of sex. Our first impulse is to say that any behavior that involves genital stimulation or orgasm is sexual, but a moment's thought leads us to reject this view. A kiss or simply the meeting of two hands can be highly erotic, although neither genital stimulation nor orgasm is involved. Under different circumstances, the same kiss may have no sexual connotation at all. A woman's hand on a man's penis is surely a sexual act. But what if the woman is a nurse inserting a catheter into a hospital patient?

To include the wide range of behavior that can be sexual and to eliminate apparently sexual behavior that has no erotic meaning, we'll cast our definition of sexual activity in terms of subjective meaning. If a person who is involved in any act thinks it is sexual, it is. This brings us right back to the topic of psychogenic stimuli and the conclusion that, for human beings, sex is mostly psychological.

Sexual behavior can be solitary, can involve men and women, only men, or only women. In the four chapters that make up Part Three, we'll investigate each of these forms of sexual behavior. After examining masturbation and other solitary activities in Chapter 7, in Chapter 8 we'll consider general patterns of sexual behavior and heterosexual intercourse. In Chapter 9 we discuss homosexual behavior patterns, noting the similarities and differences involved when both partners are of the same gender. Chapter 10 focuses on ways to communicate sexual messages, including the initiation or rejection of sexual activity.

# 7 Solitary Sexual Behavior

# *Chapter 7*

**masturba-
tion** deliber-
ate self-
stimulation
that produces
a sexual re-
sponse

No other sexual act has been so widely condemned and at the same time so widely practiced as **masturbation**—deliberate self-stimulation that produces a sexual response. Historically, medical, religious, and even sexual authorities have frowned on the practice, although
it is common in most human societies and most animal species. This difference between
what we say and what we do may be prevalent because masturbation is generally a solitary
activity. It can be performed in private and condemned in public—and no one is the wiser.

Only recently have the historical prohibitions against masturbation been reexamined,
and they now seem unconvincing. The more obvious masturbation myths have been discarded. We no longer believe that masturbation will lead to insanity or cause hair to grow
on the palms of our hands or any of those other tales that frightened generations of children. But the old warnings linger. Less than twenty years ago, when the adolescent hero of
Philip Roth's *Portnoy's Complaint* discovered a freckle on the underside of his penis, he
was certain that his incessant masturbation had given him cancer:

> All that pulling and tugging at my own flesh, all that friction, had given me an
> incurable disease. And not yet fourteen! In bed that night the tears rolled from
> my eyes. "No!" I sobbed. "I don't want to die! Please—no!" But then, because
> I would very shortly be a corpse anyway, I went ahead as usual and jerked off
> into my sock. (Roth, 1967, p. 19)

When Roth wrote this, people were more uneasy about masturbation than they are today. Even though attitudes have changed, most are still at least slightly uncomfortable about

# Solitary Sexual Behavior

discussing the subject. In the 1980s, masturbation remains an almost universal sexual activity that is surrounded by confusion, misinformation, and shame.

Masturbation is not the only solitary sexual activity. In this chapter we'll look at sexual fantasies, whether in the form of daydreams, as an accompaniment to masturbation, or during sex with a partner. And sexual responses continue during sleep, sometimes becoming so intense that the sleeper is wakened by an orgasm.

## CHANGING VIEWS OF MASTURBATION

The discomfort and shame that often surround masturbation come from the Judeo-Christian tradition, which sternly disapproves of all sexual activity that does not lead to reproduction. Many religious groups believe that bodily pleasures interfere with spiritual growth. Since masturbation provides pleasure without procreation, it has no place in such belief systems.

Although the Catholic Church adopted early Jewish taboos on masturbation, no one seemed overly concerned about the practice until the eighteenth century. In medieval Europe, masturbation was regarded as rather like scratching—a way to handle a bodily itch (Haeberle, 1978).

Then an obscure English clergyman wrote a pamphlet warning people about masturbation, which he called "onania," after the biblical Onan who was killed by God for spilling his seed on the ground. Yet Onan never masturbated. As the story in Genesis describes it, Onan's crime was withdrawal, or coitus interruptus—removing his penis before he ejaculated to keep from impregnating his sister-in-law. So began a misunderstanding that has terrorized generations. Masturbation became known as the "sin of Onan"—even though Onan didn't do it.

By the nineteenth century, the religious prohibition against masturbation received strong support from the medical profession. For example, the highly respected Swiss physician Samuel Tissot published a major textbook on the consequences of onanism, which included blindness, tuberculosis, impotence, insanity, and acne. When in the 1830s his work became available in the United States, it had a powerful impact. Medical educators maintained that masturbation led to a weakening of all bodily functions and affected the masturbator's offspring as well. In fact, masturbation became a favorite scapegoat for a variety of physical, mental, and sexual problems.

Already condemned by the church, masturbation fell into even greater disrepute when Richard von Krafft-Ebing (1840–1902) warned that it was a major factor in all unusual forms of sexual behavior, which in the nineteenth century were called "perversions." Krafft-Ebing succeeded in making sexual disorders a subject for psychiatric study, but his work was biased by a moralistic and puritanical outlook. Over the centuries, sex had often been made a sin or a crime; Krafft-Ebing added the idea of its being a disease as well (Brecher, 1969).

As a psychiatrist, Krafft-Ebing was primarily concerned with sexual "perversions," which were believed to be the result of disease or "degeneration" of the nervous system. It was supposed that either hereditary factors or some form of traumatic experience could lead to such degeneration. Because masturbation was so common among his patients, Krafft-Ebing decided that it always played a role in perversion. He was clearly unaware of the prevalence of the practice in the general population, and mistakenly assumed that it was found only among deviants.

The Victorians believed all these ideas. Masturbation was known as "the secret sin," "self-pollution," "self-abuse," and "the solitary vice." Victorians seemed to spend a good deal of their time watching to make sure their children did not masturbate. They believed it was easy to spot masturbators, who were apathetic and lazy, had shifty eyes, a pale complexion, slouching posture, and trembling hands. Once the sin had been uncovered, parents fought it with hard beds, thin blankets, cold baths, freezing rooms, and special diets (Haeberle, 1978).

Sometimes the treatment was harsh. Little boys who persisted in masturbation might be castrated, or the nerves leading to the penis might be cut. If they were lucky, their parents simply used restraining devices to keep them from handling their penis. As we saw in Chapter 4, circumcision was also a remedy. Little girls who were habitual masturbators might have their clitoris removed (Sussman, 1976).

Freud and his followers took a slightly less harsh view. They expected children to masturbate, but believed that it was an immature form of sexual behavior. Mature adults were supposed to lose interest in this solitary sexual act. In the Freudian tradition, adult masturbation was usually considered a sign of immaturity or incomplete sexual development.

This strong antimasturbation tradition was opposed by Alfred Kinsey (1948), who presented an impressive array of statistics showing that masturbation is both common and "normal." More recent sex surveys (Hunt, 1974) also show that nearly all men and most women had masturbated at some time. What's more, the view of masturbation as sinful has been steadily weakening. In the surveys, men and women under the age of thirty-five generally rejected it. Although most people now said there was nothing wrong with masturbation, many continued to feel guilty, and the thought that others might find out about their "habit" embarrassed them (Hunt, 1974). As a sixteen-year-old boy said:

> Even if you know it's normal and all that, you still lock the door! You don't go around advertising that you're doing it. . . . Everybody does it, but they sort of pretend they don't. (Bell, 1980, p. 80)

That masturbation might have beneficial effects on sexual and social adjustment is a relatively new idea. One of the first therapists to see masturbation as a positive force was Wilhelm Reich. He believed it was a useful technique for helping patients solve their sexual problems. Today, sex researchers also approve masturbation. In the past decade, many therapists have reported that teaching women how to masturbate is often successful in overcoming their orgasmic difficulties (McMullen and Rosen, 1979). There is even evidence that masturbation improves women's capacity for orgasm during intercourse (Kinsey et al., 1953), as well as reducing the pain of menstrual cramps, as mentioned in Chapter 3.

As late as 1975, however, the Catholic Church once again condemned masturbation as a "seriously disordered" act. While acknowledging that psychologists and sociologists now regarded the practice as normal, the Vatican reaffirmed the position that sexual activity must be tied to procreation and carried out in the context of "true love" and "mutual self-giving." Despite the Vatican's continuing opposition, few individuals today consider masturbation as either unnatural or immoral. Even fewer people believe the practice has negative effects on well-being. Parents no longer spy on their children or tie their hands to keep them from masturbating. But the old tradition dies hard, as one woman recalled:

> At about age four I was accused of playing with myself and was slapped with a metal spatula and made to stand up against a wall. (Athanasiou, Shaver, and Tavris, 1970, p. 49)

But many of us still wonder if masturbation is really "healthy," how it might affect our sexual and psychological relationships, and how much is "too much." A look at what is known about masturbation may help to answer these questions.

## FACTS ABOUT MASTURBATION

Until the Kinsey reports appeared in the mid-twentieth century, masturbation was generally regarded as a vile habit primarily of weak-willed male adolescents. Boy Scout manuals counseled against the practice, and it was widely assumed that, once past adolescence, the practice was dropped. The assumption was easy to make because no information about the prevalence of "the solitary vice" was available. Sex surveys have changed all that. Once researchers realized how widespread masturbation was among "normal" adults, they began to think seriously about the reasons for its prevalence.

## Who masturbates

Our most complete set of statistics on masturbation comes from Kinsey and his associates (1948; 1953). Kinsey's statistics on masturbation surprised and shocked many members of the scientific community and most of the public. Three of his findings had particular impact: that fully 93 percent of the male population mastur-

## *Table 7.1   Kinsey and Hunt findings on masturbation*

|  | MEN | | WOMEN | |
|---|---|---|---|---|
| INCIDENCE[1] | KINSEY | HUNT | KINSEY | HUNT |
| Cumulative | 93% | 94% | 62% | 63% |
| By age 13 | 45 | • 63 | 15 | • 33 |
| Unmarried | | | | |
|   Age 18–24 | 86 | 86 | 30 | • 60 |
|   Age 30+ | 80 | 90 | 50 | • 80 |
| Unmarried frequency | | | | |
|   Age 18–24 | 49 times/yr | 52 times/yr | 21 times/yr • | 37 times/yr |
|   Age 30+ | 30 times/yr | • 60 times/yr | 16 times/yr | Not rep. |
| Married | | | | |
|   Age 30+ | 40 | • 72 | 33 | • 68 |
| Married frequency | 6 times/yr | • 24 times/yr | 10 times/yr | 10 times/yr |
| Grade-school education | 89 | About same | 34 | Somewhat higher |
| College education | 96 | About same | 57 | Somewhat higher |
| Religion Regular attenders | Slightly less | 92 | Much less | 51 |
|   Nonattenders | Slightly more | 93 | Much more | 75 |

[1]Cumulative incidence refers to the total proportion who have ever masturbated; incidence refers to the proportion who still masturbated at the time of the survey. Hunt's criteria for incidence are stricter than Kinsey's, so that his increases in several categories are conservatively estimated. Where no specific figures have been given, the original researchers provided only descriptive information; asterisks indicate major differences between the two surveys.

Source: Derived from A. C. Kinsey et al., *Sexual Behavior in the Human Male*, Saunders, 1948; A. C. Kinsey et al., *Sexual Behavior in the Human Female*, Saunders, 1953; and M. Hunt, *Sexual Behavior in the 1970's*, Dell, 1974.

bated at some time, that women who masturbated were more likely to achieve orgasm in marriage, and that masturbation was most common among the well educated.

Kinsey was interested in how common masturbation was within each social class, how often it occurred in different age groups, and what proportion of total sexual activity it formed. The key question regarding masturbation in Kinsey's interview was, "Does it lead to orgasm?" Kinsey did not ask about the emotional aspects of masturbation—he was not interested in the feelings and motives surrounding it or the fantasies that frequently play an important role. From Kinsey's work we know a lot about who masturbates and how often, but not much about why.

The second major source of information about masturbation, published about twenty years after Kinsey's work, is the survey by Morton Hunt (1974). Both Kinsey and Hunt took care to break down their statistics by age, marital status, educational level, religious background, and a variety of other factors. Although there had been some changes over the years, many of the findings stayed the same, as shown in Table 7.1. For example, both Kinsey and Hunt found that more than 90 percent of men and more than 60 percent of women masturbate at some time in their lives. However, the men and women in Hunt's survey were likely to have masturbated for the first time at an earlier age than those who talked to Kinsey. In addition, Kinsey had found that many more men than women masturbated and that the men masturbated much more frequently. Hunt discovered that the gap between the sexes had narrowed. Even in Hunt's survey, however, nearly 30 percent of the women had never masturbated to orgasm.

As for the myth that young men who masturbate frequently during adolescence stop the practice once they begin to have intercourse on a regular basis, Kinsey had damaged it severely. Among the married men he talked to, 40 percent were still masturbating, although the frequency had declined to about six times a year. Hunt demolished the myth by reporting that 72 percent of the married men in his survey still masturbated and did so about twice a month.

## Why people masturbate

Although a lot is known about the incidence of masturbation, not much is known about why people masturbate. This question is usually not part of sex surveys. When it is included, people often have difficulty putting their motives into words. However, reasons for masturbation appear to fall into four broad categories: instinctive self-stimulation, the expression of unacceptable desires, the search for an altered state of consciousness, and motives that have nothing to do with sex.

**Instinctive self-stimulation** Self-stimulation of the genitals is extremely common among most mammals (Ford and Beach, 1951). In lower mammals, stimulation often takes the form of cleaning or grooming; in nonhuman primates, such as apes and monkeys, it seems to be directed toward producing orgasm. Among human beings, the manipulation and exploration of the genitals appear to be spontaneous and instinctive. When a child or adolescent fondles the genitals and is re-

# *Focus*

IS MASTURBATION
HARMFUL?

Many of us have rejected the idea that masturbation causes disease or insanity, but we may still harbor misgivings. One common fear is that masturbation can change the shape or appearance of our genitals. This belief may have originated in the work of early sexologists, some of whom thought that "excessive" masturbation caused recognizable changes in genital structure (Dickinson, 1933). However, the belief seems unfounded, for there is no evidence that masturbation alters genital appearance.

Yet the great variety in the appearance of the genitals leads some people to blame what they believe are their genital "deformities" on their masturbatory habits. A man may attribute his an-

gled penis or a woman her enlarged labia to secret masturbation. One woman reported:

I pulled one of my labia minora when I was masturbating when I was eleven. It got long and I thought that was the reason. The other got almost as large, later. . . . My mother said my labia majora were separated because I had "touched" myself. (Hite, 1976, p. 240)

Although worries over physical changes in the genitals can be dismissed, the question of psychological harm is more complex. Masturbation may be harmful if it is accompanied by anxiety or guilt. For example, boys or girls who are punished severely for masturbation can develop inhibitions about all aspects of sexual be-

havior. Anxiety and guilt can also cause people to masturbate hastily and secretly. In men, the resulting pattern of extremely rapid ejaculation may transfer to sexual activity with a partner, causing problems with intercourse. In other cases, masturbation can complicate problems with erections. Men who have erection problems sometimes learn to masturbate to orgasm with only partial erection. The habit of ejaculating without erection may lead to or worsen problems with erection during intercourse.

Men and women who develop extremely unusual methods of masturbation—such as stimulation of the urethral canal—may find it difficult to duplicate this pattern during inter-

warded by the pleasurable sensations of orgasm, masturbation becomes a source of conditioned sexual gratification. Because the pleasure of orgasm becomes associated with the act of masturbating, the youngster repeats the act. According to one woman:

> I first discovered masturbation at the young age of six. . . I was lying on my stomach and my hands took it upon themselves to drift down to my pubic area. I began feeling rhythmic sensations. I experienced an orgasm, and have masturbated ever since that wonderful day. (Wolfe, 1981, p. 161)

Among adults, the most common reason given for masturbation is the pleasurable release of sexual tension (Hunt, 1974).

2. **Expression of unacceptable desires** For many people, sexual fantasy is an important aspect of masturbation. Although most masturbation fantasies follow such conventional themes as love and romanticism, some men and women develop fantasies they cannot or will not act out in life. In such cases, masturbation be-

course. As a result, they may be unable to reach orgasm with a partner. But in none of these instances does masturbation itself appear to cause the harm. Instead, it is the learned habits that accompany the practice that create sexual problems.

Our concern over possible harm from masturbation shouldn't obscure its potentially healthful and beneficial effects. Masturbation is the way most of us learn about our own sexuality. It is an important means of relieving sexual tension, especially among men and women who have no sexual partner. Within a sexual relationship, masturbation can be an acceptable form of sexual variety or an activity that reconciles the different sexual needs of the partners. Masturbation is

a safe means of experiencing sexual pleasure because it carries no risk of pregnancy or sexually transmitted disease. As noted earlier, it is often an important and effective part of sex therapy programs.

People who don't think masturbation is harmful may abstain from the practice because they believe masturbation "uses up" sexual desire. This idea is found in many cultures. It comes from the belief that people have only a limited amount of sexual energy and that when this energy is used for masturbation, the desire for other forms of sexual contact will decline. Although many adolescents, especially boys, masturbate in order to relieve sexual tension, masturbation doesn't interfere

with other sexual activities. In fact, masturbation can be an effective means of stimulating sexual energy.

Most people regard sexual desire as like the gasoline in an automobile—the more the car is driven, the less gasoline in the tank. A better analogy would be to compare sexual desire with the battery of the automobile—if the car is left undriven in the garage, the battery will surely run down. Although the immediate effect of masturbation may be to decrease sexual desire, its long-term effect is usually a continuing and stable interest in sexual activity. Masters and Johnson (1970) have referred to this idea as "use it or lose it."

comes a way of vicariously experiencing novel or unconventional sexual activity. It serves as a "safety valve" for the expression of socially unacceptable desires.

Masturbation can also be a way of learning about sexuality (Figure 7.1). By masturbating, people who are inexperienced or inept at sexual activity can practice

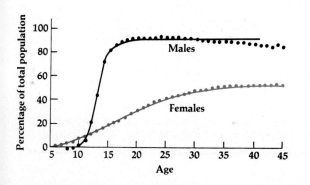

**Figure 7.1**

The cumulative incidence of masturbation to orgasm in males and females, according to data in the Kinsey studies.

their sexual skills and learn to have orgasms. Such rehearsal can increase their sexual satisfaction and make them better partners.

3 **Altered state of consciousness** All through human history, people have sought altered states of consciousness. They have used drugs, alcohol, meditation, fasting, and chanting—and perhaps masturbation. For example, it has been proposed that masturbation can produce a trancelike state (Masters, 1967). As noted in Chapter 5, psychophysiological research has shown that orgasm is accompanied by a unique set of brain waves that might indicate a special state of consciousness (Cohen et al., 1976).

4 **Nonsexual motives** Masturbation is not always practiced for sexual reasons. Some of the men in the Hunt survey masturbated to relax or to overcome insomnia. Some women masturbated in order to ease menstrual cramps. The calm and relaxation most people experience after orgasm is also an effective way of coping with tension.

Nonsexual motives for masturbation are not always positive. Masturbation can be used as a weapon or to avoid sexual interaction. For example, one partner in a relationship may masturbate in order to reject or avoid the other. Or a man who is afraid or hostile toward other people may use masturbation as a substitute for sexual relationships.

In none of these instances is masturbation itself harmful. As we'll see, however, under certain conditions the practice may have unwanted side effects.

## WHEN WOMEN MASTURBATE

Many men believe women masturbate by inserting something into the vagina. Indeed, a tour through pornography produced by males turns up candles, cucumbers, bananas, bottles, and dildos (artificial penises) as substitutes for the missing penis. Although a few women do masturbate in this way—20 percent of the group interviewed by Kinsey (Kinsey et al., 1953) used some form of vaginal insertion—most do not, and the ones who do frequently use other techniques along with vaginal penetration.

In masturbating, women usually stimulate their most sensitive areas—the clitoris and the labia. The majority of women rub the clitoral shaft with a firm and rhythmic motion that increases the pressure or intensity as orgasm approaches.

Women use a much greater variety of masturbation techniques than men. The most frequent procedure involves stimulating the outer genitals by hand while lying on the back. Some women use manual stimulation while lying face down. About one women in ten masturbates by rubbing or squeezing her thighs together and never touching her genitals with her hand (Kinsey et al., 1953). Others use vibrators, press their genitals against a soft object—such as a pillow—or run water over their genitals (Hite, 1976). Although most women adopt a favorite technique and stick to it, some use a variety of methods.

In addition to these basic techniques, different women use different body positions, sites of stimulation, and intensity of rhythm of stimulation. For example, some women want their legs apart while masturbating, some want their legs together, and others prefer to bend their knees. These preferences probably develop early and often are important throughout a woman's sexual life.

In the past decade, the use of the vibrator has increased greatly among women. At the time of the Kinsey survey (Kinsey et al., 1953), so few women used a vibrator that he could not assign a number to them. Later studies (Wolfe, 1981) have found that as many as 26 percent of women use them. Vibrators stimulate the genitals just as fingers do, but the stimulation is faster, steadier, and more intense than is possible with the hand (Heiman, LoPiccolo, and LoPiccolo, 1976). With some women, the effect is dramatic:

> I've been using the vibrator since last summer, but I never masturbated before then. . . . And would you believe it? I actually came in about three minutes after 25 years of not coming! (Dodson, 1983, p. 54)

Some therapists (Kaplan, 1974) believe that women can become "hooked" on the vibrator. Because it delivers an intense stimulation that neither she nor a partner can produce, a woman who uses a vibrator regularly may become unable to reach orgasm through manual stimulation or intercourse. This does seem to happen to a few women. For example, one woman reported:

> I'm afraid the vibrator has spoiled me a little. It's now harder to climax with a man. Also, it's even harder to climax while masturbating manually. . . . I'd like to give up my vibrator but am afraid I won't be able to do it until I'm married and in a very sexually satisfying relationship with my partner. On the other hand, I'm not sure how I'm going to accomplish this unless I give it up. (Wolfe, 1981, p. 169)

Thus, the quick, dependable vibrator-induced orgasm may lead some women to give up when orgasms in intercourse are slow to develop. Some therapists (Barbach, 1976) believe women who think they are becoming dependent on a vibrator can return to self- or partner-induced orgasms if they are truly interested. The problem arises, as it does with any form of masturbation, when a woman uses the vibrator in order to avoid or reject her partner.

For some women the problem is not dependence on a vibrator but a seeming inability to reach orgasm. Most sex therapists (Barbach, 1976; Heiman, LoPiccolo, and LoPiccolo, 1976) believe women can increase their sexual responsiveness by doing exercises in self-stimulation. In suggesting masturbation as a way to reach orgasm, therapists stress practice, time, and the right attitude.

The following exercise is similar to exercises prescribed by therapists. Once you have become comfortable with your body by practicing the body awareness exercises in Chapter 6, begin your self-stimulation in a relaxing atmosphere. The right mood can be induced with flowers, candles, incense, music, or whatever you find most sensual. After a relaxing bath, massage your body with oil and focus on the sensations you feel as you touch different areas. Caress your nipples, your stomach, your breasts, your thighs. Then, keeping the genital area moist, explore your vulva. Experiment with various strokes and pressures. Now turn your attention to your clitoris. While you stroke it, you may want to use muscle tension—perhaps doing Kegel exercises—to increase your arousal. As you feel yourself becoming aroused, relax and flow with your feelings.

Similar methods have been effective with women who never—or almost never—have orgasms. Among a group of several hundred women with orgasmic difficulties, 93 percent were consistently having masturbatory orgasms after a five-week group program featuring self-stimulation exercises. Within three months, more than half were also having orgasms with their partners (Barbach, 1976). Thus, it appears that the orgasmic responses learned during masturbation can be transferred to sexual activity with a partner.

## WHEN MEN MASTURBATE

Men have fewer techniques for masturbation than women do. Most often, men masturbate by rhythmically stroking the shaft of the penis. The variation comes in how firmly the penis is grasped, the speed of the movements, or how much of the shaft and head is stimulated. A few men masturbate without manual stimulation; for example, some lie face down and rub the penis against a sheet or bed cover while simulating the movements of intercourse. As with women, there are individual preferences as to body position—some men must lie down, others masturbate while standing.

Although virtually all men masturbate at some time, their feelings about it are usually a mixture of pleasure and discomfort. They may regard it as a necessary evil—a way of getting rid of sexual tension. One man summed up this attitude by saying:

> I really don't enjoy masturbating very much. Feel kind of deprived and angry when I have to do it. . . . But when something's got to be done. . . . (Shanor, 1978, p. 39)

Such a man may believe that masturbation indicates that he simply isn't good enough or man enough to have a sexual partner (Zilbergeld, 1978).

When carried out without guilt or shame, men's masturbation can result in improved sexual activity with a partner, just as it does for women. It can increase sexual skills, improve control over ejaculation, and help to solve problems with erection (Zilbergeld, 1978).

Exercises in self-stimulation for men are similar in many ways to those devised for women. The exercises recommended by Bernie Zilbergeld (1978) develop out of the body awareness exercises in Chapter 6 and require time, solitude, and a lack of pressure.

You can set an appropriate mood by controlling the light to suit your taste, by lighting candles or incense, or by playing music—so long as it is not distracting. Some of the body awareness techniques may be helpful in establishing your mood, as is recollecting a good sexual experience or looking at erotic material.

Begin by stroking other parts of your body before you touch your penis. As the exercise progresses, focus on the sensations in your penis, trying to discover just what sort of stroking feels best. Using a lubricant to reduce friction and enhance pleasure, spend about fifteen minutes experimenting with various strokes, pressures, and speeds. If you feel close to orgasm, stop, wait for the sensation to ebb, then begin again. After you discover new sensations and just how to evoke them, you can move on to other types of masturbation exercises developed to increase control over ejaculation and to reduce problems with erection.

For both men and women, masturbation is often accompanied and enhanced by sexual fantasy. Erotic images can initiate or heighten arousal and deepen pleasure in all kinds of sexual activity. They are an important part of most people's sexual lives.

## SEXUAL FANTASY

Sexual fantasies may accompany masturbation or sex with a partner, be a response to erotic books or movies, or be simply a form of daydreaming. This solitary sexual activity of the mind may be spontaneous, with the fantasies seeming to surface by themselves, or deliberate, with the person consciously constructing the episode. Fantasies may be fleeting images, such as one man's report of "rushing through space with no feeling of time or direction, or seeing exploding colors or fireworks" (Shanor, 1978, p. 125), or elaborate scenes that involve exotic places and detailed sexual encounters.

Freud viewed sexual fantasies as expressions of unconscious desires. Many psychologists today (Byrne and Byrne, 1977) believe that the content of sexual fantasies is the result of conditioning. The images have been associated with sexual arousal in the past and have themselves become psychogenic stimuli.

### *Fantasy during masturbation*

Fantasy is especially common during masturbation, and the proportion of women who fantasize at such times appears to be increasing. Three decades ago, only about half the women but three-fourths of the men interviewed by Kinsey (Kinsey et al., 1953) had sexual fantasies while masturbating. Kinsey concluded that fantasy played a far less important role in female arousal than it did with men. Such differences may be the result of cultural conditioning, because more recent surveys (Hunt, 1974), taken in a changed cultural climate, have found that as many women as men fantasize while masturbating.

Young people generally have a greater variety of fantasies—and fantasies of a

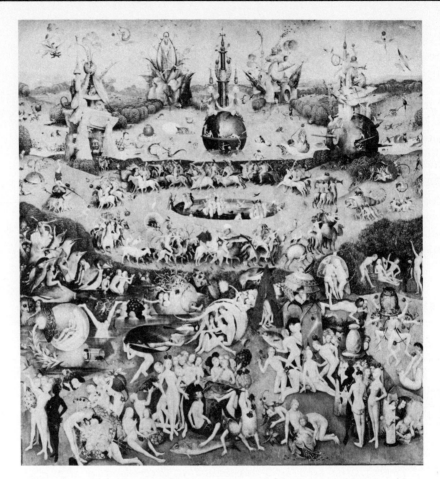

Sexual dreams and erotic fantasies take many forms, and in the 15th century Hieronymous Bosch put a variety of them into "The Garden of Delights." (EPA/Art Resource)

more daring nature—than older people (Hunt, 1974). Just why this is so is not clear. Perhaps the differences can be traced to the fact that the sexual impulse is stronger in young people. Or perhaps, having grown up in a less restrictive sexual atmosphere, young people tend to have a more experimental attitude toward sex. Or it may be that older people have become sexually conditioned to particular images.

Few generalizations can be made about masturbation fantasies. Some people are unable to masturbate without fantasy, while others have never used any fantasy during masturbation (Hite, 1976). Some people have the same fantasy whenever they masturbate; others continually invent new and different fantasies. Some fantasies are extremely elaborate and complex; others are simple images of the genitals. The most common fantasy during masturbation involves intercourse with a loved partner. Other fantasies focus on traditional positions of intercourse with partners of either sex, perhaps with strangers or with more than one person at a time. Fantasies sometimes center on socially unacceptable or forbidden acts. An adolescent boy summed up this sort of "forbidden" fantasy:

> That's almost the definition of a fantasy for me: something I'd never do. Then I feel free to do it in my mind without feeling guilty. Usually the things in my imagination would be real embarrassing to me, really humiliating if I was ever in one of those situations. (Bell, 1980, p. 77)

Forbidden fantasies may focus on sadism (sexual gratification from inflicting pain or humiliation on others), masochism (sexual gratification from receiving pain or humiliation), or rape.

## Fantasy during intercourse

Many people also fantasize from time to time during intercourse. The purpose of these fantasies varies. Some people say fantasies heighten arousal, some say they increase the attractiveness of the partner, and some say they allow imagined activities that are not part of intercourse with the partner. For some people, there seems to be no specific reason for fantasizing during sex; it may simply be a habit (Sue, 1979).

The content of intercourse fantasies resembles fantasies that accompany masturbation. Among both sexes, the most common fantasies involve oral sex or being irresistible to others, although fantasies about a former or an imaginary lover are also prevalent. Forbidden fantasies are also relatively common, as they are during masturbation (Sue, 1979).

Some therapists advise couples to share their fantasies if they can do so comfortably (Zilbergeld, 1978). Others agree that sharing fantasies about various activities or sex with celebrities may enrich intercourse, but point out that some fantasies are best kept private (Heiman, LoPiccolo, and LoPiccolo, 1976). Sharing sexual fantasies about former lovers, friends, or acquaintances may make a partner jealous. As with other aspects of sexual activity, what seems appropriate varies from couple to couple.

## Sex differences in fantasy

Although the sexual fantasies of men and women overlap a great deal in content, some consistent differences appear. Men's fantasies are just as likely to center on imaginary women as on former lovers or acquaintances. Women's fantasies tend to be about men they know. In one woman's words, her fantasies were about "old boyfriends, my friends' husbands, my husband's friends, even the paperboy" (Wolfe, 1981). But a man reported: "The woman is usually fictional or someone I don't know but have seen somewhere" (Shanor, 1978).

Women's fantasies also frequently focus on sex in which the woman is at first reluctant or fearful (Sue, 1979). In a typical report, one woman said:

> My favorite fantasies are of being overpowered, tied up, and teased until I'm begging a man to enter me. At which point, he does. There's no pain, but I am not able to resist what he is doing to me. (Wolfe, 1981, p. 190)

This sort of fantasy has nothing to do with rape; women almost never include physical abuse in these fantasies. Instead, they appear to be a way of allowing women to take sexual pleasure without feeling guilty (Crepault and Couture, 1980).

Men on the other hand, often have fantasies that center on sexual power or aggressiveness (Crepault and Couture, 1980). As one put it:

> A girl runs into my office, closes the door behind her, rips off her clothes, and begs me to have intercourse with her. (Shanor, 1978, p. 48)

It is not difficult to see cultural expectations and conditioning at work in these fantasies.

Our fantasies come from some inner stimulus to the imagination, but erotic literature can provide a stimulus from someone else's imagination (Goldstein and Kant, 1973). Although there may be important psychological differences between these two types of sexual fantasy, women's responses to erotic material indicate that traditional assumptions are probably wrong.

Sexologists had generally assumed that romance, not explicit sex, aroused women. As noted in Chapter 6, however, women and men responded similarly to erotic movies, with both most highly aroused by scenes of group sex. In a similar study (Heiman, 1975), men and women listened to tape-recorded scenes of explicit sex and romantic encounters. Both men and women responded most to straightforward explicit sex, preferring such scenes to romantic encounters without explicit sex or explicit sexual scenes in which the partners expressed affection for each other.

On the assumption that such sexual scenes might be arousing because the listening women were observers rather than participants, researchers (Mosher and White, 1980) had women imagine themselves as taking part in the sexual scenes they heard. No difference appeared in their arousal, whether the tape involved sex with "your fiance, who proposed marriage last week after a loving courtship" or with "an unusually attractive man you met in one of your classes last week."

Sex differences did appear when responses to self-generated fantasy and erotic tapes were compared. When women were asked to produce sexual fantasy in the laboratory, their arousal was not as high as when they heard tapes of explicit sexual encounters. Yet men's arousal was the same whether they produced the fantasy themselves or listened to someone else's production (Stock and Geer, 1982). However, the researchers noted that women who said they always fantasized while masturbating were more highly aroused both by their own fantasies and by the tapes than other women were. It may be that this sex difference in responsiveness to fantasy is primarily the result of experience.

# SEXUAL RESPONSE DURING
# SLEEP AND DREAMS

Solitary sexual responses are common during sleep, but their connection with dreams is uncertain. Although researchers have paid more attention to men's sexual responses during sleep, women seem to react in a similar manner.

## *Sex and sleep in men*

Almost all men have awakened in the morning with a firm erection. Because men find it difficult to urinate with an erection, many people attribute these erections to the pressure of urine in the bladder. However, there appears to be no connection between the condition of the bladder and nocturnal erections. Instead, erections occur at regular intervals during the night and are associated with a stage of sleep when most dreaming takes place.

Recordings of brain waves during sleep indicate that these waves show dramatic changes about once every ninety minutes. For about twenty minutes, breathing, heart rate, and blood pressure become irregular; muscles become limp, making movement impossible; and the eyes move rapidly beneath closed lids. Just before this rapid eye movement (REM) sleep begins, the penis usually becomes erect and often throbs. Although erection can occur in other stages of sleep and episodes of REM sleep occasionally pass without erection, about 90 percent of the time the two coincide (Karacan et al., 1972).

Since most dreaming takes place during REM sleep, it would appear that men are having sexual dreams. This is not necessarily the case. If awakened during a REM episode, men rarely report having a dream with obviously sexual content, and the erection seems to have nothing to do with sexual tension. Nocturnal erections have been measured in men who had ejaculated only a few hours earlier (Fisher et al., 1965). Yet there appears to be some connection between these erections and male hormones. Measurements of blood hormone levels during sleep indicate that testosterone levels often climb during REM sleep (Schiavi et al., 1982). We do not yet know just what causes either the increase in testosterone or the nocturnal erections.

The dependability of these nightly erections has been used by sex therapists to determine whether a man's inability to have an erection is due to physiological or psychological causes. An instrument that measures erection is placed over the penis before a man goes to sleep, and any erections are recorded. (See Figure 7.2.) If erections occur during sleep, the therapist is likely to assume that the man's problem is psychogenic.

Men's sexual responses in sleep are not limited to nocturnal erections. Most men also ejaculate in sleep from time to time. This **nocturnal emission,** or "wet dream," is most common among adolescents, whose first ejaculation may take place in this manner. Adolescents generally have nocturnal emissions about once each month. Once a man is in his twenties their frequency declines, but they can

**nocturnal emission**
ejaculation during sleep; also known as a "wet dream"

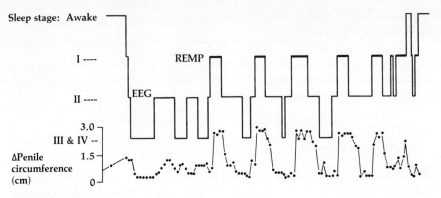

## Figure 7.2

A graph showing the relationship between erections (lower line) and REM sleep (upper line) in a healthy male.

take place at any age and have occurred in eighty-year-old men (Kinsey, Pomeroy, and Martin, 1948).

The nocturnal emission may be a way of releasing sexual tension. The sleeper usually feels sexually aroused, but his dream may not seem especially sexy. One man who had a nocturnal emission in the sleep laboratory said he dreamed he had had touched a woman's hand (Fisher et al., 1965).

## Sex and sleep in women

Although little research has been done, it appears that women may go through a cycle similar to that observed in men. Measures of blood flow in the vaginal walls indicate increased flow and pulse pressure—typical signs of sexual arousal—during periods of REM sleep (Abel et al., 1979).

Some women also have the equivalent of a wet dream. Although there is no emission, a woman is wakened by the vaginal contractions that accompany orgasm. A woman who said she had no sexual fantasies during her waking hours reported that her sleep was often sexy:

> I have experienced some incredible sexual fantasies in my dreams. I can't remember exactly what I fantasized about, but I do remember having a great orgasm. (Wolfe, 1981, p. 184)

This nocturnal orgasm is not as common in women as in men; less than 40 percent of the women in one study had experienced them (Kinsey et al., 1953). But one young woman reported having them from the time she was six years old (Sorenson, 1973).

Since the function of sleep itself is not completely understood and the role of REM sleep continues to puzzle researchers, our ignorance about the role of sexual responses during sleep should come as no surprise. That nocturnal arousal and orgasm commonly occur is established; *why* they occur is unknown.

Our solitary sexual activities are only a part of human sexuality, and they often involve images of activity with others. In our interactions with a partner, sexuality becomes social; now the wishes and responses of another affect what we do and how we feel about it.

# Summary

**1** **Masturbation** is any delibrate self-stimulation that produces a sexual response. Although it is practiced by almost everyone, the activity is often surrounded by confusion, misinformation, and shame.

**2** Both religious and medical authorities traditionally condemned masturbation. Psychoanalysts believed that it was common in children but a sign of immaturity in adults. Since the Kinsey surveys, however, people have come to understand that masturbation is common and "normal." Today sex researchers regard masturbation in a positive light.

**3** Almost all men and the vast majority of women have masturbated at some time in their lives. People generally masturbate for one of four reasons: instinctive self-stimulation, the expression of unacceptable desires, the search for an altered state of consciousness, or nonsexual reasons, such as the relief of tension or menstrual cramps. Masturbation can also be used to avoid sexual interaction or to reject a partner.

**4** There is no evidence that masturbation alters the appearance of the genitals or that it "uses up" sexual desire. Masturbation itself appears to be harmless, although the learned habits that accompany it can create sexual problems.

**5** Women use a wide variety of techniques when masturbating, although only a minority use any kind of vaginal penetration. In recent years, the use of the vibrator has increased among women, since it provides fast, steady, and intense stimulation. Many sex therapists believe that masturbation can help women to become orgasmic and that the response often transfers to sex with a partner.

**6** Men have fewer masturbatory techniques. Although almost all men masturbate, many feel discomfort about the practice as well as pleasure. However, when carried out without guilt or shame, masturbation can improve a man's sexual activity with a partner.

**7** Sexual fantasies are common during masturbation. Today it appears that about as many women as men fantasize during masturbation, although in the past such fantasies were more common among men. Many people also fantasize during intercourse, saying that it heightens arousal, increases the attractiveness of a partner, and allows imaginary participation in activities that are not part of intercourse with a partner. Sometimes, however, such fantasies appear to be simply habit. Although male and female sex fantasies overlap in content, men are more likely to fantasize about an imaginary partner, while women are more likely to fantasize about someone they know. Like men, women show higher arousal to explicit sex than to romantic interaction without explicit sex or to explicit sex with affection.

**8** About every ninety minutes during sleep, men enter a period of rapid eye movement (REM) sleep and develop an erection. Although they are usually dreaming, the dreams rarely have sexual content. However, testosterone levels generally climb during REM sleep. Men sometimes have **nocturnal emissions,** or "wet dreams," and report sexual arousal but dreams without much sexual content. Women appear to go through a similar cycle, with increased blood flow and pulse pressure in the vaginal walls during REM sleep. Some women also have orgasms during sleep, although such orgasms are less common than nocturnal emissions among men.

# 8 Sexual Interaction

# Chapter 8

Our sexual behavior is primarily the product of past experience; it is shaped by learning and by decisions we have made. At each stage in the life cycle we are exposed to a wide range of sexual options. Often without being aware that we are making a choice, we select from among these options. Our choices can be influenced by many factors—by what we learn about our sexual selves, by what we learn from our partners, and by what the culture says is acceptable or unacceptable. Attitudes, beliefs, emotions, and moods affect the way we interpret sexual situations, what we do in them, and how we react to what a partner does.

In the last chapter, we saw the great variety of solitary sexual behavior. Although masturbation can be satisfying, sex with a partner is the choice of most people. The possibilities for sexual interaction are limited only by our imaginations. The touches, kisses, caresses, and juxtaposition of body parts that make up sexual experience are combined by each of us in individual ways. Given the complexity of human behavior and the vast differences in individual experience, it's not surprising that no one has been able to count all the ways in which sexuality can be expressed.

The work of most sex researchers emphasizes the observable aspects of sexual behavior—type of behavior, number of orgasms—but often ignores its emotional significance. Yet human sexual behavior has nonsexual as well as sexual aspects and can communicate complex emotions. When sex communicates love, it becomes the focus of an intimate exchange that often brings out intense emotions. When sex is primarily recreational, it focuses on physical pleasure. And when sex is carried out primarily for reproductive purposes, it expresses our basic biological roles.

# Sexual Interaction

Depending on whether a person prefers to have sex with someone of the other sex or the same sex, behavior patterns are considered heterosexual or homosexual. Except for genital intercourse, there is a wide overlap between these patterns, and most of the other activities discussed in this chapter are as important in homosexual relationships as they are in relationships between heterosexuals.

We'll begin by considering the way sexual scripts influence behavior. We'll then take up a range of sexual behavior, looking first at touching and kissing. Oral sex, we'll discover, has become increasingly common, with greater changes in sexual practice than in attitudes. Next we'll investigate intercourse, discussing its evolution and general frequency, as well as discussing the common positions. After a consideration of anal sex, we'll close with a look at afterplay.

## SEXUAL SCRIPTS FOR MEN AND WOMEN

In our sexual activities, each of us has a sexual script, or pattern, consisting of various acts that generally take a similar order (Gagnon and Simon, 1973). The words or gestures we use to initiate a sexual encounter begin the script by inviting a partner to participate. When no coercion is involved, acceptance begins a sexual exchange.

**foreplay** kissing, hugging, stroking and oral stimulation that may precede intercourse or may make up the entire sexual encounter

The next stage of sexual interaction is often called **foreplay**. In most Western societies, caressing, kissing, undressing, and touching the nongenital areas set the stage for genital contact. Foreplay is important in establishing trust and intimacy, and in overcoming inhibitions against touching or being touched. Some people become aroused during the early stages of foreplay; others prefer more extended contact. Many people enjoy foreplay for its own sake and feel no necessity to proceed further. At times, the sexual script ends here.

The words we use often have a powerful influence on the way we interpret our actions. When called "foreplay," kissing, hugging, stroking, and oral stimulation are generally seen as minor events that precede the main act of intercourse. According to Bernie Zilbergeld (1978), men are particularly susceptible to the myth that foreplay is a relatively unimportant preliminary. Since men are brought up to be goal-oriented, and since most men see the goal of sex as intercourse and orgasm, many either ignore or slight foreplay. As a result, they miss many stimulating and pleasurable experiences.

Amount and type of foreplay vary greatly among cultures. In some societies foreplay is minimal, with almost no contact or embracing before intercourse; in others, foreplay may last for several hours. Prolonged stimulation of the woman's breast is common among a number of tribal societies, but virtually unknown in others. Among some groups, men are forbidden to touch female genitals, but women are free to handle male genitals (Ford and Beach, 1951).

Manual or oral stimulation of the genitals can be seen as advanced foreplay or the focus of sexual interaction. A person who wishes to avoid intercourse, pregnancy, or the loss of virginity might find such stimulation a satisfactory alternative to genital intercourse. When used as foreplay, these techniques can provide the man with a firm erection and the woman with vaginal lubrication, preparing them both for intercourse.

For most heterosexuals, penile-vaginal intercourse is the central act of the sexual script. Indeed, for some people, sex *is* intercourse. As one woman said:

> If only I could get over this feeling of wanting the "real thing." There seems to be so much pressure to have intercourse every time we make love. (Authors' files)

In every culture studied, genital intercourse is the most preferred sexual activity, although position, timing, and technique vary from one society to another (Ford and Beach, 1951).

Most people define the end of the sexual script as male orgasm. However, as male and female roles are redefined, this definition is changing. Many couples incorporate a period of **afterplay** into their pattern of sexual activity, in which sexual contact continues after one or both partners have reached orgasm. Afterplay usually takes the form of touching and kissing.

This sequence of sexual behavior—initiation, foreplay, intercourse, and afterplay—is the most typical and socially approved sexual script. But people often vary its sequence, and the variation may be as obvious as a new technique or as subtle as a change in the feelings associated with a particular technique (Gagnon, Rosen, and Leiblum, 1982). But no matter what form or sequence sexual activity takes, touching is likely to play a major role.

# THE SEXUAL TOUCH—FROM PETTING TO FOREPLAY

Many of us have felt the sudden shock, like a jolt of electricity, that comes at the mere brush of the fingertips of a highly desired partner. Touching and being touched, it seems, are a primary way of expressing our sexual feelings. In a sense, all sexual behavior, from kissing to intercourse, is based on the sense of touch. In fact, the skin may be the basic organ of perception and communication (Montagu, 1971). Although we usually think of the sexual touch as arousing, skin contact can also convey feelings of intimacy, comfort, safety, and love. Touch is so important that our language is filled with expressions based on it, such as "rubbing people the wrong way," "getting in touch," "different strokes for different folks," "making contact," and "being thick-skinned."

Among animals, touching often takes the form of grooming. In this case, touch improves health and cleanliness while it strengthens social bonds. Apes and monkeys spend considerable amounts of time scratching and licking one another and removing insects or dirt from fur. Sometimes grooming leads to intercourse. For instance, the female baboon in estrus frequently grooms the male as a way of ensuring his sexual attention. A low-status male chimpanzee may groom a female in order to curry favor with her (Ford and Beach, 1951). Grooming as a sexual prelude is not confined to animals. In some cultures, couples spend hours cleaning, primping, and touching before sexual intercourse begins.

In American culture, sexual touching can be viewed as an end in itself or as a prelude to intercourse. When sexual touching stops short of intercourse, it's called

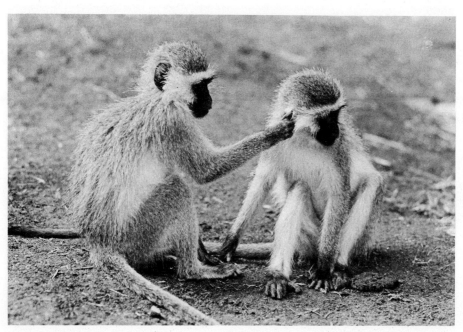

Among primates, grooming serves several important functions. It maintains cleanliness, strengthens social bonds, and may lead to intercourse. (© Ira Kirschenbaum/ Stock, Boston)

necking or petting. When that same touching leads to intercourse, it's generally called foreplay. Although most people think of petting as adolescent behavior and foreplay as typical of adults, there are many exceptions. Adults with long-standing sexual relationships may sometimes enjoy petting without intercourse, and some adolescents use touch only as foreplay.

## Petting

**petting** tactile stimulation of any part of the body that stops short of intercourse

Petting can be defined as the tactile stimulation of any part of the body, but it usually involves the face, hair, neck, breasts, and genitals. Such behavior may be viewed as an American compromise between pressure for premarital chastity and the sexual liberalism that developed in the 1920s (Hunt, 1974).

By midcentury, petting was both common and frequent and women were more likely than men to have had petting experience, perhaps because the double standard of sexual morality made women more likely to postpone intercourse. The highest incidence and frequency of petting was found among the youngest women and those with advanced education (Kinsey et al., 1953). Twenty-five years later, petting had become even more acceptable. One young woman described her own experience:

> We used to make out almost every night after my parents went to bed. I knew he wanted to go all the way, but I wasn't ready yet, even though I knew the time would come. (Authors' files)

"Making out" is an important phase of sexual experimentation and development. It helps teenagers to establish trust and intimacy and to overcome inhibitions. (© Joan Liftin/Archive)

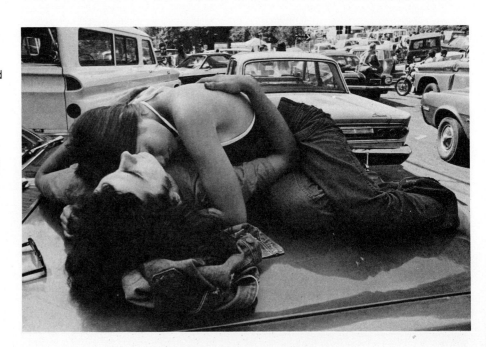

Most people now approved of petting, particularly in an affectionate relationship, and both men and women were much more likely to pet to orgasm than they had been in the 1950s (Hunt, 1974).

Despite the prevalence of petting, Alfred Kinsey (Kinsey, Pomeroy, and Martin, 1948) had mixed feelings about it. He found that adolescent petting experience tended to be followed by good sexual adjustment in marriage—perhaps because petting teaches sexual communication. This was especially true of women. Women with no petting experience, he believed, might find sex after marriage a traumatic experience. Yet Kinsey was concerned that arousal from lengthy petting that did not lead to orgasm might seriously disturb some people by leaving them in an extended nervous state. Some men in his study reported pain unless they masturbated soon after the end of a long petting session.

The specific feeling of tension or pain that some men feel in their genitals after prolonged petting or intercourse without ejaculation is often called "blue balls." Many people believe that the sensation comes from a buildup of semen, but it is actually produced by vasocongestion and muscle tension. The feeling can easily be relieved by masturbation, but men sometimes use their discomfort to pressure partners into intercourse. We hear a great deal about "blue balls," but not much about the fact that women may also feel pain or tension after prolonged petting. Some women say they experience abdominal discomfort after lengthy petting or intercourse without orgasm.

## Types of touching

Whether we experience touch as pleasurable or exciting depends to a large extent on learning. A particular touch—say, anal stimulation—may be arousing to someone who sees this activity as "normal," and unpleasant to someone who sees it as "abnormal." Men and women often develop preferences for a pattern of touching that is associated with past sexual experiences or that closely duplicates the stimulation they use during masturbation. These individual differences highlight the importance of communication during foreplay.

The need for communication is especially important in genital stimulation. Women, for example, prefer very different patterns of clitoral stimulation. Some like a soft touch, others want firm pressure; some like direct clitoral stimulation, other find direct touching to be uncomfortable or painful. One woman complained:

> So many men hurt me when they rub my clitoris. I can come with the
> slightest amount of clitoral pressure, but when a man starts to rub me hard
> there, the way *they* like to be rubbed hard, I want to scream with pain, not
> pleasure. (Wolfe, 1981, p. 100)

In the same way, men learn to prefer particular patterns of penile or other stimulation, and unless they tell their partners, they may not get the sort of touching they like. One man volunteered:

> During foreplay, I like to have my partner scratch the underneath part of my
> testicles. She pulls my balls up toward my penis and scratches the underneath
> part—not in a painful, hurting way—but in a stimulating way as someone
> might scratch a dog. (Shanor, 1978, p. 216)

In Chapter 10, we'll consider ways of communicating these preferences.

Most people think of sexual touching as soft movements of the hands over a
partner's body, but some individuals are aroused by scratching, tickling, and biting.
Although a positive response to painful stimulation is generally considered masochistic, conventional sexual patterns in some societies include pinching, scratching, and biting by both partners.

Human beings are born with the physiological capacity to respond erotically
to mild degrees of pain, and this capacity can be shaped by childhood experiences.
When a culture teaches its children that biting or pinching can bring sexual satisfaction, and when such behavior is seen as an essential part of the sexual script, it will
generally be perceived as sexual pleasure. However, cultures that encourage mild
pain as part of their sexual patterns also emphasize mutuality and lack of coercion.
The woman who allows her partner to bite her usually enjoys the opportunity to
bite back (Ford and Beach, 1951).

Tickling is another form of touch that can be arousing or inhibiting, depending on a person's past experiences. No one understands why some people are ticklish and others are not, but there are clearly large individual differences in erotic
responses to tickling. Perhaps the giggles, laughter, and playful struggles that often
accompany tickling are ways of building emotional intimacy and thus work to enhance sexual desire and arousal. A very ticklish person, however, may find the
sense of being out of control so uncomfortable that it inhibits sexual response.

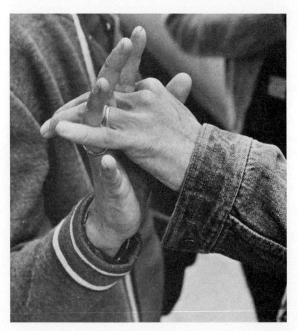

Touching is a basic way of
expressing intimacy, and the
context of the touch
determines whether it is
perceived as sexual.
(© Bohdan Hrynewych/
Stock, Boston)

Touch can be sexual in other ways as well. Simply exploring the skin and the contours of a partner's body with no other goal than to enjoy the tactile perceptions can be a high form of sensual pleasure (Masters and Johnson, 1970). It can be even more pleasurable for the partner. One man described his feelings:

> When I'm hot and horny, my entire body is super-sensitive, especially my back
> and feet. I love to massage and be massaged during this period, before
> heavier things. (Hite, 1981, p. 551)

Whatever sort of touching partners prefer or use, touch is a primary form of sexual communication. Kissing, an activity we associate with sex in many forms, can be seen as a special form of touching.

# KISSING

Kissing is probably the most widely accepted sexual act in Western society and the only one that can be performed in public without causing raised eyebrows. Indeed, the assumption that all sexual relationships include kissing is so strong that most recent sex surveys don't even bother to ask about it. Kissing seems such a normal, instinctive, pleasurable, and desirable way of expressing affection that most of us take it for granted.

Yet a look at the customs of other cultures reveals that there is nothing "natural" about the kiss. Like most other sexual behavior, the sexual value of the kiss is more a matter of learning than of instinct. Among 190 tribal societies, only 21 have any form of kissing. Among the rest, many societies consider mouth-to-mouth contact to be unpleasant, unhealthy, even disgusting. At their first sight of Europeans kissing, the Thonga laughed, saying: "Look at them—they eat each other's saliva and dirt" (Ford and Beach, 1951).

Some societies that approve of kissing use techniques that are not common in Western cultures. For example, the Arapesh touch lips and inhale, while the Lapps kiss the nose and mouth at the same time (Tiefer, 1978). The absence of kissing doesn't necessarily mean that a society is sexually restrictive. The Mangaian people of Polynesia are sexually permissive and train young women to reach orgasm, but kissing was unknown before they encountered Western culture (Marshall, 1971).

Human beings learn to associate sexual pleasure with kissing, and the learning may begin in the cradle, when the child learns that the mouth is a source of pleasure. The growing child learns that society connects kissing with sex, and games like "Spin the Bottle" and "Post Office" give children and young adolescents an opportunity to exchange mouth-to-mouth kisses in an otherwise nonsexual situation. Such games are marked more by giggles, blushes, and derision than by sexual desire. Although kissing games may not provide much sexual pleasure, their social rewards ensure continued practice in the art of kissing (Tiefer, 1978).

Kissing is usually the first step toward adolescent petting, and kissing games usually begin with closed lips and no tongue contact. With time, the pattern of petting broadens to include deep kissing, in which one partner thrusts the tongue into

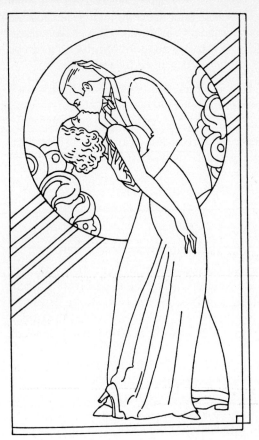

In the early 20th century, when sexual contact before marriage was frowned upon, the sexual kiss held enormous significance. This illustration is from a popular 1936 manual, *The Art of Kissing.*

the other's mouth, and kissing other parts of the body. As with most aspects of human behavior, individual preferences develop out of such experiences. Some people prefer light, soft contact; others prefer more pressure.

The sexual kiss has many variations—so many that the German language has about thirty words to describe its different types. For example, the word *abkussen* means giving little kisses to different parts of the face. In English, "soul kissing" or "French kissing" describes deep kisses with the tongue active, while the "butterfly kiss" refers to fluttering movements of the eyelashes against a lover's cheek.

Not all kisses are sexual. When a kiss is exchanged, its meaning depends on the context and the script involved. But when the kiss is set within the sexual interaction, it can be highly arousing. As one woman wrote:

> Two or three minutes of tongue-kissing is almost all the foreplay I need. After that, I'm extremely well-lubricated. (Wolfe, 1981, p. 98)

Kissing may be the most widely known and accepted act in Western societies, but oral sex appears to be widely practiced yet often unaccepted. As lovers, we expect to kiss; we don't always expect to have oral sex.

# ORAL SEX

Oral sex, or sexual contact between the mouth, lips, or tongue of one person and the genitals of the other, is an optional element in sex with a partner. It may be the main act or part of foreplay or afterplay. But despite its popularity among both homosexuals and heterosexuals, the practice of oral sex is often controversial.

There are enormous differences in the degree to which oral sex is accepted from one culture to another. Even within the same culture, there are strong differences in how people feel about it. Husbands and wives have had bitter conflicts over this issue, and wives have murdered their husbands because they insisted on oral sex (Kinsey, Pomeroy, and Martin, 1948). Yet attitudes can change, as one woman found out:

> I used to feel that there was something dirty about oral sex. Now that I'm with someone who really enjoys it, my feelings have changed. In fact, I'm starting to realize how much I've been missing all these years. (Authors' files)

A culture's attitude toward oral sex is revealed by the words it uses to describe the practice. In the United States, the technical terms for oral sex come from Latin: **fellatio** (from *fellare,* meaning "to suck") for oral stimulation of the penis, and **cunnilingus** (from *cunnus,* meaning "vulva" and *lingere,* meaning "to lick") for oral stimulation of the female genitals. Numerous slang expressions, such as "blowjob," "giving head," and "going down," are part of the common vocabulary.

**fellatio** oral stimulation of the penis

**cunnilingus** oral stimulation of the female genitals

Most of the slang terms convey a negative attitude. In an attempt to avoid negative terms, Theodore Van de Velde (1926) coined the expression "genital kiss," which has been adopted by some sex educators (Comfort, 1972). Other cultures use positive terms to describe oral sex. Perhaps the most beautiful description of cunnilingus is the Sanskrit "licking a lotus blossom" and of fellatio, the Japanese "playing the flute" (Edwardes and Masters, 1962).

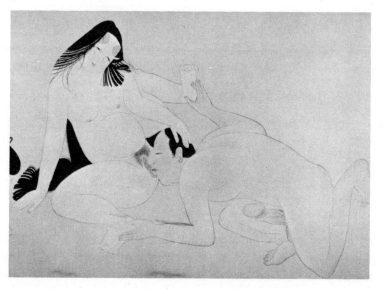

The view of Eastern cultures toward oral sex is revealed by their positive terms for the practice. In Sanskrit, cunnilingus is called "licking a lotus blossom," and the Japanese refer to fellatio as "playing the flute." (From EROTIC ART by Phyllis and Eberhard Kronhausen, Bell Publishing Company, 1968.)

*Focus*

The Judeo-Christian tradition contains powerful prohibitions against oral sex, and in some states oral-genital contact, even between husband and wife, is illegal. However, information from sex surveys shows that oral sex is practiced by a great number of Americans.

The first systematic survey with evidence on oral sex came from Alfred Kinsey (Kinsey, Pomeroy and Martin, 1948; Kinsey et al., 1953). He believed taboos against oral sex probably led some of the people he interviewed to lie about the practice. Nevertheless, among the men, close to 60 percent had given or received oral sex. The practice was related to educational level, with 72 percent of the college-educated men but only 40 percent of those with a grade-school education having experience with oral sex. Among women, about 50 percent had participated in cunnilingus and fellatio. Educa-

tional level was also related to the practice among women: 62 percent of the college-educated women reported giving fellatio, and 46 percent reported receiving cunnilingus.

In the years since the Kinsey survey, oral sex has become more generally accepted in American society. In fact, recent surveys among readers of *Redbook* and *Cosmopolitan* have found it part of standard sexual practices among younger people. In the *Redbook* survey, for example, more than 90 percent of the women had tried oral sex. Even among religious women—a group Kinsey had found unlikely to engage in the practice—more than 80 percent said they had experienced oral-genital contact (Tavris and Sadd, 1977). In the *Cosmopolitan* survey, 84 percent of the women reported regular participation in cunnilingus and fellatio (Wolfe, 1981).

In most instances, women reacted positively to oral sex. Only 10 percent of the women who had experienced cunnilingus found it neutral or unpleasant (Tavris and Sadd, 1977). Other surveys found that some women who cannot reach orgasm through genital intercourse do have orgasms during cunnilingus (Hite, 1976). Among women who had tried fellatio, 72 percent enjoyed the experience (Tavris and Sadd, 1977).

Women who enjoyed oral sex and practiced it frequently were most likely to rate their marriages and sex lives as excellent. Conversely, women who strongly rejected oral sex often reported less satisfactory sex lives and more sexual inhibition. It may be a general willingness to experiment rather than the specific practice of oral sex that contributes to satisfying sexual relations (Tavris and Sadd, 1977).

## Attitudes toward oral sex

American attitudes toward oral sex have not kept pace with our dramatic shift in behavior. Although oral sex has become a relatively common part of the sexual script, remnants of the Victorian heritage linger.

Some people regard oral sex as unclean, unsanitary, or a health risk. Such people are often concerned with taking such bodily fluids as urine, semen, or vaginal lubrication into their mouths. Thus, some women are reluctant to perform fellatio for fear that the man might ejaculate. Others worry about what to do with the semen should ejaculation occur. They don't want to swallow it but fear that spitting it out will offend their partners.

However, there is no need to worry on sanitary grounds. Such fluids are harmless in a healthy individual and present a danger only when the partner already has some sexually transmitted disease. Oral sex transmits fewer germs than does kissing.

Some people object on religious, moral, or esthetic grounds. The Judeo-Christian emphasis on sex for procreation led to the labeling of oral sex as "unnatural" or "immoral." Indeed, studies generally find a lower acceptance of oral sex among people who regularly attend religious services. Among students at a private church-related college, the incidence of fellatio and cunnilingus among male students was at about the same level that Kinsey had found thirty years before—just over half. Among female students, less than a third had tried fellatio and less than half had experienced cunnilingus (Young, 1980).

Objections to oral sex have been answered by those who see such behavior as normal and acceptable. According to the biological argument, the mouth and genitals are the most erotically sensitive parts of the body, so oral sex may be a simple, instinctive sexual act that has been inhibited by cultural restrictions (Kinsey, Pomeroy, and Martin, 1948). There are also practical arguments in favor of oral sex. For example, since it both stimulates the genitals and provides the natural lubricant of saliva, oral sex is an effective form of foreplay. In addition, oral sex carries no risk of pregnancy.

Individuals who are experiencing sexual problems may find oral sex satisfying because it requires neither a male erection nor female vaginal lubrication. For similar reasons, older couples who want to maintain an active sex life and who encounter the diminished vaginal lubrication and the occasional erectile failures that are a normal part of aging may find oral sex a good addition to their sexual activities. Finally, oral sex provides variety. Some people find that when sex is limited to intercourse, it becomes boring; in such cases, oral sex can help to stimulate renewed sexual interest.

## The pleasures of oral sex

Oral sex is almost always pleasurable when practiced by people who are free of cultural inhibitions and who use careful and considerate techniques. Beyond the physical pleasure of oral stimulation is the psychological meaning of the act. As a woman explained:

> The reason I enjoy cunnilingus so much is that it is such an intimate act. I feel totally accepted and appreciated—all of me! (Authors' files)

Not everyone feels this way. Some people find oral sex less intimate than genital intercourse. One man reported:

> Usually I'll stop her short and try for intercourse since there isn't a feeling of oneness with oral sex. I want to hold on to someone when I'm close to coming. (Hite, 1981, p. 531)

And a woman reported similar feelings:

> My lovers always want to go down on me. But I don't like it. It seems so impersonal. They're so far away. I don't mind doing it to a man, but I don't like it when they do it to me and I get excited and there's no one to hold in my arms. (Wolfe, 1981, p. 103)

Yet for many men and women, receiving oral stimulation is full of emotional meaning because it shows the partner's love and caring.

Sharing oral sex can also be intrinsically pleasurable, and some men and women become highly aroused when they perform the act. They may also derive pleasure from watching the partner as he or she responds to the stimulation.

Is the pleasure of oral sex a matter of instinct or of learning? Those who stress the importance of instinct point out that oral-genital contacts are prevalent in most mammals, especially the higher apes (Ford and Beach, 1951). Odors released from the genitals of either sex may stimulate a reflexive licking response in animals and human beings. However, oral sex may be a nonsexual grooming response in other mammals, despite the fact that it has an erotic meaning among human beings.

As noted earlier, Kinsey speculated that cultural inhibitions had overpowered instinct in this case. By teaching us that the genitals are dirty, learning plays a role in creating those inhibitions. However, learning can also help us to overcome cultural inhibitions. When we learn that proficiency in oral sex is expected of competent and mature individuals, we begin to experiment with oral sex. Rewards from the partner—in the form of feedback that oral sex is enjoyable—help us to overcome our learned aversion (Gagnon and Simon, 1973).

Once the notion that the pleasures of oral sex are learned is accepted, the value of learning specific techniques becomes apparent (Figure 8.1). Sexual anatomy and preferred patterns of stimulation vary from one person to the next. In giving fellatio, slow, firm, and steady movements of the lips and tongue are generally most effective. In giving cunnilingus, gentle tongue movements over the labia and clitoral shaft provide the most effective stimulation (Hite, 1976).

*Figure 8.1*

A common position for simultaneous oral-genital stimulation, sometimes referred to as the "69" position.

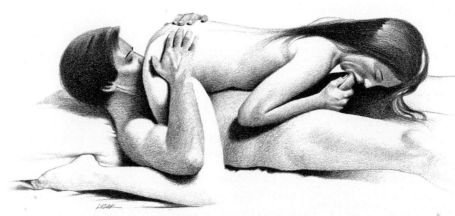

It's important, however, to fit the technique of oral sex to a partner's needs. What is pleasurable to one person may well be unpleasant to another. For example, many authorities advise never letting the teeth touch the penis during fellatio. Yet one man says:

> I enjoy having my penis gently skimmed with my partner's teeth as she's on the up motions. (Shanor, 1978, p. 217)

And other authorities advise sucking the shaft of the clitoris (Haeberle, 1978), although some women find this sort of stimulation too intense and even unpleasant.

So there is no one "right" way to perform oral sex, and the ability to learn from experience is probably the key to developing effective techniques. Communication between partners is just as important in oral sex as in other aspects of the sexual relationship, as we'll see in Chapter 10.

There is, however, one shadow over the new acceptance of oral sex. Therapists caution that this acceptance may lead to a new set of performance demands. Performance and failure are two sides of the same coin, and demands for perfect performance often lead to stress. But when oral sex is viewed as an expression of intimate feelings, it can do much to enhance a sexual relationship, whether it is the major sexual activity or a prelude to intercourse.

# INTERCOURSE

Intercourse, when used without a qualifying adjective such as "oral" or "anal," generally refers to genital intercourse, or **coitus**, in which the penis is inserted in the vagina. Coitus, the scientific term, has never caught on with the public, perhaps because as Eric Berne suggests, it "sounds sticky, like walking through molasses in a pair of sneakers" (1970, p. 3). But there's no misunderstanding when the popular word, "fuck," is used. Fuck as a term for coitus has been with us since the sixteenth century and probably comes from an old Germanic verb for penetrate.

**coitus** genital intercourse, in which the penis is inserted into the vagina

Intercourse occupies center stage in most sexual interaction, as the adolescent expression "going all the way" indicates. The major reason for its importance is that genital intercourse—unlike other forms of sexual behavior—has an obvious connection with reproduction.

## *Intercourse and evolution*

This link between sexual intercourse and reproduction makes the effect of natural selection on patterns of intercourse an important consideration. From an evolutionary perspective, the central point is how any pattern of intercourse contributes to reproductive success.

When human beings lost the dependence on the estrus cycle that controls intercourse in lower mammals (see Chapter 3), human intercourse became inefficient. Freed from hormonal control, human beings often had intercourse when there was no possibility of pregnancy. This meant that unless men and women were motivated to have frequent intercourse, they might not produce enough offspring to maintain the species.

The loss of human reproductive efficiency led psychologist Frank Beach (1976) to conclude that intercourse patterns evolved as a way of coping. For example, people compensate for the loss of hormonal signals for sex with symbols. Words, pictures, sounds, and gestures can arouse human beings. Another way of meeting this need for more frequent intercourse was the development of a nuclear family based on bonding between a woman and a man. The intensified and prolonged bond increased the frequency of intercourse. A third evolutionary development was the female orgasm. Since orgasm does not depend on the hormone cycle, it continually motivates women to have intercourse.

Not all experts agree that human intercourse patterns evolved in order to compensate for the lack of estrus control. In fact, psychiatrist Mary Jane Sherfey (1973) believes that the effect of civilization and the development of the nuclear family do not promote frequency of intercourse, but instead restrain and control the potentially "insatiable" demands of female sexuality. Sherfey maintains that a highly developed sexual capacity, the freedom from direct hormonal control, and the potential for multiple orgasms have contributed to the evolution of an inordinate sexual drive in women. To support her claims, she presents evidence that in preagricultural times it was not uncommon for women to dominate society and to engage in much higher rates of intercourse than are found today. In her view, modern patriarchal societies are based on the suppression of female sexuality.

More recently, sociobiologist Sarah Blaffer Hrdy (1981), who agrees with Sherfey that orgasm makes women sexually assertive, has proposed that female orgasms contributed to evolutionary success—but not in a monogamous context. By making women more likely to have multiple sexual partners, female orgasm made males uncertain about the paternity of offspring. Each male who had intercourse with a female could be expected to protect, care for, or at least tolerate the infant she bore. Such protection increased the likelihood that offspring would survive. Hrdy sees the political and sexual control of women as male attempts to keep from being tricked into supporting some other man's child.

## How often do people have intercourse?

If evolution has guaranteed frequent intercourse, how often does it occur? Among human beings, no "standard" frequency exists. Although biology and the aging process can limit a person's potential for intercourse and orgasm, the major influences on frequency appear to be social. Cultural expectations probably influenced this man's experience:

> I used to think that we should be having sex every night of the week. It got to
> be a tremendous pressure after a while. Now I realize that it's quality and not
> quantity that counts. (Authors' files)

Different cultures have vastly different expectations about the "normal" frequency of intercourse. Among the Mangaians of Polynesia, for example, young men report having intercourse from five to seven nights per week, with an average of two or three orgasms per night. Older men report one orgasm per night, but have intercourse from two to four nights per week (Marshall, 1971). In contrast, the Capaya tribe of Latin America appears to operate at diminished sexual levels. Although the Capaya admire male virility, newly married Capayan men say they usually have intercourse no more than once or twice a week (Altschuler, 1971).

In most tribal societies, adults generally engage in intercourse once a day during periods when sex is permitted. Some groups expect that young men and women will have intercourse many times on the same day. Among polygamous tribes, a man may be expected to have intercourse with each of his wives in a single night. Even in the most sexually active societies, however, intercourse is often taboo. Some cultures forbid intercourse with a woman who is menstruating or nursing a child. Some forbid intercourse in connection with religious rites, during wartime, or while preparing for occupational roles (Ford and Beach, 1951).

Compared with most tribal societies, intercourse frequencies in the United States are low. Married couples have intercourse about two and a half times a week, although younger couples have intercourse more often and older couples less often than average (Hunt, 1974). As we'll see in Chapter 13, age, length of marriage, and religious conviction all seem to affect rate of intercourse. But these factors do not explain why American rates are only about one-third of those found in Polynesia.

Perhaps the way our culture prepares us for marital sex and the condition of sexual life within marriage provide a better explanation (Gagnon, 1977). Although Americans spend a great deal of time learning to find and attract a mate, they pay relatively little attention to remaining attractive after marriage. The presence of children may also complicate marital sexuality: Parents may find they have little privacy and little time for each other. They may also find it difficult to reconcile their roles as sexual partner and parent. Repetition of the same sexual script may lead to boredom and reduce activity among some couples, although others may find repetition comfortable and satisfying. For whatever reason, Americans seem to be less sexually active than human beings in some other cultures. One man apparently spoke for a number of Americans when he said:

> I am ashamed to tell you how often I have intercourse, it is so infrequent. The only time we have frequent and satisfactory intercourse is when we are away together on vacation, or when we are free from family stresses. (Hite, 1981, p. 378)

Since there is no "normal" coital frequency and since human sexuality shows such wide individual differences, what seems like "too often" for one person will seem like "not often enough" for another. People seem to vary as much in the frequency of intercourse as they do in the time they devote to it.

## Intercourse positions

Although there may be more than 600 possible ways in which a man and woman can arrange their bodies during intercourse, all are variations on a few basic positions (Comfort, 1972). The couple can sit, stand, lie down, face each other, or the

# Focus

## HOW LONG DOES INTERCOURSE LAST?

**intromission** insertion of the penis into the vagina

Among most mammals, the amount of time spent in the act of intercourse depends primarily on how long it takes the male to ejaculate after **intromission,** or the insertion of the penis. Among apes and chimpanzees, it usually takes place in less than thirty seconds, although in some primate species, the male delays ejaculation by dismounting from time to time. The prize for the longest intercourse seems to go to the mink and the sable. These animals may continue intercourse for as long as eight hours. Although the males ejaculate a number of times during this period, the penis is not withdrawn (Ford and Beach, 1951).

The duration of intercourse also varies among human societies. The men of Ifugao, an island in the South Pacific, ejaculate almost immediately after penetration, but the people of Bali believe that hasty intercourse produces deformed children. Traditional sexual patterns in China and India place considerable emphasis on prolonging intercourse through techniques that delay ejaculation (Edwardes and Masters, 1962). The factors that determine the duration of intercourse have little connection with physiology; instead, they seem closely linked to social conventions and cultural expectations.

In American society there is an emerging trend toward prolonged intercourse. Among the factors that account for the trend are recognition of the sexual rights of women, increased variety in conventional sexual scripts, and a tendency to view a man's ability to control ejaculation as an indication of sexual competence. One man expressed this belief by saying:

If only I could begin to hold out a bit longer before I come. It's so frustrating to lose it every time just when things are really getting going. (Authors' files)

Although it's difficult to make precise comparisons, length of intercourse among American men appears to have increased considerably since the time of the Kinsey survey, when many men reported that they ejaculated within two minutes (Kinsey, Pomeroy, and Martin, 1948). Men in all classes of society now report that intercourse lasts about ten

---

woman can turn her back; either partner can be on top, or both can lie on their sides.

Individual preferences play some role in the choice of position. A person's sexual architecture may make some positions more comfortable or satisfying than others. Physical constraints, such as pregnancy or physical handicap, may also influence the choice. But the most important influence may come from the culture. In both subtle and blatant ways, a culture sends messages about which positions are "natural" and which "unnatural," which are "sexy," which awkward, which comfortable, which approved, and which forbidden.

**The basic positions** Most people use four or five variations out of the 600 possible positions for intercourse. Searches for the "ideal" position are likely to result in different solutions, since the most desirable position for any couple is largely a matter of personal preference.

minutes from intromission to ejaculation, with younger men taking about three minutes longer than older men (Hunt, 1974).

However, information about the duration of intercourse that comes from surveys should be taken with several grains of salt. Few people have actually timed themselves in the act, and estimates of its duration are always based on what people can recall. The experience of one group of medical students shows how inaccurate such recall may be. These students saw a film of a young couple engaged in sexual activity. The next day each student was asked to estimate how long the foreplay and intercourse portions of the film had lasted. Students estimated the length of foreplay in the movie with much greater accuracy than the length of intercourse. Both men and women significantly *overestimated* the duration of intercourse (Levitt and Duffy, 1977).

How do we explain these results? People's estimates of time are easily affected by intense emotion. If the act of intercourse had greater emotional impact that the aspects of foreplay, the students' overestimation is understandable. People who rate the duration of their own intercourse may overestimate it even more than these medical students did, since people are likely to experience more intense emotion while engaging in intercourse than while watching a film.

The desire to prolong intercourse often sends couples in search of ways to delay ejaculation. They try distraction techniques, ranging from mental mathematics to sudden applications of ice, anesthetic creams, and a variety of sex therapy treatments to counter what they believe is premature ejaculation. In Chapter 14, we'll discuss some of these treatments. Such methods are often helpful, but an exaggerated concern with this aspect of sexual performance might lead some people to pay too much attention to "staying power" and to neglect other aspects of sexuality (Rosen and Rosen, 1977). Either partner knows when a sexual experience has been gratifying, and satisfaction is rarely just a matter of timing.

**Face-to-face, man-above** The face-to-face, man-above position is called the "matrimonial position" (Figure 8.2) by Alex Comfort (1972), who recommends it because it adapts to any mood: tough or tender, long or quick, deep or shallow. A major advantage of this position is the opportunity it provides for eye contact, kissing, and other forms of intimacy during intercourse.

Numerous variations can add to the comfort or intensity of stimulation—the woman's legs can be wide apart and the knees drawn up for deeper penetration, or the woman's legs can be close together when less penetration is desired. If the man fails to support his weight ("A gentleman always leans on his elbows"), the woman may be uncomfortable. The position is not recommended for pregnant women.

It was once believed that the technique of "riding high"—elevating the man's pelvis to press against the woman's pubic mound—increased clitoral stimulation and made female orgasm more likely. Yet many women find this technique not especially effective, and some people may even find it uncomfortable.

**Figure 8.2**

Face-to-face, man above intercourse position. This is the most common intercourse position in our own and most other societies.

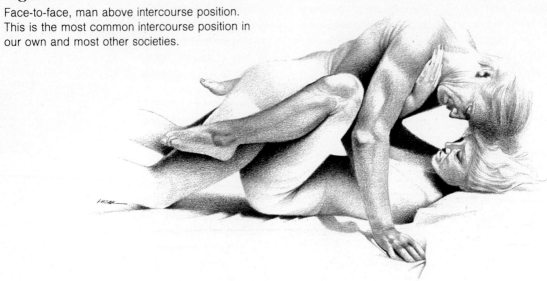

**Figure 8.3**

Face-to-face, women above position. This position may facilitate orgasm for the female partner.

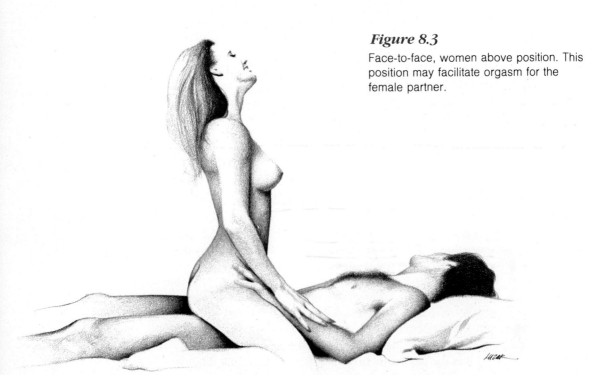

**Face-to-face, woman-above**  Many couples prefer the face-to-face, woman-above position (Figure 8.3) because they find that it helps the man to delay ejaculation and the woman to reach orgasm. According to one woman:

> Being on top means getting my clitoris right wherever I want it. . . . Being on top means never having to cope with a man who is trying to get in deeper and deeper while you are struggling to keep sensations on your clitoris and vaginal lips (Wolfe, 1981, p. 111)

Some men like the position as well as women do:

> I like all positions but especially with my partner straddling me, touching my balls, my penis hitting her vagina front and back as she moves back and forth. (Shanor, 1978, p. 214)

As with the man-above variation, numerous options are possible. The woman may face toward her partner's head or toward his feet; she may lie flat, bend forward from the waist, or sit in an upright position. An important advantage of this position is that it allows the man relatively free use of his hands. Kissing and eye contact are possible. The position is often recommended by therapists for couples with sexual problems.

**Rear-entry**  The major recommendation for the rear-entry position is the intense stimulation it can provide for the man—the tactile stimulation of deep penetration and the contact with the woman's buttocks. However, the position sometimes evokes negative feelings because it seems too "animal-like." In fact, a common name for this position is "doggy-style." Its advantage for the woman is that in this position either partner can stimulate the clitoris manually. The position is sometimes recommended for the late stages of pregnancy.

**Side-by-side**  When using the side-by-side position, a couple can lie facing each other or (Figure 8.4) take a rear-entry approach—the "spoons" position. When lying face to face, kissing and eye contact are possible, and some of the advantages of the woman-above position apply. In the "spoons" variation, the man

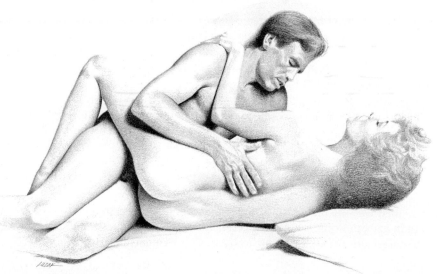

*Figure 8.4*

Face-to-face, side-by-side intercourse position.

achieves penetration from a rear-entry position, with both partners lying on their sides. The side-by-side positions can be very relaxed, and some couples enjoy remaining in them as they fall asleep after intercourse. These positions are also recommended for the late stages of pregnancy.

Side-by-side positions can be further varied by having either the man or woman lift one leg up and over the hips of the other. When the woman is half on her side and half on top of the man with one of his thighs between her legs, the position is called *flanquette*. Some women enjoy additional clitoral pressure from the man's thigh in this position. When the man enters from the rear, with one of the woman's legs drawn up so that he can insert a thigh between her legs, the position is called *cuissade* (Comfort, 1972).

**Sitting and standing positions**   Erotic illustrations from India often show intercourse positions in which the man and woman are seated facing each other. These illustrations are meant to demonstrate the Tantric yoga goal of minimizing body movement during intercourse. The woman is supposed to have such skillful control of her vaginal muscles that she can stimulate the penis without moving any part of her body.

Active thrusting may be difficult in either of these positions, which may explain why they are rarely used in the United States. Although some people become enthusiastic about them, a standing position may be difficult to maintain for long.

**Other cultures, other positions**   The value of other positions and the importance of using them have varied through history and across cultures. Among "sex-positive" ancient cultures, such as the Hindus of ancient India and the Buddhists of ancient China, great emphasis was placed on appropriate variations in position. Since these cultures viewed sex as important to physical and spiritual health, they instructed members in the full range of possibilities. For example, the most famous sex manual of ancient India is Vatsyayana's *Kama-sutra*. This book describes eighty-four different positions. Each is named after an animal, and couples are encouraged to make appropriate animal noises while using them. Positions are also categorized according to posture and accompanying movements. In "spinning the top," for example, the woman is on top and spun around like a wheel. Couples are encouraged to attain the more difficult positions through exercise and practice.

In China, a group of sex manuals called *fung-chung-shu*—literally "art of the bedchamber"—were popular. These books described and illustrated positions with such exotic names as "silkworm spinning a cocoon" and "bamboos near the altar." The man-above, woman-below position was preferred for philosophical reasons, but the Chinese recognized that other positions were natural, acceptable, and desirable (Bullough, 1978).

Like the Chinese, every culture appears to have one basic intercourse position that in some way reflects the concerns of the society—for example, the relative status of men and women. In ancient Greece, where a platonic relationship between two men was the highest form of love, rear entry was the preferred coital position. But in ancient Rome, where women had considerable power within the home, the most frequent position appears to have been woman above (Marks, 1978).

**Changes in American society**   In the United States, changes in attitude toward coital positions have taken place in recent decades. Although the Judeo-Christian tradition does not prohibit the use of any posture, its emphasis on procreation has had considerable influence on behavior. For many centuries, the man-above position was considered the only "correct" position for intercourse. Since women were expected to be sexually passive and indifferent, this position dominated the Victorian era. It came to be called the "missionary position" when missionaries working in the South Pacific during the last century taught Polynesians that it was the only proper and moral coital technique.

This attitude persisted into the twentieth century. Although sex manuals describing a variety of positions appeared during the 1920s, few members of the general population accepted the view that variations were normal or desirable. When Kinsey (Kinsey, Pomeroy, and Martin, 1948; Kinsey et al., 1953) interviewed Americans at midcentury, the man-above position was the only position used by as many as 70 percent of the population.

Two decades later, however, nearly 75 percent of the couples in Hunt's (1974) survey at least occasionally used the woman-above position, and more than half used the side-by-side position. Positions that were rare at midcentury—sitting or rear entry—had become more common. Unlike Kinsey, Hunt found no relationship between willingness to try new positions and education. Although both Kinsey and Hunt found that the younger generations were more likely than the older to use a variety of positions, the women who responded to a recent *Cosmopolitan* survey showed no difference between generations (Wolfe, 1981). Table 8.1 and Table 8.2 show results from these surveys.

## Table 8.1   *White married couples' use of variant positions*

| POSITION | AGE | | |
|---|---|---|---|
| | 18–24 | 35–44 | 55+ |
| Woman above | 37% | 29% | 17% |
| Side by side | 21 | 15 | 15 |
| Rear entry | 20 | 8 | 1 |
| Sitting | 4 | 2 | 1 |

Adapted from Morton Hunt, *Sexual Behavior in the 1970's.* Dell, 1974, p. 203.

## Table 8.2   *Women's preferred coital positions*

| | |
|---|---|
| Man above | 61% |
| Woman above | 26 |
| Side by side | 8 |
| Rear entry | 8 |

Source: From Linda Wolfe, *The Cosmo Report.* Arbor House, 1981.

**The benefits of variety** If a couple always has intercourse in the same position with the same pattern of movements, they may come to find sexual activity boring. Couples sometimes complain that their intercourse patterns have become mechanical or predictable, and that routine has replaced spontaneity. Other people use intercourse as a form of athletic competition, with the goal of ever more unusual and demanding techniques. It appears that either too little or too much experimentation can detract from the full enjoyment and emotional intimacy of sexual intercourse.

Couples don't necessarily have to keep trying new positions in order to avoid monotony; varying movements can also keep alive a feeling of spontaneity. The rhythm, pressure, or speed of pelvic thrusting can be altered to increase stimulation for either partner. Although most men tend to concentrate on in-and-out motions and deep thrusting, women often report great pleasure from the slow rotation of the penis inside the vagina. Another common preference of women is to rub or grind the pubic bone against the partner during intercourse, stimulating the clitoris. Just as habitual use of the same position can lead to monotonous lovemaking, an unvarying movement during intercourse can detract from the pleasure of the experience. So can rigid requirements made by one partner on another, as one man complained:

> The main demands made of me during sex are to hold off ejaculation and to
> stimulate the right "spot" on my partner without much trying on her part. I
> feel a woman has to concentrate on stimulation and learn to receive it as well
> as the man performing it. (Hite, 1981, p. 368)

The ideal intercourse script is one in which positions and movements are varied and adapted to the mutual needs of the partners. Couples may fail to achieve this ideal if they believe sexual initiative is the man's prerogative. In such cases, men may continue to use deep thrusting throughout intercourse even though their partner does not care for it at all. And women may cling to the idea that they should not initiate change in either position or movement, and wait in vain for the man to find the right approach. In Chapter 10, we'll see how sexual communication can solve many of these problems.

## Orgasm during intercourse

Most Western societies have long expected men to experience orgasm and ejaculation during intercourse. But the notion that women should also have orgasms during intercourse is relatively new. As most sexual surveys show, however, a large proportion of women do not reach orgasm during coitus.

These findings have created concern and are regarded as a sign of widespread dissatisfaction among women. Blame for this "failure" has been placed on sexual inhibition among women, faulty sexual techniques among men, and sexual misinformation. As we'll see, however, the notion that in a sexually healthy individual intercourse and orgasm always go together is simply an assumption.

In the United States, female orgasm has become a preoccupation, and some researchers (Hunt, 1974) have argued that it is synonymous with women's sexual pleasure and satisfaction. Since women expect to have an orgasm, many are disappointed and disturbed if they do not. Further, many men accept responsibility for their partner's orgasm—or its absence. It seems that the goal of female orgasm during intercourse can lead to tension, doubt, anxiety, and unhappiness for both sexes. One man summed up the problem this way:

> Sex is getting too complicated. Sometimes I just go and pay a prostitute so I don't have to worry about "fulfilling" the woman. . . . Suddenly having an orgasm has become so important to many women that they expect you to do anything you can—standing on your head if you have to—to make sure they get off. (Shanor, 1978, p. 210–211)

The situation does seem to be improving. Over the past fifty years, an increasing number of women say they always—or almost always—reach orgasm during intercourse. Among a group of married women studied in 1931, less than half reported having an orgasm during intercourse (Dickinson and Beam, 1931). But by midcentury, half of the newly married women interviewed and nearly two-thirds of the women who had been married for twenty years regularly had coital orgasms (Kinsey et al., 1953). In addition, younger women were more likely than older women to be orgasmic. By the 1970s, as many as three-fourths of the married women surveyed had regular orgasms during intercourse (Hunt, 1974).

Most single women don't appear to fare nearly as well. In studies that include a large number of single women, only about a third or less have orgasm from intercourse alone (Hite, 1976; Wolfe, 1981). When manual stimulation of the clitoris is added during intercourse, however, the proportion rises to about half of all women (Hite, 1976). Some women who do reach orgasm during intercourse say that they use the woman-above position, that they have intense clitoral stimulation during foreplay, that they fantasize during coitus, or that a previous orgasm during foreplay ensures a later orgasm during intercourse (Wolfe, 1981).

In the view of Shere Hite (1976), female orgasm during intercourse is a political issue, and not simply a reflection of a woman's sexual or psychological adjustment. Hite believes that a woman's sexual architecture is not designed for orgasm without the addition of direct clitoral stimulation to intercourse. But continual striving for the elusive coital orgasm sets the stage for disappointment and sexual failure, and can breed anger and insecurity.

Not all women accept the notion that they may not be able to have orgasm from penile thrusting alone. Years of emphasis, in sex manuals and the media, on orgasm from penile stimulation have made many women reluctant to accept anything less. In response to their needs, a variety of sex therapy programs have been developed that teach women to duplicate, during intercourse, the pattern of stimulation that brings them to orgasm during masturbation. These methods will be discussed in Chapter 14. Using such techniques, many women can learn to experience coital orgasm; there is some question, however, as to whether such orgasm is always necessary or meaningful. Many women enjoy coitus even if they generally reach orgasm in other ways:

I rarely have orgasms during intercourse, but I love it anyway because I love the way men are so intense during it. As long as they've gotten me excited before they start, and as long as they're willing to make me come manually afterwards, then I find it a wonderful, close, thrilling thing. Nothing beats it for intimacy. (Wolfe, 1981, p. 107)

In some cultures, orgasm is not the goal of intercourse for men or women. Among the Taoists of ancient China, ejaculation was seen as both stressful and fatiguing for the male, particularly for men of advanced age. In contrast with the Western view that ejaculation brings relaxation and calm, Taoists believed that it brought only fatigue and was simply a brief sensation followed by hours of weariness (Chang, 1977). This very different view of ejaculation makes the Western belief that orgasm during intercourse is good and necessary simply one possible attitude among many. Perhaps emphasizing the experience rather than the goal of orgasm would lead to more satisfying sexual relationships.

## ANAL SEX

Although attitudes have changed greatly over the past decades, anal sex, or stimulation of the anus of one person by the mouth or sex organs of another, remains a source of conflict and confusion for many men and women. Anal sex is condemned in the Judeo-Christian tradition and is illegal in many states. Religion and law are not the only barriers: In order to engage in anal sex, American concerns with body odor and cleanliness must be overcome. Health authorities have done much to bolster the belief that anal sex presents serious health risks. Warning against infections, most sex educators strongly emphasize the practice of washing the penis before switching from anal to genital intercourse. These admonitions probably intensify an existing reluctance, although the risk of transferring bacteria from the anus to the vagina has not been clearly demonstrated.

In spite of these problems, anal sex seems to have become more acceptable than it was at the time of Kinsey's surveys. Kinsey (Kinsey, Pomeroy, and Martin, 1948) reported that there was some anal play—in the form of touching the anus—among married couples, but that anal intercourse was infrequent. It was so rare, in fact, that he didn't bother to ask women about it. A quarter of a century later, anal intercourse was still uncommon among heterosexual couples, although it is often practiced by male homosexuals. Despite the fact that only about 25 percent of the men and women interviewed by Morton Hunt (1974) agreed with the statement "Anal intercourse is wrong," only 6 percent said that they had anal intercourse sometimes or often.

In the *Redbook* survey, less than half of the women said they had tried anal sex, but among those who had tried it, 41 percent said they enjoyed it. The rest rated it as neutral to unpleasant (Tavris and Sadd, 1977). Although 21 percent of the *Redbook* readers engaged in anal intercourse sometimes or often, only 13 percent of the *Cosmopolitan* readers said it was a regular part of their sexual activity

(Wolfe, 1981). Like other variations in sexual techniques, anal intercourse was more likely to be tried by younger than by older women. As with oral sex, women who were willing to experiment with anal sex were more likely to rate their sex lives as very good than women who were not willing to try it (Tavris and Sadd, 1977). A woman's major motives for performing anal intercourse were curiosity and a strong desire to please her partner. Some women also say they enjoy anal sex because they feel it is an extremely intimate form of sexual expression.

Stimulation or penetration of the anus can be perceived as pleasurable for both physiological and psychological reasons. Physiologically, the anal entrance is much more sensitive than its interior, for the entrance is richly supplied with nerve endings. Since the anal and genital areas share certain muscles, stimulation of one area may arouse the other. For instance, contractions of the anal sphincter—the tight ring of muscle that holds the rectum closed—also produce contractions in the male and female genitals (Kinsey et al., 1953). For this reason, some heterosexual men also enjoy anal stimulation during foreplay or intercourse.

Psychologically, it is probably a person's attitude that primarily determines whether anal sex is perceived as pleasant or unpleasant. Some people are strongly attracted to the practice because it has been forbidden. Others may be repelled because of the linkage of the anus to the expulsion of feces.

Anal intercourse is generally performed with the woman on her stomach, although she can also lie on her back with her knees raised to her chest (Haeberle, 1978). We have little information about the number of women who reach orgasm during anal intercourse. Although some women may have orgasms, they are more likely to occur among men (Gagnon and Simon, 1973). A woman's chances of orgasm during anal sex are improved if she also has clitoral or breast stimulation. As one man described his experiences:

> I always orgasm and ejaculate when I make rectal love to a woman. But only one lover has ever desired anal intercourse. To make her climax I stimulated her clitoris manually while moving in her anus. (Hite, 1981, p. 590)

Even among women who find anal intercourse erotically appealing, there may be difficulties in its practice. If the anal muscles are not relaxed, penetration may cause discomfort or pain. For example, a woman reported:

> My boyfriend and I have tried anal sex. But even though he was very slow and gentle, we gave up on the idea. It was just too painful. (Wolfe, 1981, p. 112)

Since the anus provides no lubricant of its own, either saliva or K-Y Jelly applied to the anus before any penetration is attempted may eliminate pain. If the penis is inserted violently or without lubrication, anal intercourse may even injure tissues in the anal area. Because of this concern, some sex educators urge caution and extreme gentleness when experimenting with anal sex (Comfort, 1972).

Whether a couple focuses on anal, oral, or genital sex, the encounter generally ends with afterplay.

# AFTERPLAY

**afterplay** touching and kissing that follow sexual activity

**Afterplay** can be called the last act of the sexual script. Just as the final scene of a play or movie often leaves a lasting impression on the audience, the way people wind down after intercourse has a strong influence on the way they feel about the experience. When afterplay is perfunctory, a feeling of distance can arise at a time when most people have a strong need for intimacy and closeness. Words of affection and gentle expressions of tenderness are important. In the words of one woman:

> There doesn't have to be a lot of conversation, just a few tender words, some physical intimacy, some contact that tells me that the closeness is still there even after the orgasm is over. (Zilbergeld, 1978, p. 192)

The exertions of intercourse may leave one or both partners feeling anything from slight weariness to exhaustion, so the need to rest and relax during afterplay is also important. But instead of falling asleep immediately, cuddling, relaxed talk, and relating without a goal can increase satisfaction (Zilbergeld, 1978).

The feelings men and women experience after intercourse can be greatly affected by whether or not they have reached orgasm. For one thing, as we saw in Chapter 5, the physiological afterglow of orgasm can produce a special feeling of satisfaction. But the temporary loss of control during orgasm may also make some people feel embarrassed or vulnerable, feelings that increase the need for intimacy and affection during afterplay. A man or woman who is unable to reach orgasm may feel frustrated or disappointed and crave words of reassurance and comfort. For some people, orgasm never lives up to expectations. According to one man:

Affection and tenderness between lovers during afterplay can increase feelings of intimacy and enhance the way partners feel about their experience. (© Barbara Alper)

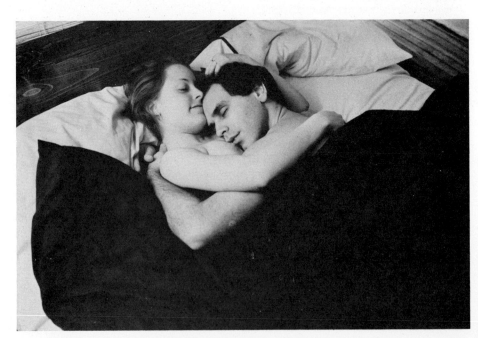

Sometimes I get depressed, and have feelings of failure and self-hatred. It could have been longer, bigger, better, etc. (Hite, 1981, p. 339)

It's often said that men tend to be selfish or insensitive during this period. The man who simply rolls over and falls asleep may arouse resentment and hostility in his partner. She may feel rejected at a time when she most desires her partner's affection. The urge some men feel to sleep may be learned, not physiological. Many men find the time after intercourse difficult to handle because there's nothing specific to do. They may feel uncomfortable simply being with another person with no goal in mind (Zilbergeld, 1978).

A sexual encounter need not end when the man ejaculates. Some couples view afterplay as an intermission between acts instead of as the final curtain (Gagnon, Rosen, and Leiblum, 1982). If the woman has not reached orgasm, the man can continue manual or oral stimulation after he has ejaculated. Sometimes a couple may desire further intercourse, especially if the man is soon able to regain an erection. When both partners feel satisfied and relaxed, however, the focus of attention will naturally shift away from sexual interaction, leaving behind the warm afterglow of emotional intimacy.

# Summary

**1**  Each of us has a sexual script consisting of various acts that generally take a similar order. The script begins with an invitation, then moves into **foreplay,** kissing, hugging, stroking, and oral stimulation. Although a sexual encounter can be limited to foreplay, in most heterosexual activity intercourse is the central act. Intercourse is generally followed by **afterplay.**

**2**  Touch is one of the primary ways of expressing sexual feelings. The American practice of **petting** (which stops short of intercourse) may have developed as a compromise between pressure for premarital chastity and sexual liberalism. There are wide individual differences in preferred patterns of touching, and people can learn to enjoy painful stimulation or tickling.

**3**  Although kissing is widely accepted in Western societies, the sexual value of the kiss is in large part learned. In some societies kissing is virtually unknown. Kissing usually begins with closed lips, but the pattern of petting soon broadens to include deep kissing and kissing other parts of the body.

**4**  Oral sex, or sexual contact between the mouth, lips, or tongue of one person and the genitals of the other, can be the central part of sexual activity, foreplay, or afterplay. Its acceptance varies greatly both among and within cultures. **Fellatio,** or oral stimulation of the penis, and **cunnilingus,** or oral stimulation of the female genitals, are the technical terms for oral sex, although some sex educators prefer the term "genital kiss." Although oral sex seems to be becoming a standard part of sexual activity, some people still have negative attitudes toward it. Oral stimulation of the genitals appears to be instinctive in many animals, and it has been suggested that cultural inhibitions may have overpowered a natural human tendency to engage in oral sex.

**5** In genital intercourse, or **coitus,** the penis is inserted in the vagina. Since human intercourse is free from hormonal control, coitus often takes place when a woman cannot conceive, making it inefficient from the standpoint of species reproduction. It's been proposed that sexual symbols, the nuclear family, and female orgasm compensate for inefficient intercourse by motivating people to have coitus more often. Some disagree, saying that the nuclear family restrains female sexuality and that modern patriarchal societies, instead of increasing the frequency of intercourse, suppress female sexuality.

**6** There is no "normal" frequency of intercourse among human beings, and the standard varies from culture to culture. Intercourse frequencies in the United States appear to be lower than in most tribal societies, perhaps because of the way Americans are prepared for sexual life within marriage. The amount of time spent in intercourse depends primarily on how long it takes from **intromission** (the insertion of the penis) to ejaculation. The duration of intercourse varies among human societies, and in the United States a trend toward longer intercourse seems to be developing. Today most men say that intercourse lasts about ten minutes, although their estimates may be highly inaccurate.

**7** Individual preference, sexual architecture, physical constraints, and cultural attitudes all play a part in the choice of intercourse position. There are five basic positions: face-to-face, man-above; face-to-face, woman-above; rear entry; side by side; and sitting or standing positions. Each culture seems to have a favorite position, and sex-positive cultures emphasize variations. Although the man-above position once was considered the only "normal" position in the United States, today men and women use a variety of positions. Varying position or coital movements can help to keep a feeling of spontaneity in a sexual relationship.

**8** A preoccupation with female orgasm during intercourse has led some couples to be anxious or upset if the woman does not reach orgasm. Although the proportion of women reaching orgasm during coitus has been rising over the past fifty years, many women require additional clitoral stimulation. However, intercourse can be enjoyable without coital orgasm, and some cultures deliberately avoid it.

**9** Anal sex, or stimulation of the anus of one person by the mouth or sex organs of another, has become more prevalent and more acceptable in the past few decades. The anal entrance is extremely sensitive, and because anal and genital areas share muscles, anal stimulation may cause genital arousal. The perception of anal sex as pleasurable probably depends upon a person's attitude.

**10** The atmosphere and quality of afterplay have a strong influence on the way people feel about a sexual experience. A need for intimacy and affection at this time is fairly common, and afterplay can increase sexual satisfaction.

## a lesbian's experience

There has never been any doubt in my mind that I was gay. From my first high-school crush to my present lover, it's been only women that I cared about. Men are all right as friends, but I can't imagine going to bed with one. (Authors' files)

## a man's first homosexual experience

It was a friend from school who spent the night at my house. We were talking about sex, and pretty soon we were feeling each other's hard-ons. It was exciting, but afterward I felt I'd done something wrong, very bad. (Bell, Weinberg, and Hammersmith, 1981, p. 98)

# 9 Homosexual and Bisexual Patterns

# Chapter 9

Although most human sexual activity is between partners of different sexes, men and women often have sexual experiences with others of their own gender. Sexual activity with a partner of the same gender is known as **homosexuality**. The prefix "homo" is simply Greek for "same." It has nothing to do with the "Homo" in Homo sapiens, which comes from the Latin word for man. Homosexual is the scientific term for both men and women.

Many homosexual women, however, prefer to be called **lesbians**, a traditional name for female homosexuals derived from the island of Lesbos, where the Greek poet Sappho was born. Sappho was married and had a child, but her poetry is full of her sexual feelings for other women. Many male homosexuals also dislike the term homosexual and call themselves "gays," a word that was at one time applied to prostitutes (Bullough, 1979). The term was picked up by homosexuals, who used it among themselves for many years before the general public took it up about twenty years ago.

In most parts of the United States, homosexual is not a neutral term describing sexual preference. To be labeled as a homosexual can lead to almost every manner of discrimination and result in the loss of job, friends, and housing. As one American man said:

> In our society you can go to war and kill a guy, but God help you if you're caught in bed with one. (Hite, 1981, p. 799)

In order to understand the experience of being homosexual, we'll explore the social context within which homosexuality takes place. The chapter begins with a look at homosexuality in other times and other places and an exploration of historical background of

**homosexuality** sexual activity with a partner of the same sex

**lesbian** female homosexual

**gay** male homosexual, although the term is sometimes applied to female homosexuals

# *Homosexual and Bisexual Patterns*

American attitudes. After a brief description of today's gay experience, we'll investigate various theories of homosexuality. Next, following a description of the homosexual style of life, we'll consider techniques used in homosexual lovemaking. We'll close with a look at **bisexuality** ("two sexes"), for a number of women and men in the center of the sexual continuum seem equally aroused by and have sexual experiences with both genders.

**bisexuality**
sexual activity with both men and women

## HOMOSEXUALITY IN PERSPECTIVE

Homosexuality appears to have been practiced at least as long as human beings have been on the earth—perhaps longer. Many animals engage in homosexual activity, and it is found in most, if not all, human societies (Marmor, 1976). Our own attitudes toward homosexuality may be easier to understand if we first see just how it is treated in other societies.

### *Homosexuality in other cultures*

In other cultures and other historical periods, attitudes and customs surrounding homosexual activity have ranged from acceptance and encouragement to severe disapproval and punishment. Some societies allow homosexual behavior but limit the circumstances in which it may be practiced. Among the Big Nambas of the New Hebrides, for example, homosexuality was part of the rites of circumcision. An older man acted as guardian and lover of the young boy before circumcision and again thirty days after removal of his foreskin. This custom was believed to strengthen the boy's penis (Bullough, 1976).

Among seventy-six tribal societies, 64 percent accepted homosexual behavior or approved of it under certain circumstances (Ford and Beach, 1951). When homosexual activity was relatively rare, there were usually strong and specific sanctions against it; when a society condoned homosexual behavior, approval was often limited to adolescents. In all these societies, homosexuality appeared to be far less prevalent among women than among men. This difference may reflect a true contrast in sexual behavior, or it may simply indicate that a culture pays less attention to female homosexuality.

Over the ages, Western societies have displayed a wide variety of attitudes toward homosexuality. Among the ancient Greeks, sexual pleasure was seen as a valuable goal, and the naked male body symbolized the ideal of both physical and emotional love. Homosexual love was acceptable for a young man from the time he had his first haircut (at about age sixteen). Although erotic relationships between such youths and older men are best known, they seem to have been common among Greek men of all ages. The Greeks tended to regard homosexual feelings as "natural" and so made no attempt to explain why one man was sexually attracted to another (Boswell, 1980).

In ancient Greece, homosexual relationships were regarded as "natural" and seemed to have been common among men of all ages. (Editorial Photocolor Archives, Inc.)

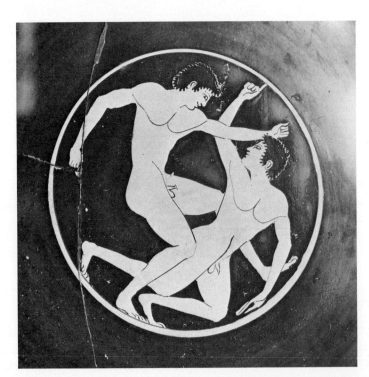

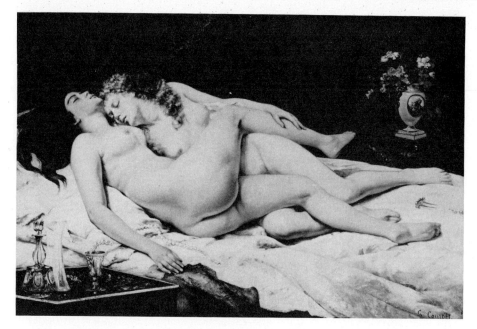

Through history, male homosexuality has generally received public attention while female homosexuals have tended to blend into the wider community. (EPA/Art Resource)

This elevation of male homosexuality occurred in a society that assigned a low status to women and discouraged love or friendship between husband and wife. The family unit was highly esteemed, but its primary function was the production of children. Except for the poetry of Sappho, little is known about female homosexuality among the ancient Greeks, probably because most of the writers were men.

Among the Romans, homosexuality appears to have been common, and the capacity for homosexual feelings was assumed to be universal. Neither religion nor law distinguished between homosexual and heterosexual activity. The same rules applied to both, and the gender of a sexual partner seems to have been a matter of indifference (Boswell, 1980).

## The roots of antihomosexual bias

American society is the heir of two widely differing cultural and sexual heritages—that of the ancient Greeks and that of Judeo-Christian religious thought. Although the Greek tradition was generally positive, the religious traditions are strongly anti-homosexual. The Old Testament does not equivocate: "If a man also lie with man-kind as he lieth with a woman, both of them have committed an abomination: they shall surely be put to death; their blood shall be upon them" (Leviticus 20:13).

Early Christianity saw all physical pleasure as interfering with spiritual growth. Within this framework, sexual abstinence was the highest form of human existence. Sex for procreation within marriage was permitted, but all other forms of sexual contact, whether homosexual or heterosexual, were condemned. Despite the law of Leviticus, there are relatively few references to homosexuality in the Old

Testament and the New Testament fails to mention it. Strong religious hostility came later, when Jewish and Christian scholars wrote commentaries on the scriptures.

During the early Middle Ages, homosexuality was tolerated and regarded as no worse than heterosexual activity between unmarried partners. As strong governments began to develop, pressures for social conformity of all kinds increased. By the end of the twelfth century, society had become actively hostile toward homosexuality (Boswell, 1980). The notion that it is sinful or immoral was incorporated into the legal system. In medieval England, church laws against sodomy, or anal intercourse, became part of English civil law. Such "crimes against nature," as they were called, were punishable by death. English immigrants to the United States brought these laws with them, and the Pilgrims of Massachusetts declared homosexual activity to be a capital offense.

The legacy of this tradition is evident in present sexual laws. In many states, laws do not specifically prohibit homosexual activity; instead they outlaw "crimes against nature" or "unnatural acts"—terms that are interpreted as including homosexual behavior. Only in recent years have states begun to grant legal protection to homosexual activity between consenting adults. In many communities, attempts to pass laws protecting homosexuals from job or housing discrimination have met with great resistance, but in a few places homosexuals are gaining legal rights. In San Francisco, for example, the homosexual lover of an assassinated city supervisor was officially recognized as a "partial dependent" and awarded death benefits as a survivor (*New York Times,* 1982), although the ruling was later reversed. Despite such signs, it is likely that the battle for legal protection will continue for some years.

## The gay experience in contemporary society

In recent years there has been a marked shift in both scientific and public views of homosexuality. After World War II, many people ceased to regard homosexuality as a sin or a crime and came to consider it a disease. This change does not mean that homosexual activity was suddenly considered normal, only that Americans came to see the homosexual as someone who needed treatment, not punishment. In response to this view, numerous forms of therapy—most of which had little success—were developed. Psychiatrist Thomas Szasz (1965) saw no progress for the homosexual in this changed classification. Being labeled sick rather than criminal simply substituted one set of sanctions—such as hospitalization or compulsory treatment—for another.

In response to their low status within the social, legal, and psychiatric establishments, American homosexuals began to organize. Seeing themselves as members of a repressed minority, they sought to assert their rights to pursue their own way of life without legal or social interference. The result was the gay liberation movement, which became active during the 1950s.

Although homosexual groups had existed for decades, they had tended to be secret and to have little influence (Bullough, 1979). Then, with the publication of

Kinsey's research (Kinsey, Pomeroy, and Martin, 1948; Kinsey et al., 1953), attitudes began to change. Such a large proportion of the public had apparently had homosexual experiences that it became increasingly difficult to label the practice abnormal. By 1956, the research of psychologist Evelyn Hooker attacked the premise that homosexuality was a "disease" by showing that homosexuals were just as psychologically healthy as heterosexuals (Hooker, 1975).

Partly as a result of information discovered by sex researchers, homosexuals became more open about their sexual orientation. The turning point of the gay liberation movement came in June 1969, when New York City police raided the Stonewall Inn, a gay bar in Greenwich Village (Bullough, 1979). Instead of meekly submitting, the gays resisted and battled the police on that night and for several nights thereafter. With homosexuals willing to speak out and with a dawning public recognition that homosexuals were subjected to police harassment, the movement's goals received widespread attention.

As the movement grew, its attempts to change traditional psychiatric views on homosexuality were partially successful. In 1973 the Association for the Advancement of Behavior Therapy recognized the right of homosexuals to live as they pleased. In the same year, the American Psychiatric Association voted to drop the category "homosexuality" from its classification of mental disorders. However, it substituted a new subcategory, "sexual orientation disturbance," which applies to individuals troubled by their homosexuality. Other professional organizations, such as the American Psychological Association, have stated that homosexuality is neither pathological nor the sign of personality disturbance. But these new per-

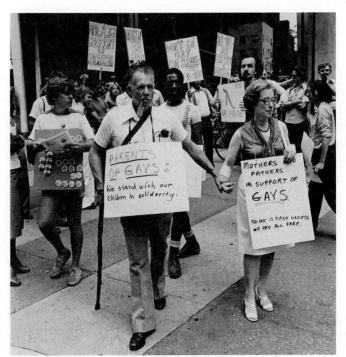

Twenty years ago, few parents would acknowledge the sexual orientation of their gay children. Today many parents are openly supporting their children's right to live as they please. (© Peter Southwick/ Stock, Boston)

spectives do not reflect the views of all professionals. Many of them continue to see homosexuality as a personality problem, as do many of the general public.

Although there has also been some liberalization of public attitudes, a considerable number of people retain traditional moral or religious views. Others accept homosexuals' right to follow their own way of life but are unable to shake off the legacy of the culture's sexual heritage. One such man was puzzled about his own feelings:

> Why do I still feel uncomfortable around gays? Even though I've accepted it intellectually, it still bothers me to be around them. (Authors' files)

**homophobia** an irrational fear of homosexuality

The attitude of many people has been characterized as **homophobia**—an irrational fear of homosexuality that can affect heterosexuals and homosexuals alike. This fear can have negative consequences for homosexuals if it makes them dislike themselves or feel that they must hide or deny their sexual preferences.

Homophobia also limits the behavior of heterosexuals. For example, heterosexual men often refrain from expressing physical or emotional closeness with other men because they fear being labeled as homosexuals. As one man said:

> Just because you look or act a certain way, it doesn't mean you're gay. But it's hard to be close to another man without causing suspicions. (Authors' files)

Apparently, homophobia limits social behavior in much the same way as claustrophobia can limit a person's use of elevators.

 According to some authorities (Haeberle, 1978), the effects of the gay liberation movement have been mixed. On the positive side, the movement has allowed homosexuals to claim their civil rights, and its militancy may push the "straight," or heterosexual, world into a state of peaceful coexistence. The movement has also encouraged many gays to come to terms with themselves, to be, in Stephen Morin's (1977) words, "proud, angry, open, visible, political, and healthy."

The movement's negative effect has been an increase in labeling, as more people have felt psychological pressure to identify themselves as "gay" or "straight." And once a person declares that he or she is gay, a new stereotype—that of the gay subculture—may follow. As we'll see, however, homosexuals are not necessarily any more alike than heterosexuals.

## THEORIES OF HOMOSEXUALITY

We tend to see heterosexuality as the "natural" course of development, and so a good deal of effort has gone into explaining why some people prefer sexual activity with members of their own sex. None of the explanations, whether biological or psychological, has been completely satisfactory, and some gays have quit trying to find a cause:

> I used to think a lot about why I was gay and what was "wrong" with me. Now I just accept it. (Authors' files)

One reason an explanation has eluded our grasp is the difficulty in agreeing on just what the term homosexuality means.

## *Who is homosexual?*

Deciding when to label an individual as homosexual is perhaps the most troubling question confronting researchers. The problem may become clearer to you if you try to label the sexual orientation of the men and women in the following case studies from our files:

**1** John is married and has three children. His only experiences with sexual intercourse have been with his wife. When he masturbates, John fantasizes only about men. Although he does not intend to act out his fantasies, he is sexually attracted to several of his male friends.

**2** Sally is a college student who had a two-year sexual relationship with her female roommate. When the relationship broke up, she began dating a male student. She has married him and enjoys their sex life.

**3** After an adolescence that included dating and sex with girls, Donald joined the army and was stationed at an isolated research base. There he developed a close and loving relationship with another man that included sexual contact. When he was transferred nearer to his home, he began dating women again.

**4** Michael is a young man who earns money as a homosexual prostitute. He accepts money from older men who want to perform oral sex on him. When he goes home to the woman with whom he lives, Michael speaks derisively about these men.

**5** After twenty years of marriage and two children, Ginny divorced her husband under bitter and hostile circumstances. She moved in with another divorced woman and, after several months, the two of them began a loving sexual relationship that has continued for several years. Before this experience, Ginny had never fantasized about sex with another woman or considered the possibility.

**6** Mark says that by the time he was seven or eight years old, he knew he was different from other boys. Now middle-aged, he has never had sex with a woman, although many of his friends are women. Since adolescence he has been involved in a series of sexual relationships with men.

How did you label each of these individuals? Agreeing that Mark is a homosexual probably presented no problem, but it was undoubtedly more difficult to categorize the other cases. Except for Mark, John may be the only one of the group who considers himself homosexual. Yet if homosexuality is defined simply as any sexual activity with a partner of the same sex, all but John would be labeled homosexual.

Such a definition would, according to Alfred Kinsey and his colleagues (1953), include a large proportion of men and a sizable group of women. Kinsey found that, sometime between adolescence and old age, about 37 percent of men and 13 percent of women had at least one sexual experience leading to orgasm with a partner of the same sex. Among those who never married, the proportions were even higher: about 50 percent of the men and 25 percent of the women. What's more, although the proportion of men with any homosexual experience remained steady whether the men had been born before 1900 or after 1930, the amount of homosexual activity increased in the younger generations. Among older men, homosexuality was likely to be a fleeting experience confined to adolescence, but more of the younger men tended to keep up such activities during their twenties—at least on a casual basis (Downey, 1980).

Among the people interviewed by Kinsey, only 4 percent of the men and only about half that percentage of the women were exclusively homosexual. To label as homosexual anyone who has ever experienced a homosexual contact distorts the picture, since the vast majority of such people have also had satisfactory heterosexual experiences. As a result, Kinsey concluded that the term homosexual had almost no value in describing a particular type or personality or sexual identity. The word "homosexual" was only a way to describe behavior. Thus, Kinsey might speak of homosexual acts, but he would not talk about homosexual people or homosexual personality.

In response to the dilemma of describing homosexual activity, Kinsey developed a 7-point scale of sexual orientation that has been widely accepted. At the zero end of the scale are those individuals who are exclusively heterosexual in both fantasy and behavior; at the other end are those whose behavior and fantasies are exclusively homosexual. In the middle are men and women who show equal amounts of heterosexual and homosexual activity (see Figure 9.1). Looking at homosexuality in this way was a radical departure from conventional thinking, as we saw in Chapter 1.

Although Kinsey's contribution has been influential, there are problems with

## Figure 9.1

The Kinsey scale presents sexual orientation on a continuum from 0 (exclusively heterosexual) to 6 (exclusively homosexual). The scale illustrates the fact that sexual preference may be a matter of degree for many individuals.

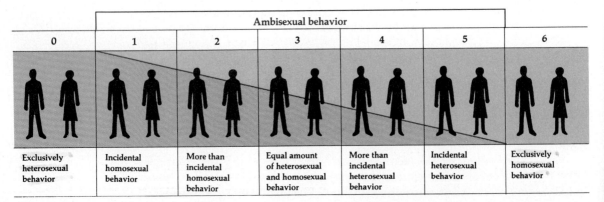

| | Ambisexual behavior | | | | | |
|---|---|---|---|---|---|---|
| 0 | 1 | 2 | 3 | 4 | 5 | 6 |
| Exclusively heterosexual behavior | Incidental homosexual behavior | More than incidental homosexual behavior | Equal amount of heterosexual and homosexual behavior | More than incidental heterosexual behavior | Incidental heterosexual behavior | Exclusively homosexual behavior |

the concept. Kinsey paid no attention to the way people viewed their own behavior, a dimension of homosexuality that we'll explore in the section on identity. So the problem of deciding whether a person is or is not "homosexual" is still complicated.

## Biological theories of homosexuality

Homosexuals frequently say they have "always" been drawn to members of their own sex. According to one man:

> As long as I can remember I've been attracted to guys. When I was in high school I tried dating girls for a while, but it wasn't the same. (Authors' files)

Although many homosexuals are convinced they are "born" and not "made," no biological cause of homosexuality has yet been firmly established. If biology does influence the development of homosexuality, hormones are a likely path, and researchers have begun to investigate it. One way hormones could be involved is through prenatal exposure to certain hormones. Another possible way is through the effects of hormones after birth.

**Prenatal exposure** As we saw in Chapter 3, without prenatal androgen, a fetus cannot develop into a physically normal boy. There is nothing unusual about a male homosexual's body, however, so some researchers have suggested that temporary androgen deficiencies *after* the sexual system has formed may predispose a boy to become homosexual. This proposal has not been ruled out, but neither has it been strongly supported (Meyer-Bahlburg, 1977). Similarly, in the case of women, prenatal exposure to androgens may be linked with bisexuality, but again the connection is weak and most such women are exclusively heterosexual (Meyer-Bahlburg, 1979).

**Hormone levels** Some researchers suggest that hormone levels influence sexual orientation, with male homosexuals having lower than normal testosterone levels and female homosexuals having low estrogen and high androgen levels. Although this proposal seems an easy one to check, research has produced only confusion.

Some studies find clear hormonal differences between heterosexual and homosexual men, others find no difference at all. Most studies find a great deal of overlap in the hormone levels of the two groups: Some homosexual men have lower testosterone levels than heterosexuals, and some heterosexual men have lower testosterone levels than homosexuals. But the overwhelming majority of homosexual men have testosterone levels well within the normal range (Meyer-Bahlburg, 1977).

Low testosterone levels and high estrogen levels do not seem to predict homosexual arousal or behavior among men. However, one problem with such studies is that we can't be certain that the comparisons are reliable. As noted in Chapter 4, testosterone levels vary so that one blood sample cannot establish true differences—yet most of these studies rely on a single blood sample from each individual.

One group of researchers (Kolodny et al., 1971) compared testosterone levels with men's rankings on the Kinsey 7-point scale. Men who were rated 2, 3, and 4 on the Kinsey scale had testosterone levels just like those of heterosexuals who were rated at 0 to 1 on the scale. But men who were rated 5 or 6, indicating virtually exclusive homosexual activity, had significantly lower testosterone levels than the rest. The researchers did not propose that homosexuality is caused by low hormone levels or that homosexual men have a hormone abnormality. Instead, they suggested that depressed testosterone levels may be a result of the stress and anxiety that accompany an openly homosexual life in this society.

When blood samples from lesbians are compared with blood from heterosexual women, the majority of lesbians have hormone levels well within the normal range. However, about a third of the lesbians have a higher than normal level of male hormones (Meyer-Bahlburg, 1979). Again, hormonal levels do not seem to predict homosexual arousal or behavior among women.

The search for a relationship between hormones and homosexuality is based on the assumption that the direction of the sexual drive depends on a person's balance of hormones, with male hormones leading to a preference for female partners and female hormones to a preference for men. Yet connecting sexual activity with hormones has been a difficult task.

Giving female hormones to a heterosexual man doesn't make him homosexual. Instead, he seems to lose interest in any form of sexual activity. Low levels of testosterone imply nothing about a man's sexual orientation, although they may indicate a general disinterest in sexuality. In fact, when homosexual men are given testosterone, their *homosexual* desires and behavior intensify. Giving androgens to a heterosexual woman doesn't make her a lesbian. Instead, her interest in heterosexual activity generally intensifies (Bancroft, 1981).

The sex drive seems to be neither male nor female, but simply an urge for close body contact and the juxtaposition of genitals (Money and Ehrhardt, 1972). Perhaps any approach to sexuality that focuses solely on physiology is bound to produce confusing results. Hormones may intensify sexual interest, but the way that interest is expressed is primarily the result of learning and experience. As we'll see in the discussion of psychological theories, homosexuality—like heterosexuality—is primarily psychological.

## Psychological theories of homosexuality

Psychoanalytic and social learning theories agree that the development of homosexuality is a matter of psychology, not biology, but they disagree over the way that development takes place. Psychoanalytic theorists point to the parents and look for family relationships that produce a "homosexual personality." Learning theorists believe people learn to prefer homosexuality just as they learn anything else, from a preference for lemon pie or rock music to a passion for politics.

**Psychoanalytic theories**   In the psychoanalytic view, homosexuality is generally seen as the product of abnormal development. Some deep conflict arises in a child over emotional responses to experiences within the family (Gadpaille, 1981). Freud believed all people are born with a potential for bisexuality. The usual resolution of the Oedipus complex (discussed in Chapter 11) is the child's identification with the parent of the same sex, which psychoanalysts believe is crucial to the development of heterosexuality. When the child fails to identify in this way, he or she becomes an adult who fears sexual contact with the opposite sex.

Among a group of homosexual men who were psychoanalytic patients, the mothers tended to be overprotective and excessively intimate with their young sons, while the fathers were distant or passive (Bieber et al., 1962). However, since these men had sought therapy, there is no reason to assume they were typical homosexuals. Among one group of lesbians, the mothers were hostile toward their daughters and the fathers were overprotective and emotionally distant; in another group, the mothers rejected their daughters in favor of their sons and the fathers were withdrawn (Kaye et al., 1967). As the discussion of sexual preference will indicate, however, no consistent family pattern appears among homosexuals who have not sought therapy.

**Social learning theory**   In the learning view, homosexuality is not a case of "abnormal" development, but simply a matter of conditioning. Each person is born with the ability to respond to stimuli from males or females. If pleasure is consistently associated with homosexual experiences and unpleasantness with heterosexual experiences, homosexuality develops.

Others (Feldman and MacCullough, 1971) have suggested two learning paths to homosexuality. People who travel the path of "pure" learning develop in a conventional heterosexual manner until adolescence. Then, because of some negative experience with the other sex, these adolescents begin to fear and avoid them. If such people also have pleasant sexual experiences with members of their own sex, they may become homosexuals.

The second path to homosexuality mixes learning with biology. Before birth, prenatal hormones influence the brain so that a baby is born with a predisposition to develop interests and behavior associated with the other sex. As a lesbian recalled her childhood:

> I liked sports and would take dares that most of the girls didn't. I didn't like dolls or cooking and all that. I liked playing outdoors, football and baseball, and sort of ended up with the boys because of that. (Bell, Weinberg, and Hammersmith, 1981, p. 145)

If the parents encourage the child and if the youngster also has pleasant sexual experiences in childhood or adolescence with members of the same sex, the person will come to prefer homosexuality. Some studies (Gadpaille, 1981) have indicated that two-thirds of adult homosexuals recall preferring the activities and interests of the opposite sex during childhood.

## *Homosexuality and sexual identity*

As the contrast between the psychoanalytic and learning views indicates, the controversy about the nature of homosexuality continues. If homosexuality is the result of a failure to identify with the parent of the same sex, we'd expect male homosexuals to have adopted elements of female identity and female homosexuals to have adopted elements of masculine identity. There would be a "homosexual personality." But if homosexuality is the result of conditioning, we'd expect homosexuals to differ little from heterosexuals except in sexual orientation.

The "homosexual personality" failed to appear in a group of college men and women. Personality tests given students who had rated themselves as homosexual, bisexual, or heterosexual turned up no significant differences on any measures of masculinity or femininity (Storms, 1980). In fact, scales of masculinity and femininity have never been successful in detecting homosexuals (Singer, 1970). The erotic fantasies of these students were the best indication of their sexual orientation. Homosexuals fantasized a great deal about their own sex; heterosexuals fantasized a great deal about the other sex; bisexuals fantasized a lot about both sexes. Although no one knows what produces erotic fantasies, it seems that the sexual fantasies of these students were clearly separate from their sex-role orientations (Storms, 1980).

Homosexuals can meet at dances or social gatherings sponsored by gay and lesbian organizations or in the less personal atmosphere of gay bars. (© Alon Reininger 1981/Contact Press Images)

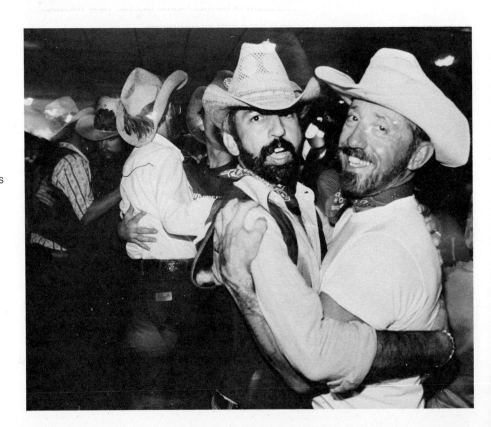

Grouping people into personality categories on the basis of sexual activity may be like grouping everyone who drinks coffee into a single personality type. All coffee drinkers may become upset if they must go without coffee, but they have little else in common. Although homosexuals are as different from one another as heterosexuals, the outside world expects them to look, act, and respond in certain ways.

Once people are considered members of this special group, cultural expectations are likely to have real effects on behavior and identity. In fact, the main experience (other than sexual choice) that homosexually oriented people have in common may be social pressure (Tripp, 1975). For example, certain important decisions, such as whether to "come out" or remain "in the closet," are a common part of the homosexual experience. In addition, since homosexually oriented people have grown up in a "straight" world, many have adopted society's negative judgments about their behavior and way of life.

People also label themselves. Although the extent of homosexual behavior may fall along a continuum, as Kinsey's scale indicates, when people attach a label to their sexual behavior, it is often of the either-or variety. Michael, the homosexual prostitute in the case studies, was actively engaged in homosexual behavior but did not see himself as homosexual. In contrast, John, who never engaged in homosexual acts, probably saw himself as homosexual because of his fantasies and his attraction to other men. To complicate matters further, some people view themselves as heterosexual at some times in their lives and as homosexual at other times.

Given these differing perspectives on what it means to be homosexual, some researchers have defined the experience in a way that stresses variety (Bell and Weinberg, 1978). Being homosexual may sometimes be very important to a person's decisions, thoughts, and behavior; at other times, sexual orientation is irrelevant (Gagnon, 1977).

## HOMOSEXUAL RELATIONSHIPS AND LIFE STYLES

It's difficult for us to escape the stereotypes about homosexual life styles and homosexual roles that permeate the culture. The media tend to focus on homosexuals who live in predominantly gay communities in such large cities as New York and San Francisco. Their reports emphasize homosexual "promiscuity" and "cruising," as well as the militancy and flamboyance of a small minority of homosexual groups. This distorted image reflects only a small proportion of the homosexually oriented population and may produce the same sort of distortion that would emerge from surveys of heterosexuality based on people who frequent singles bars. People who choose to disguise their homosexuality usually lead a very different sort of life. Because homosexuals who have decided to remain in the closet rarely participate in research, most of what is known about homosexual life describes the lives of those who have come out. There seems no way to find out how the majority of homosexuals conduct their lives.

*Focus*

THE
DEVELOPMENT
OF SEXUAL
PREFERENCE

Since there is no homosexual personality, how do people become homosexually oriented? A team of researchers from the Kinsey Institute tried to find out. Alan Bell, Martin Weinberg, and Sue Hammersmith (1981) interviewed nearly a thousand homosexuals and nearly five hundred heterosexuals living in the San Francisco Bay area, and probed deeply into their recollections of childhood.

If the memories of these 1,500 people are correct, the proposal that parents play an important role in the development of homosexuality fall apart. There was no evidence for the "mother is to blame" theory of male homosexuality, and homosexual and heterosexual men did not

differ in how positively or negatively they described their mothers. Homosexual men were no likelier to identify with their mothers than were heterosexual men. As for women, lesbians were less, not more, likely to identify with their fathers than were heterosexual women. No matter what their sexual preference, women were likely to identify with their mothers.

Although no consistent family background divided homosexuals from heterosexuals, researchers did find some evidence for an early lack of conformity to traditional sex roles. As boys, about half of the male homosexuals studied tended to dislike typical boys' activities, to enjoy girls' activities, and to

have a weak sense of masculine identity. One man recalled:

I was never a real boy. I was afraid of fighting. I was easily bullied and have never forgiven myself for it. (Bell, Weinberg, and Hammersmith, 1981, p. 78)

As girls, lesbians tended to dislike girls' activities, to enjoy boys' activities, and to have a weak sense of feminine identity. "I didn't cry a lot," said one woman. "The other girls seemed to cry a lot" (p. 148). Yet more than half of the heterosexual women in the study also reported that as girls they had not always felt or acted very feminine. Since gender nonconformity is more common among girls, its relationship with

---

The same homosexuals who participated in the study of sexual preference discussed earlier also described their sexual roles, their relationships, and their way of life (Bell and Weinberg, 1978). The life styles of these San Francisco homosexuals fell into five general categories: close-coupled, open-coupled, functional, dysfunctional, and asexual (see Table 9.1). As will become apparent, similar life styles can be found among heterosexuals.

Most close-coupled homosexuals regarded themselves as "happily married." They maintained a close relationship with one partner and appeared to be the best-adjusted group. Lesbians tended to prefer this kind of relationship:

My love and I have been together for twelve years. She's very different from me in a lot of ways, and I suppose that's part of the attraction. (Authors' files)

Open-coupled homosexuals maintained a stable relationship with one partner but also engaged in sexual relationships with others. This way of life was most prevalent among male homosexuals.

Functional homosexuals were the counterpart of the swinging singles of the

sexual preference may not be important.

Nothing in what these researchers called "childhood gender nonconformity" seemed strongly linked to family background. For this reason, the researchers propose that biology is somehow involved in the development of homosexuality. Children, they believe, are born predisposed to become homosexual.

They note that although heterosexuals and homosexuals had similar homosexual experiences in childhood, they interpreted the experiences differently. Early sexual attraction to the other sex was apparent, and sexual preference appeared to be determined by early adolescence, whether or not the individual had been sexually active. Crucial to the development of homosexual preference, the investigators conclude, is "a pattern of feelings and reactions within the child that cannot be traced back to a single social or psychological root" (p. 192).

Has this research team firmly established a biological basis for homosexuality? No. No hormonal, biochemical, or other biological measures were taken. Biology emerged by a process of elimination, but the eliminating was done on the basis of retrospective accounts. Memory is tricky, and we often reshape our memories to make them harmonize with the present (Loftus, 1980). Although the process is unintentional, it is deeply human. Yet this study (Bell, Weinberg, and Hammersmith, 1981) should give pause to those who see family relationships as the cradle of homosexuality, since the data that indicate family influence are mostly based on the recollections of homosexuals who were so unhappy they sought therapy. Because Bell's team compared recollections of homosexuals and heterosexuals, many of whom were not in therapy, we have taken an important step forward. We have also been given some indication of the importance of early sex-role behavior as a possible predictor of later sexual orientation.

## Table 9.1 Homosexual life style

| | CLOSE-COUPLED | OPEN-COUPLED | FUNCTIONAL | DYSFUNCTIONAL | ASEXUAL | UNCLASSIFIABLE |
|---|---|---|---|---|---|---|
| Lesbians | 28% | 17% | 10% | 5% | 11% | 28% |
| Male homosexuals | 10% | 18% | 15% | 12% | 16% | 29% |

From A. P. Bell and M. S. Weinberg, *Homosexualities.* Simon and Schuster, 1978.

heterosexual world. They tended to be active in meeting new sexual partners and showed little interest in settling down.

Dysfunctional homosexuals were either deeply dissatisfied with their way of life or had major problems with their sexual performance. Men and women in this group were most susceptible to deep emotional conflicts and often had serious problems in social adjustment.

Asexual homosexuals were essentially loners—either through choice or because they couldn't find a partner. Many of the men in this group were closet homosexuals who seldom interacted with other homosexual men.

## *Coming out*

More and more homosexuals are making their sexual orientation clear to other members of society. However, coming out to others is the last step in what can be a lengthy process.

As we've seen, many people are aware of their sexual orientation by early adolescence. Since American society approves of heterosexuality, sexual attraction to the other sex is encouraged, making it easy to establish a heterosexual identity. But teenagers who are sexually attracted to their own gender generally go through a stage of discovering that their feelings conflict with the messages they get at home, at school, and from the media.

For some, the conflict is slight and the awareness of homosexual feelings is handled in a positive way. For example, a seventeen-year-old lesbian said:

> I never went through a thing like, "These feelings I have are gay feelings, so I better go talk to somebody like a shrink about them." I always thought that it was natural. I just followed my feelings and went along with them, and everything was fine. I never had any head problems about them. (Bell, 1980, p. 114)

For others, who may have accepted the cultural messages that their sexual feelings are "wrong," the establishment of a homosexual identity can be a lengthy process that often begins with denial. One young gay recalled:

Lesbians are much more likely than gays to live in a close-coupled relationship and to confine their sexual activities to their partner. (© Cynthia Copple)

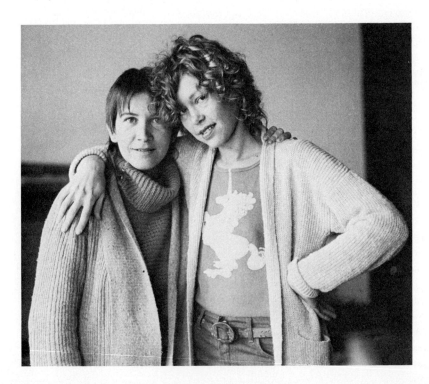

By the time I was twelve, I realized that men were a part of my sexual
fantasies. I liked guys, you know? And once, around that same time, out of a
clear blue sky, someone said to me, "Hey, man, if you don't watch it you're
going to be a homosexual." And I said to myself, Nah, not me. That's the last
thing I'll ever be. I'll never be a homosexual. So from about the age of twelve
to sixteen I squashed those feelings whenever they came to me. (Bell, 1980, p.
115)

Young people who deny their homosexual feelings often date members of the
other sex. Sometimes their denial is so successful that they become homophobic.
Once they have begun to accept themselves, some may go through phases of anger, bargaining (in which they strike bargains with God or with themselves in an
attempt to rid themselves of homosexual feelings), and depression before their homosexual identity is established (Bullough, 1979).

With full acceptance of their homosexual preferences, men and women have
come out to themselves. However, they may continue to conceal their sexual orientation from others. This sort of existence has been called "wearing a mask" (Boyd,
1978) and requires homosexuals to live a double life, in which they can be open
only among other members of the gay community.

Coming out to others is the final phase of establishing a gay identity and involves the decision to stop hiding homosexual feelings. A gay described the experience:

After a long struggle with myself, I finally made the big decision. Coming
out was a slow process, though. And my parents were the last to know.
(Authors' files)

The decision to come out does not require gays to become active in the gay
liberation movement—although some do—or to announce their sexual orientation
to everyone they meet. Instead, it involves being open, refusing to lie, and living
the same life in public and private. The decision to come out is one that can be
made by the individual involved only after careful consideration of its effects. Although coming out is often stressful, its ultimate effects may be beneficial for the
individual.

## The multiplicity of partners

Although a substantial number of homosexuals live in coupled relationships, many
homosexual men have developed a pattern of impersonal sexual activity with a
large number of partners. About 50 percent of the homosexual men in the study by
Bell and Weinberg (1978) had had more than 500 sexual partners; in fact, 28 percent had had at least 1,000 partners. Despite this large number of partners, many of
these men said they usually spent time with their partners and exchanged personal
information, which suggests that their relationships were not entirely impersonal.

For years little attention was paid to this aspect of the gay experience, but it
has recently become an issue that may have significance for the health of gay
males. As we'll see in Chapter 17, reports of acquired immunity deficiency syn-

drome (AIDS), a disease that has been linked to frequent sexual contacts among homosexual men, have been growing rapidly (U.S. Public Health Service, 1982).

*Question* In contrast to the male pattern, the majority of lesbians in Bell and Weinberg's study (1978) had had fewer than ten sexual partners. Moreover, most of these women said they had never had "impersonal sex," in the sense of sexual contact with a stranger. About 75 percent were involved in a stable, long-term relationship with another woman.

Why do homosexual men tend to have so many more sex partners than lesbians or heterosexual men and women? A common explanation is that the number of sex partners has less to do with sexual orientation than with childhood socialization (Gagnon and Simon, 1973). Women, whether heterosexual or homosexual, are brought up in ways that stress the formation of long-term emotional commitments, so the lesbian is likely to have a strong interest in love and affection. Lesbian relationships tend to be full of warmth, tenderness, and caring and, if anything, may suffer from emotional overinvolvement (Nicholas and Leiblum, in press).

*Reason* → Men are often socialized in ways that permit them to separate sexual expression from emotion and long-term commitment. Heterosexual men are limited in their ability to have casual sexual relationships by the relative scarcity of like-minded female partners, but no such limitation restricts homosexual men. In fact, it has been suggested that the high rate of sexual contacts may help to bind the gay male community together (Gagnon, 1979).

Regardless of the reason, homosexual men do have access to a number of meeting places where they can make contacts with possible partners. For example, there are many "gay bars," which are known to members of the homosexual community. The character, the atmosphere, and the clientele of gay bars reflect the local surroundings. In the South, farmhands listen to country and Western music in gay bars; in the Midwest, truck drivers stop over in gay bars on cross-country hauls; in the East, a social elite dominates many gay bars (Sage, 1979).

Gay bars may be even more important in the social life of lesbians, since lesbians don't seem to "cruise," or solicit impersonal sex in public places. Although gay bars are not the lesbian's only source of social or sexual contact, they provide a protected setting where women who maintain a straight front in their daily lives can be open about their homosexuality (Hedblom and Hartman, 1980).

Some homosexual men also cruise. They use public baths and toilets (or "tearooms") to make sexual contacts. Such places provide an opportunity for impersonal sexual activity. The sexual script of the gay bath, another meeting place for gay men, differs radically from that of the public toilet. The physical environment of the bath is designed to make sexual contact comfortable, relaxed, and sensuous. In contrast, sexual contact in public toilets is usually hasty and filled with apprehension; it often seems sordid to one or both participants (Humphreys, 1970).

Dances and social gatherings sponsored by homosexual organizations also provide places for homosexuals to meet. These events create a personal, less stigmatized atmosphere in which male and female homosexuals can meet new people without the need for sexual contact. The recent growth of gay social, cultural, and religious organizations has provided greater opportunities for homosexuals to meet. In these organizations, the focus is less on the search for sexual partners than on sharing mutual interests and activities.

According to the stereotype, when male homosexuals grow old, they are always unhappy: The aging gay male who wants a sexual partner must pay a prostitute. This picture did not describe male homosexuals studied in the Los Angeles area. Although older men tended to have fewer partners than younger men, many of them maintained an active relationship with someone in their own age group and did not appear to be sexually dissatisfied (Kelly, 1979). When other homosexual men from different age groups were compared, older men were not significantly less happy than younger men. In fact, the older men appeared to have fewer conflicts about their sexual orientation and to have attained greater self-acceptance (Weinberg and Williams, 1974). Like other aspects of homosexual life, the image of the unhappy aging homosexual appears to be more myth than fact.

## HOMOSEXUAL INTERACTIONS

In a culture where "sex" is equated with placing the penis in the vagina, some of us wonder what homosexuals do. The sexual techniques used by homosexuals are essentially the same as those described in the last chapter as heterosexual foreplay. The primary difference is that these acts are performed by two persons of the same sex (Hunt, 1977). The sexuality of homosexual men and women is as varied as is the sexuality of hetereosexuals, and sexual scripts are just as individualistic. One young man said:

> A lot of straight people think every gay guy does every gay sex act, including anal intercourse. That's not true. I've only done it once. What my lover and I do depends on what we're both wanting and feeling at the time. (Bell, 1980, p. 122)

As with heterosexuals, interactions are affected by a variety of factors, including age, sexual experience, duration of the relationship, and individual sexual preference.

Among male homosexuals in one national study (Hunt, 1974), reciprocal masturbation was the most popular and widely used technique. About two-thirds of this group had performed fellatio, and half had received it. About the same number had experienced anal intercourse. Among homosexuals in the San Francisco Bay area, however, fellatio was the most popular and widely used technique, followed by reciprocal masturbation, anal intercourse, and body rubbing (Bell and Weinberg, 1978).

Lesbians use many techniques similar to heterosexual petting. One young lesbian said:

> I don't try to do it right. I just feel this flood of affection and excitement and I somehow know how I want to touch her. (Bell, 1980, p. 122)

The most popular and widely used technique in a national study (Hunt, 1974) was general body contact, with many lesbians also engaging in reciprocal masturbation, cunnilingus, and oral stimulation of the breasts. Contrary to popular myths, few had ever used a dildo (an artificial penis). Among lesbians in the San Francisco Bay area, mutual masturbation was the most common and most frequently used technique, although cunnilingus was the most highly preferred (Bell and Weinberg, 1978).

Among both men and women, the relationship between age and sexual behavior was the same as among heterosexuals; the younger the person, the wider the range of sexual practices. Younger homosexuals, like their heterosexual counterparts, seemed more willing to experiment and less sexually inhibited than older homosexuals. Of course, it may be that the older group had used a greater variety of techniques in the past but with increasing age practiced only a few favorite techniques (Bell and Weinberg, 1978).

Kinsey (Kinsey et al., 1953) found that experienced homosexual women were more likely to have orgasms during sexual encounters than heterosexual women who had been married for five years. He suggested that the difference might be partly due to the fact that two people of the same sex understand each other's sexual and emotional needs better than two people of different gender. The approach of one gay male supported this belief:

> I work on the theory that if *I* like something, he may like it, too—I try to give the kinds of pleasure I'd like to receive. (Hite, 1981, p. 814)

Observations of homosexual activity in the laboratory by Masters and Johnson (1979) also support the suggestion. A major difference between homosexual and heterosexual techniques was that committed homosexual couples took their time during sexual activity. They seemed more relaxed and involved in the activity than did heterosexuals. This difference led Masters and Johnson to propose that heterosexuals are primarily "goal-oriented"—preoccupied with reaching orgasm—but that homosexuals focus more on "the exchange of pleasure." For example, male homosexual couples spent considerable time stimulating the partner's entire body before touching the genitals, and when genital stimulation began, it was prolonged with "teasing" techniques. One homosexual explained:

> I love feeling his body all over, front and back, head to toe, and at the same time he feels me (except I do not touch his cock during foreplay and he doesn't touch mine). (Hite, 1981, p. 812)

The traditional view of heterosexual encounters has been that the man plays the "active" role and the female the "passive" role. Although this notion of rigid roles has become much less common among heterosexuals, many people still believe homosexual partners play rigid sexual roles. Straight people often assume that one homosexual partner always plays the masculine role and the other the feminine role. Although such roles do exist in some homosexual relationships, they appear to be the exception. Reported one male homosexual:

> My preferences depend a lot on who I'm with. With some of my lovers I'm definitely more into giving than receiving, and I don't usually care for penetration. (Authors' files)

Another common myth is that people prefer homosexuality because they are either afraid of heterosexual lovemaking or incompetent at it. On the contrary, many gay men and women have had extensive heterosexual experience at some time in their lives. Although most homosexuals say they feel uncomfortable when engaging in heterosexual activity, this does not necessarily mean they are unable to perform. In fact, some individuals seem equally responsive to men or women, as we'll see next.

## BISEXUALITY

Bisexuality is even more difficult to define and explain than homosexuality. For one thing, some people regard the concept of bisexuality with deep skepticism, as one bisexual man found out:

> Straight people are more or less dubious about bisexuality. You are either one way or the other, and that's it. And in some instances you have trouble convincing the gay person. [They say] you can't enjoy sexual relationships with men and women. (Blumstein and Schwartz, 1977, p. 85)

If a bisexual is anyone whose sexual experience is neither exclusively homosexual nor exclusively heterosexual, then the group is extremely large. It would include some individuals in conventional heterosexual marriages as well as committed homosexuals, for the standard of bisexuality would simply be sexual contact with members of both sexes at some time.

Among a group of students who rated themselves as either heterosexual, homosexual, or bisexual, however, all the bisexual students placed themselves in categories 2, 3, and 4 on Kinsey's scale. No student in category 1 or 5, which denoted "incidental" sexual activity with a second gender, considered him- or herself bisex-

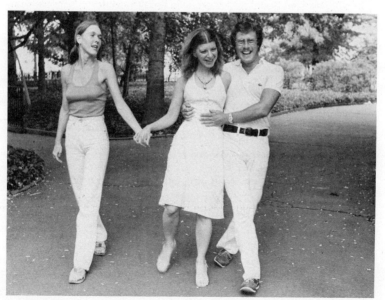

Most bisexuals have more than "incidental" sexual activity with both genders, but often feel pressure from the straight and gay communities to choose between the genders. (© Leonard Speier 1980)

*Focus*

THE QUESTION
OF TREATMENT

Once society began to regard homosexuality as a disease, many homosexuals entered treatment with psychologists or psychiatrists. For example, among more than a thousand homosexual men, 43 percent had received psychiatric treatment at some time (Weinberg and Williams, 1974). The goal of treatment was generally a change in sexual orientation.

During the past fifty years, therapists have used many forms of treatment to "convert" homosexuals to heterosexuality. The most common treatments have been psychoanalysis and behavior therapy, although brain surgery, electroconvulsive shock treatment (ECT), and various forms of drug therapy have also been used (Katz, 1976). In psychoanalytic therapy, the therapist guides the homosexual in a search for the childhood origins of his or her sexual orientation. In behavior therapy, attempts are made to

change the nature of the stimuli the person finds arousing. Homosexual stimuli (such as the sight of a nude male in the case of gay men) may be associated with nausea or electric shocks, while heterosexual stimuli (such as the sight of a nude woman) are associated with orgasm. None of these methods have succeeded with more than 40 percent of the homosexuals who have sought treatment (Masters and Johnson, 1979).

Changing attitudes toward homosexuality have decreased the proportion of homosexuals who seek treatment. Homosexuals who are troubled by their sexual orientation still enter therapy, but the goal is likely to be different. Many therapists today work toward helping homosexuals to become comfortable with their sexual orientation and to come to terms with their life style (McWhirter and Mattison, 1980).

In fact, during the past

ten years a controversy over the ethics of changing sexual orientation has developed. Spokespersons for the gay community (Katz, 1976) have argued that such therapy is a form of social repression. Psychologists (Davison, 1976; 1978) have argued that the mere existence of such programs strengthens prejudices against homosexuality and that, given the attitude of society, homosexuals are under so much pressure that a "free choice" to change their sexual orientation is virtually impossible. In this view, attempts to change a person's sexual preference are unethical.

Not all therapists agree. Some psychiatrists (Bieber, 1976) regard homosexuality as the result of serious disturbances during childhood and believe that even if all social pressure were removed, some homosexuals would still want to change their sexual orientation. Therapists who feel this way

---

ual. This standard seems reasonable, and gives us a way of talking about bisexuality as distinguished from homosexuality or heterosexuality.

A different approach has been used by Masters and Johnson (1979), who prefer the term **ambisexual**, which refers to people who have approximately equal interest and enjoyment in sexual encounters with men and women and who have no interest in a continuing relationship with one person. In sexual activity, the ambisexuals studied by Masters and Johnson responded physiologically just as did heterosexuals or homosexuals, but their emotional responses were different. Ambisexuals made their sexual choices simply on the basis of an opportunity to

**ambisexual** a bisexual with no interest in a continuing relationship with one person

say that homosexuals who want to develop a hetero-sexual orientation should have the opportunity, while those who do not wish to change can be helped to make a better adjustment of homosex-uality.

Psychiatrist Seymour Halleck (1976), who be-lieves that therapists' per-sonal values always influence their advice to patients, urges caution. He says that before at-tempting to change a pa-tient's sexual orientation, therapist and patient should conduct a lengthy dialogue so that the pa-tient understands his or her motivations and the consequences of making a change. When this is done, says Halleck, most homosexuals reject het-erosexuality as a goal. For example, one gay man said:

I entered analysis, volun-tarily I thought, with the idea that my "problem" was my homosexuality, and my goal a heterosex-ual "cure." . . . Paradoxi-cally, my experience in

therapy turned out to be an extremely good one, helping me to know and affirm positive parts of my-self, among them my ho-mosexuality. By accident I had found a therapist who helped people to find and be themselves, who did not view my "problem" as I did myself. (Katz, 1976, p. 131)

Masters and Johnson (1979) remain willing to help change sexual orien-tation, but only after a careful screening of appli-cants and only if the ho-mosexual has a cooperative partner of the other sex. Their goal is to help the homosexual ar-rive at a place where an unpressured decision be-tween homosexuality and heterosexuality can be made. They offer "conver-sion therapy" for individ-uals who are primarily homosexual but who wish to function in a heterosex-ual relationship and "re-version therapy" for individuals who have had sexual experience with both genders but wish to return to a predominantly

heterosexual orientation. Despite the screenings and the requirement that a partner be available, Masters and Johnson re-port that about 30 percent of the gays and lesbians who have gone through their program have failed to switch sexual orienta-tion.

Homosexuals who are content with their sexual orientation may still need therapy in order to func-tion better with their ho-mosexual partners. The sexual problems of homo-sexuals are similar to those found in heterosex-uals (see Chapter 14), and homosexuals respond as well—if not better—to sex therapy. Using techniques that have proved success-ful with heterosexual cou-ples, Masters and Johnson have been able to help about 90 percent of their gay and lesbian clients with such problems as erectile failure or inabil-ity to reach orgasm.

engage in sexual activity with someone they perceived as physically attractive; gen-der had nothing to do with it. These ambisexuals seemed lonely and lacked direct involvement in close love or family relationships.

This definition of ambisexuals as people who have difficulty in making emo-tional commitments is a restricted one, and eliminates many people who regard themselves as bisexual. Some bisexuals have only one sexual relationship at any one time, but alternate between male and female lovers (Klein, 1978). For some, their bisexuality is a transitional phase, usually between a heterosexual and a ho-mosexual way of life. Others view bisexuality differently. Bisexuals have been seen as people in the vanguard of sexual liberation—men and women who can express their sexuality without regard to gender preference. Bisexuals have also been seen as uncommitted homosexuals—"fence sitters" who lack the courage to admit their true sexual orientation.

Observers of bisexuality are forced to the conclusion we've reached concerning heterosexuals and homosexuals: there is no "bisexual personality" or single bisexual way of life. Among a large number of bisexual women, researchers (Blumstein and Schwartz, 1976) identified four main groups. One group said they had a variety of emotional needs, some that could be met only by men and others only by women. Another group seemed to have become bisexual because of unique circumstances, such as life in a prison, although these women had a history of sexual fantasy or involvement with both sexes. A third group seemed to have found bisexuality a way of establishing an identity, and many of these women had come to the position through involvement in the women's movement.

The last group were simply libertarians and regarded sexual experiences as needing no justification. They felt all varieties of sex were equally good as long as they did not exploit others and believed that a failure to experience the varieties was psychologically limiting. Some of this last group became bisexual because of a conscious decision to experiment. The rest became bisexual through experiences in sexual trios, in which a man with whom they were involved arranged a "threesome" with another woman.

As the experience of these women indicates, the paths to bisexuality are diverse. They also seem lengthy, for many people adopt the label late in their development. Although most heterosexuals and homosexuals identify their sexual preference during adolescence, the average age at which men and women in one group of bisexuals adopted the label was twenty-four years. Before this time, most had considered themselves to be predominantly heterosexual (Klein, 1978). Similar results have been found among bisexuals in the San Francisco Bay area (Bell, Weinberg, and Hammersmith, 1981), and in Seattle, New York, and Berkeley (Blumstein and Schwartz, 1976). In all these groups, bisexuality emerged during adulthood and seemed to be the result of adult social experiences. From what is known, the childhoods of bisexuals seem no different from those of heterosexuals or homosexuals.

Men appear to have more trouble than women in establishing and maintaining a bisexual identity. Some researchers (Blumstein and Schwartz, 1977) believe this difference is partly due to the ways in which men and women are socialized. They point to the general female preference for love and commitment in a relationship and the preference for impersonal sex among many men. Some men who routinely engage in impersonal homosexual activities, whether in prisons or in public rest rooms, regard themselves as heterosexuals.

Although some men with bisexual identities have predominantly heterosexual or homosexual experience, many have nearly equal experience with both sexes. As one man said:

> I love my wife. But I think I like sex a lot more than her, and anyhow I'm on the road a lot. It's easy just to get some sex along the way and it's easier with men. I never spend the night. . . . I never kiss them. It's just sex, and they do all the work. (Blumstein and Schwartz, 1977, p. 95)

This man's strictly impersonal attitude toward his homosexual partners was not typical of men with extensive heterosexual and homosexual experience studied by these same researchers. Most men adopted a bisexual identity only after their sexual interactions with other men went beyond impersonal sex. A large minority had never learned to attach any stigma to homosexual activities, and many had had a pattern of bisexual experience during adolescence, exclusively heterosexual experience during early adulthood, followed by a reawakened interest in homosexuality. Unlike bisexual women, men rarely became bisexual through group sex.

Bisexual men and women face problems that confront neither heterosexuals nor homosexuals. Unlike the heterosexual, the bisexual gets no support from social conventions and traditional moral standards. And unlike the homosexual, the bisexual has no support from an organized community of like-minded men and women. In fact, bisexual men and women often feel considerable pressure to choose between the genders and to identify with a well-established sexual preference and life style.

Bisexual women say that lesbian communities in large cities treat them with hostility and mistrust, making it difficult to maintain a bisexual identity. As a result, the women must choose among rejecting the lesbian community, rejecting their heterosexual interests, or disguising them (Blumstein and Schwartz, 1976). Bisexual men have somewhat similar problems. They discover that the gay community often regards them with suspicion, seeing the "failure" to admit to a homosexual identity as a rejection of gay liberation or fearing that social stigma or pressures on homosexuality may lead the bisexual man to retreat to the safety of the heterosexual world (Blumstein and Schwartz, 1977).

Studies of bisexuality seem to support the heavily psychological nature of human sexuality. Sexual identity, whether heterosexual, homosexual, or bisexual, doesn't always correspond to sexual behavior. And people's places on the continuum of sexual orientation may shift considerably during a lifetime.

# Summary

**1** Sexual activity with a partner of the same sex is known as **homosexuality**, although many homosexual women prefer to be called **lesbians** and many homosexual men prefer to be called **gays**. Some people are **bisexual**: they are aroused by and have sexual experiences with both men and women.

**2** Attitudes toward homosexuality vary across cultures. In some societies, homosexuality is allowed under certain circumstances; in some cultures it is limited to adolescents. In some cultures, it is forbidden and punished. In most cultures, homosexuality seems to be more prevalent among men than among women.

**3** American society has both a positive homosexual tradition (from the Greek heritage) and a negative homosexual tradition (from the Judeo-Christian heritage). Laws and customs tend to reflect the Judeo-Christian heritage, and homosexual activity has been illegal in many states. In recent years, however, legal rights have been extended to homosexuals in a number of states. In the Judeo-Christian tradition, homosexuality was a sin; after World War II, it came to be seen as a disease; today, partly as a result of data gathered by sex researchers, it is coming to be seen as a "normal" sexual variation. However, many people are **homophobic**—they have an irrational fear of homosexuality.

**4** A great many people are neither exclusively homosexual nor exclusively heterosexual, so it is very difficult to classify people by sexual orientation. Kinsey's scale of sexual orientation, which places people on a continuum, has been widely accepted. According to biological theories, hormones—either by exposure before birth or by effects after birth—probably play a role in the development of homosexuality. According to psychoanalytic theories, emotional conflicts within the family that keep a child from identifying with the parent of the same sex are primarily responsible. According to social learning theory, homosexuality develops through conditioning: a person learns to prefer sexual partners of the same gender. Some believe that homosexuality develops from prenatal exposure to hormones combined with learning. Researchers have been unable to find a "homosexual personality," and it appears that the only thing homosexuals have in common is their sexual orientation.

**5** In a study of 1,500 homosexuals, researchers could find no consistent family background that distinguished homosexuals from heterosexuals. However, they did find a lack of conformity to sex roles during childhood among both lesbians and gays, with each preferring the activities of the other sex. Although both heterosexuals and homosexuals often had childhood homosexual experiences, they interpreted those experiences differently.

**6** Homosexuals have different life styles: some are close-coupled, with exclusive relationships; some are open-coupled, with a stable relationship but engaging in sexual relationships with others; some are functional, much like heterosexual "swinging singles"; some are dysfunctional, with major problems in social adjustment; and some are asexual, without partners either by choice or circumstance. Coming out, or making their sexual orientation known to others, begins for homosexuals with the development of a homosexual identity, a process that may include denial, anger, bargaining, and depression before the identity is established. Although coming out is often stressful, it can be beneficial.

**7** Many homosexual men tend to follow a pattern of impersonal sexual activity with a large number of partners, a practice that has recently been linked to AIDS, a serious disease. The pattern may be the result of socialization practices in which men are permitted to separate sex from emotion and commitment, and it is rarely found among lesbians.

**8** Homosexuals use essentially the same sexual techniques found in heterosexual foreplay, and the sexuality of homosexual men and women is as varied as the sexuality of heterosexuals.

**9** There is no bisexual personality or a single bisexual way of life. People become bisexual by many paths, and generally adopt a bisexual identity during adulthood. The childhoods of bisexuals seem identical with the childhoods of heterosexuals. Bisexual men and women may have problems maintaining their sexual identity because they have neither support from social convention and traditional moral standards, as heterosexuals do, nor support from an organized community, as homosexuals do.

*a man's view*

Making the first move is always the hardest. No one likes to be rejected, and I'm no exception. Sex would be a lot easier if people could read each other's minds, or maybe we could learn to do it by numbers! (Authors' files)

*a woman's view*

One of the things I liked was having my breasts fondled. This was something I had to ask for specifically with my ex-husband and it was very hard for me to do. I felt the man was supposed to know what would satisfy me, so I rarely made any requests. I guess I felt embarrassed or ashamed to ask for anything specific. (Barbach and Levine, 1981, pp. 179–180)

# 10 Sexual Communication

*Chapter 10*

We may have learned all about sexual anatomy and mastered the techniques of intercourse, but unless we can convey our wishes to a potential partner, we're limited to the solitary pleasures of fantasy and masturbation. Whether we are heterosexual, homosexual, or bisexual, unless we can establish communication, there can be no shared sexual activity.

Communicating our sexual intentions can be done with words or with gestures and signs. We can exchange glances, smile, take a seat beside a desirable partner, use a lingering touch in a social situation that calls for fleeting contact. Most of these messages are vague, easy to misunderstand, and hard to describe.

The vagueness of a preliminary sexual invitation is no accident. Vague invitations bind neither party and allow offers to be withdrawn or refused without offending the person who sent the sign or the one who received it. Even when the intent is clear, as when gaze is met and held, or else prolonged and then broken off so eyes can travel over the possible partner's body, as long as there is no stated commitment, the "courtship" can be ended at any time (Cook and McHenry, 1978).

Once a sexual partner is found, the communication problem does not disappear. Timing, individual preferences, and personal problems can interfere with satisfaction in an established sexual relationship. In this chapter, we'll study how sexual intentions are expressed in various cultures. Then we'll look at emotional communication in sexual relationships, examining the feelings that can build emotional barriers as well as common roadblocks to sexual communication. After exploring the art of sexual assertiveness and

# Sexual Communication

how to initiate sex or decline a partner's advances, we'll look at nonverbal communication in sexual relationships. Finally, we'll explore the limits of sexual communication.

## CULTURAL VARIATION

In most human societies sexual signals are indirect, but in a few tribal societies they can be blatant. A Lesu or Dahomean woman may display her sexual organs to the man of her choice, and among the Kurtachi, a woman may lie down in the man's presence and part her legs—an exposure of the genitals that is considered indecent in any other situation. Such cultures are rare, however; most societies exercise rigid control over genital displays. A society is far more likely to insist that the vulva be concealed than to demand that the penis be covered (Ford and Beach, 1951).

Most societies are also likely to insist that the man initiate sexual advances. Although a few cultures permit a woman to make the first sexual move, the majority resemble traditional American society: The man takes the initiative. With this custom, human beings differ from animals. In most animal species, both male and female actively solicit sex. Among chimpanzees, it is generally the female who initiates sexual activity (Ford and Beach, 1951).

As noted earlier, most bids for sexual activity are indirect. A simple verbal request is

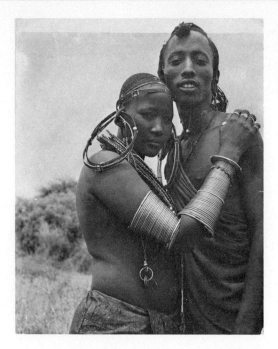

Although the specific signals differ from one society to another, every culture has ways to indicate sexual interest and establish intimacy. (© Hector R. Acebes/Photo Researchers, Inc.)

acceptable in some societies (which may insist that the question be whispered), but far more common is a wordless signal. In the South Pacific Caroline Islands, a simple gesture is enough. The man asks and the woman accepts by putting a hand to the forehead and moving it slowly downward over the face (Ford and Beach, 1951). Among the Hottentots, a man creeps into the woman's hut at night and lies beside her. On that first visit—and until she makes up her mind—the woman gets up and leaves. The midnight visits continue until the woman sends her own signal. A woman who decides to accept the invitation stays with her suitor and has intercourse. A woman who decides to reject the suitor is already gone one night when he comes into the hut (Cook and McHenry, 1978).

In some societies, an object is used to request sexual activity. Men of the Yungar use a stick covered with yellow clay. Each stick is carved in a unique manner, and Yungar men carry their sticks about so that all women know the pattern of each young man's stick. At night the man slips his stick through the wall of the chosen woman's hut and nudges her with it. She runs her hand over the carving, identifies the owner, and decides whether to accept the invitation (Cook and McHenry, 1978).

Although custom has discouraged women from initiating sexual activity in American culture, most have learned subtle ways of indicating their interest. One woman listed the kinds of flirtation she uses to indicate her sexual availability: brushing by the potential partner's body; holding his glance longer than necessary; retaining a handshake; altering the tone of her voice; saying something provocative that can be taken in more than one way (Barbach and Levine, 1981). But once contact has been made and the partner won, communication must continue if the relationship is to be satisfying.

# EMOTIONAL COMMUNICATION
# IN A SEXUAL RELATIONSHIP

For most of us, the sexual script depends on an emotional involvement with a partner. If we can establish intimacy and learn to exchange positive feelings with a partner and to resolve our emotional differences, the way is paved for a satisfying sexual relationship. A woman described the importance of emotional communication to her:

> We must have talked for hours before we finally made love. It made me feel so much closer to him, and sex has never been better. (Authors' files)

Sexual intimacy may also require the solution of basic conflicts in the relationship and the dispelling of myths about the communication.

## Establishing intimacy

Intimacy means sharing another person's feelings and experiences. Since intimacy runs both ways, it involves acceptance of the partner as well as personal openness—an openness that leaves each partner vulnerable.

The problem of establishing intimacy is complicated because relationships often begin on a false note. Each partner presents him- or herself in a flattering light and sees the other in a romantic haze. False impressions are made and barriers thrown up that must be broken down if the relationship is to last. The exciting job turns out to be low-paid drudgery. The jaded world traveler turns out to have spent a single cut-rate weekend in Jamaica. The proficient tennis player turns out to be clumsy on the court. The wine connoisseur turns out to have drunk nothing but jug wines. The Ferrari turns out to be a Volkswagen. In short, neither partner is the idealized lover who gazes sexily from the screen in television commercials.

But it doesn't stop there. Each partner is also human, with weaknesses and annoying habits. "He" leaves the top off the toothpaste. "She" sheds hair, clogging drains and combs. "He" automatically reaches for the salt before tasting food. "She" can never remember to pay her bills. "He" ejaculates before she has an orgasm. "She" adheres rigidly to her sexual script and refuses to try anything new.

As intimacy slowly develops, each partner accepts the other's flaws, one at a time. Acceptance can be conveyed by word and by act. A smile, a hug, a kiss, a caress, a compliment can all indicate acceptance. In fact, nothing deepens intimacy and increases communication faster than compliments. Partners need to know that they are cared about, admired, and needed, and open expressions of caring encourage free communication (Alberti and Emmons, 1978).

Acceptance of a partner involves offering empathy instead of criticism, listening to opinions and ideas, wishes and secrets, without putting the other person down. It is actually establishing a friendship, for a sexual relationship that lacks friendship is usually fated to fail (Phillips and Judd, 1982).

Hand in hand with acceptance goes vulnerability. Partners who do not feel accepted, who think that their confidences will be ridiculed or that their secrets are not safe, tend to hold back, keeping up the barriers. When a partner feels accepted and becomes open, he or she risks being hurt. For that reason, some authorities (Phillips and Judd, 1982) recommend disclosing vulnerabilities slowly. If a partner reacts by moralizing, criticizing, or becoming hostile, the hurt is small. But if the disclosure evokes warmth, compliments, or understanding, the relationship has become stronger.

Although the first sign of sexual intent is often purposefully vague, communication between a pair of established partners needs to be clear and nonthreatening. Information should always be placed in context so that misunderstanding becomes less likely (Buscaglia, 1978). If this is not done, couples often wind up trying to decode each other's actions and intentions. Instead of abandoning themselves to lovemaking, they're trying to figure out their partner's needs, wishes, and reactions. Since this sort of analysis combines ignorance and mind-reading, the conclusions drawn—especially by an insecure partner—can be disastrous. As one woman said:

> It's so hard to know what he really wants. I can't stop wondering if I'm doing the right thing. (Authors' files)

Partners who accept each other and feel able to say what they think can reveal their fears and their fantasies. They will be able to "let go" in sex, abandoning themselves to pleasure without fretting over their sexual performance, for they don't have to worry about being judged (Bach and Torbet, 1982).

## Resolving basic conflicts

Many couples are unable to achieve sexual intimacy because they have not resolved basic conflicts in their relationship. Feelings of anger, resentment, or mistrust can build emotional barriers that make sexual intimacy almost impossible. When partners avoid communicating their feelings, secrets, and desires, it's usually because they are covering up some problem they are afraid to face. For example, although it had been six years since Philip had had an affair with Beth's best friend, he still felt guilty and could not shake his fear that Beth would one day find out about it. His unresolved feelings made it increasingly difficult for him to approach Beth for sex, or to enjoy their sexual relationship in a free and spontaneous manner. Being unaware of Philip's feelings, Beth blamed herself for the coldness between them. She decided it had developed because she had not maintained her youthful good looks. In order to regain her husband's interest, Beth tried one diet after another.

The most frequent problem behind an emotional barrier is a fear of rejection, but other things can also stop communication: overdependence, a feeling of being exploited, or a sense that the partner is extremely hostile (Bach and Wyden, 1968). The fears are often groundless, and learning to communicate more effectively can help to resolve many emotional conflicts that would otherwise spill over into the sexual side of the relationship.

When couples fail to express their feelings, intimacy usually withers. A person who can't state dissatisfaction over trivial matters often becomes unable to speak up over important matters that may be causing great pain. Tension builds until an explosion destroys the partnership, or feelings shrivel until two people are living together in a dead relationship. The question is not "whether" to talk about distressing situations, but "how" and "when" (Fensterheim and Baer, 1975).

Speaking up requires each partner to be **assertive**—to act in his or her best interest, expressing honest feelings and exercising personal rights without denying the rights of others (Alberti and Emmons, 1978). For assertive communications to be effective, impact must equal intent. But because any message must pass through the filter of both speaker and listener, the message often becomes distorted. The mood of either partner can change, even reverse, the impact of the words (Gottman et al., 1976).

Suppose Brian and Mary are going out to dinner, and Brian, who has had a hard day, looks at Mary and says: "You're wearing your red dress." What he means is, "You always look so sexy in that dress that, tired as I am, you excite me." His weariness filters his words, however, so that Mary, who's also had a long, tiring day, interprets the message as "Wearing that old dress again? Why can't you make an effort to look nice when we go out?" Instead of initiating a loving exchange, Brian has inadvertently put a temporary chill on the relationship. Because such incidents are so common, many authorities (Gottman et al., 1976) suggest that partners ask each other for feedback—information about the message's impact—when their statements seem to have gone astray.

When the impact of a communication differs from its intent, there's often a lot of mind-reading going on. Two people in a long-standing sexual relationship generally believe that each knows what the other is feeling or thinking. Mind-reading can build its own unnecessary barriers. Because she never initiates sex, Joel believes Julia has a low level of sexual interest. Acting on his belief, he sometimes masturbates when he'd rather be enjoying sex with her. Actually, Julia's sexual desire is just as high as Joel's but she believes that "nice girls" don't show an active interest in sex. She reads Joel's mind, too, and assumes that whenever Joel feels sexy, he will approach her. Neither Julia nor Joel is satisfied with their once-a-week sexual encounters, but each mind-reader tries to accommodate him- or herself to the other's wishes, and each assumes the other is content.

Successful communication between partners requires two basic skills: leveling and editing (Gottman et al., 1976). **Leveling** means expressing feelings in clear, simple language; it doesn't mean pointing out what the partner is doing wrong. There is no place in leveling for character assassination ("You're a mamma's boy") or insults ("You simply can't be on time"). The purpose of leveling is to make clear partners' expectations of each other, their likes and dislikes, what binds them together and what pulls them apart.

Constructive leveling follows this form: When you do X in situation Y, I feel Z. Suppose your partner has a habit of leaving you alone at parties while he or she goes off to talk animatedly with members of the other sex. In order to level about the subject, you might say: "When you leave me at parties to spend your time with

**assertive** able to act in one's personal interest, expressing honest feelings and exercising personal rights without denying the rights of others

**leveling** expressing feelings in clear, simple language in order to clarify expectations, likes, and dislikes

*Focus*

ROADBLOCKS
TO SEXUAL
COMMUNICATION

Most people have no trouble at all telling their partner that they love liver or loathe limburger, but when it comes to communicating about sex, they freeze. Yet many of these same people can trade "dirty" jokes, discourse at length about specific findings in the latest sex survey, or speculate about the sexual basis of their neighbors' divorce. Talk about sex in the abstract may have invaded the classroom and the parlor, but personal sex—talk about one's own sexual needs and desires—is generally still taboo. Sex therapists report that even people who consider themselves swingers and who have "had sex in every conceivable way with almost everyone in town" find it difficult to discuss with their partners their own

thoughts, feelings, and actions during sex (Zilbergeld, 1978).

So most people come to a sexual relationship with no practice in discussing personal sex. And any impulse to begin talking about it immediately runs into a pair of myths that block the path of sexual communication. These myths are "sex should be natural and spontaneous," and "if my partner loved me, he (she) would know what I want."

Why sexual techniques should come naturally and spontaneously to each human being who has had to learn how to talk, eat, read, swim, drive a car, or play a piano is never explained. In learning all these other human actions, models are available—people whose behavior can be observed

and imitated. But when the bedroom door closes, people are on their own.

Spontaneity in any other field, from painting and ballet dancing to tennis, comes from knowing the skills so well that they are used without thought. Yet spontaneity in sex is supposed to be as natural as breathing. One woman summed up the prevalent attitude, saying:

I bought into the myth that you don't need to talk about sex. If it's all right, if it's really love, it will just go smoothly and everybody will know what they like and enjoy (Barbach and Levine, 1981, p. 176)

Not until after she was divorced did this woman learn to communicate her own sexual preferences.

There is no reason, of course, why talking about sex cannot be spontaneous. "I'd like it if you

other women (or men), I feel rejected and lonely." You talk about your feelings. You don't say, "You always desert me at parties."

In fact, two words that invariably tag a statement as a put-down or an insult are "always" and "never." They have no place in leveling.

Leveling is one side of effective communication. The other side is editing. **Editing** means being polite to your partner, eliminating comments that are rude, offensive, or snide. It means leaving out complaints in favor of specific requests and making honest statements you think your partner will like. Properly used, editing neither distorts the truth in order to avoid repercussions nor withholds information in order to be tactful. Suppose a man enjoys anal stimulation during intercourse, but fails to say so because he thinks he might offend his partner or she might believe he was "perverted." (Notice that he edited his behavior because he read his partner's mind.) Not only will his editing result in a failure to get anal stimulation, but he may also build up resentment against his partner for not initiating anal play

**editing** leaving out complaints and rude, offensive, or snide comments in favor of specific requests and honest statements

would . . .'' could be as natural as ''I love you'' or ''Look at the beautiful sunset.'' But such statements are rare, because it's not ''nice'' to talk about sex. Statements about sexual preferences are also rare becaus^ they make people vulnerable. Talking about sexual joys, anxieties, preferences, and dislikes opens a person to possible hurt, rejection, and a powerful intimacy (Zilbergeld, 1978). And as we've seen, vulnerability is one aspect of intimacy.

The second myth, ''if my partner really loved me, he (she) would know what I want,'' is a demand for mind-reading. But as Joel and Julia's relationship showed, sexual mind-reading is often just plain wrong. Many couples who consult sex therapists are

there because they believed that love, sensitivity, and consideration naturally produce a mind-reading partner. Since sex is mostly psychological and since psychogenic stimuli—which are learned—are both extremely powerful and differ from person to person, it's no wonder that mind-reading frequently goes astray.

Each gender also has its own problems that stand in the way of sexual communication. Many women have so absorbed the cultural stereotype of female purity and chastity that they feel any expression of preference either reveals a vast sexual experience or betrays a base desire women should not possess (Barbach and Levine, 1981). Men are permitted to have sexual

preferences, but they are also—according to cultural stereotypes—supposed to be so experienced that no one needs to tell them anything about sex. As a result, women worry that expressing sexual preferences will damage a male ego, and men worry that if they ask about their partner's preferences, they will reveal an ignorance in an area where ''real men'' are wise. One woman explained:

I felt the man was supposed to know what would satisfy me, so I rarely made any requests. I guess I felt embarrassed or ashamed to ask for anything specific. (Barbach and Levine, 1981, p. 180)

But difficult as it is to talk about sexual likes and dislikes, such communication can greatly enhance a sexual relationship.

on her own. This kind of editing is often the result of some common roadblocks that stand in the way of emotional communication.

## VERBAL COMMUNICATION

For most people, sex is a time of silence broken only by sighs, grunts, and moans. The roadblocks to sexual communication effectively strike them dumb at a time when a few words might make all the difference. Talking openly about sex is bound to make most lovers uncomfortable at first, but the increased pleasure that it brings is well worth the discomfort that surrounds initial attempts to tell a partner about feelings or wishes. As a man said:

Since I started asking for what I want, our whole relationship has changed. I'm not saying it's easy, but it sure has been worth it. (Authors' files)

## *The art of sexual assertiveness*

Sexual assertiveness increases pleasure in three ways. First, if you ask for something pleasurable, you're more likely to get it. Second, when you're assertive, you're unlikely to be anxious. The two feelings cannot coexist. Third, expressing your honest feelings and desires increases intimacy between partners (Phillips and Judd, 1982).

Being sexually assertive does not mean being rude or dominating. It means paying attention to your own needs as well as to the needs of your partner. It means expressing your desires directly. Sexually assertive people can do more than tell a partner how to stimulate them effectively. They can also decline a sexual invitation, make it clear when they'd prefer some activity besides genital intercourse, indicate when they'd like to stop in the middle of sexual activity, speak up when nonsexual emotions are interfering with their sexual functioning, and ask a partner how he (or she) would like to be stimulated. Aggressive or dominating people can also do these things, but the sexually assertive person can do them in a way that doesn't humiliate or reject a partner, or make a partner feel undesirable (Zilbergeld, 1978). Sexually assertive people are willing to give as well as take.

Once you know what gives you most pleasure during sex, there are only three reasons for feeling dissatisfied. Either you are having sex when you don't really want to, you are not letting your partner know about your sexual preferences, or you've told your partner but she (or he) has ignored your requests (Nowinski, 1980). If you can develop your ability at sexual communication, at least the first two situations can be avoided.

The first step toward sexual assertiveness needn't be eloquent. Just a simple statement about a small sexual worry will start to drive away anxiety and eliminate the resentment that often grows from silence (Phillips and Judd, 1982).

It's important to communicate without hurting a partner's feelings. There are techniques that can ease, if not eliminate, a partner's pain on being told that his (or her) sexual technique is not perfect. First, put yourself in your partner's place and imagine how you would want your partner to tell you the same thing (empathy). Second, communicate as much positive information as possible (reinforcement). Being told about all the good things she (or he) does makes a request easier to take and ensures that your partner will keep on stimulating you in ways you like.

Some people find it easiest to speak up during sexual activity, especially if it's to increase pleasure. "Talking not only gets me the kind of touching I want but turns me on as well," said one woman (Barbach and Levine, 1981, p. 195). Others prefer to wait, on the grounds that calling signals to your partner during sex introduces the atmosphere of instruction from a sex manual and breaks the sexual spell.

Brief comments are best during lovemaking: "Touch me here" or "Would you rub my balls?" or "Higher up" or "That feels good." Because a lengthy discussion is likely to destroy the mood, many people find it easier to set aside a specific time to share their feelings about sex. By choosing a time in advance, a couple can talk when neither partner is tired, when they have privacy, and when no television can distract them or provide them with an excuse for not listening (Gochros and Fisher, 1980).

## *Developing sexual assertiveness*

Because talking about sex is so difficult for most people, a little practice before-hand is likely to ease any attempt to talk to your partner. When using this technique, called **behavioral rehearsal**, you imagine a scene with your lover, saying out loud the things you plan to say.

**behavioral rehearsal** imaginativepractice of a planned interaction, saying aloud planned statements

The first exercise is meant for brief communication during sexual activities, although it can be adapted to other forms of sexual communication. It is a version of the exercises developed by Joseph Nowinski (1980), and it provides practice in various types of sexual communication.

Begin by imagining you are in bed with your partner. You are caressing your lover's body. As you visualize yourself touching your partner, say, "Does that feel good?" Say it again. Your voice should be soft, not demanding. While imagining the same scene, say gently: "If I'm doing anything you don't like, just tell me." Say it again.

After you feel comfortable in these two situations, say to your imaginary partner: "I'd like to have you touch me now." Keep saying this line over until you can say it smoothly, without any nervous edge in your voice.

Now visualize your partner caressing you in a way you especially like. Practice telling your lover about your feelings, saying, "I like that" or "That feels good" or "Wonderful!" several times.

Perhaps there is a certain kind of stimulation you'd like that your partner hasn't given you. Practice asking for it in a gentle but uncritical voice. Imagine that your partner is still caressing you and say: "That's great. Now I'd like to have you (whatever you'd like)."

People's sexual preferences differ, and a particular kind of stimulation that is highly desirable to one person is distasteful to another. Through behavioral rehearsal, you can learn to stop stimulation you don't like or refuse a particular activity that you find unpleasant.

Suppose you are touched in a way you find unpleasant or even painful. Imagine such a situation, and practice asking your lover to stop. Say, "I'd like it better if you would (substitute some other kind of stimulation)." Repeat this line until you can say it without sounding tense or forceful.

On occasion a partner will ask for some kind of stimulation that you find distasteful. Practice a gentle refusal that has no overtones of disapproval. Say, "I'm sorry, but I don't want to do that. Can I do something else for you instead?" In either of these situations, neither you nor your partner should feel guilt or embarrassment because your sexual preferences differ.

Sometimes brief comments are not enough. You and your partner may need to communicate about sex in a way that requires detailed messages, or you may simply prefer to avoid sexual instruction during lovemaking. Bernie Zilbergeld (1978) has developed an exercise for such occasions. In carrying out this exercise, make an appointment with your partner for a "talk-and-listen" session so your discussion can take place without distraction. The discussion should take no longer that fifteen minutes and should be limited to one main point. Presenting a lengthy bill of particulars is threatening and may do more harm than good.

Suppose your partner has refused your last few attempts to initiate sex, and you are feeling rejected. Before the session begins, you might use the technique of behavioral rehearsal to make certain you can present the problem without sounding angry or tense.

The ground rules for a talk-and-listen session are simple. The person who asked for the session says what he (or she) has to say without interruption from the partner. The partner agrees not to present a defense, to answer you, or to comfort you—the job is to understand the problem in your relationship.

When you have presented the issue, your partner gives you feedback, stating your point in his (or her) own words. In this instance, the partner might say, "I hear that you are upset because I didn't want to have sex the last few times you asked me. You think that means I no longer love you."

If your partner has understood your point, say so. If she (or he) has misunderstood you, restate the problem and again have the partner put it into her (or his) own words. Keep this exchange up until your partner understands your point.

Now, if your partner wishes to reply, he (or she) can make a point, using the same format, with you restating his (or her) point. Since sexual matters are so closely tied to emotion and self-esteem, it's best to wait for a few minutes after your point has been understood before your partner attempts a reply.

Although this talk-and-listen method is extremely effective at eliminating mind-reading and developing understanding, it does not guarantee that you'll get what you want. Suppose your point has been that you'd like to add oral sex to your lovemaking, and the burden of your partner's reply is that oral sex is highly distasteful to him (or her). Oral sex may still be out of bounds in your partner's sexual script, but you'll each understand the other's feelings.

Discussing your relationship with your partner may be uncomfortable at first, but speaking openly about feelings and wishes can deepen intimacy and increase sexual pleasure. (© Frank Siteman/Stock, Boston)

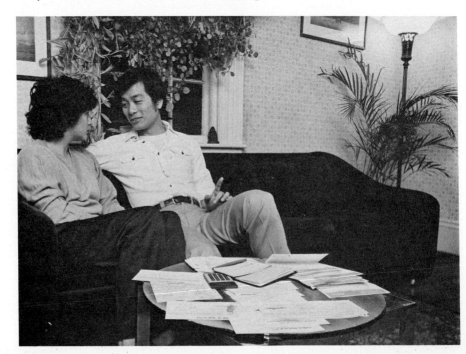

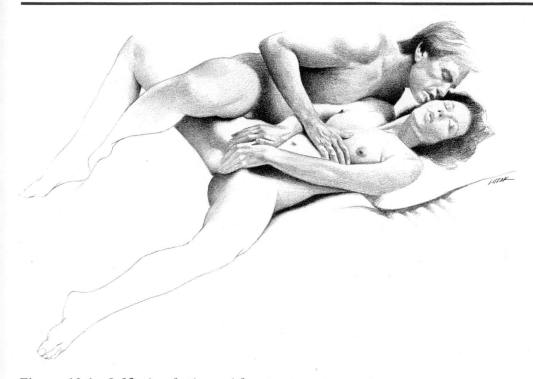

***Figure 10.1   Self-stimulation with a partner present.***
This can be an effective way for demonstrating sexual arousal techniques to one's partner.

## Initiating and rejecting sex

Indicating an interest in having sex with a partner or declining a partner's advances presents a particular problem in sexual relationships. It's a problem that can be handled best by regarding it as a time for assertive communication—expressing feelings openly without being insensitive to a partner's needs.

**Initiating sex**   In American culture, men have traditionally been expected to initiate sexual activity. The presumption is so strong that many women have trouble letting a partner know they'd like to make love. Some believe that "nice" women don't show any active sexual interest, some believe they will seem aggressive or unfeminine, and many fear their partners will reject them.

Instead of openly stating their wishes, they tend to disguise them, simply being warm and available in the hope that the partner will decode the message. Other women use nonverbal signals (see Figure 10.1), such as massaging a partner's neck, touching him in a lingering, sensuous way, or engaging in intense eye contact. One woman removes her underwear while leaving on her outer garments, and then hugs and kisses her partner. She says:

He gets really surprised and excited, and it's a neat lead-in to sex. (Barbach and Levine, 1981, p. 207)

For both men and women, a direct request can be more effective than a subtle or an ambiguous signal. It avoids unenthusiastic lovemaking sessions that may be initiated when one partner either misunderstands an expression of caring or an indirect request or erroneously reads a partner's mind. Mind-reading can cause trouble in all aspects of a sexual relationship. Besides being direct, the request should be caring, seductive, and romantic. "I want to make love with you," "Would you come to bed with me?" or "Would you like to make love" leave no doubt (Phillips and Judd, 1982).

**Rejecting sex** A direct invitation to sexual activity may be turned down, but such invitations are refused less often than they ought to be. Both men and women find it hard to say "no" to a regular partner. Many men consider it unmanly to refuse a sexual invitation. And so they enthusiastically carry through, or else they pretend to be busy or tired or angry—perhaps even picking a fight in order to avoid sex (Zilbergeld, 1978). Despite the traditional "I have a headache, dear" joke, many women are unable to reject a partner's advances. They believe sex is a male privilege, so instead of refusing, they "endure" intercourse.

A sexually assertive "no" to a partner's advances should be phrased so the partner's feelings are not hurt and he (or she) does not feel rejected or angry. It's possible to say simply, "I really care about you, but I'm not in the mood" (Phillips and Judd, 1982). However, therapists suggest offering alternatives to intercourse. Either some sensual but nonsexual contact—a massage, cuddling, or holding—or verbal contact—talking together—can provide a gentle, nonrejecting refusal.

Sometimes partners who are not in the mood themselves can offer other sexual pleasure to a lover. Sex need not always include intercourse, nor need it always be reciprocal (Zilbergeld, 1978). If one partner strongly desires sexual contact and the other is not interested, the uninterested partner can touch and kiss the aroused partner, using mouth and hands to provide sexual pleasure. In such instances, the partner who is not in the mood should make clear the fact that she (or he) has no desire for genital intercourse. However, this sort of compromise requires partners who feel no anxiety or resentment at the prospect of giving or receiving one-sided sexual activity (Phillips and Judd, 1982). It's always possible, of course, that a partner who feels no interest in sexual contact will become aroused as she (or he) stimulates the other. If so, any mutual activity that results will be free from resentment.

Just as important as being able to turn down an invitation is the ability to accept a refusal. The response should be without anger, without resentment, but with a loving, "I'm sorry that you're not in the mood." If your partner is not interested in nonreciprocal sex and you would still like some physical contact, it's all right to say: "I understand. But I'd like you simply to hold me" (Barbach and Levine, 1981).

Some couples have worked out a "sexual responsiveness scale" that runs from

0 to 10, with 0 indicating no interest at all in sex and 10 indicating an overpowering interest. In order to accommodate the wishes of both partners, they agree that whenever the couple's sexual desire totals 10, they will have sex. This method is flexible, and since it rates the intensity of desire, a partner knows when a refusal would be a real hardship and when it would be only a mild disappointment. As a woman who uses the scale said:

> If one was a ten and the other a one, just on good faith we'd have sex. . . . If I come up and kiss him in a certain way, he may then say, "Hmm, what's your number?" and I'll say, "See you in the bedroom," or I'll say "No, that was an innocent kiss. That was only a three." . . . The scale cuts through a lot, it gets right to the point. (Barbach and Levine, 1981, p. 217)

Although verbal communication can be highly effective, it's not the only way to be sexually assertive, as we'll see in the next section.

## NONVERBAL COMMUNICATION

Although most people equate communication with speech, there are many ways to express feelings without using words. Emotions can be conveyed by facial expressions, eye contact, body language, and by such vocalizations as sighs, moans, chuckles, and snorts. A man whose partner was good at sending nonverbal signals said:

> She only has to look at me in a certain way and things get started. It's hard to describe it exactly, but it works every time! (Authors' files)

Nonverbal communication can establish intimacy as effectively as words—or it can cause as many problems as the wrong words.

As we've seen, many women rely on nonverbal means to initiate sex. Sexual preferences can also be indicated without words. When a certain kind of stimulation displeases one partner, a stiffening of the body sometimes effectively signals the other. At times, simply presenting the part of the body that is to be stimulated works. One woman said that she turned her body around when she wanted oral sex, and another reported of her husband:

> It turns him off to talk about it too much. So I pretty much have to use my body to get what I want. (Barbach and Levine, 1981, p. 198)

Sometimes modeling, or showing a partner the desired technique, successfully communicates sexual preferences. There are several ways to model sexual stimulation. You can demonstrate your own sexual preferences by stimulating yourself while your partner watches, by putting your hand over your partner's and guiding it so that the partner knows where and how to touch you, or by placing your partner's hand on top of your own while you stimulate yourself. Similarly, you can dis-

# *Focus*

THE ART
OF SENSUAL
MASSAGE

Sensual massage is a form of touch that can increase pleasure in physical stimulation and awareness of a partner's responses. In addition to improving sensual and sexual communication, it can be a form of foreplay or relaxation. Massage can help men overcome their goal-oriented attitudes about foreplay (Zilbergeld, 1978). It need not lead to sexual activities, although it may.

The establishment of massage parlors that line city streets has made it more difficult for people to understand that sensual massage need not involve sex. Since these parlors are intended for the sale of sex, not massage, they have reinforced the myth that all touching leads to sex or orgasm.

In sensual massage, the person giving the massage should derive as much satisfaction from the experience as the person who gets it. Receiving a massage can be as much of an art as giving one. Some people are uncomfortable whenever they are expected to relax and let go. But if a massage is to be successful, the receiver must trust the giver, and accept rather than resist the sensations. For those who can let go, the feeling of being in touch with bodily sensations is rewarding, and the experience of trust and intimacy can enhance and strengthen a relationship.

Before the massage begins, the proper mood should be set. The absence of glaring lights, a temperature that makes

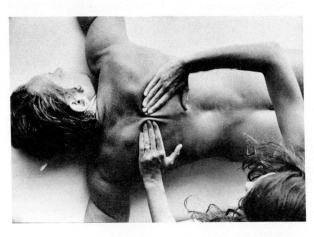

Sensual massage can improve a sexual relationship in several ways. It can increase an awareness of a partner's responses, deepen the pleasure of physical stimulation, induce relaxation, and develop trust and intimacy. (© Paul Fusco/Magnum Photos, Inc.)

cover a partner's preferences by watching your partner stimulate her- or himself, by placing your hand on top of your partner's during such self-stimulation, or by having your partner use your hand to stroke him- or herself (Nowinski, 1980).

Nonverbal communication probably works best when supplemented by words, because actions alone may send the wrong signal. One woman who liked to have her ears kissed tried to communicate her wish by kissing her partner's ears. But it just didn't work. The more often she kissed his ears, the less often he kissed hers. Then she finally asked him about it and discovered that he found having his ears kissed extremely unpleasant. He had been avoiding her ears as a nonverbal sign that he disliked the practice. The discussion cleared the air: She stopped kissing his ears, and he began kissing hers (Barbach and Levine, 1981).

nudity comfortable, and relaxing music can help to establish a relaxed or romantic mood. Talk, a glass of wine, or a shared bath can increase the pleasure of a massage; fatigue can decrease it (Heiman, LoPiccolo, and LoPiccolo, 1976).

There are many correct forms of massagé, but some of the best guidelines have been provided by George Downing (1972), whose recommendations follow:

1 Apply gentle pressure as you massage, unless your partner complains that it hurts or feels too sensitive.

2 Relax your hands—sometimes a difficult task when you are applying pressure.

3 Mold your hands to fit the contours over which they are moving. The fingers and palms of the hands should try to remain in contact with the body.

4 Maintain an even speed and pressure—jerking or any sudden movement can be distracting.

5 Don't be afraid to vary speed and pressure—too little variety can be monotonous.

6 Use your weight rather than your muscles to apply pressure. To increase pressure, lean your body weight forward instead of straining your hand or arm muscles.

7 Try to maintain contact throughout the massage.

8 Pay attention to your own position, whether you are standing, sitting, or kneeling. Although any of these positions can be used, some offer greater freedom of movement and less strain on the person giving the massage.

9 Remember that you are massaging a person and not a machine. Massage is a form of communication, and the needs and feelings of the receiver should be considered at all times.

Certain aids can be used to enhance or vary the experience of massage. Oil or cream is useful in reducing friction and increasing sensitivity. Natural oils, such as coconut oil, have the added advantage of conditioning the skin. Electric vibrators may be included in the massage as a way of increasing sensation and relaxing the muscles.

Sex therapists have recommended a form of sensual massage to develop relaxation, trust, and intimacy in a sexual relationship (Masters and Johnson, 1970). It can be particularly effective for men and women who are troubled by sexual inhibitions or anxious over their sexual performance.

Although touch is often considered only in terms of foreplay, it is much more than a nonverbal request for intercourse or an attempt to stimulate a partner sexually. Touch certainly belongs in foreplay, but too many couples relegate it to that role. For them, touch is merely a means to the end of genital intercourse. They never touch each other unless they intend to have sex.

Partners who feel this way about touch miss out on a sensual pleasure that can strengthen the relationship between two people. Touch as an end in itself is a primary way of expressing pleasure and love. When there is no goal beyond the enjoyment of tactile perceptions, the pleasure of both partners is intensified and the bond between them deepens (Masters and Johnson, 1975). One way to discover this pleasure is by practice in touch that has no direct sexual goal.

# THE LIMITS OF SEXUAL COMMUNICATION

Communication can't solve all sexual problems. Despite their honest attempts to discuss problems openly, some couples find that their needs or interests remain far apart. Partners may have very different ideas about permissible types of sexual activity, and if one partner's sexual script is extremely rigid, open communication may bring no change at all.

One common problem is a major discrepancy between the partners' level of sexual desire, a problem whose causes and treatment we'll explore in Chapter 14. Whether for physiological or psychological reasons, one partner may have an extremely low sex drive, and infrequent sexual activity causes chronic discord in the relationship. The partner with low sex drive may feel inadequate, depressed, or abnormal; the other partner may feel unloved, rejected, and threatened (Rosen and Leiblum, 1976).

In such a situation, it's important to clarify the differences between the partners. What does the partner with a normal sex drive want more of—touching, oral sex, masturbation, genital intercourse, or orgasm? If she (or he) would be content with some kind of sexual activity besides genital intercourse, a compromise may be reached that will reduce, if not end, the friction (Zilbergeld, 1978).

For example, Dave and Alice, who had been married for five years, spent their days in constant conflict over sexual activity. Alice wanted long, lazy—and frequent—amorous dalliance; Dave's idea of sex was a brief encounter on the weekend. When Alice threatened divorce, the couple—with the aid of sex therapists—worked out their compromise. Dave had a low sex drive and little interest in intercourse, but he learned to give Alice the sexual activity she desired in the form of caresses and oral stimulation. She, in turn, learned to communicate her needs clearly and directly (Rosen and Leiblum, 1976).

One way of negotiating the compromise is to ask the partner with the complaint what it would mean if he (or she) got what was requested. Sometimes it's not the physical act itself that is important, but the symbolic meaning. A partner to whom meaning is important may be satisfied with increased attention and affection shown in ways that do not involve sexual activity (Zilbergeld, 1978). For example, the offer of sensual massage or a bath may at times substitute for intercourse.

Resolving the discrepancy also requires action from the dissatisfied partner. Nagging, crying, or wheedling only makes sexual activity less likely. Once the dissatisfied partner realizes that low sex drive is not a sign of malice or hostility, she (or he) may be able to accept the responsibility for her (or his) own sexual satisfaction. Such an acceptance means that the dissatisfied partner will have to initiate sexual activity.

Compromise is not always possible. In the case of Bill and Sharon, Bill's avoidance of sex was not simply the result of a low sex drive. Bill found it difficult to express his emotions by word or deed. He disliked his own body, did not enjoy kissing or displays of affection, and avoided sexual fantasy. Although Bill and Sharon had similar interests and enjoyed each other's company, and although Bill understood Sharon's feelings of rejection, he was unable to sustain any active sexual expression (Rosen and Leiblum, 1976).

In such a situation, each partner must consider how important the sexual issue is. Sometimes changes in the sexual area will create ill will in other parts of the relationship. In other cases, the issue is not really sex at all, but something more fundamental that will destroy the relationship if professional help is not sought (Zilbergeld, 1978).

Communication about sex is vital to a sexual relationship. Our hesitation in speaking up about sex is mostly the result of the way we are socialized. In the next unit, we'll trace sexual development through the life cycle and see the roots of some of our habits and customs.

## Summary

**1** In most cultures, sexual invitations are indirect, and custom insists that the man initiate them. The specific signs that signal a request for sexual activity vary widely from culture to culture and may be in the form of words, gestures, eye contact, or objects.

**2** Satisfying sexual relationships are generally characterized by intimacy; feelings and experiences are shared. In intimate relationships, partners accept each other's flaws and provide empathy. They establish an atmosphere in which the partners can abandon themselves to the pleasures of sexual activity without worrying about performance. If a relationship has unresolved conflicts, emotional barriers are likely to make intimacy almost impossible. Learning to communicate effectively and becoming sexually **assertive** are important. Good communication is characterized by **leveling** (expressing feelings in clear, simple language) and **editing** (eliminating rudeness and complaints). Two myths can block sexual communication: the belief that sex should be natural and spontaneous, and the belief that a loving partner always knows what the other partner wants.

**3** Sexual assertiveness makes it more likely that a person will receive the sort of stimulation he or she likes, decreases anxiety, and increases intimacy between partners. Sexually assertive comments should be characterized by empathy and reinforcement. Sexual assertiveness can be developed through **behavioral rehearsal**, which consists of imaginative practice of planned interactions. When lengthy sexual communication is called for, talk-and-listen sessions are often helpful. In American culture, men have traditionally been expected to initiate sexual activity. As a result, many women find it difficult to indicate their desire for sex. However, direct requests—by both men and women—are generally more effective than ambiguous signals. Both men and women find it difficult to say "no" to a partner, but a sexually assertive "no," phrased so the partner does not feel hurt, angry, or rejected, is often called for. Partners who are not in the mood for intercourse can offer sensual but nonsexual contact, or they can stimulate the partner with mouth and hands.

**4** Nonverbal communication can establish intimacy as effectively as words—and cause just as many problems. Modeling, or showing a partner a desired technique, is a good method of nonverbal communication. Nonverbal communication often works best when supplemented with words. Sensual massage can increase pleasure in physical stimulation and awareness of a partner's response. Massage need not lead to sexual activities.

**5** Communication cannot solve all sexual problems. Sometimes there is a major discrepancy between the partners' level of sexual desire. In such cases, it is important to clarify the differences between the partners so some sort of compromise can be negotiated. Sometimes changes in the sexual area create problems in other parts of the relationship, and sometimes the problem is not really sexual at all, but something fundamental in the relationship that requires professional help.

# Part Four

# The Human Life Cycle

From birth until death, sexuality is a continually evolving part of us. Although at one time children were believed to lack sexual feelings or impulses, we now know that babies are born with the capacity to respond to sexual stimuli. In early infancy, sexual response is at first just a reflex. Because psychogenic stimuli—the most powerful aspect of sexuality—are the result of experience and accumulate very slowly, stimulation of a baby boy's penis or a baby girl's clitoris has a very different meaning for the infant than it does for an adult. To the baby, it is pure sensation.

Sexuality is also a part of aging. At one time, older people were thought to be sexless. As men and women aged, they were expected to lose not only the capability to respond sexually, but all interest in sex as well. Today we know there is no reason for a healthy adult to cease sexual activity because of age. In order to understand human sexuality, we need to look at the entire human life cycle.

The sexuality of any woman or man is the result of a lengthy and complex process. Chromosomes, hormones, and learning all affect its development. Sexuality is shaped by family, by peers, and by society; it is influenced by gender identity and by sex roles. And as we'll see, the power of sex roles fluctuates. Instead of becoming increasingly rigid and stereotypical in their behavior, people adhere more or less to the roles prescribed by society at various—and predictable—stages in the life cycle.

In the four chapters that make up this unit, we'll explore sexuality throughout the life cycle. We begin with a chapter on infancy and childhood and discover that we can learn something about normal sexual development by looking at the results of mistakes in chromosomes and hormone levels. After tracing the development of gender identity and sex roles during childhood, we'll investigate adolescent sexuality in the second chapter. The chapter on sexuality in the adult years will cover various sexual life styles, and the final chapter will explore common sexual problems and their solutions.

## a female experience

I want my child to know there's nothing wrong with being seen naked. There's nothing to be ashamed of. I think a child will grow up much more prepared for life when there's a feeling in the family of being proud of your body. (Roberts, 1982, p. 66)

## a male experience

Sex was always a taboo subject in our family. One time I remember asking my father what a condom was. He gave me this real serious look and then told me to finish eating my dinner. (Authors' files)

# 11 Sexual Development in Childhood

# Chapter 11

When you were born, you had no idea whether you were a girl or a boy. Today, even if you are androgynous, you have developed a feminine or masculine gender identity—your private sense of being female or male—and a feminine or masculine sex role—the attitudes, behavior, and beliefs your culture prescribes for women and men. Your sexual orientation is probably well established, and you know whether you find men, women, or both sexually appealing.

As you traveled this path from an unawareness of your own gender to adult sexuality, you went through a lengthy, complex process that mixed biology with learning, a process that made you psychologically male or female. Becoming male or female is known as **sexual differentiation**. It progresses through a series of stages, and at each stage a person's development can proceed in a male or female direction. Although most of us consistently follow the same direction, some individuals develop inconsistently, taking both male and female paths. The study of such people can help us to understand the factors that affect gender identity.

**sexual differentiation** the process of becoming male or female

In this chapter, we'll describe the initial steps in the process and examine the effects of chromosomes and prenatal hormones. As we look at the development of sex differences and sexuality in infancy, the relative contribution of biology and learning will be a major concern. Next we'll explore the development of gender identity and sex roles in childhood. Finally, we'll consider sex education in the schools, taking note of its controversial nature and examining the sources of children's knowledge about sex.

# Sexual Development in Childhood

## BECOMING MALE OR FEMALE

According to psychiatrist Richard Green (1974), an adult with a clearly male or female gender identity has successfully negotiated a sevenfold path of development made up of genetic sex, gonadal sex, hormonal secretions, internal sex organs, external genitals, the sex label given at birth, and gender identity formed early in childhood. The woman has an XX chromosome pattern, ovaries that secrete feminizing hormones, and the internal and external organs of a female. At birth she was labeled a girl, and she soon developed a female gender identity. Similarly, the man has an XY chromosome pattern, testes that secrete masculinizing hormones, and the internal and external organs of a male. He was labeled a boy at birth and developed a male gender identity.

When this happens smoothly, there is a steady progression toward an adult sexuality that is consistently male or female in appearance, function, and identity. But the progression can be disrupted in several ways. A genetic defect may alter the biological components of development so that the child's reproductive system is ambiguous—neither completely male nor completely female. For example, hormones given to maintain a precarious pregnancy may result in a child whose external genitals are sexually ambiguous. In such cases, the judgment of the attending physician may determine whether the child is reared as a girl or a boy.

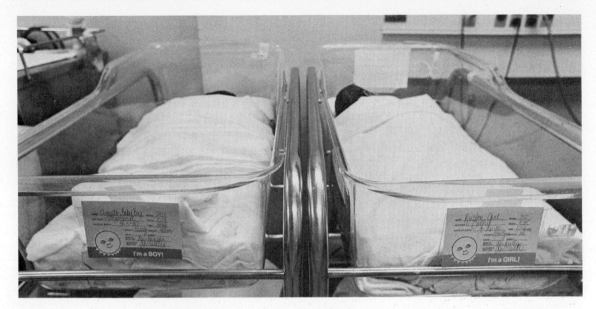

Children are classified by sex the moment they enter the world. Although the label means nothing to the infants, it has a powerful effect on the way others treat them. (© Shelly Rusten 1980)

Even when the biological aspects of the program unfold smoothly, environmental factors may disrupt the path toward gender identity. It's been suggested, for example, that when parents have mixed emotions about their child's sex, their feelings can cause problems for the child (Green, 1974). However, human beings are so adaptive that a firm gender identity often develops even when the program has been disrupted.

The importance of learning in the establishment of gender identity has generally been illustrated by a well-known study of a pair of identical twins who were born and at first reared as males. At seven months the boys were circumcised, and the penis of one twin was accidentally destroyed. Since there was no hope of reconstructing it, a consulting physician recommended that this twin be reared as a girl and that through surgery his genitals be reconstructed into female form. After almost a year of indecision, the parents consented. The baby's birth certificate was changed, its clothing and hair style altered, and surgical reconstruction begun. This baby boy was turned into a girl.

The parents learned to treat their former son as a daughter, and she began to act in feminine ways. Several years later, the child seemed to have developed a female gender identity. She neither looked nor acted like her twin brother. Because her testes had been removed, she did not develop male secondary sex characteristics at puberty. The administration of feminizing hormones stimulated the development of breasts. The girl did not menstruate and would never be able to bear children, but her physical appearance was that of an adolescent girl (Money and Ehrhardt, 1972).

Although this case has been widely used to demonstrate that sex roles and gender identity are basically learned, the fate of this twin after puberty indicates that becoming male or female is not solely the result of experience. By early adolescence, the girl had developed a masculine walk, had difficulty making friends with peers, who called her "the cavewoman," and seemed unhappy. She also seemed to have trouble adjusting to a female role, felt that boys had a better life, and looked forward to becoming a mechanic (Diamond, 1982). Whether therapy will solidify her identity as a woman remains to be seen.

Although environmental factors obviously play a major role in sexual differentiation, it would appear that the role of biology cannot be ignored. Biological influences on sexual differentiation can come from chromosomes or prenatal hormones.

## The role of chromosomes

As we saw in Chapter 3, each cell in the body of a male contains an X chromosome from the mother and a Y chromosome from the father. Each cell in the body of a female contains an X chromosome from each parent. These chromosomes have a powerful effect, for they determine whether the fetal gonads will develop into testes or ovaries. They also influence nonsexual aspects of development.

Some of the genes on the larger X chromosome protect the female against a variety of noninfectious disorders, such as color blindness, the blood-clotting disorder known as hemophilia, and rickets, which are resistant to treatment with vitamin D (Hamburg and Lunde, 1966). The possession of a pair of X chromosomes also seems to make females sturdier than males. Although about 140 males are conceived for every 100 females, only about 105 males are born for every 100 female births. (See Table 11.1.) Females also seem to be more resistant to infectious diseases and to the effects of physical deprivation. Males, who lack the protection of

**Table 11.1   Ratio of males to females by age group (1920–1980)**  (Represents number of males per 100 females)

| AGE (YEARS) | 1920 | 1940 | 1960 | 1980 |
|---|---|---|---|---|
| | BIRTH RATE APPROXIMATELY 105 MALES FOR EVERY 100 FEMALES | | | |
| Under 14 | 102.1 | 103.0 | 103.4 | 104.6 |
| 14–24 | 97.3 | 98.9 | 98.7 | 101.7 |
| 25–44 | 105.1 | 98.5 | 95.7 | 97.4 |
| 45–64 | 115.2 | 105.2 | 95.7 | 90.7 |
| 65 and over | 101.3 | 95.5 | 82.8 | 67.6 |
| All ages | 104.1 | 100.7 | 97.1 | 94.5 |

The ratio of males to females at birth nowadays is reversed by age 25. Note that the overall ratio of males to females has also reversed historically since 1920.

*Source:* Statistical Abstract of the United States, 1982–1983. U.S. Bureau of the Census (1982).

the second X chromosome, have higher mortality rates at all stages of life (Fryer and Ashford, 1972).

Although their X chromosome makes females generally sturdier than males, they are just as susceptible to abnormalities that develop when cell division in the parents results in the loss or addition of a sex chromosome in the child. By tracing the influence of such errors on an individual's sexuality, researchers hope to gain a deeper understanding of the sex chromosomes' role in human development.

In **Turner's syndrome**, girls are born with only one X chromosome, so that the genetic pattern of each cell is XO (one female chromosome, no male chromosome). Such girls have apparently normal external genitals. Because they have no ovaries, they are sterile and will not develop secondary sex characteristics at puberty unless they take supplemental hormones. Their gender identity is firmly female. No parallel condition (a YO pattern) exists for males. Apparently, an individual cannot develop without at least one X chromosome.

When girls are born with an extra X chromosome (XXX pattern), they have a complete female reproductive system but their fertility is diminished. Such girls develop a normal female gender identity (Money and Ehrhardt, 1972).

There are two abnormal chromosomal patterns for boys. In **Klinefelter's syndrome** there is an extra female chromosome (XXY pattern). These genetic males have small external genitals, low testosterone, and are sterile. They seem passive, dependent, and have a diminished sex drive (Rubin, Reinisch, and Haskett, 1981).

Men with an extra male chromosome (XYY) do not differ from normal males in appearance, although they are often more than six feet tall. At one time it was believed that these "supermales" were likely to become criminals. In fact, they may be impulsive or aggressive, but their aggressiveness does not seem to take the form of physical violence toward others. Their sexuality appears to be normal (Rubin, Reinisch, and Haskett, 1981).

In all these cases of chromosomal error, the Y chromosome is the key. No matter how many X chromosomes in a fertilized egg, it will become male if there is one Y chromosome present. Without the Y chromosome, the egg develops into a female.

**Turner's syndrome** a condition in which girls are born with only one X chromosome in each body cell, no ovaries, but apparently normal external genitals

**Klinefelter's syndrome** a condition in which boys are born with an extra X chromosome in each body cell, resulting in small external genitals, sterility, and a diminished sex drive

## The role of prenatal hormones

During the first six weeks of development, there is no difference in the sexual systems of males and females. As noted in Chapter 3, only when the Y chromosome instructs the gonads to secrete male hormones does the development of the sexes diverge. In the absence of such instructions, the fetus is female. From this moment, hormones control the development of sexual differences.

Hormones are not only responsible for the development of sexual organs, they influence the brain as well. They determine whether it will be responsive to androgens or estrogens during later life, and the pattern of hormone release during adulthood. Testosterone, an androgen produced by the fetal testes, sets the brain in a male pattern in which hormone levels rise and fall, but there is no clear monthly cycle. In the absence of testosterone, the brain is set in a female pattern, so that the types and proportions of hormones circulating in the body vary in a regular month-ly cycle.

Clues about the lasting effects of prenatal hormone on personality or behavior can be found in the behavior of people who were exposed to abnormal hormone levels while in the uterus. Sometimes a genetic male secretes adequate amounts of the correct hormone mixture, but his tissues are unable to use the hormone. This condition is called the **androgen insensitivity syndrome**. At birth, the baby appears to be a female. The external genitals develop as if there were no androgens present, forming a clitoris, labia minora, and labia majora. But the fetal tissues have re-sponded to the Mullerian inhibiting substance secreted by the fully functioning but undescended testes, so there are no internal female organs. The child is labeled a girl and is reared like one. The condition may not be discovered until puberty, when the absence of menstruation leads to a physical examination.

Such individuals usually develop a female gender identity. They are sexually attracted to males and though they can never bear children, they can lead the life of a woman. These genetic males show no traces of masculinization from prenatal hormones; their interests and behavior are typically feminine. Yet because they were reared as girls, we cannot separate the effects of hormones and environment (Ehrhardt and Meyer-Bahlburg, 1981).

Sometimes genetic females are exposed to large amounts of androgens before birth. In the **andrenogenital syndrome**, the source of the excess androgen is the adrenal cortex, a hormone-producing gland located just above the kidney. When the adrenal cortex secretes an improper form of cortisone, the defective hormone acts like androgen in the body. In other cases excess androgen comes from the mother, because in the past women were given synthetic hormones to prevent mis-carriage.

In both conditions, the effect of androgens is to masculinize a genetic female. In most cases, the internal organs are female, but the external genitals have a mas-culine appearance. The exposure to androgens seems to affect behavior. When reared as girls after surgical correction of the genitals, these females are generally tomboys. They prefer male playmates and body contact sports, have a high level of physical energy, a minimal interest in dolls and baby care, and find careers much more interesting than motherhood. Yet they develop a secure female gender identi-ty, and the majority of them (who are normally given hormonal supplements at puberty to ensure female sexual development) are sexually attracted to men (Ehr-hardt and Meyer-Bahlburg, 1981). When reared as boys, they develop male gender identities.

Research on the role of prenatal hormones in shaping personality is particular-ly controversial. Many girls without prenatal exposure to androgens also behave like tomboys. However, androgenized girls show much more tomboy behavior than girls who have had no exposure to androgens. As we saw in Chapter 1, prena-tal exposure to androgens in girls and to extra androgens in boys seems to make both sexes more physically aggressive than girls and boys who were not exposed to the hormone (Reinisch, 1981).

Such research has been important. It has led to treatments that have benefited individuals affected by the various conditions. In addition, the research has re-

**andrenogenital syn-drome** a condition in which a genetic fe-male's adrenal cortex produces an improper form of cortisone which masculinizes the ap-pearance of her exter-nal genitals

**androgen insensi-tivity syndrome** a condition in which a genetic male cannot use the androgen se-creted by his testes; his external genitals are female but his in-ternal genitals are male

duced the number of afflicted individuals by leading to a reevaluation of the once-common practice of giving hormones to pregnant women. Finally, the research has shown that hormones play an important role in the process of sexual differentiation, and that in extreme cases the process can be radically disrupted. However, even if abnormal levels of hormones before birth are related to differences in the behavior or personality of boys and girls, this tells us little about the degree of sex differences among normal boys and girls.

## SEXUAL DEVELOPMENT IN INFANCY

Boys and girls behave differently from birth, but at first the differences are not very impressive. Behavior with a biological basis need not be present the moment a child enters the world. Walking is based on biology, but requires time to develop. Prenatal hormones probably dispose boys and girls to behave in certain ways, but hormones cannot act in isolation. The interaction of biology, the physical environment, and social forces is at work in every aspect of development.

It is particularly difficult to trace a direct connection between sex hormones and behavior because an infant's genitals signal gender to the world, ensuring that boys and girls are treated differently from the instant of birth (Lamb and Campos, 1982). As a result, the differences that have been found in infancy could easily be the result of learning. The continuous interaction between biology and culture is especially apparent in the development of sexuality, as the radically different sexual customs of various societies show.

The course of sexual development is not smooth, but is characterized by important transitions and stages and by numerous bumps in the road from infancy to old age. Yet it can be viewed as a continuous process, in the sense that important events and experiences take place from the moment of birth and continue throughout the life cycle. It was Sigmund Freud who dispelled the Victorian myth of the "sexual innocence" of children. In the nineteenth century, experts and public alike believed that sexuality first manifested itself during adolescence and that children could be reared as asexual beings. Today, despite disagreement about the specific events and psychological significance of childhood sexuality, the continuous nature of sexual development is widely accepted.

The course of sexual development in infancy may become clearer if we consider it in the light of differences in behavior, overt sexuality, and emotional development.

### Sex differences in infancy

Among newborn infants, boys seem more restless from the first day of life. Although newborn boys cry no more than girls, they are awake more—scowling, wriggling, twitching, and jerking much more than girls do (Phillips, King, and Du-Bois, 1978). By the time they are three months old, boys fuss more than girls do,

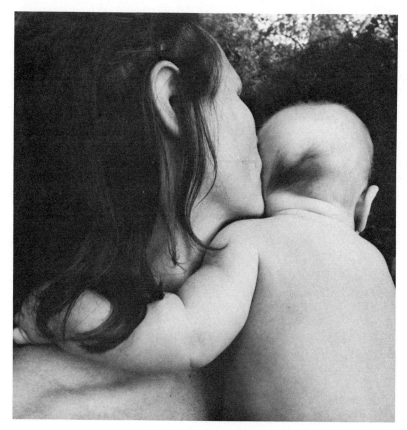

Babies' first emotional bonds are with their parents, and the quality of the attachment can have an enduring effect on later emotional development. ("Edith and Issac, Newtown, Pennsylvania 1974." Photo by Emmet Gowin, Courtesy Light Gallery, N.Y.)

and once they are upset they are harder to calm down. However, boys' behavior changes less in the first three months (Yang and Moss, 1978). Researchers have concluded that infant boys function at a less organized and less efficient level than girls, and that boys are less responsive to the social signals around them. Baby girls seem to be more receptive to environmental influence and to learn faster (Moss, 1974).

Boys and girls may also learn differently, with boys being more responsive to sights and girls to sounds. In a suggestive experiment, three-month-old boys learned to look at the correct spot fastest when they were rewarded with a red light. Given the same task, girls learned fastest when the reward was a low tone instead of a light (Watson et al., 1980). Although this research is preliminary, if supported the difference could subtly affect the way adults treat infants and the way the babies respond.

These differences in behavior may affect the way a mother interacts with a baby. (See Figure 11.1) Perhaps responding to a girl's preference for sounds, mothers are more likely to talk to their infant daughters, to reward their vocaliza-

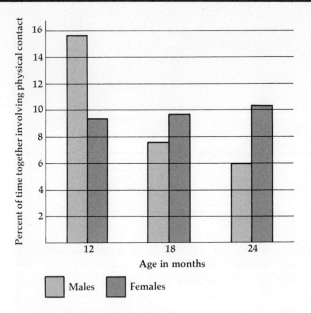

*Figure 11.1   Physical Contact Between Mothers and Children of Different Ages.*

The barriers that keep American men from expressing physical affection may be built in the home. Mothers of twelve-month-old infants touched their sons more than they touched their daughters, but within six months the same mothers sharply curtailed physical contact with their sons. (Adapted from K. A. Clarke-Stewart and C. M. Hevey, Longitudinal relations in repeated observations of mother-child interaction from 1½ to 2½ Years. *Developmental Psychology,* 1981, *17,* 127–145.

tions, and to play quietly with them. And perhaps responding to a boy's restlessness, irritability, and preference for sights, mothers play more boisterously with their infant sons, tickling them, throwing them in the air, and rubbing their tummies (Kagan, 1978).

In line with their greater restlessness at birth, boys may be predisposed to action when faced with uncertainty. Girls may act more cautiously as a result of their advanced physical development, for a newborn girl's central nervous system, bones, and muscles are slightly more developed than those of a boy.

Although a biological basis for some sex differences in infancy may exist, rearing and socialization processes may emphasize and exaggerate them. For example, in our culture the male tendency to act and the female tendency toward caution are in line with adult sexual scripts in which the man initiates and the woman sets limits. Infants' great responsiveness to experience means that biological influences need not determine behavior.

## Infant sexuality

We know from the evidence of an erect penis that baby boys are sexually responsive from birth. In fact, many male babies actually have erections at the moment of birth. Infants apparently find stimulation of the penis quite pleasurable. In many cultures, fretting baby boys are quieted by stroking and tickling the penis. Although at first the baby probably can't localize the pleasant sensation, its relaxing effect and his pleasure are plainly visible (Gadpaille, 1975).

A baby can develop an erection without direct stimulation of his penis. Almost any intense emotion, as well as the sensuous pleasure of nursing, is often accompanied by an erection. Erections also occur regularly during sleep, just as they do in men. Although baby girls lack such external evidence of genital arousal, they begin to touch and explore their genitals as soon as they have the necessary muscular coordination.

Both male and female infants have been observed having orgasms. Orgasm has been seen in baby boys as young as five months and baby girls as young as four months (Kinsey, Pomeroy, and Martin, 1948). Infant orgasms seem to have many of the same characteristics as their adult counterparts, including rapid pelvic thrusting in the male and a buildup of body tension to the point of climax, followed by a period of calm and relaxation.

Although infants have the capacity for erection and orgasm, such behavior shouldn't be equated with adult orgasm (Gagnon, 1977). Sexual responses in infants demonstrate the very early development of the reflex pathways involved in sexual arousal and orgasm. But until the higher brain centers that control thoughts and perceptions develop, the baby's experience of arousal and orgasm will bear little resemblance to the adult's experience, since the baby cannot interpret the sensations involved.

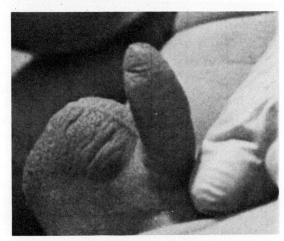

A baby boy's penis often becomes erect, whether he is awake or asleep, lying quietly or nursing. Some boys have penile erections at birth. (Courtesy, Gorm Wagner, M.D., and Focus International, Inc.)

When infants masturbate, parents respond in a variety of ways. Some are shocked or dismayed to see obviously sexual behavior in their baby and are likely to remove the offending hand or distract the infant each time it occurs. Some have learned that infant masturbation is a normal and healthy part of development and accept it without interfering. Others—probably the largest group—have intellectually accepted the normality of infant masturbation, but still disapprove of the practice and generally manage to convey their negative feelings to the child (Gadpaille, 1975). As one man said:

> What are you supposed to do when you find your kid playing with himself? I know it's normal, but I don't think it should be encouraged. (Authors' files)

If parents who feel as this man did could learn to become truly accepting of their baby's masturbation, they could probably help their child to develop with a minimum of sexual guilt. This means neither interfering nor trying to distract the infant's attention each time a small hand strays to the genitals. By reacting negatively, parents may interfere with the normal process of self-exploration.

## Emotional development

Sexual development builds a psychological structure on early responses to stimulation. The emotional bonds established during infancy and the baby's emerging personality are part of that structure.

At birth, the human infant is a vulnerable and totally dependent organism. The nervous system is not fully developed, and the baby's only coordinated responses are sucking and swallowing, perhaps because the sensory nerves are more highly developed in the lips, tongue, and mouth than in any other part of the body (Gadpaille, 1975).

The mouth of the infant plays such a major role during the first year that Freud called this period the **oral stage** of psychosexual development. He pointed out that the baby's sensual pleasure comes from stimulation of the mouth. Babies seek oral stimulation, and any object that brushes cheeks or lips goes into the mouth.

**oral stage** the first stage in Freud's scheme of psychosexual development, which lasts through the first year of life; the lips and mouth are the focus of sensual pleasure

A major need during the first few months of life is to be touched and held (Montagu, 1971). Babies are born willing to accept cuddling, milk, and care from anyone. By the time they are six to eight months old, however, they become attached to their parents and establish their first emotional bonds. They become distressed when separated and eagerly seek contact when reunited.

At one time it was believed that babies developed emotional bonds because their parents fed them, but most authorities now believe that being touched and held—the pleasure of close human contact—forms the basis of this attachment. This became clear when psychologists Harry and Margaret Harlow (1966, 1969) raised infant monkeys with two surrogate mothers, one made of wire and equipped with a feeding mechanism, and another of soft terrycloth. The monkeys spent most of the time clinging to the terrycloth mother—just as infant monkeys cling to their own mothers—and developed what looked like a genuine attachment for the soft mother. When anything frightened the little monkeys, they ran to the comfort of the terrycloth mother. After the young monkeys had become adults and were reunited with their mothers after a year's separation, they ran to embrace the terrycloth mother but showed little interest in the wire mother who had fed them. From these reactions, we might speculate that being fed in a positive emotional context might heighten attachment, but that being fed by a mother who is cold, holds the baby stiffly, and provides little comforting contact is like taking nourishment from a wire mother.

According to psychoanalyst Erik Erikson (1963), the quality of babies' first emotional relationships with their mothers makes a permanent impression. A baby who experiences constant, reliable care develops a basic sense of trust that makes it possible for him or her to tolerate frustration and to delay the immediate satisfaction of needs. Babies whose needs are not met become people who are mistrustful of others and are anxious and upset when frustrated.

It's clear that early experiences with caregivers affect the warmth, trust, and degree of positive expectation with which babies approach other people (Hall, Lamb, and Perlmutter, 1982). It's also easy to see how mistrust and demands for instant gratification could interfere with the development of committed sexual relationships. A person who cannot trust a partner is likely to find it extremely difficult to develop intimacy.

We might even speculate that the establishment of this first emotional relationship plays a role in an adult's level of sexual desire. Therapists report that men and

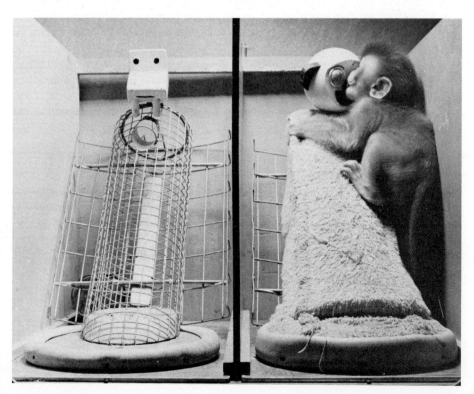

The need for human infants to be touched and held was supported by research with young monkeys, who sought the warmth and protection of the cuddly terrycloth "mother," while ignoring the wire "mother" that fed them milk. (© Harry F. Harlow, University of Wisconsin Primate Laboratory)

women who seem to lack sexual desire or to have very low levels sometimes report that for as long as they can remember, they got little affection from their mothers or fathers (Rosen and Leiblum, 1982b).

# SEXUAL DEVELOPMENT IN CHILDHOOD

The time between a youngster's first steps and puberty is a period that covers enormous leaps in physical, emotional, and intellectual development. During the first part of this period, the preschool years, children learn sex roles and develop gender identity. During the school years they build on that basic knowledge, learning about reproduction, perhaps exploring sex with their peers, and deepening their understanding of what it means to be male or female.

## *The preschool years*

Once a child begins to walk and talk, infancy is shed and forces outside the family begin to affect sexual development. Peers, other adults, and the media—especially television—join parents in providing continual instruction in proper male and female behavior, in the way emotions are expressed, and in what is *not* permitted. This informal instruction in behavior, attitudes, values, and sex roles is known as **socialization.**

**socialization** the process of absorbing a culture's behavior, attitudes, values, and sex roles

Emotional development in childhood is sometimes seen as a series of stages. For example, Freud clearly divided childhood into stages of psychosexual development. Because Freud's ideas have had an enormous impact on American society, we'll explain his concepts. But remember that most authorities today take many of Freud's ideas with a grain of salt.

**Personality in the preschool years** As children become more competent, parents begin to insist on some growth in responsibility. During the second or third year, for example, most children go through toilet training. Freud was so impressed with the influence of toilet training on personality development that he referred to this time as the **anal stage.** He believed that during this period—from about the first birthday until children are three years old—pleasurable feelings center in the rectum. Although oral pleasures do not fade, expelling and retaining feces becomes satisfying.

**anal stage** the second of Freud's psychosexual stages of development, occupying the second and third years of life; the rectum is the focus of sensual pleasure

Freud speculated that children who experience very strict toilet training are likely to become excessively orderly, obstinate, and stingy, and perhaps to develop chronic sexual inhibitions in later life. It appears, however, that toilet training itself does not affect personality; the influence is in the way toilet training reflects the parent-child relationship. An extremely rigid mother who is emotionally undemonstrative may be teaching her child the characteristics Freud described as "anal" in all areas of life (Finney, 1963).

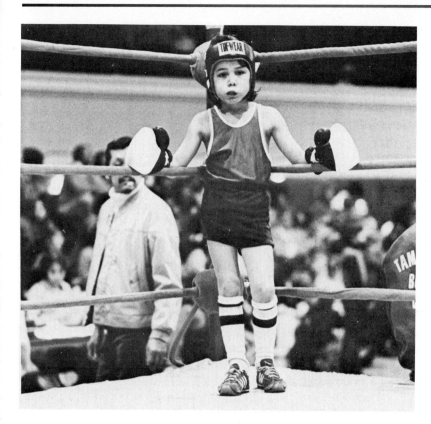

Through socialization, children absorb their ideas of male and female roles. This boy, who is adhering so closely to the traditional male role, would probably be shocked to find himself facing a girl in the ring. (© Lawrence Frank 1978)

Toilet training is only one area of socialization. With increasing frequency, parents restrain or limit the toddler's activities, both for the child's own protection (keeping the child out of the streets) and for the well-being of the family (making mealtime pleasant or conversation possible). In their attempts to promote socially accepted behavior, many parents place increasing restrictions on masturbation, nudity, and other expressions of the toddler's curiosity in the body and its functions. In a study of Cleveland, Ohio, parents, the majority told their children that nudity was bad and warned them to be careful about exposing their bodies. Said one father:

> I don't feel my daughter should see me naked. I cannot give you a more intelligent answer than that. I just would rather not. (Roberts, 1982, p. 71)

Once children are toilet trained, they enter what Freud called the **phallic stage**, a period that begins at about three and ends when children are about six years old. Now the genitals are the source of pleasure, and youngsters enjoy fondling them. According to Freud, as a boy discovers the pleasure of his penis, his love for

**phallic stage** the third of Freud's psychosexual stages of development, occupying the years from three to six; the genitals are the focus of sensual pleasure

his mother develops into a strong incestuous wish to take his father's place. This wish to do away with his father and marry his mother is known as the Oedipus complex, after the Greek myth about Oedipus, who did just that. But since a small boy knows his father is too powerful to replace, he fears his father may retaliate. His fear becomes a fear of castration. In Freud's view, every little boy is faced with an inevitable conflict between sexual desire for his mother and fear of castration by his father. This conflict is resolved when the boy represses his desire for his mother. Gradually, the boy identifies with his father, vicariously sharing the father's sexual relationship with the mother.

Freud believed that girls go through a parallel but slightly different Oedipal struggle (once known as the Electra complex). When the little girl discovers that she lacks a penis, she believes she has already been castrated. She blames her mother for the act, and her "penis envy" weakens the loving bond with the mother in favor of a growing preference for the father, who has the organ she is missing. For her, the Oedipus complex results in sexual desire for the father and jealousy of the mother. As the conflict is resolved, a girl identifies with her mother so she can vicariously bear the father's baby.

Freud proposed that this difference in the outcome of the Oedipus complex was the basis of major sex differences in adulthood. In little boys, a permanent male sex role and heterosexual orientation are established, and a conscience develops. Because little girls are not threatened by castration anxiety, they supposedly develop a weaker conscience than boys, so that as women they are more intuitive and less principled than men.

Freud's controversial theory was developed largely from observations of his patients and from introspection. Little scientific evidence has been found to support it—and some aspects of it have been contradicted. The theory has been criticized as unscientific and as sexist for explaining psychosexual development in terms of the penis. Male and female personality development are not as different as Freud supposed, and his description of female personality has not held up (Fisher and Greenberg, 1977).

Yet, as we'll see, the concept of identification with the parent of the same sex has been adopted in some form by most researchers, although they have generally rejected fear or jealousy as its basis. The notion of the Oedipus complex performed one important service: It made us aware that children have sexual feelings and that childhood sexuality can have an important influence on later sexual expressions.

**Learning sex roles** Before a child can adopt the culture's male or female sex role, the child must discover whether it's a girl or a boy. About the time they are eighteen months old, children learn such gender labels as "boy" and "girl," "mommy" and "daddy," apparently on the basis of dress and hair style. Yet most two-year-olds are not certain of their own gender, and many often give the wrong answer when asked "Are you a girl?" or "Are you a boy?" (Thompson, 1975). By thirty months, most know their own sex, and by the time they are three, they are aware that all people are either males or females. (See Table 11.2.) As we saw in Chapter 1, gender identity, the private sense of being male or female, is an important aspect of gender.

## Table 11.2  *Understanding gender*

| TASK | PERCENT ANSWERING CORRECTLY | | |
| --- | --- | --- | --- |
| | 24 MONTHS | 30 MONTHS | 36 MONTHS |
| Identify own picture | 82 | 100 | 100 |
| Apply gender labels to stereotypical pictures of people | 76 | 83 | 90 |
| Stereotype objects and clothes by gender | 61 | 78 | 86 |
| Answer gender questions about self | 44 | 70 | 79 |

(From Thompson, 1975)

Long before gender identity develops, children are being steered into their sex roles. Two-year-old girls and boys are treated differently for the same behavior. Girls tend to be discouraged when they manipulate objects and encouraged to be helpers and to ask for assistance. Boys aren't discouraged when they manipulate objects and are not encouraged to give help or to ask for it. In most cases, parents have no idea that they are teaching their daughters to be dependent and their sons to be independent and to explore the world (Fagot, 1978). Mothers also tend to discourage their toddler sons from following them around the house, but they encourage their daughters to stay near them (Fagot, 1974). As one mother said:

> You know how little girls are. . . . They're so sweet and helpful. And you just love to have them around. (Authors' files)

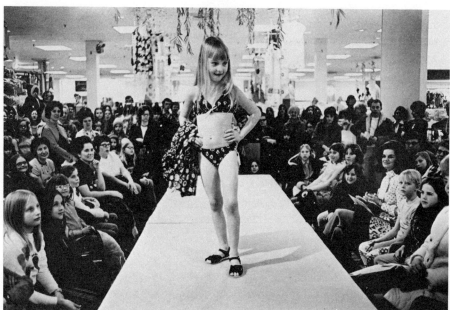

In subtle—and not so subtle—ways, the culture teaches children to follow its sex roles. This little girl has already entered the world of the beauty pageant queen. (© J. Berndt/Stock, Boston)

At first, three-year-olds may believe that they can switch their gender. Most think that changing clothes and hair style is all that is needed. By the time they are five, however, children generally understand that gender will never change—boys always grow up to become men, and girls always grow up to become women. Once they realize this, sex-role behavior takes on a new dimension.

Four- to six-year-olds watched television commercials in which a sexually neutral toy—a Fisher-Price Movie Viewer—was portrayed as being either a boy's toy or a girl's toy. No matter how the toy was depicted, youngsters who did not yet understand that gender was permanent played with it afterward. But children who understood that they would always remain male or female shunned the toy when it was depicted as belonging to the other sex (Ruble, Balaban, and Cooper, 1981).

This sense of gender constancy has been proposed by psychologist Lawrence Kohlberg (1966) as the basis for identification with the parent of the same sex. Although Freud saw identification as the outcome of the stormy Oedipal conflict, Kohlberg sees it as an intellectual step. Once children understand that gender does not change, they identify with the same-sex parent and seek out the behavior and attitudes that go along with that gender.

Other psychologists believe rewards are more important than the realization that gender is permanent. After children have associated their parents with the satis-

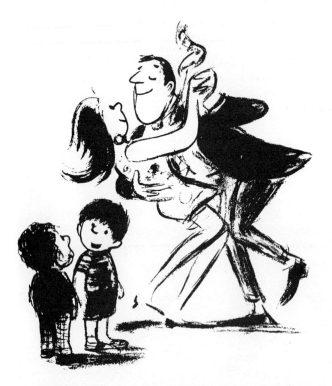

"The big difference between men and women is that women dance backwards."

faction of needs, they soon associate any typical parental behavior with satisfaction. By imitating a parent, they reward themselves (Miller and Dollard, 1941).

More recently, Albert Bandura (1977) has proposed that learning from a parent is more than simple imitation. Children observe parents, and as they watch, they think about what they see. They form concepts that later guide their own actions, and they can change these concepts as they try out the behavior and discover what happens to them. In this view, parents are not the only models a child imitates. Other people—children as well as adults, television characters as well as people they encounter in the flesh—can also serve as models.

Despite disagreements concerning how and why children come to behave like adults of their own gender, it is clear that some sort of observation and imitation are involved in the process. It also appears that the process begins early and is well developed—perhaps irreversibly—before the onset of puberty.

Children not only learn their sex roles from models, but the role of the other sex as well. When a little boy observes his father automatically slip behind the wheel each time the family goes for a drive, he learns aspects of two complementary sex roles—males are expected to take charge, and females, who may drive the car at other times, are expected to defer to males when they are present. By learning what the other sex is supposed to do, children learn how *not* to behave, think, or feel. They also learn what to expect from members of the other sex (Money, 1977).

During these years, parents begin to pay increasing attention to the child's adoption of a sex role, and those who overlook it when their infants stray from prescribed sex roles begin to insist that their preschoolers stay within bounds. As one mother of a three-year-old boy said:

> It's time for Joey to start acting like a boy. I used to think it was cute when he played with his sister's things, but now it's starting to bother me. (Authors' files)

Although boys may show more physical aggression than girls, in the United States they become men who often have trouble expressing physical affection. This male reluctance may have its roots in body contact with parents. In one study (Clarke-Stewart and Hevey, 1981), mothers of twelve-month-olds were more likely to initiate physical contact with their sons than with their daughters, but by the time their offspring were eighteen months old, the same mothers were more likely to touch their daughters. The change was due entirely to a drop in physical contact between mothers and sons.

Among five-year-olds, girls are hugged and touched more than boys by both parents—but for different reasons. Mothers don't want to be overly seductive with their growing sons, and fathers may fear that too much physical affection from men will cause their sons to become homosexual (Montagu, 1971). The gradual withdrawal from physical contact with boys may help to explain an important aspect of differences in adult sex roles.

However, part of the difference probably comes about as children watch their parents interact with friends. Among the 1,500 Cleveland parents, 60 percent of the mothers said they often hugged their female friends, but 75 percent of the fathers said they never—or rarely—hugged their close male friends (Roberts, 1982). In such ways children learn who gets to express emotions and who is supposed to keep them under control.

As adult sex roles change and fathers take a more active role in child care, boys may learn to be more comfortable with physical affection and girls may learn to become more assertive and confident. These changes showed in the Cleveland study, in which 90 percent of the fathers said they wanted their children to learn that it was good for men to cry, and some fathers were consciously trying to become emotionally expressive.

**Sexual interest among preschoolers** A natural consequence of the toddler's explorations is the observation of parents in the act of sexual intercourse. This witnessing of the "primal scene," as psychoanalysts call it, was once thought to be a traumatic experience that left lasting emotional scars on a child, but views have changed. Today experts believe that the effects vary widely, depending on the circumstances under which it occurs, and that the sight is not always harmful. As one man recalled:

> I didn't know what was happening at the time, but I could tell something was wrong from the way they reacted. My father seemed really embarrassed, and I couldn't understand why. (Authors' files)

Although little evidence exists, it appears that nearly 20 percent of children either see or hear their parents' sexual activity. Among a group of college students, those who as children had seen or heard their parents having intercourse had reacted negatively at the time or with disbelief and uncertainty. In some cases the experience appeared to stimulate sexual feelings in the child, but it had no effect on their sexuality as college students. Neither the frequency of their sexual activity nor their sexual satisfaction differed from that of students who had neither seen nor heard their parents' sexual activity (Hoyt, 1979).

In many societies, sexual activity is not hidden from children, and its observation is part of every child's experience. All members of a family sleep in the same room, so that even if parents are discreet, children are well aware of what is taking place. It is the sexual privacy that is so deeply engrained in American society that leads people to believe the experience is invariably harmful.

Their natural interest in the body also leads toddlers into sex play with other children. Such play usually begins some time during the third year, depending upon the opportunity to interact with other children and the child's level of maturity. Acceptance of sex play also varies greatly from one society to another. In cultures that place few restrictions on such behavior, children's inspection of one another's genitals and some mutual masturbation are extremely common. Such sex play is so prevalent among human children and among young monkeys and apes that some researchers believe an underlying drive toward such play is built into the human species (Ford and Beach, 1951).

Cultures that are tolerant of sex play often allow youngsters to observe adult sexual behavior and give young children frank and honest information about sexual matters. Children in these societies generally grow up with fewer inhibitions and problems than children who are deprived of such early sexual learning.

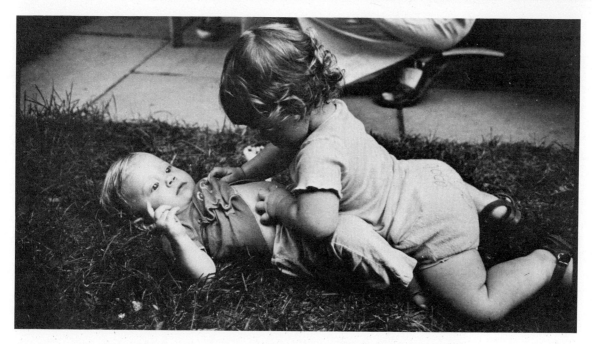

Their natural curiosity leads young children to explore one another's bodies in sex play that may include genital inspection and mutual masturbation. (Susan Shapiro)

In the United States, parental uneasiness about sexuality often comes through, even when parents are attempting to be open and permissive. Among the parents in the Cleveland study, more than 80 percent acknowledged that most children masturbate, but 40 percent said that such behavior was immoral, wrong for religious reasons, or could be harmful (Roberts, 1982). Many of these parents, who could be permissive about infant masturbation because it was "natural," found themselves anxious when their own preschoolers masturbated. One mother told how she had reacted:

> I noticed that my five-year-old daughter was doing it [masturbating] last night. I just explained to her that there were germs and that she would get the germs on her fingers and I would appreciate it if she would wash her hands after she was done playing with herself because she could get sick from it. (Roberts, 1982, p. 70)

Instead of being reassured, this little girl probably got the message that masturbation was a bad thing that spread disease.

Although there may be a general increase in sexual interest among most four- or five-year-olds, children differ widely in their activity. Many children show no sexual activity or interest until adolescence (Kinsey et al., 1953). And much sexual activity among preschoolers escapes adult attention. When adolescents were asked about their childhood activity, one boy said he couldn't remember a time when he did not masturbate, and a girl recalled that she used to rub the nose of a stuffed animal against her vulva:

I would go around rubbing this animal against me all the time. I don't think I really had an orgasm, it was more like after a while I would just get tired and stop. (Bell, 1980, p. 79)

It seems that as children become aware that masturbation or sex play is socially unacceptable, they keep their sexual explorations private.

## Sexual development in the school years

Just as parents are extremely important during infancy and early childhood, so peers are vital to emotional and sexual development during later childhood. Peers apparently provide social experiences that are not available within today's small family.

This first became apparent when researchers experimented with monkeys (Suomi and Harlow, 1975). Monkeys raised with only their mothers but no other monkey contact seem slightly abnormal in their emotional expression. As adolescents they make poor playmates, for they are aggressive and show less affection toward their peers than monkeys raised with the companionship of other young monkeys. Monkeys raised in isolation are even more disturbed. They are extremely aggressive and sexually incompetent as adults. Yet monkeys who have no contact with their mothers but are allowed to play for two hours a day with peers can spend all the rest of their time in isolation and emerge as relatively normal adults. Play with peers seems to go a long way toward laying the foundation for a healthy emotional and sexual life.

Contact with peers is also an important aspect of human socialization. During the school years, children rehearse the occupational and social roles available in adult society. Such role playing reinforces gender identity, because boys tend to rehearse masculine roles and girls feminine roles. Exposure to television, movies, and books greatly stimulates these activities by providing children with an endless source of role models (Gagnon and Roberts, 1980).

In their play, children have an opportunity to express their feelings about what it is like to fall in love. This kind of role playing often leads to the development of crushes on schoolteachers, popular peers, or music idols. Such feelings in a boy or girl may be intense, although in most cases they are not explicitly sexual.

The years from first grade to puberty form what Freud called the **latency period**. He believed that once a child had successfully resolved the Oedipus complex, the sex drive was repressed until puberty. Although the Freudian concept of latency has been influential and is still used as an argument against sex education in the elementary schools, it has not been supported by studies of childhood sexuality.

Instead of living a bland, sexless existence, children steadily increase their sex play with peers. The number of girls and boys who have experienced orgasm also increases gradually but steadily (Kinsey et al., 1953). One boy described his sexual explorations by saying:

We started by playing doctor and nurse games. It was a lot of fun poking and touching each other all over. I remember a lot of giggling at the time. (Authors' files)

**latency period** the fourth of Freud's psychosexual stages of development, lasting from age six until puberty; the sex drive is supposedly repressed during this period

As they learned to do with masturbation as preschoolers, children apparently keep their sexual activity private. They play by adult sexual rules, behaving around adults in the sexless manner that leads observers to believe they are sexually inactive.

Sex play with peers occurs about equally with the same and the other sex. As one girl recalled:

> I had my first sexual experience when I was seven years old. It was with my best friend. . . . One day we started fooling around and touching each other all over. For about a year, we'd sleep over at each other's houses and do this. (Bell, 1980, p. 85)

As puberty draws near, the experiences of girls tend to differ markedly from those of boys. Parents tend to be more protective of little girls and insist that they show "modesty." As a result, boys generally initiate sex play with other boys more often than girls engage in similar activities. When children are sexually inactive, they are apparently not going through a latency period, but are instead adhering to the culture's demand that they abstain from sexual expression, a demand that is especially strong on girls (Kinsey et al., 1953). A look at childhood sexuality in other cultures supports this view. Where childhood sexual activity is permitted, children gradually increase their sexual activities as they approach puberty. Among the Trobrianders, for example, children receive explicit sexual instructions from older companions whom they watch and imitate. Sex play includes masturbation, heterosexual and homosexual oral sex, and heterosexual intercourse. Prolonged sex play between a Trobriander boy and girl has the full approval of their parents (Ford and Beach, 1951).

Although Americans are obviously much less permissive than Trobriand Islanders, sex play with peers is an important source of sexual information in American society. The basic notions of privacy and secrecy that characterize sex life in the United States are acquired during this period. Thus, as researchers (Gadpaille, 1975) have noted, the most private aspect of sexual experience—sexual fantasies—increases markedly during childhood.

## SEX EDUCATION IN ELEMENTARY SCHOOLS

Sex education goes far beyond an understanding of physiology. By now it's clear that attitudes, emotions, and social roles cannot be separated from biology. Attitudes are so important that the home has been called "a continuous school for sex" (Schiller, 1977, p. 34). In fact, William Masters once said:

> The greatest form of sex education is Pop walking past Mom in the kitchen and patting her on the fanny and Mom obviously liking it. The kids take a good look at this action and think, "Boy, that's for me." (Masters and Johnson, 1969, p. 56)

Although the seemingly nonsexual aspects of life—including the way a baby is touched and handled, the gentle (and not so gentle) pushes into sex role, the way

*Focus*

TALKING
TO CHILDREN
ABOUT SEX

Many parents become uncomfortable when asked such questions as "Where do babies come from?" or "Where did mommy's penis go?" When a group of American mothers were asked how they handled such questions from their five-year-olds, most reported giving replies that probably confused their children. Although the days of deliveries by stork and finding babies under cabbage leaves have passed, some mothers still gave false information, and some gave no information at all (Sears, Maccoby, and Levin, 1957). None was free and open in the discussion of sex. Twenty-five years later, the situation showed little improvement. Asked whether he'd talked to his children about sex, one father said:

Talk to the kids? Are you kidding? My kids aren't old enough yet. Of course I'll talk to them when they're ready, but they aren't ready yet. They're only eleven and twelve. (Roberts, 1982, p. 91)

Even when parents give careful answers to children's questions, the youngsters often do not understand. One four-year-old who had been given a picture book about sex education said, "To get a baby, go to the store and buy a duck" (Bernstein, 1978, p. 9). The book told about reproduction in other species before showing human reproduction. The child assumed that since the picture of a duck came before the picture of the baby in her book, the duck must have turned into a baby.

Not to answer children's questions about sex gives them the message that sex is not to be talked about and that the child is wrong—or bad—to bring up the subject.

Perhaps as a result of their parents' reticence or embarrassment or perhaps because they have absorbed American taboos on sexual discussions, by the time they are nine or ten years old, most children stop asking their parents about sex. Once the questions stop, few parents initiate sexual discussions. Among the Cleveland families, this tendency meant that children often learned about pregnancy, birth, love, nudity, and the dangers of sexual molestations from their parents, but rarely heard about intercourse, abortion, homosexuality, prostitution, premarital sex, sexually transmitted disease, or contraception (Roberts, 1982). It ap-

pears that most children aren't getting from their parents the information they need to make decisions in the sexual situations they are likely to encounter during adolescence.

When children do ask questions, parents can minimize confusion by answering honestly and simply, and by matching the reply to the child's level of understanding. After carefully interviewing more than a hundred children, Anne Bernstein (1978) discovered that children go through six levels in reaching an understanding of sex, and that the levels correspond to the child's general stage of intellectual development (see Table 11.3).

Not all children go through the levels at the same age, but all pass through them in the same order. By asking "What do you think?" before answering, a parent can establish a child's present level of understanding and build on it. The secret is to give information that is not more than one level above the child's present grasp of the process.

The same six levels of understanding appeared when nearly a thousand five- to fifteen-year-old children in five countries were interviewed. Children from the United States and Canada were slowest at grasping the elements of sex, falling behind the middle-class children Bernstein interviewed in San Francisco, as well as behind children in Australia, England, and Sweden. The interviewers (Goldman and Goldman, 1982) believe that the level of school sex education programs is primarily responsible for the lagging performance of North American children. In Sweden, where children learn fastest, extensive sex education begins in the schools for all eight-year-olds. In the upstate New York area of the United States, where the American interviews were conducted, sex was such a controversial topic that it was difficult to persuade parents to allow their children to take part in the interviews.

## Table 11.3  *Understanding sex*

| LEVEL | AGE | INTELLECTUAL STAGE | TYPICAL BELIEF | READY TO LEARN |
|---|---|---|---|---|
| I | 3–5 | Geographer | Babies have always existed. Having a baby is a matter of transporting it home. | Babies are made by putting together a sperm from the father's body with an egg in the mother's body. |
| II | 4–8 | Manufacturer | Babies are manufactured by assembly-line techniques, putting together skin, bones, "head stuff," and so on. | Babies are made from ingredients in the parents' bodies. Daddy's sperm enters Mommy's vagina (a tunnel leading to the egg) through his penis. |
| III | 5–10 | Transitional | A contradictory mixture of technology and physiology. | An accurate, but simple, physiological explanation. |
| IV | 7–12 | Reporter | Conception cannot occur without marriage. Doesn't know the role of sperm and egg and is reluctant to speculate. | An accurate, but simple, physiological explanation. |
| V | 7–12 | Theoretician | Understands intercourse, but believes a baby is preformed. | The role of genetic contribution from each parent. |
| VI | 7–12 | Informed | Understands reproduction and parents' roles, including the contribution of genetic material. | |

Based on information in A. C. Bernstein. *The Flight of the Stork*. Delacorte Press, 1978.

emotions are expressed within the family, and silence or embarrassment when the forbidden subject is mentioned—have powerful effects on a child's understanding of sexuality, children must pick up the basic information somewhere. And most do.

Their source of explicit sex education is generally the peer group (Gagnon and Simon, 1969). What children are not taught at home or in the school they pick up in the street, in the form of facts embedded in a web of rumor, distortion, and outright lies. The often garbled stories children get from peer group gossip are digested in the context of information provided by the media: news stories about rape, incest, abortion, and personal scandal; dramas with sexual themes; explicitly sexual lyrics of popular songs; and outright pornography (Schiller, 1977).

Faced with this knowledge and aware of the rising tide of teenage pregnancy (which we'll discuss in the next chapter), many educators have been developing sex education programs for preadolescents. The programs are controversial in many parts of the country, as researchers in upstate New York discovered when they tried to find out just how much American children know about sex. Such classes are effective only when teachers themselves are comfortable and secure about their own sexual feelings and when the information covered is suited to the intellectual level of the children (Gagnon and Simon, 1969).

The school program devised by Patricia Schiller (1977) of the American Association of Sex Educators, Counselors, and Therapists (AASECT) is designed to meet those conditions. It begins in kindergarten, with the aim of imparting basic facts within a framework of human relationships. By the time children have completed the third grade, the goal is that they:

**1** Have a healthy attitude toward all parts of the body.

**2** Appreciate and are aware of the physical sex differences in girls and boys and are confident and proud of being a boy or a girl.

**3** Use universally understood and accepted words for all body parts (such as penis, vagina, urinate, bowel movement, toilet).

**4** Know the meaning of being a cooperating member of a family with specific roles and relationships.

**5** Know the elementary facts of human reproduction.

**6** Can ask questions and participate in group discussions without embarrassment.

For example, kindergarten children learn that the family is the basic unit of social life, that all living beings produce their own likeness, that there are individual differences in patterns of growth, and that all parts of the body are healthy and have a name. Each year the course of study spirals back over some of the same material, building on previous knowledge and giving new information at an appropriate intellectual level.

Without such classes, the pattern discovered in the study (Goldman and Goldman, 1982) described earlier is likely to continue, with 36 percent of the thirteen-year-olds and 13 percent of the fifteen-year-olds still at level four in Bernstein's scale of sexual understanding. These adolescent "reporters" are confused about many aspects of sex—some of them believe that conception cannot occur without marriage—yet most are capable of reproduction. In the next chapter, we'll see how adolescents tend to handle the demands and opportunities of sexual maturation.

# Summary

**1** In order to become male or female, each baby goes through **sexual differentiation**, a lengthy, complex process that mixes biology with learning. At each stage in the process, development can proceed in a male or a female direction; in most people it consistently takes the same direction.

**2** An adult with a clearly male or female gender identity has gone through a path of development made up of genetic sex, gonadal sex, hormonal secretions, internal sex organs, external genitals, the sex label given at birth, and gender identity formed early in childhood. Either biology or environment can disrupt the process. Girls with **Turner's syndrome** have only one X chromosome (pattern XO); they have female external genitals but no ovaries; their gender identity is female. Girls with an extra X chromosome (pattern XXX) have a complete female reproductive system and a female gender identity, but their fertility is diminished. Boys with **Klinefelter's syndrome** have an extra female chromosome (pattern XXY); they have male genitals but are sterile and have a low sex drive. Boys with an extra male chromosome (XYY) may be impulsive or aggressive, but their physiology and sexuality appear to be normal.

**3** In the **androgen insensitivity syndrome**, a genetic male is unable to use hormones secreted by his testes. He appears female when born, but his internal genitals are male. He is usually labeled a girl, develops a female gender identity, and leads the life of a woman. In the **andrenogenital syndrome**, a genetic female is exposed before birth to an improper form of cortisone that acts like androgens in her body. Her internal organs are female, but her external organs appear masculine. (A similar condition develops when a pregnant woman carrying a female fetus is given androgens.) In either case, the child's gender identity generally depends on the sex of rearing.

**4** From birth, boys seem more restless, fussier, and harder to calm down than girls; they may also be more responsive to sights, while girls are more responsive to sounds. These sex differences may influence the way their mothers treat them, as well as predisposing boys to action and girls to caution. Rearing and the socialization process exaggerate such sex differences. Babies are sexually responsive from birth and have been observed having orgasms. Because the baby lacks the basis for a sexual interpretation of such sensations, the infant experience is very different from that of adults. Masturbation is apparently a normal process of infant self-exploration. The first year of life was called the **oral stage** by Freud, who believed that the baby's sensual pleasure comes from stimulation of the mouth. A baby's first emotional bond with parents may make a permanent impression on later emotional and sexual development.

**5** The preschool child goes through an informal instruction in the culture's beliefs, attitudes, values, and sex roles that is known as **socialization**. During the second and third years of life, the child is in Freud's **anal stage**, in which the rectum is the center of sensual pleasure. As parents socialize their children, many also restrict masturbation, nudity, and expressions of curiosity about the body and its functions. From age three until six, children are in Freud's **phallic stage**, in which the genitals are the center of sensual pleasure. During this period, children supposedly work through the Oedipus complex, in which they feel sexual desire for the parent of the other sex and resolve it by identifying with the parent of the same sex. The Oedipal theory has been criticized as both unscientific and sexist.

**6** Most children are about thirty months old before they know for certain whether they are boys or girls, but almost from birth their parents steer them into their sex roles. Various psychological theories have been proposed to replace the Oedipal complex as a basis for identification with the parent of the same sex. Some psychologists believe it is the child's knowledge that gender will never change; some believe it is parental rewards and satisfaction of the child's needs; and some believe it is the concepts the child forms while observing the actions of parents and other adults, children, and media characters.

**7** Although experts once believed that witnessing parents in the act of sexual intercourse (the primal scene) invariably left emotional scars, it now appears that the sight is not always harmful. Sex play is prevalent among children of all cultures, but some societies tolerate or encourage it, while others attempt to suppress it. As children become aware of adult disapproval, they learn to keep their sex play private.

**8** During the school years, peers are important in both emotional and sexual development. With peers, children rehearse adult social roles and express their feelings about falling in love. This time was called the **latency period** by Freud, for he believed that after the Oedipus complex was resolved, the sex drive was repressed until puberty. However, it appears that children steadily increase their sex play and that such sex play occurs about equally with the same and the other sex. Because parents tend to be more protective of daughters, boys generally initiate more same-sex sex play than do girls. The amount of sex play during childhood depends in part on the degree of sexual permissiveness in a society.

**9** Most parents apparently find it difficult to talk to their children about sex, and young children often distort the information they are given. By the time children are nine or ten, most stop asking sexual questions of their parents. When answering a child's questions, parents can answer honestly, giving the child only as much information as he or she can handle and matching the reply to the child's level of understanding. Children apparently go through six intellectual levels in reaching an understanding of sex, but not all pass through the levels at the same age.

**10** Most children get their explicit sexual information from the peer group. This information is set in the context of sexual information provided by the media. Sex education classes in the schools are effective when the teachers are comfortable with their own sexual feelings and when the information provided is suited to the child's intellectual level. Sex education programs have been designed to impart basic facts within a framework of human relationships, covering the same basic topics in each grade, but each year building on previous knowledge with additional information at the child's new intellectual level.

## a male experience

My first ejaculation came as quite a shock. I'd heard some of the guys making jokes about it, but I had no idea what to expect. It really blew me away! (Authors' files)

## a female experience

Mother talked to me about menstruation like it was something on the moon. She was looking up at the ceiling. I won't forget that as long as I live. Boy, I knew everything she was talking about and I was saying to myself, this is too late now. I don't want my child to grow up that way. (Roberts, 1982, p. 74)

# 12 Sexual Development in Adolescence

# *Chapter 12*

**adolescence**
transitional
phase of life
between pu-
berty and
adulthood

With adolescence, the body's sexual motor shifts into high gear. Hormones transform the straight child's body into a physique that is obviously male or female. Before they assume the roles of men and women, however, children in most industrialized societies must go through a period of **adolescence**, a transitional phase in which they are regarded as sexually mature but socially and psychologically immature (Miller and Simon, 1980). This public definition of the adolescent as a person who is simultaneously mature and immature often creates tension, since society attempts to restrict the sexual status of individuals who may be sexually active.

This sort of tension did not develop in tribal societies, where adolescence was brief—if it existed at all. As they became sexually mature, children went through rituals that made them adults in the eyes of the community.

Adolescence as a phase of life is a relatively new invention. In early Western cultures, biological maturity received little attention. Most children had joined the labor force and were learning adult behavior and responsibilities long before sexuality maturity. It required a series of social, economic, and historical changes to create adolescence. The rising economic productivity that followed industrialization freed young people from farm and factory labor. New laws forbade full time employment of young teenagers, and society could afford to educate all its members. As society became more complex, education became more important. The period of adolescence, when most young people are free to pursue psychological growth, refers to the person's social status and generally is considered to end when she or he assumes adult responsibilities.

The challenges of adolescence today are demanding: adjusting to a new body, estab-

# Sexual Development in Adolescence

lishing an identity, deciding on a vocation, becoming independent of family, coming to terms with sexuality—all within a situation full of contradictions between individual freedom and outside control. In this chapter, we begin by tracing the physical changes that accompany sexual maturation. We look at sex roles during adolescence and investigate teenage sexuality. Sexuality in late adolescence is often developed within a college setting, so we study sex on campus. We look briefly at two current issues, teenage pregnancy and childbirth, and conclude by exploring the interaction between sex education and sexual decision making.

## SEXUAL MATURATION

The period of early adolescence, when a sequence of physical events transforms children into sexually mature adults, is known as **puberty**, a term that once referred to the appearance of pubic hair (Tanner, 1978).

The exact mechanism that sets the process in motion is unknown. There may be a "biological clock" in the brain, programmed to signal the hypothalamus to send messages to the pituitary gland, a tiny structure at the base of the brain (Money and Ehrhardt, 1972). The pituitary responds by producing sex hormones known as **gonadotropins**. The gonadotropins in turn signal the gonads to produce androgens or estrogens.

The messages go out several years before any physical change is apparent, because es-

**puberty** period of early adolescence when biological changes are transforming children into sexually mature adults

**gonadotropins** sex hormones produced by the pituitary gland

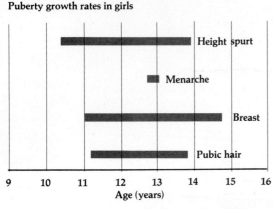

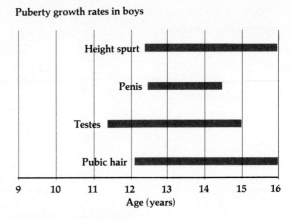

**Figure 12.1  *Physical Changes During Puberty.***
The height spurt reaches a peak at about age 12 in girls and about age 14 in boys. The bars represent the duration (average ages for beginning and end) of the events of puberty. (Tanner, 1973, p. 40)

trogens and androgens may reappear in a child's urine when the youngster is eight or nine years old. Both sexes produce estrogens and androgens, but in different balance, with boys secreting a larger proportion of androgens and girls, a larger proportions of estrogens.

As these hormones circulate through the bloodstream, the child's body responds—not only with the obvious characteristics of maleness and femaleness, but with the adolescent growth spurt as well. Both boys and girls shoot up spectacularly in height and weight. Their growth may show **asynchrony**; different body parts may grow at different rates. (See Figure 12.1.) Because of this disproportionate growth, adolescents' hands and feet may seem too big for their bodies, or the nose or jaw may seem too prominent. This is only temporary, however; soon the various parts of the body regain their harmony.

**asynchrony** the maturation of different body parts at different rates, a growth characteristic typical of adolescence

## *Puberty: girls*

When the hypothalamus stimulates a girl's pituitary, it releases the gonadotropic hormones FSH and LH. FSH stimulates ovulation. In response to LH, the ovaries produce and release estrogens. Estrogens are carried by the bloodstream to the breasts, uterus, vagina, pelvic bones, and fatty tissue, where they begin their work of transforming the girl's body. Small amounts of androgens are produced by the adrenal glands, and these male hormones lead to the growth of pubic and armpit hair and the enlargement of the clitoris. At about the time of menarche, or first menstruation, the levels of various hormones begin to rise and fall in the rhythmic pattern described in Chapter 3. Once established, this pattern continues until menopause.

The first visible changes of puberty appear when girls are about eleven years old, but individual differences are so wide that the event can occur at any time between eight and thirteen (Tanner, 1978). The first sign of puberty is usually the appearance of the "breast bud," a slight enlargement of the breast and nipple, although in about a third of girls, pubic hair develops first. Underarm hair becomes visible. A girl's growth spurt typically peaks early in puberty, at about the age of twelve. Menarche generally takes place about two years after the first sign of puberty. Menstruation indicates that the internal sexual organs are almost mature.

The average age of menarche has been decreasing over the past century (Figure 12.2), but not nearly so much as had been supposed. Scattered data from Scandinavian countries had indicated that in 1840, menstruation began at the age of seventeen and that between 1880 and 1960 the average age dropped four months every decade, finally slowing—if not stopping—within the past few years (Tanner, 1978). It now appears, however, that the drop has been much less sharp. Although in the United States the average age is now between 12.3 and 12.6 years, it probably was never more than 15. Indeed, in medieval Europe, authorities assumed that girls would begin to menstruate between the ages of twelve and fourteen (Bullough, 1981).

One popular explanation for the drop that has occurred is better nutrition, especially more protein and calories in early infancy. Less exposure to infectious disease has also been suggested (Tanner, 1978). These factors are undoubtedly important, since even today African girls in poor areas begin menstruating between the ages of fifteen and seventeen, but girls in more prosperous areas begin at the same age as European girls (Brooks-Gunn and Matthews, 1979). The onset of puberty in any girl, however, is probably determined by a complex interaction among heredity, individual physiology, and the external environment.

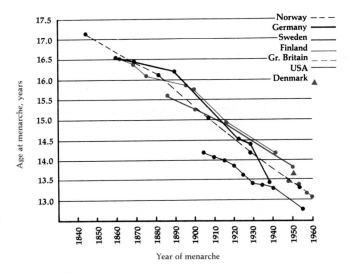

*Figure 12.2*
This graph shows the decline in the age of the first menstruation (menarche) in various Western countries. (Tanner, 1962)

## *Puberty: boys*

The gonadotropic hormones released by a boy's hypothalamus are ICSH and FSH, which were discussed in Chapter 4. ICSH stimulates the testes to produce testosterone, and FSH, which stimulates ovulation in girls, stimulates sperm production in boys.

As the testes enlarge under the influence of these hormones, they can produce even more testosterone. As testosterone levels in the bloodstream rise, physical changes begin. The testes and penis enlarge further, and pubic hair appears. The voice becomes deeper, and the chest and shoulders take on a masculine contour. Only later do armpit hair and a beard appear. Height and weight increase rapidly during the growth spurt, but may keep increasing at a slow pace until about age twenty.

The technical marker of puberty in boys is the appearance of sperm in the urine. But since this signal can be detected only in the laboratory, the official sign is generally the first ejaculation, which has been called **spermache**. Spermache usually takes place at about twelve or thirteen, but as with girls, individual differences are wide. The first nocturnal emission, or wet dream, usually takes place about a year after the penis begins to grow, and that growth can begin as early as ten or as late as fifteen (Tanner, 1978). The boy's growth spurt peaks later in puberty than does the girl's—at about fourteen years. By the time a boy is about fifteen, his semen contains mature sperm.

**spermache** the first ejaculation, a sign of puberty in boys

## *Timing problems*

Puberty doesn't always proceed smoothly and according to schedule. For various reasons, it may be early, late, or incomplete.

If puberty begins before a girl is eight or a boy is nine years old, the condition is called **precocious puberty** (Ehrhardt and Meyer-Bahlburg, 1975). Precocious puberty can begin shortly after birth, but more often appears when children are six to eight years old. The condition may be the result of the adrenogenital syndrome in girls or of a tumor in the hypothalamus, gonads, or adrenal glands—or its cause may never be discovered. Although precocious puberty sometimes runs in families, it generally affects only one child.

**precocious puberty** puberty that appears before the age of eight in girls or the age of nine in boys

These very young children may develop typical secondary sex characteristics—pubic hair and either breasts or enlarged genitals, a beard, and a deep voice. They may undergo menarche or spermache.

Precocious puberty presents special problems for child and parents. Sex education and frank communication are important for such a child, who is deprived of the usual sort of peer exchange on these matters. In addition to handling the problems of an ill-timed sexual development, the child has the additional problem of being much larger than his or her peers.

When a girl's precocious puberty is due to the adrenogenital syndrome, the drug cortisone can help delay maturation. For most cases of precocious puberty, however, there is no simple medical treatment for either girls or boys. Specialists recom-

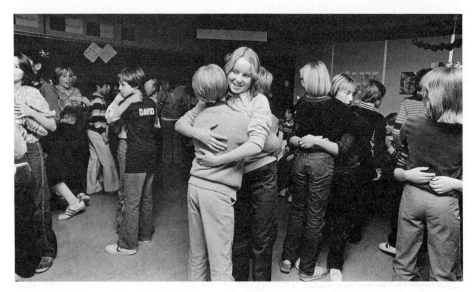

Twelve-year-old girls often tower over their male peers, but the disparity in height, weight, and sexual development will disappear in about two years when boys begin the adolescent growth spurt. (© Donald Deitz/Stock, Boston)

mend extensive psychological counseling for child and parents (Ehrhardt and Meyer-Bahlburg, 1975).

In delayed puberty, the lack of sex hormones—or a failure to respond to them—stops or markedly slows physical changes. A girl with Turner's syndrome will not show any pubertal development because she has no ovaries to secrete estrogens. Although she can never bear children, hormonal supplements will cause secondary sex characteristics to develop. A boy who is castrated or who suffers from androgen-insensitivity syndrome doesn't follow the usual course. His voice remains high, his genitals remain small, no beard develops, and his arms and legs are disproportionately long. He is likely to have little interest in sexual activity. He will, however, grow pubic and armpit hair, since these changes are caused by hormones secreted by the adrenal glands. If the delay has some other cause, hormonal supplements will speed the pubertal process.

## ADJUSTING TO PUBERTY

Although infants also go through enormous physical changes during the first two years of life, they don't have to deal with the self-consciousness that accompanies the physical changes of puberty. Adolescents watch the entire process, and as many observe their altered bodies, their feelings shift among fascination, delight, and horror. The physical changes of adolescence have social and psychological consequences. In coming to terms with the changes in their bodies, adolescents have to handle their reactions to menstruation or ejaculation, the disparity in growth between boys and girls, uneven growth rates, and their concern about their own looks.

### Reactions to menstruation

Depending on the attitude of her parents and peer group and the way she has been prepared for menarche, a girl may react with fear, pride, embarrassment, or shame. At one time few girls were told about menstruation ahead of time, so many were frightened by their first menstrual flow. A girl who hadn't been told said:

> I started to scream. I thought I was bleeding to death. Nobody told me about periods, nobody told me about anything. I was in the fifth grade and I still thought babies grew in your stomach and came out your belly button. (Bell, 1980, p. 31)

Girls who are not prepared for menstruation tend to have more menstrual symptoms, including pain, and their symptoms are more severe than in girls who know what to expect (Ruble and Brooks-Gunn, 1982). Today most girls are prepared in advance, and some are proud when they begin to menstruate because they see it as a badge of womanhood:

> I told everybody when I got my period. Everybody! I celebrated and went out and bought myself a present. (Bell, 1980, p. 32)

The reaction of pride is more likely today than a generation ago. Among a group of women who were interviewed in the late 1950s, only 15 percent recalled that their mothers had reacted to their daughters' menarche with pleasure or excitement, but among a group of adolescents interviewed in the late 1970s, most said their mothers had been happy (Brooks-Gunn and Ruble, 1980).

As girls get older, most become more comfortable about menstruation and much less embarrassed. Despite the fact that girls today generally find menstruation much less of an ordeal than they had anticipated, as time goes on many become more negative about the process. Researchers (Brooks-Gunn and Ruble, 1982a) who studied the attitudes of nearly 700 teenage girls suggest that the increasingly negative attitude is in part the result of learning. As girls become more knowledgeable, the initial pride may fade as they realize they must cope with menstruation each and every month for several decades.

The way a girl deals with her period may also affect her feelings about menstruation. Among these same girls, those who used tampons tended to be less self-conscious about menstruation than girls who used napkins (Brooks-Gunn and Ruble, 1982b). They were also less concerned about menstrual accidents and less likely to find that menstruation interfered with their sports activities.

### Reactions to ejaculation

Although most boys know about menstruation, few are told in advance about ejaculation. Unlike other aspects of puberty, ejaculation is explicitly sexual, making it a difficult topic for many parents to handle.

Among a large group of Cleveland parents, for example, only 2 percent had discussed the subject with their sons (Gagnon and Roberts, 1980). Ejaculation's sexual nature also makes it unlikely that boys will ask their parents about it, for as we saw in Chapter 11, few children older than ten ask their parents about sexual matters. This means that most boys rely on their peers for information about ejaculation, and the word doesn't always get to them.

As a result, 20 percent of the boys in one group were frightened by their first experience. Those whose first ejaculation came as a nocturnal emission were ashamed because they thought they had wet their beds. Those who had first ejaculated while masturbating felt they had done something wrong. Boys who are not frightened may be surprised at the experience. Only 6 percent of these boys reacted with pleasure (Shipman, 1971). But when a boy knows what to expect and reacts positively, he may respond as one boy did:

> I'd heard about it from friends and read about it in books. So it was no big surprise to me. All I can remember is feeling very proud of myself—like scoring a touchdown or something! (Authors' files)

## Variations in development

As they go through the normal changes of adolescence, boys and girls temporarily seem to inhabit two different worlds. Since girls generally experience the first effects of puberty about two years before boys show any signs of sexual maturity, the twelve-year-old girl is likely to be taller, heavier, and more sexually developed than her male counterpart. When her breasts begin to show, she may be set apart from former male friends who are not yet able to cope with this symbol of sexual maturity.

As a result, girls of this age often adopt an attitude of dominance or superiority toward their male peers, who still seem to be "silly little boys" at a time when girls are experiencing the first signs of womanhood. Boys typically deal with the anxiety this situation creates by joining together in all-male groups that stay as far away from girls and their activities as possible (Gadpaille, 1975).

At the time when girls and boys are restructuring their relationships with one another, they must also adjust to uneven rates of growth among members of their own sex. Young girls and boys almost invariably compare their own growth with that of members of their peer group. The girl whose breasts develop first may be envied by her classmates, or she may feel awkward and strange. Similarly, a boy whose growth spurt is delayed a year or so longer than that of his friends generally feels at a disadvantage. Normal variations in development may lead an adolescent to worry that he or she is abnormal.

## Adjusting to appearance

Like adults, adolescents compare their bodies to the images they see on television or in movies and magazines. But because they have not yet come to terms with the changes in their appearance, they are even more insecure than adults about what they see in the mirror. Nearly half of young adolescent girls and a quarter of the boys say they often feel "ugly and unattractive" (Offer, Ostrov, and Howard, 1981). No matter what they weigh, girls think they are too fat, that their breasts are too small or too large, that their hips, their thighs, their hands, their feet, are all wrong. They want to be slim but curvaceous, with flawless skin. Boys think they are scrawny, underweight, and lack muscles. They want to be tall and muscular, with broad shoulders and flawless skin.

The struggle to come to terms with their new bodies seems easier for boys than for girls. As one man recalled:

> When the first dark hairs sprouted on my upper lip, it was a big event. It meant I got my own razor and a personal lesson from Dad in how to use it. There was a lot of kidding around, but it made me feel sort of proud and masculine—like I was on my way to becoming a real man. (Authors' files)

Boys are much more likely than girls to be proud of their bodies, to take satisfaction in the physical changes they have undergone, and to believe that members of the other sex find them attractive (Offer, Ostrov, and Howard, 1981). This difference is probably in good part a reflection of the culture's stress on female beauty and of the traditional female role, which depended upon attracting a mate. Until sex roles broaden, girls will continue to feel such pressure.

In addition to cultural standards, the reactions of parents and peers and the adolescent's own personality affect the degree of concern adolescents feel about

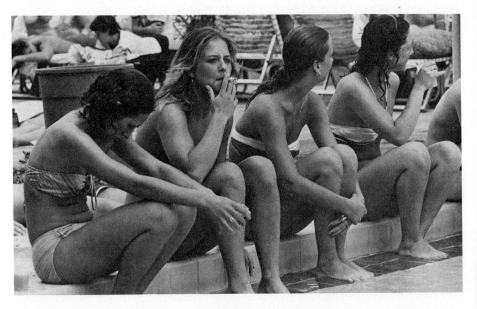

Adjusting to their new bodies is a struggle for many adolescents, and because of the culture's stress on female beauty it is often harder for girls than for boys. (© Frank Siteman/Stock, Boston)

their changing bodies. A chance remark by a parent ("You have your father's big feet") or a friend ("Your nose looks like Bob Hope's") can be devastating. Teenagers who already have a low estimate of themselves may become especially anxious about their appearance, even though they look perfectly normal to others (Peterson and Taylor, 1980). By late adolescence, the image they have of their own bodies has a strong relationship with the way adolescents judge themselves as people (Lerner and Spanier, 1980).

Anxiety over appearance usually fades by late adolescence as teenagers become less self-conscious and their body proportions come back into balance. In the meantime, adolescents need more than a simple reassurance that they look fine or that they'll "grow out of it." Factual information about maturation may help ease the pain for some youngsters. For others, the realization that most adolescents share their feelings of self-consciousness may dispel some of their anxiety.

The worried adolescent may also be reassured to learn that the masculinity or femininity of his or her body bears no relationship to adult sexual behavior or orientation (Money and Ehrhardt, 1972). The broad-shouldered, muscular adolescent boy will not necessarily grow up to become a virile lover, and the thin, effeminate boy will not necessarily become a sexually indifferent man. Similarly, the size of a girl's breasts or a boy's penis tells us nothing about her or his future sexual activities.

## SEXUAL BEHAVIOR

As children become adolescents, they tend to retreat to traditional sex roles. About the time they are fourteen, girls and boys begin to see the world in stereotypical terms. Most girls are as careful to be "feminine" as boys are to be "masculine." The retreat is only temporary. Although hormones may play a part in the change, its primary sources are probably uncertainty about a new sexual self and social pressures to conform to traditional sex roles.

Gender differences are not as rigid as they once were, but the expectations attached to sex roles are probably the most powerful force shaping the sexual behavior of adolescents (Miller and Simon, 1980). They always have been, but today's teenagers develop their sexual scripts in a changed adult world. When sex was never mentioned, divorce almost unthinkable, and people expected sexual interest and capacity to wane during middle adulthood, young people had few overtly sexual models. Now, they observe the swinging singles and the divorced in search of new partners. Whatever they don't see in their neighborhood is shown on movie and television screens and described in books and magazines.

As might be expected, more teenagers are sexually active at younger ages than ever before. In response, society has begun to accept adolescent sexual experimentation as normal. But there is concern over rising pregnancy rates among teenagers and the consequences of abortion or illegitimate birth, along with sharp increases in rape and sexually transmitted disease among young people.

## Masturbation

Masturbation is an important aspect of adolescent sexuality. Various surveys have found different rates of activity, but all find that masturbation to orgasm is much more common among adolescent boys than girls. Surveys also agree that young people of both sexes are masturbating at an earlier age today than they did a generation ago. As we saw in Chapter 7, within twenty-five years the incidence of masturbation among thirteen-year-old boys rose from 45 to 63 percent and among thirteen-year-old girls from 15 to 33 percent (Kinsey, Pomeroy and Martin, 1948; Kinsey et al., 1953; Hunt, 1974). The numbers climb throughout adolescence.

Teenagers who have experienced intercourse are more likely to masturbate than are "virgins," whether male or female. Reaching an orgasm through petting or sexual intercourse leads many adolescents to masturbate for the first time. A sixteen-year-old boy said that he learned to masturbate:

> From the girl I was with. When she did it to me I thought I would do it to myself. (Hass, 1979, p. 89)

A girl of the same age reported:

> When my boyfriend would touch my vagina, I usually had to help him find the clitoris. After a while I found that I could please myself the same way by myself. (Hass, 1979, p. 90)

Although more young people seem to be masturbating at earlier ages, the activity still makes many feel guilty and embarrassed (Sorenson, 1973; Hunt, 1974). Masturbation is more difficult for teenagers to discuss than any other topic (Gadpaille, 1975). Many adolescents regard masturbation as an immature and socially unacceptable outlet, even if they understand that it is essentially normal. Although the attitudes toward masturbation have shifted, the stigma still lingers (Hunt, 1974). According to one youth:

> When I was about thirteen, I masturbated a couple of times but then I heard from the other guys that it would sap your strength and that it leads to becoming a pervert. So I sort of gave it up. (Bell, 1980, p. 80)

After children reach puberty, masturbation changes more for boys than for girls. Although both sexes can masturbate to orgasm before puberty, boys' new capacity to ejaculate significantly affects their experience. Ejaculation typically becomes the goal for the adolescent boy, and the release of tension associated with orgasm and ejaculation is soon a major source of satisfaction.

A second difference between the sexes is the use of sexual fantasies during masturbation, which is almost universal among adolescent boys but somewhat less common among girls (Hunt, 1974). Many teenagers who fantasize during masturbation think of explicit sexual images. Others—usually those with less sexual experience—have vague, almost dreamlike images (Hass, 1979). Sexual fantasies are still a major source of sexual conditioning for adolescent boys, and perhaps males are more easily conditioned to a variety of sexual stimuli than are females (Kinsey et al., 1953). Or perhaps American boys are given more permission than girls to experiment sexually. In addition, most erotic stimuli that can fuel fantasies (books and magazines) are designed with a male audience in mind.

## *Homosexual experience*

As noted in Chapter 11, sex play with members of the same gender is one way children learn about sex. Such play may extend into adolescence among some young people whose adult experience will be primarily—if not exclusively—heterosexual. But the homosexual experiences of adolescent boys and girls differ in several ways.

**Boys** For some boys, homosexual activity during early adolescence is a natural continuation of childhood sex play. Other boys have their first homosexual experience then. Among the men interviewed by Kinsey, 27 percent had had some homosexual experience after puberty but before their sixteenth birthday (Kinsey, Pomeroy, and Martin, 1948). Yet only 11 percent of the adolescent boys in another group had experienced any homosexual activity (Sorenson, 1973).

This difference may be the result of social changes. During puberty, the maturational gap between boys and girls reaches its peak, and many boys who may feel threatened by sex play with girls of the same age experiment with boys. With increased availability of sexually available teenage girls, the incentive for sexual experiences with their own sex may have decreased. This apparent decrease in homosexual experience has been confirmed in later studies done on the subject (Hass, 1979).

In most cases, the homosexual relationships of adolescence are nothing more than a passing phase, after which the individual adopts a heterosexual life style. As youngsters move into their late teens, many become more conscious of social reaction to such contacts and adjust to society's heterosexual standard (Kinsey, Pomeroy, and Martin, 1948). The experience described by an eighteen-year-old boy is fairly common:

> I used to have sex with my best friends, who were guys, all the time. This was until I was fourteen or so. And I never thought it was wrong or anything like that. (Bell, 1980, p. 114)

In some boys, however, the homosexual preference continues into adulthood, as we saw in Chapter 9.

Among the men interviewed by Kinsey, adolescent homosexual activity was most frequent among those who matured early, masturbated more often before puberty, and were less religious. Although a few adolescents—less than 5 percent—go on to develop an exclusively homosexual orientation, most young men make a gradual transition from homosexual experiences to predominantly heterosexual relationships.

The transition probably happens easily because many teenage boys don't regard their sexual contact with other boys as "homosexuality" in the adult sense. As a result, it does not become incorporated into their sexual scripts (Gagnon and Simon, 1973). If adolescents worry that they will become homosexuals, the experiences may provoke a crisis. But the vast majority pass through both the crisis and the homosexuality (Manaster, 1977). Even boys who prostitute themselves to older homosexual "clients" usually see themselves as heterosexuals who are using sex only to get money (Reiss, 1961).

**Girls** Homosexual experiences are much less common among adolescent girls than among boys. Only about 3 percent of the women interviewed by Kinsey had had homosexual relations during adolescence that resulted in orgasm. A much larger percentage, however, had homosexual feelings as adolescents but didn't act upon them (Kinsey et al., 1953). In a later study (Sorenson, 1973) the rate of homosexual experience among adolescent girls had doubled. Perhaps attitudes toward homosexuality had begun to shift by the time of the second survey. Most adolescents now tend to accept the idea that others will have homosexual experiences, although they are certain they will never have such experiences themselves (Hass, 1979).

The lower rate of homosexual activity among girls may be the result of sex-role learning. Most women are socialized into a relatively passive sexual role and are less likely than men to initiate sexual behavior in any situation. They are also less likely than men to go into a relationship without an emotional commitment. As one girl said:

> We were best friends. She was the first person I was able to talk to about my emotions. First we kissed and necked and fondled each other. Then we got into mutual masturbation. I felt I loved her, but I was scared because I didn't want to be gay. In fact we tried to stop seeing each other. (Bell, Weinberg, and Hammersmith, 1981, p. 165)

Sex-role learning could easily account for the difference in homosexual experiences, since girls in reformatories or penal institutions frequently have homosexual relationships. These institutions are societies of their own where scripts followed in the outside world may lose their power.

## Heterosexual experience

With the security blanket of sex roles wrapped around them, young adolescents venture into heterosexual relationships. In one large survey (Offer, Ostrov, and Howard, 1981), most of the boys and about half of the girls said they often thought about sex, but a substantial minority said that it's very hard for a teenager to know how to handle sex. A more sexually open society may add to the worry by changing expectations and attitudes. In the 1960s, only 7 percent of American teenagers thought they were behind their peers in sexual experience; by the 1970s, 21 percent felt that way (Offer, Ostrov, and Howard, 1981).

**Dating and petting scripts** The usual goal of courtship or dating is the formation of heterosexual pair bonds, which were discussed in Chapter 2. Dating as we know it is a relatively recent development; it first appeared on college campuses about fifty years ago. Until that time, contact between courting couples was mostly limited to general social occasions or to the front parlor of the girl's home, perhaps under the watchful eye of a chaperone. Unlike courting in most animal species, whose only purpose is to find a mate, dating serves a variety of additional functions: It affirms masculinity and femininity by permitting young men and women to demonstrate their attractiveness to the other sex; it provides a semistructured social situation for the learning and rehearsal of basic social and sexual skills; and it allows young people to share entertainment and recreation away from home and parents.

The rules of today's dating game reflect traditional sex roles (Brooks-Gunn and Matthews, 1979). The socialization of girls has stressed interpersonal skills and a capacity for intimacy. So in their heterosexual relations, girls are friendly but passive, concerned with "catching" a boy. Although some girls are beginning to make the first move, most still feel it is up to the boy. One sixteen-year-old girl complained:

> Sitting around waiting for the phone to ring is a big part of my life. (Bell, 1980, p. 66)

Boys are socialized to be active and assertive. They are expected to take the initiative in asking for dates and in petting. Since adolescents see sex roles as moral absolutes, they view behavior that violates the roles as immoral (Miller and Simon, 1980). One girl who shattered her date's expectations discovered how adolescents may rush to judgment:

> I really liked this guy, and so I went all the way on our first date. It really shocked him. Afterward he said he kept expecting me to stop him. He thought I was a "nice" girl. (Authors' files)

Dating relationships pass through several stages. During casual dating, the partners are either too young or not interested enough for more than a short-term, limited involvement. But despite their lack of interest, adolescents can't ignore the dating game. Those who don't date are dropped by their peer group. Chronological age, not sexual maturation, predicts entry into the dating game, and many prepubertal youngsters date in order to stay in their group (Dornbusch et al., 1981).

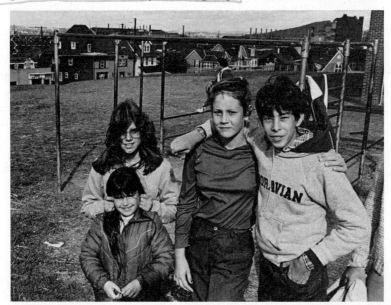

Dating can teach adolescents a great deal about the formation of mature relationships between men and women and about emotional intimacy. (© Joan Liftin/ Archive)

Among high school and college students, dating sometimes provides partners for relatively impersonal sexual encounters. At a later stage, couples who have been dating for some time may decide to "go steady." This more or less exclusive relationship is important, because it shows commitment and the formation of a pair bond. On some campuses, the next step is "pinning," when the boy gives the girl a pin or lavalier. The last important dating stage is engagement, which signifies the couple's intention to marry.

Perhaps the most striking change in American dating practices has been in attitudes toward sexual activity. The official religious and moral position has always required abstinence before marriage for both males and females. Men have been expected to push for sexual contact, and women to resist the pressure. Only recently has a permissive standard that applies equally to males and females been suggested.

When a group of older adolescents was asked to rate the various strategies used in influencing a partner, their judgments conformed to stereotypes. All the strategies meant to persuade a date to have sex were described as used mostly by men, and all the strategies designed to avoid sex were described as used mostly by women. What's more, the students said their own behavior followed this script. Whether students were "liberated" or "conservative" in their general view of sex roles, they clung to the stereotype (La Plante et al., 1980).

Several factors affect permissiveness among young people. Parental attitudes, family ties, and religious commitment limit permissiveness, while the attitudes of peers and friends increase it (Reiss, 1977).

As a result of permissiveness, petting now includes every technique described as foreplay, including oral sex. The traditional labels of virgin or nonvirgin have less meaning than they once did. Many young people today are "technical virgins," in that the only heterosexual experience they lack is putting the penis into the vagina. For many technical virgins, sex is sacred and powerful, and they believe it should be reserved for a deeply committed relationship. They may believe that premarital genital intercourse is ill-advised, stupid, or immoral (Kiniery, 1982). Technical virginity seems linked to religious attitudes, with the depth of religious belief apparently affecting males more strongly than females. A sixteen-year-old boy who described himself and his girlfriend as "very religious" said:

> Both of us agree that we'd rather wait until we're married to do some things, because we just feel that you make more of a deep commitment to each other if you wait. (Bell, 1980, p. 89)

At one college, religious male students were likely to be technical virgins, with experience in oral sex but not with intercourse. Among other students, whether male or female, genital intercourse was more common (Mahoney, 1980).

**Sexual intercourse**  In line with increased permissiveness in society, the rate of premarital intercourse among American teenagers is higher than it ever has been. But the increase is mostly accounted for by more girls becoming sexually active at an earlier age. Since there has been little increase among boys since the days of the Kinsey reports, males and females now have quite similar rates of premarital inter-

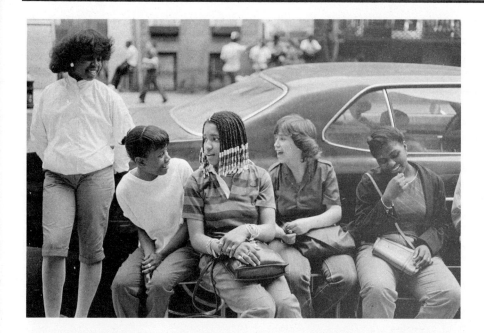

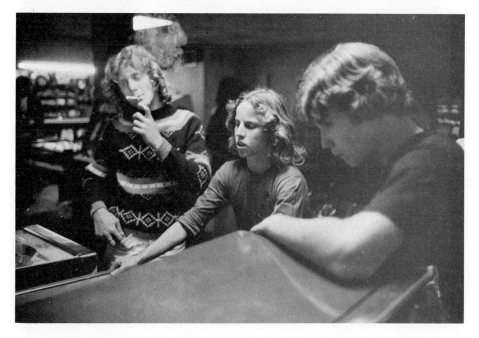

Sex roles affect all social relationships, and girls and boys have different standards for their interactions. Girls are ''allowed'' to express their emotions and friendships openly and directly. Boys are often so concerned with maintaining a strong male image that they have difficulty expressing their feelings of friendship. (© Hazel Hankin 1983; © Paul Fusco/Magnum)

course (Miller and Simon, 1980). The most reliable information comes from two national studies in which thousands of girls were interviewed (Zelnick, Kantner, and Ford, 1981). Among fifteen-year-olds, 19 percent had coital experience, with the rate steadily rising until among unmarried nineteen-year-olds, 60 percent had experienced intercourse, up from 50 percent just five years before.

Although the double standard appears to be waning, the sexual experience of adolescent boys and girls is still fall apart. A boy's first experience is typically with a partner he does not love, and it will be a one-time experience or he will have intercourse with that girl no more than a few times. A girl's first experience is typically with a partner she loves and intends to marry. Boys tend to talk about their experience afterward with others; girls do not (Miller and Simon, 1980).

As boys get older, however, they are less occupied with "scoring" and more interested in an extended relationship. In a study of more than 600 teenagers (Hass, 1979), nearly 23 percent of fifteen- and sixteen-year-old boys wanted to have intercourse on the first or second date (see Table 12.1), compared with 13 percent of seventeen- to eighteen-year-olds. Less than 1 percent of adolescent girls felt this way.

How much this urge to score is the result of peer pressure is uncertain. One boy summed up the pressure he felt by saying:

> Every time I'm out on a date it feels like I have to prove myself. The guys always ask afterwards if you made out, and how far did you go, and did you score? Sometimes it makes me really mad. (Authors' files)

The increase in intercourse does not mean that adolescents are becoming promiscuous. Despite their greater permissiveness, most adolescents insist on a relatively stable and affectionate relationship before having intercourse (Reiss, 1977). A sixteen-year-old boy declared:

> Before I'd do it with some girl I'd want to know her really well. I'd want to respect her and I'd want her to respect me. If you're going to be that close to someone . . . you really want to care for each other. (Bell, 1980, p. 99)

## Table 12.1   *Adolescent sexual partners by age group*

|  |  | PERCENTAGES | |
| --- | --- | --- | --- |
|  | AGE GROUP | BOYS | GIRLS |
| Sexual experience with one partner only | 15–16 | 23 | 41 |
|  | 17–18 | 19 | 52 |
| 1 to 5 partners | 15–16 | 54 | 85 |
|  | 17–18 | 60 | 83 |
| More than 10 partners | 15–16 | 28 | 7 |
|  | 17–18 | 19 | 5 |

*Source:* Adapted from Aaron Hass. 1979. *Teenage Sexuality,* New York: Macmillan, pp. 67–68.

A fifteen-year-old girl agreed, saying:

> Making love means something to me. It means really loving the person you're doing it with and it means not feeling bad that you did it even if the two of you break up. (Bell, 1980, p. 98)

It seems that love has replaced marriage as the major justification for sexual experimentation.

The experience of sexual intercourse during adolescence can have positive or negative effects—or both. On the positive side are the results of several studies, starting with the Kinsey report (Kinsey et al., 1953), which show that premarital sexual experience is linked with a woman's sexual satisfaction during marriage. This relationship makes many young couples unwilling to marry before testing their sexual compatibility. In addition, premarital sex can increase intimacy and strengthen a relationship, whereas abstinence can build tension and frustration. Finally, although young people are dating earlier, they are marrying later; to expect abstinence for so many years may just be unrealistic.

On the negative side is the ever-present possibility of pregnancy. Although effective contraception is easily available, many dating couples use no birth control techniques at all (Zelnick et al., 1981). (In Chapter 19, we'll investigate the circumstances that affect adolescent's use—or nonuse—of contraceptives.) In addition, premarital sex may be a source of psychological strain. Boys may feel pressure to score, and girls may feel mature only if they are sexually active. Finally, young people often feel caught between the conflicting values of parents and peers. By pleasing one group, they risk rejection by the other.

Some authorities (Kinsey et al., 1953) suggest that when an adolescent who believes sex is morally wrong becomes sexually active, the young person risks psychological damage and may find marital adjustment difficult. Whether such psychological conflict arises may depend upon the way an adolescent interprets the experience. In one study (Antonovsky et al., 1978), girls who were sexually active despite their belief that it was wrong were just as likely to feel love, pride, physical satisfaction, or a sense of being grown up as they were to feel guilty, ashamed, or confused.

**Restraints on sexual activity** When students come to college, they bring their emotional baggage along with them. Students who feel guilt or shame about sexual behavior are less likely than others to engage in petting, advanced foreplay, or intercourse, and they also have conservative views about the expression of sexuality within marriage (Mosher and Cross, 1971). Students who experience guilt concerning sex tend to believe that sex is dangerous and to hold a number of myths that can interfere with their later sex lives (Table 12.2). The deeper their guilt, the more myths they believe.

Earlier we saw that religious convictions sometimes lead males to become "technical virgins." Religious female students tend to have more conservative sexual attitudes than their nonreligious counterparts, but at one college, the two groups did not differ in their sexual behavior (Zuckerman et al., 1976).

*Focus*

SEX
ON THE
COLLEGE
CAMPUS

Students enter college after as many as six years' apprenticeship in the dating game. The intention to go to college seems to affect the high school experience of males and females differently. Boys who go on to college progress through the various petting activities to intercourse more slowly than do boys whose education stops at high school. For girls, however, those who go on to college move along toward intercourse more rapidly than girls whose education is over at high school (Clayton and Bokemeier, 1980).

Although the rate of intercourse among college students has risen sharply over the past few decades, it is difficult to pin down. Surveys taken in community colleges, elite private institutions, large state universities, and religious colleges produce quite different pictures of sexual activity.

In the college environment, students are exposed—often for the first time—to issues and influences such as contraception, abortion, sex roles and feminism, homosexual rights, and comprehensive sex education. At the same time, they have increased opportunity to experiment with sexual activities and the pressure

of making sexual decisions. The resulting stress in their social and sexual relationships may overshadow their academic lives. As one student put it:

By the end of my freshman year, I was much more concerned and involved with my sex life than with grades. (Authors' files)

Some of these stresses appeared in small group discussions held as part of a human sexuality course taught by one of the authors at a large university. As students shared their experiences and problems, common themes appeared.

A major issue was contraception. A sophomore told of her humiliation and resentment at the way she was treated when she asked for oral contraceptives from the college health service:

I can't understand why they needed to know how many different sexual partners I had, and the nurse's look when she asked what I wanted made me feel so embarrassed. (Authors' files)

A freshman said that although she was sexually active, she was too frightened by the idea of a gynecological exam to request contraceptives. Another freshman told about the time he went to

a drugstore to purchase condoms—and left with a box of cough drops.

Another issue that concerned the students was homosexuality. One student told about her brother's recent "coming out" and the problems it had created in her family. Another student described his surprise and conflict when his roommate came out as gay:

Mike is still my friend, but I look at him differently now—there are certain things we just can't talk about, and I guess I'm always a bit concerned about how he feels about me. (Authors' files)

Male and female students agreed that the college atmosphere pressured them to increase their sexual experience. One young woman confessed:

I'm afraid to admit that I'm still a virgin, since I assume that I'm the only one left in my dorm. (Authors' files)

Fears of being sexually inadequate—of not reaching orgasm at the "right time," for example, or being unable to have an erection—were also common. Many students admitted that their sexual activity conflicted with their religious views, family upbringing, or romantic notions about love and commitment.

## Table 12.2   Sex myths and college students

While it is very rare, humans can get "hung up" during sexual intercourse as dogs more commonly do.

The more sexually active a person is and the earlier the age at which such activity begins, the sooner sexual life is over in old age.

*When women masturbate, they most commonly insert foreign objects into the vagina.

If a man urinates after sexual intercourse, it does nothing to reduce his chances of contracting some venereal disease.

A person can experience orgasm or ejaculation too often.

*Conception is most likely to occur if the man and woman experience a simultaneous climax.

*Women ejaculate when they experience orgasm.

*Aphrodisiacs ("spanish fly," oysters, etc.) increase sexual desire.

*The man does not determine the sex of the child.

Women never have nocturnal orgasms which accompany erotic dreams.

Most men have had at least one sexual experience with a prostitute.

*Sexual intercourse should be avoided during pregnancy to ensure the health of the infant and mother.

*Significantly more college men than women believed these myths.

*Among students at one university, about a third believed these myths about sex, and men believed more of them than did women. Students with sexual experience believed just as many of the myths as did virgins, which seemed to indicate that some of these students were not learning from their sexual activity—just doing it.

From: D. L. Mosher. "Sex Guilt and Sex Myths in College Men and Women," *Journal of Sex Research,* 15 (1979), 228–229.

Yet among students at one university, the rate of intercourse among students with little religious interest was far higher than the rate among religious students. Nearly half of the religious women and men had experienced genital intercourse, but more than three-fourths of the nonreligious women and nearly all the nonreligious men had such experiences (Mahoney, 1980). Perhaps religiosity—not church attendance—influences sexual behavior. If membership continues to grow in fundamentalist religions across the country, the group of sexually conservative students may increase (Chilman, 1979).

In addition to religious or moral convictions and sex guilt, other factors may be involved in a decision to abstain from intercourse. The absence of a strong relationship as well as fear of pregnancy or sexually transmitted disease can be important. For these students, the notion of a campus sexual revolution can result in uncomfortable pressures and performance demands (King and Sobel, 1975). Students who see their own behavior as neither liberated nor revolutionary may develop uneasy feelings.

**Cohabitation among college students** Sexual standards on today's college campuses are not promiscuous, for that implies multiple sexual partners with minimal emotional involvement. Most college students have liberal attitudes toward sexual behavior—but mostly when the behavior is that of others. Among both men and women, sexual experience is clearly related to an emotional involvement in the context of dating or a steady relationship (King and Sobel, 1975).

**cohabitation** the sharing of living quarters by unmarried heterosexual couples

The increase in campus sexual activity, together with attempts to establish meaningful relationships, has led to a rise in **cohabitation,** or the sharing of living quarters by unmarried students. Contributing to the increase is the availability of effective contraceptives and the tendency for students to live off campus instead of in dormitories (Peterman et al., 1974).

Although it has been suggested by researchers that cohabitation is simply another step in the courtship process, women students who are cohabiting seem to see it differently. On one university campus, cohabiting women tended to have negative views of marriage and of marital roles. In fact, their views of marriage resembled those of men more than those of dating, engaged, or married women (Abernathy, 1981).

The experience of cohabitation seems generally positive. Most students who have been involved in such arrangements say it promoted their own personal growth. But as with any intense relationship, cohabitation can lead to conflict as well as to harmony (Chilman, 1979). Like the experience of sexual intercourse, the effects of living together vary according to individual attitudes and interpretations of the experience.

## PREGNANCY AND CHILDBIRTH

With more adolescent girls sexually active at younger ages, the inevitable result is an increase in pregnancy among teenagers (Figure 12.3). Each year in the United States, 600,000 babies are born to adolescent mothers and another 300,000 are aborted, while 100,000 girls have miscarriages. Nearly a third of all girls who become sexually active are pregnant before their twentieth birthday (Zelnick, Kantner, and Ford, 1981).

Some believe it can never happen to them. A sixteen-year-old who became pregnant recalled saying every night:

"This can't be happening to me. Go away. Leave me alone. I can't handle this.". . . I was so frightened I just thought I'd force my body not to be pregnant. (Bell, 1980, p. 190)

Becoming pregnant is a serious problem for teenagers, one that forces them to make decisions that can change the course of their lives. The first decision concerns abortion. No matter which way young people decide, they often regret their choice. A girl who had an abortion said two years later:

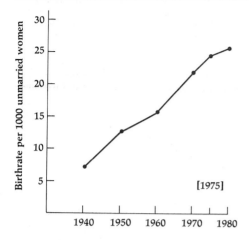

***Figure 12.3 Number of Births per
1000 Unmarried Women Aged 15–19
in the U.S.***

(Statistical Abstract of the United States
1982–1983, U.S. Bureau of the Census [1982])

> I wish I had thought more about my decision to have that abortion. . . . I was
> only fifteen. But I don't think it's right to say that abortion isn't killing just
> because the fetus is too small to live outside the mother. (Bell, 1980, p. 200)

Another couple who married and had their baby were separated within five
years. The young father said:

> It's hard to think about abortion now because I can't wish Luke wasn't here,
> but Becky and I really weren't ready for marriage. (Bell, 1980, p. 208)

If she decides against abortion, a pregnant adolescent faces other choices. She
must decide whether to give up her baby for adoption, to marry her partner, to go
it alone and attempt to support the baby, or to live at home and try, as mother of
an infant, to resume her former life. As we'll see in Chapter 20, the decision to have
a baby does not end the problems.

Adolescent mothers have a death rate 60 percent higher than the rate among
older women (Thorburg, 1979). The baby also faces increased risks. Babies born
to teenage mothers are more likely than other babies to be born too soon, too
small, mentally retarded, or with birth defects (Bolton, 1980). The social and economic risks can be enormous. Among girls who keep their babies, only two out of
every ten marry the father (Bolton, 1980). Whether a girl marries the father of her
child appears to have less effect on her life than whether she drops out of school
(Zelnick, Kantner, and Ford, 1981). Girls who drop out find themselves unem-
ployed or trapped in low-paying jobs and responsible for the physical and emo-

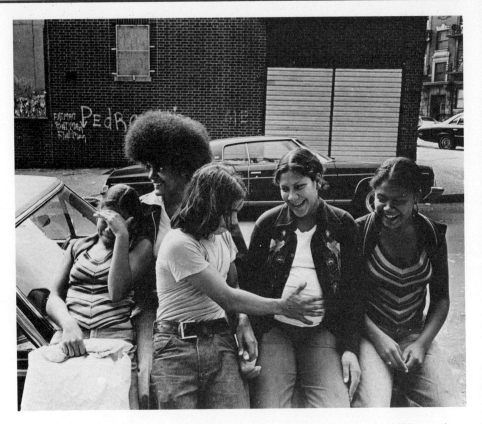

Few of the teenagers who give birth each year are aware of the responsibilities and restrictions that will close in upon them when they assume the care of a baby.
(© Sepp Seitz/Woodfin Camp & Assoc.)

tional care of an infant. Suddenly, the adolescent who had visions of cuddling a sweet-smelling baby who would love her discovers a world of wet diapers, 2 A.M. feedings, sour milk, and colic. Babies born to adolescent mothers also run the greatest risk of child abuse (Field et al., 1980).

One authority (Furstenberg, 1976) believes that the worst thing an adolescent with a baby can do is to try to rear the child by herself. Getting married seems to be slightly better, but still risky. The most advantageous course appears to be staying at home with parents and resuming her education. Adolescent mothers who go back to school generally come out on top psychologically and economically. They are also less likely to have another illegitimate baby. Within two years, 65 percent of the adolescents who stay out of school are pregnant again (Bolton, 1980).

But adolescent pregnancy is not simply a result of losing a gamble. In Denmark and Sweden, two societies that are more sexually permissive than the United States, the rate of adolescent pregnancy is less than half that among American teenagers (Zelnick, Kantner, and Ford, 1981). The problem is that most American teenagers either never use contraceptives at all or use them only "sometimes." Comprehensive sex education is a partial solution, for studies (Zelnick and Kim, 1982) have shown that it seems to reduce the proportion of adolescents who have intercourse without contraceptives.

Even with increased sex education, the wave of adolescent pregnancies is not likely to recede soon. As permissiveness with affection becomes the standard for adolescents, as women insist on making decisions about their own lives, and as single parenthood becomes increasingly accepted among professional women, adolescents will continue to have more babies.

# DECISION MAKING AND SEX EDUCATION

All adolescents are faced with sexual choices, and many of them make their decisions based on misinformation or ignorance. Some adolescents get pregnant because they believe that if a girl doesn't have an orgasm, or if they have intercourse standing up, or if the girl squirts a cola drink into her vagina after intercourse, they don't have to worry.

Responsible sexual decisions require more than knowing about contraceptives. They require knowing the emotional and moral sides of sexuality as well. Today's American adolescents have grown up in a society that has told them by way of advertisements, magazines, films, novels, and television that intercourse is the only real expression of love (Gordon, 1973). When their parental guidance has been limited to "Don't!" or "Sex before marriage is always wrong," they are making decisions on as shaky a basis as the couple who believe that without female orgasm conception can't occur. Some adolescents get confusing signals: "Don't mess around, but if you do, be sure to be careful" (Furstenberg, 1980).

Just how do adolescents find out about sex? Ideally, their information comes from their parents. Indeed, most parents do seem to provide information about fetal growth and birth, but only 15 percent of the mothers and less than 5 percent of the fathers in one large study ever mentioned the connection between intercourse and pregnancy. And only 5 to 10 percent of the parents ever discussed any explicitly sexual behavior or its social consequences (Roberts, Kline, and Gagnon, 1978).

The sort of information provided by parents is most likely to cover topics *children* are interested in: maturation, reproduction, and perhaps intercourse. But *adolescents* want to know about the interpersonal aspects of sex and about the possible consequences of sexuality and their own behavior (Gilbert and Bailis, 1980). These are the topics parents generally avoid. As one sixteen-year-old boy said:

What they told me was too little and too late. (Authors' files)

Like children, teenagers pick up a good deal of their information from friends. Most also get more information from school than from their parents, and learn about as much from books and magazines as they do at home (Davis and Harris, 1982). This may mean that the Playboy Advisor is a major source of sex education and advice for a good many adolescent boys.

Despite the fact that the culture expects the male to have more sexual knowledge than the female, studies show that adolescent girls know a good deal more about all aspects of sex than boys do (Davis and Harris, 1982). The adolescent girls in this study were more likely to be informed about rape and abortion than about ejaculation, erection, or masturbation.

Schools are certainly a better source of information for adolescents than peers, even though many people believe that formal sex education encourages sexual activity among adolescents. Such fears seem groundless. Two extensive national surveys have shown that young people who have courses in sex education are no more likely to have premarital intercourse than young people without such courses. But sex education does affect behavior in one important way: Young people who have had such courses are more likely to use contraceptives (Zelnick and Kim, 1982). As one authority (Gordon, 1973) points out, ignorance of birth control does not prevent adolescents from having sex, and ignorance about sex itself seems highest among those who are most active.

When adolescents make sexual decisions, they balance the various influences on them—parents, peers, the media, their religious attitudes and beliefs, their own needs, and their own standards (Bell, 1980). The more reliable information they have, the more intelligent their decisions are likely to be.

# *Summary*

**1** American teenagers go through a phase called **adolescence** in which they are regarded as sexually mature, but socially and psychologically immature. Adolescence as a phase of life developed in most industrialized societies as economic productivity and affluence enabled society to free young people from farm and factory labor and to support them in school.

**2** The period of early adolescence is known as **puberty**. Its exact trigger is unknown, but it begins when the pituitary produces sex hormones known as **gonadotropins**, which stimulate the gonads to produce androgens or estrogens. As boys and girls go through the adolescent growth spurt they may show **asynchrony**, a state in which different body parts grow at different rates. In girls, the first visible signs of puberty usually appear at about eleven, in the form of the breast bud or pubic hair. Menarche usually takes place at about twelve or thirteen. In boys, the official sign of puberty is generally first ejaculation, or **spermache**, and it usually occurs at about twelve or thirteen. If puberty begins before a girl is eight or a boy is nine years old, the condition is called **precocious puberty**.

**3** A girl may react to menarche with fear, pride, embarrassment, or shame, depending on the way she has been prepared. Most girls find menstruation much less of an ordeal than they had anticipated, although they later become more negative about it, a change that may be due to learning. Boys may react to ejaculation with fear, surprise, or pleasure, depending upon their preparation.

Because girls enter puberty about two years before boys show any signs of sexual maturity, boys and girls appear to live in different worlds during early adolescence. Both boys and girls are insecure about their body changes and must adjust to their new appearance, a task that seems easier for boys than for girls. Anxiety over appearance usually fades by late adolescence.

**4** As young adolescents, boys and girls generally see the world in stereotypical terms. Although gender differences are not as rigid as they once were, sex-role expectations are probably the most powerful force shaping sexual behavior. Masturbation is much more common among adolescent boys than among girls, with teenagers who have experienced intercourse being more likely to masturbate than are virgins. Many young people feel guilty about masturbating, even if they understand that it is normal. The goal of ejaculation and the more frequent use of fantasies distinguish the masturbation of boys from that of girls.

**5** Homosexual experience in adolescent boys is a continuation of childhood sex play. In most cases, adolescent homosexuality is a passing phase, although about 5 percent of boys go on to develop an exclusively homosexual orientation. Homosexual experience is much less common among adolescent girls, although its rate appears to be rising. Lower homosexual activity among girls may be due to sex-role learning, which makes women tend to be relatively passive in sexual situations and unlikely to enter a relationship without an emotional commitment.

**6** The usual role of dating is the formation of heterosexual pair bonds. Dating reflects traditional sex roles. Although some adolescents use dating for relatively impersonal sexual encounters, for most, relationships pass through several stages (casual, steady, pinning, and engagement) before leading to marriage. Despite the new sexual permissiveness, most adolescents seem to follow traditional sex roles, with the male pushing toward intercourse and the female setting limits. Although premarital intercourse is higher among teenagers than ever before, the increase is primarily among girls, who are becoming active at an earlier age. A boy's first experience is typically with a partner he does not love, while a girl's first experience is typically with a partner she loves and intends to marry. The experience of sexual intercourse during adolescence can have positive or negative effects, and the effect may depend on the way the adolescent interprets the experience.

**7** Guilt, shame, religious or moral convictions, the absence of a strong relationship, and the fear of pregnancy or of sexually transmitted disease can restrain young people from sexual intercourse. The increase in sexual activity combined with attempts to establish meaningful relationships has led to a rise in **cohabitation,** or the sharing of living quarters by unmarried heterosexual couples. The experience of cohabitation seems generally positive.

**8** Nearly a third of all girls who become sexually active are pregnant before their twentieth birthday. Pregnancy forces a girl to choose, first, whether to get an abortion. Depending on that decision, she must decide whether to give up her baby for adoption, marry her partner, go it alone, or live at home and try to resume her former life. Both adolescent mothers and their babies face much higher physical risks than when pregnancy occurs after adolescence. The social and economic risks for the pregnant teenager are also great. The greatest negative effect on later life occurs when the adolescent drops out of school. The adolescent who goes back to school does better psychologically and economically, and is less likely to have another illegitimate baby.

**9** Adolescents often have little information on which to base sexual decisions. Adolescent girls appear to be better informed about sex than boys. Although some people believe sex education encourages sexual activity, surveys indicate that it does not and that teenagers who have had such classes are more likely to use contraceptives if they do become sexually active.

*a man's view*

Getting married was the biggest decision of my life. After three years of going together, I felt sure that she was the right person for me. But still I couldn't make up my mind and put off the decision for as long as I could. I can't understand how other people just get married without even thinking about it. (Authors' files)

*a woman's view*

The first few years of my marriage were definitely the hardest. Looking back on it, I don't think we were ready for all the adjustments we had to make. Even though we came close to separating more than once, something kept us together and we stuck it out. Who says marriage is easy? (Authors' files)

# 13 Sexual Development in Adulthood

**THE MARITAL RELATIONSHIP**     *Choosing a mate*     *Marital satisfaction*     *Sex in marriage*     *Keeping sex alive*
FOCUS: SEXUAL SATISFACTION AND A "HAPPY" MARRIAGE
**EXTRAMARITAL SEX**     *Changes in American standards*     *Why people have*

# Chapter 13

As we've seen in earlier chapters, social ceremonies mark the passage into adulthood in some societies. In the United States there is no public "ceremony," only a blurred territory in which adolescence gradually fades as we become independent, choose a vocation, and select a stable sexual partner. Sexual relationships encompass much more than our choice of bed partner. They touch on some of the deepest questions of personal identity, social roles, and interpersonal values. From the nature of sexual relationships and life styles come the greatest rewards and disappointments of human sexuality.

Some authorities believe that the quality of our sexual relationships changes as we become adults. According to Erik Erikson (1980), truly intimate sexual relationships are reserved for adulthood, for in adolescence we are so concerned with establishing a firm sense of personal identity that our sexual relationships necessarily lack the mutual intimacy that can mark the adult sexual relationship.

A major task of adulthood is to develop significant relationships and select a life style. These choices carry enormous consequences for the individual, yet they are choices for which most of us are not prepared and which we often make with little reflection. The decision to marry, for example, drastically shapes our future, but a marriage license is much easier to get than a driver's license, which at least requires some demonstration of proficiency.

Sexual relationships and life styles are extremely sensitive to cultural variation. Because American society endorses sexual relationships based on love, more Americans marry for love than for any other reason. As we saw in Chapter 2, many cultures regard love as having

*affairs*    *Incorporating the affair into marriage*    *Swinging and group marriage*
ALTERNATIVE LIFE STYLES    *The single life*    *Celibacy*    *Divorce and remarriage*
SEX AND AGING    *Myths about aging*    *Physiological changes with aging*    *Sexual behavior and aging*

# Sexual Development in Adulthood

little to do with mate selection: The family, children, economic considerations, or social needs dictate the choice of a partner. Some societies insist on monogamy, others favor polygyny; some demand strict marital fidelity, others support and encourage extramarital relationships; some forbid homosexuality, others allow its open practice.

Since the overwhelming majority of Americans marry at some time in their lives, we'll begin this chapter by considering marriage, the basic sexual life style in the United States. We'll also look at such variations as extramarital sex, swinging, and group marriage. Next we'll examine some other options: celibacy, staying single, divorce. We'll close with an exploration of sexuality in later adulthood and consider the effect of aging on sexual expression.

## THE MARITAL RELATIONSHIP

Getting married is considered a major milestone of adult life in American society. When this century began, marriage marked the transition to independent adulthood, for it was at this time that the young first left their parents' home. Today young people often move out and establish independent lives without first marrying, but most people still regard marriage as signaling the assumption of responsible adulthood. As one woman said:

I felt the time had come to settle down. Making a commitment scared me, but I knew I was ready for it and the time was right. (Authors' files)

Critics have charged that marriage is a sterile and growth-inhibiting relationship, but it remains the preferred and most desirable life style. More than 90 percent of Americans marry at some time, and 96 percent of them believe marriage is the ideal way of life (Yankelovich, 1981). This belief that life's greatest satisfactions are to be found in marriage has not prevented a rise in divorce rates and an escalation in the number of people who live alone. Perhaps the disparity between the ideal and the reality has something to do with our expectations about marriage and sex.

## Choosing a mate

Traditional marriage had four basic functions: It provided economic security; it ensured reproduction of a family line; it provided for psychological security and a place in society; and it socialized children. When Americans demanded that it also provide romantic love, personal growth, and self-fulfillment for both partners, they made it more difficult to select the right mate and placed new emotional demands on the institution (Laws and Schwartz, 1977).

Today we tend to assume that each person decides for him- or herself just whom to marry—or whether to marry at all. The idea of having a mate chosen for us seems distasteful. But in many societies today and not long ago in the United States, the parents did most of the choosing. When marriage plays an important economic or social role in a society, marriages are often arranged by families. The partners' inclinations have little bearing on the final choice.

Parents are, of course, free to influence their children's mate selection, and many do. In some families, parents still have a veto, and although they cannot tell a child whom to marry, they can reject a mate as clearly unsuitable. Parental influence is likely to be strongest if children stray across ethnic or socioeconomic boundaries or if they are fairly young. The older a child, the less influence a parent is likely to have on the choice (Gagnon and Greenblatt, 1978).

The "right" time for marriage seems to change with changing social conditions. In the United States, the "right age" has been getting older for the past two decades. In 1960, 53 percent of American men and 28 percent of American women between the ages of 20 and 24 were single (Figure 13.1); by 1980, these percentages had increased to 69 percent for men and 50 percent for women (U.S. Bureau of the Census, 1981).

Several factors have probably had a major influence on the trend toward delayed marriage. Cohabitation has reduced the pressure to marry, since couples can experiment with shared living quarters in order to test their personal as well as their sexual compatibility. Because of effective contraceptives and safe abortion, couples are also less likely to marry in order to legitimize a baby. Finally, the emphasis on careers for women has led many young women to postpone marriage until they have completed their education and established themselves.

When they finally select a mate, few men or women make the choice on the basis of sexual compatibility alone. Although many couples are sexually active be-

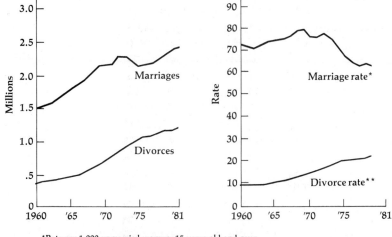

**Figure 13.1
Marriages and
Divorces:
1960–1988.**

While the total number of marriages and divorces have gone up since 1960, the average rate of marriage for persons fifteen and over has declined slightly. (Statistical Abstract of the United States 1982–1983, U.S. Bureau of the Census [1982])

fore marriage, other factors usually govern the decision to marry. One man explained:

> I got married for the most part because I was in love, partly because I wanted companionship, partly because most of my friends and acquaintances were married and it seemed the "normal" thing to do . . . and partly, I suppose, because I needed a regular sexual outlet. (Hite, 1981, p. 215)

Love, companionship, social conformity, and sexual opportunity made this man decide to marry. But what made him fall in love? Studies have consistently shown that men and women tend to choose people who are like themselves in education, intelligence, and attractiveness. They also tend to marry individuals who are about their own age and socioeconomic level and who live near them. At one time, similarity of ethnic background, race, and religion were also powerful elements in mate selection. Although still strong, these factors are less important than they once were (Murstein, 1980).

The postponement of marriage, together with the increase in sexual freedom, could have a positive effect on the quality of marriage. As more people remain single or decide to cohabit, the result could be more satisfying marriages. When neither marriage nor childbearing is seen as required, more people may marry only when they both "like" and "love" their partners.

## Marital satisfaction

Watching marriages collapse about them, some people have begun to question the belief that marriage can meet social, sexual, and personal needs. The expectation that marriage will provide lifelong intimacy, security, excitement, and stability seems an impossible dream.

It may be that the higher the expectations, the lower the marital satisfaction. A person's satisfaction may be determined by the comparison of the expectations with which the marriage began and the actual outcome. But a gulf between the two does not necessarily predict divorce. The stability of a marriage depends on the partner's comparison of his or her own marriage with the best available alternative. If nothing better seems possible, people may stick with a marriage that provides little satisfaction (Spanier and Lewis, 1980).

Once married, both partners find that their freedom is reduced, that their financial situation has changed, and that their partner has personality characteristics which either went unnoticed or were soft-pedaled during courtship. The way wife and husband adjust to this new situation has an important influence on marital satisfaction.

Another important influence on the quality of a marriage is children. When the first child is born, marital satisfaction often drops sharply, especially among women (Spanier and Lewis, 1980). Couples whose marriage is primarily based on "loving" may feel the strain more than couples whose marriage is based on "liking" (Belsky, 1981).

One reason for the drop in satisfaction following the birth of a child may be the decrease in communication that commonly occurs. Husband and wife talk less, which means that the couple's feeling of intimacy may diminish. When a couple can communicate openly about all aspects of marriage, satisfaction is more likely to remain high (Calderone and Johnson, 1981). The public seems to have become aware of this fact. Asked about a "perfect lover," the majority of people in one national survey chose "someone to be totally open and honest with"—twice as many as chose "someone who is sexually exciting" (Yankelovich, 1981).

Some authorities believe marital satisfaction depends heavily on the way a couple handles decision making (Scanzoni and Szinovacz, 1980). When couples share a high level of empathy and trust, and each feels the other is cooperative and fair, sharp differences over educational plans, occupational goals, and decisions to have children can be made in a way that strengthens the marriage. Partners become willing to compromise and can reach a consensus both find comfortable.

As sex roles have become less traditional, the process of decision making has become an even more important factor in marital satisfaction. When sex roles were rigid, men made all the decisions and tradition dictated the division of work. Now that sex roles are more flexible, couples share decisions as well as responsibilities. When both partners adapt to changing sex roles, they may find that the greater flexibility is an advantage, since it allows wives to pursue career goals and husbands to be more involved in rearing children. As one woman said:

> Our relationship has changed a lot in the seven years we've been married. Things are much more equal between us today and we're trying to share in all the responsibilities of the marriage. I especially appreciate his involvement in raising our two children. (Authors' files)

Indeed, many couples do have happy marriages. When couples who considered themselves happily married were surveyed, women of all ages said that emotional security and intimacy were extremely important factors in their marital

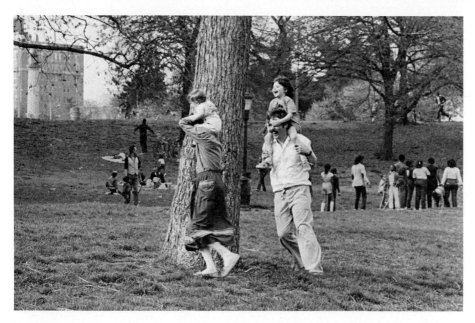

The birth of children affects a marriage, sometimes increasing the pleasure of the relationship and sometimes decreasing the level of marital satisfaction. (© Hazel Hankin 1983)

satisfaction, while men of all ages valued loyalty and a commitment to the future of the relationship (Reedy, Birren, and Schaie, 1981). Among the young happily married couples, ability to communicate openly and honestly and to express their sexual feelings freely were vital to marital satisfaction.

## *Sex in marriage*

During the nineteenth century, when reproduction and not pleasure was the goal of sexual activity, married couples were expected to limit the frequency of their "sexual indulgence." A marriage manual published at midcentury advised couples to have intercourse no more than once each month (Alcott, 1866). Since women were not expected to enjoy intercourse, the notion that they were capable of orgasm was considered improper. In the twentieth century, ideas about marital sexuality changed. Female orgasm was recognized and came to be seen as an important part of marital satisfaction. Standards went up. Instead of being permitted to enjoy their orgasms, couples felt obligated to join the quest for the elusive **simultaneous orgasm,** in which husband and wife reached orgasm at the same moment. Before long, with the discovery of the multiple orgasm in females, women were made to feel inadequate if they stopped with only one. Couples were told that sex should be varied, creative, and frequent throughout marriage.

    Faced with rising expectations, many couples may have become disappointed

**simultaneous orgasm** an orgasm in which both partners climax at the same time

with sex lives that do not meet these standards. The numerous books, magazine articles, and television programs dealing with sexual problems, together with the spread of sex therapy clinics across the country, might lead us to conclude that marital sexuality is in serious trouble in the United States. This appears to be the conclusion of William Masters and Virginia Johnson (1970), who have estimated that as many as half of all marriages have some kind of sexual problem. But this conclusion may be wrong. Perhaps we are not beset with new sexual problems; perhaps we are simply more willing to discuss our problems openly and to seek help for them.

As we saw in Chapter 8, American couples are having sex more effectively, using a greater variety of foreplay and intercourse techniques, than the generation interviewed by Kinsey. Some people clearly are enjoying marital sex, and this married man may be typical of them:

> Sex with the same partner is beautiful. We each know what the other likes. Communication during sex is usually only a touch of the hand. It's great.
> (Hite, 1981, p. 206)

Although recent surveys may be slanted by replies from more sexually open-minded people, some aspects of marriage have shown little change in the past few decades. Among Kinsey's males, for example, the frequency of marital coitus among married men under thirty remained steady across the generations, dropping from about four times a week among married men under twenty to just over 2½ times a week among married men in their late twenties. Date of birth had no effect on these rates (Downey, 1980).

Recent surveys show similar results: The frequency of marital coitus declines with age, and the average rate among married couples in their late twenties is about what Kinsey found—2½ times per week. The factors that affect premarital intercourse—social class, education, and religion—seem to have little effect on married couples. Whether rich or poor, highly educated or not, religious or nonreligious, the decline with age and the average rate of intercourse remain constant (Gagnon and Greenblatt, 1978).

Religion does appear to affect marital sex in one way. Religious women seem to be more satisfied with their sex lives than nonreligious women. Since their rates of intercourse are about the same, it may be that religious women demand less from marital sex and hence are not faced with unfulfilled demands (Tavris and Sadd, 1977).

When a group of young married couples were followed over a four-year period, the initial rate of 2½ times per week dropped to twice a week for most couples. Individual differences were quite apparent, and not all couples showed similar declines. A third of the couples reported an increase in intercourse during the four-year period, and about a tenth reported no change at all. Rates of intercourse climbed among couples when they used effective contraception, wanted no more children, and the wife did not work outside the home (Udry, 1980).

Perhaps the greatest problem most couples face is how to avoid turning marital sex into a dull routine. Among people who find the excitement of sex primarily

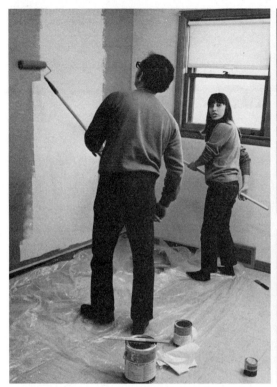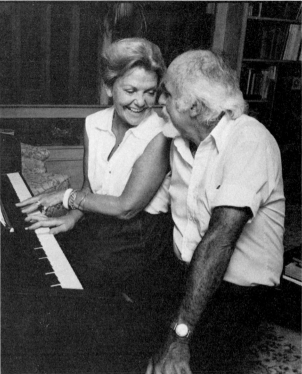

Whether sex within marriage remains "beautiful" or becomes dull or disappointing may depend upon a couple's expectations, fears, family and career concerns, and their response to aging. (© Suzanne Szasz/Photo Researchers, Inc.)

in the chase and conquest, marital sex will inevitably become boring (Bernard, 1975). If most married couples have intercourse about twice a week, then after a decade of marriage, they have had a thousand sexual encounters with the same person—a repetitive experience that some might find dull.

Boredom is not the only problem married lovers face. Other factors associated with marriage also work to lessen the frequency of intercourse. Sexual activity may be given a low priority when it competes with the demands of pregnancy, child-rearing, home care, career concerns, and financial pressures. In addition, aging in a youth-oriented culture leads to a decline in perceived physical attractiveness.

Some people may get tired of negotiating sexual encounters. Fearing rejection, they wait for the partner to make a move or else routinize sex by setting aside a specific time each week for it. When sex is a Saturday night ritual the rate of intercourse drops, but neither partner has to worry about a rebuff.

Among women and men who hold nineteenth-century views of sex—and they have not vanished—intercourse is primarily procreative. When either partner is sterilized or the wife reaches menopause, they lose interest in sex. If their views define mothers as "nonsexual," the arrival of children may be enough to cool sexual interest. As one man said:

> After the kids were born I couldn't relate to my wife sexually. She was a good wife and mother, but I began to look for sex outside the marriage. (Authors' files)

### Keeping sex alive

The boredom that sometimes plagues marriages and lengthy cohabitations can often be dispelled by putting the same sort of time and attention into the relationship that we apply to our jobs, our hobbies, and our community activities. If you feel that the magic is going out of a long-standing sexual relationship, following these suggestions may restore your interest.

Keep the lines of communication open between you and your partner, perhaps using some of the techniques described in Chapter 10. The problems that affect the frequency or enjoyment of marital sex often respond to communication. Among one group of young, educated married women, 80 percent of those who described their sexual relationships as "good" or "excellent" said they could talk openly with their partners about sex. And women who could assert their rights and talk about their feelings when arguing with their partners tended to have good or excellent sex lives. Women who withdrew emotionally after an argument were generally dissatisfied with their sex lives (Sarrel and Sarrel, 1980).

Remember that when you first began dating, you set aside time for each other that was free from the pressures of work, school, or home. The same kind of care and attention to a long-standing relationship sometimes revitalizes sexual interaction. You may find that you and your partner have almost no private time together and that your sexual activity is limited to brief encounters late at night, when you are both tired. You may bring back excitement to your relationship, suggests Lonnie Barbach (1982), if you and your partner will set aside regular periods of at least an hour once or twice each week when you can be together. The time can be devoted to sexual encounter or to some other intimate activity. The important thing is to get away from telephones, family responsibilities, and household or business chores. One couple found that such a policy succeeded in keeping their feelings alive:

*Case*  Harold and Mimi would schedule a date every week to counteract their busy lives. They would write the appointment into their appointment books and consider it as sacred as any of their other meetings. On this special evening they would hire a babysitter or take the children to their grandparents. Then, after a romantic dinner together, they would return home, build a fire, drink some cognac, and often make love in front of the fireplace. They looked forward to this weekly ritual and felt that it was, in large part, responsible for their close, loving relationship. (Barbach, 1982, p. 265)

You might add spice to your relationship by using massage or sharing a shower or bubble bath before you make love. You might take a page out of Harold and Mimi's book and hire a babysitter, then go off to a local motel for an afternoon, an evening, or a weekend.

Look at sexual activity with the same partner as an opportunity to practice various sexual techniques, to try new positions, and to adjust to each other's sexual needs and rhythms. You may find that increased proficiency in sexual stimulation and orgasmic ability compensates for the lack of novelty. As your sexual relationship becomes more comfortable and relaxed, you and your partner may be more willing to experiment with the sharing of sexual fantasies—perhaps even acting them out (Gagnon, Rosen, and Leiblum, 1982).

Finally, some couples have found that an extramarital sexual experience by either wife or husband has heightened the quality of the sexual relationship within marriage. As we'll soon see, however, this strategy can also create major risks for the marriage.

# EXTRAMARITAL SEX

Most of us marry without any intention of engaging in extramarital sex, but a sharp conflict exists between our attitudes and practices. An overwhelming majority of Americans disapprove of extramarital sex, yet many of those who voice their disapproval practice it (Sprenkle and Weiss, 1978).

Adultery is regarded as a primary legal justification for divorce. Opposition comes not only from the Judeo-Christian religious tradition, but also from a view of marriage as a form of property rights. Sexual infidelity is seen as a violation of ownership. Other disapproval is grounded in a view of adultery as a violation of a deep personal commitment. Indeed, the words we use to describe extramarital sex—"cheating," "unfaithfulness," "adultery"—are all pejorative terms.

Not all cultures share these attitudes. When adultery is tolerated, however, it is usually the man who is permitted additional sexual partners. Among 139 tribal societies, a solid majority restricted the extramarital liaisons of women, but tended to accept male activity. In some societies that officially disapproved of extramarital sex, the practice was punished only when the participants were indiscreet. In other societies, the custom of "wife lending" was socially regulated and approved. For example, when traveling, Chukchee men of Siberia arrange a sexual liaison with their host's mate in each of the communities they visit. In return, the hosts are given the same privilege when they visit the traveler's community (Ford and Beach, 1951).

Less common are tribes that permit a woman several lovers. One society that does, the Toda of India, has no word for adultery. Among the Bena of Africa, when

## *Focus*

SEXUAL
SATISFACTION
AND A
"HAPPY"
MARRIAGE

If the experiences of a hundred Pennsylvania couples are typical of American marriage, happiness in marriage depends more on the emotional tone of the relationship than on peak performance in the bedroom. The sex lives of these couples fell far short of the idealized American standard, yet 83 percent of the wives and husbands described their marriages as "happy" or "very happy." Given a chance to relive their lives, about 90 percent of them would marry the same person again (Frank, Anderson, and Rubinstein, 1978).

Nearly a third of these couples were having sex two to three times a week, with about a quarter having sex once a week, and another quarter two to three times a month. Although most of the couples found their own sex lives "satisfying" or "very satisfying," more than a third of the men complained of premature ejaculation, and nearly half the women found it difficult to reach orgasm—with about one woman in seven being unable to have an orgasm at all.

These problems were less likely to detract from sexual satisfaction than were minor "difficulties," such as too little foreplay, disinterest, or having sex at an inconvenient time. What's more, awareness of a spouse's problem or difficulty was more likely to affect the degree of sexual satisfaction than a problem of one's own.

Wives had more sexual complaints than husbands. Nearly half the women found it difficult to become aroused, and about a third found it difficult to stay that way. Women tended to complain of disinterest in sex, of being "turned off," of an inability to relax, of sex at inconvenient times, of too little foreplay, and too little tenderness afterward. In short, their traditional complaints sounded as if the sexual revolution had passed them by, except for the one woman in ten who said she "reached orgasm too quickly." Husbands consistently underestimated their wives' complaints, following the hallowed but dubious American assumption that everything's fine as long as the wife doesn't complain or withhold sex.

Men had few complaints besides premature ejaculation. Not many had trouble getting or maintaining an erection. Minor male difficulties included too little foreplay and serious attraction to another woman.

Only a few of these problems were strongly connected to sexual dissatisfaction. Among the women, difficulty in arousal, disinterest, and being "turned off" were the most devastating complaints. Such difficulties probably reflected interpersonal problems to which both husband and wife contribute—problems that can spill over into the sexual area. Among the men, disinterest and a disparity between sexual practices of husband and wife led to their dissatisfaction.

The experiences of these couples indicate that not sexual performance, but the way a couple perceives the relationship, is the primary influence on satisfaction in marriage. As partners live together, they apparently learn to adapt to their sexual incompatibilities. Couples can enjoy sex even when their own or their partner's performance does not measure up to some idealized standard. When partners do not adapt, one partner—or both—may become involved in extramarital sex.

extramarital affairs are discovered, the only censure is a brief outburst of temper from the aggrieved husband or wife.

## Changes in American standards

The double standard that characterized the late nineteenth century in England and the United States resembles the standard of those tribal societies that accept male infidelity but forbid women to stray. Although marriage and the family were held in high regard, a man with money or power often kept a mistress or patronized prostitutes. But adultery by a married woman was severely condemned.

The legacy of the Victorian double standard lasted far into the twentieth century. At midcentury, Kinsey discovered that about half of American men had experienced an extramarital relationship by the time they were forty years old, but that only about a quarter of the women had done so. And when a spouse's activity was discovered, the double standard prevailed. Men were twice as likely as women to cite a spouse's extramarital activities as a prime factor in divorce.

A good deal of change has taken place since Kinsey's time. The shift toward more tolerant sexual attitudes and the increased attention being paid to extramarital sex have been accompanied by two major shifts: The first extramarital encounter is occurring at a younger age, and among middle-class, educated women the rate of extramarital sex is approaching the level found among men (Macklin, 1980).

In a recent survey (Petersen et al., 1983) by *Playboy* magazine of its middle-class readers, 48 percent of the men and 38 percent of the women said they had had at least one extramarital affair. Among couples in their twenties, however, the women were significantly more likely than the men to have had an affair. Although *Playboy* readers—especially the women—probably don't resemble the general population, the social trend is quite apparent: among readers over fifty, about 70 percent of the men but just over 30 percent of the women had had affairs.

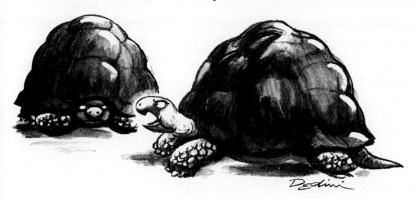

*"All right, I was unfaithful. But, damn it, that was over <u>one</u> <u>hundred</u> <u>years</u> ago!"*

Not everyone who is attracted by the idea of extramarital sex actually takes a lover. It is one thing for people to discuss the topic openly and quite another to risk endangering a marriage. When people are asked why they are *not* engaging in extramarital sex, they are much less likely to give legal or religious reasons than they are to say that such behavior would threaten their marriage (Hunt, 1974). A married woman expressed her feelings this way:

> I can't say that I haven't been tempted. I've often thought of having an affair, but I'm afraid of what it would do to my marriage. It just doesn't seem worth it. (Authors' files)

A married man echoed her sentiments:

> I've often fantasized about having an affair, but that's as far as it goes. My marriage means too much to me to take that kind of a risk. (Authors' files)

This dangerous aspect of extramarital sex is generally taken for granted. In novels and films, the affair is typically a highly secret activity involving elaborate deception and certain to lead to divorce. Sometimes this stereotype is accurate, but often it is not. The extramarital script can be developed in many ways, depending on such factors as whether the spouse knows about the relationship, the quality of the marriage, and whether one or both partners have lovers (Sprenkle and Weiss, 1978).

## Why people have affairs

Marital dissatisfaction is often the motive for extramarital sex, but not always. The motives behind such behavior are almost endless. Among the common ones are an interest in varied sexual experience, pressure from a friend or spouse, status seeking, a need for greater independence, and a desire to punish the spouse.

People who begin an affair motivated by a desire for greater sexual satisfaction often find an extramarital affair something of a disappointment. Among one group of women with extramarital experience, 35 percent failed to have orgasm with their lovers, as compared with only 7 percent who failed most of the time with their husbands (Hunt, 1974).

But orgasm is only one aspect of sexual satisfaction; extramarital sex may give some people a renewed sense of personal desirability, the illusion of recaptured youth, or the rediscovery of passion. The guilt that often accompanies extramarital activity can also be exciting—until the liaison is discovered. For others, the game may not be worth the trouble. Guilt and the nagging fear of discovery can be a heavy burden.

## Incorporating the affair into marriage

Although extramarital relationships can disrupt a marriage, many experts have begun to argue that such relationships can sometimes benefit the individuals involved and their marriage. When extramarital affairs are beneficial, they are generally part of an **open marriage**, in which husband and wife agree that each is free to form outside sexual liaisons. In such arrangements, fidelity shifts from sexual faithfulness to placing the partner first in an open, egalitarian relationship (Macklin, 1980). Behind the concept of open marriage is the premise that life has become so complex that one person can no longer satisfy all a partner's needs (Francoeur and Francoeur, 1977).

A former president of the American Association of Marriage Counselors, Gerhard Neubeck (1969), believes that since it is natural for married people to be attracted to outside relationships, it is possible to negotiate acceptable ground rules for extramarital affairs. When such affairs are covered by the rules governing a marriage, they are known as **consensual** or **comarital relationships**. But such relationships can be successful only when there is a high degree of mutual affection, respect, and understanding in a marriage; when the partners have a high degree of interpersonal skill and the ability to handle potentially stressful relationships; and when the comarital partner does not try to compete with the marital partner for primacy (Macklin, 1980).

Despite such relatively positive testimony, extramarital affairs sometimes have strongly negative effects. As one man reported:

> The extramarital activity on both sides hurt us both a lot, and eventually created an atmosphere of hurt so deep-seated that the relationship was impossible, in spite of the love which persisted. It was always complicated and very painful. (Hite, 1981, p. 194)

When couples view sexual infidelity as the ultimate transgression—a view that is extremely common in the United States—the discovery that a spouse has had an affair can end all marital trust and intimacy. Although comarital arrangements can help to end guilt and the fear of discovery, few couples are emotionally attuned to a frank airing of the topic. Most discussions of extramarital liaisons stimulate jealousy and possessiveness, not cooperation and openness. American religious, moral, and legal traditions all strongly support sexual monogamy—an ideal that has a major influence on our *attitudes* toward extramarital sex, but a minor impact on our *behavior*. All too often, it is the gap between what we think and what we do that causes marital distress.

## Swinging and group marriage

A number of couples have attempted to eliminate the hurt involved in extramarital affairs by experimenting with unconventional forms of marital sexuality, such as swinging and group marriage. For some, these activities are one-time events or occasional sexual adventures; for others, they become a new way of life.

**Swinging** Sexual novelties and fads receive a great deal of publicity: Newspapers carry advertisements for "like-minded couples," and certain clubs and hotels cater to **swingers**, or those interested in group sex. No one knows just how many people are involved in such activities, but it has been estimated that 2 percent of

**open marriage** a marriage in which husband and wife agree that each is free to form outside sexual liaisons, so that fidelity shifts from faithfulness to placing the partner first

**comarital relationship** an extramarital relationship that is allowed under the marriage rules established by both partners

**swinger** person who engages in group sex

married couples have experienced this sort of mate-swapping at some time (Hunt, 1974), and that about 75 percent of those who try it drop out within a year (Murstein, 1978). In the recent survey of *Playboy* readers (Petersen et al., 1983), about a third of the men and women said they had engaged in public sex at least once; however, in a study of swingers, 99 percent of the men were *Playboy* readers (Bartel, 1974). The majority of swingers belong to a conventional, middle-class segment of society, and many are professionals.

When 200 actively swinging California couples were compared with nonswinging couples like themselves in age, education, and socioeconomic level, a number of differences appeared (Gilmartin, 1977). Swingers had less happy childhoods, more distant relationships with their parents, and a greater incidence of separated or divorced parents than nonswingers. Although the religious and political affiliations of the two groups were similar, the swingers were less active in organized religion and politics. In general, the swingers had begun dating at an earlier age, had gone steady with more partners before marriage, and had married earlier than nonswingers. They also had their first intercourse at an earlier age and had had more premarital experience.

Swingers said they were more satisfied with their marriages than were nonswingers. They also reported less boredom with marriage and more frequent sexual relations with their spouses. Most couples began swinging when the husband discovered literature about the practice and persuaded the wife to become involved.

Swinging appears to have both positive and negative effects on a marriage. Among the positive effects are increased sexual interest in the spouse, increased sexual excitement, a shedding of sexual inhibitions, and shared interests. Among the negative effects of swinging are the inability of swingers to live up to their sexual illusions about themselves, sexual jealousy, and personal jealousy of the partner's popularity. As one man said:

> My wife and I tried swinging sex with other couples. The effect on me was that I liked it. My wife, on the other hand, says she didn't like it. . . . She is strictly a one-man woman she says. Swinging almost separated us. (Hite, 1981, p. 198)

Couples who stop swinging appear to do so because of the generally impersonal nature of the swinging scene (Bartel, 1974). One of the swinger's rules is to avoid any personal involvement with other swingers, and most swingers see other couples only once. Swinging thus leads to maximum sexual involvement with minimal personal involvement, a situation that can greatly reduce sexual satisfaction.

**group marriage**
marriage in which three or more partners each considers him- or herself married to more than one of the other partners

**Group marriage** A radical American expression of sexual liberation is **group marriage**, in which three or more partners each considers him- or herself married to more than one of the other partners (Constantine and Constantine, 1977). Experiments in group living have marked American history, and they are usually founded as an idealistic attempt to replace the nuclear family. In the nineteenth century, the Oneida Community, set up by John Humphrey Noyes in Oneida, New York, practiced group marriage for thirty years. Public disapproval finally forced it to disband. In the 1960s and early 1970s, thousands of communes, which practiced various forms of group marriage, mushroomed and then died out.

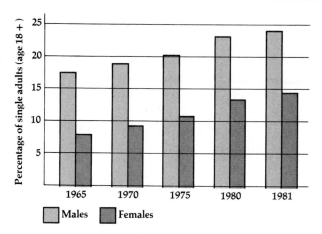

**Figure 13.2   Singles: Percentage of the Population, Aged 18 and Over.**

The average number of males and females who remain single has increased steadily from 1965 to the present. (Statistical Abstract of the United States, 1982–1983 U.S. Bureau of the Census [1982])

The average group marriage consists of four or more adults and their children. The marriage partners tend to be relatively young, highly educated, and liberal. They feel a need for independence and change, lack guilt, and seem not to need order (Macklin, 1980).

An extensive study of group marriages found that sex was an important determinant in both the formation and the collapse of a group marriage, but that it was not the crucial factor (Constantine and Constantine, 1977). Jealousy was a problem in group marriages, and most groups devised strategies to control the pairing of partners. For example, in one group women controlled the sleeping arrangements one month and men controlled them the next.

Most group marriages break up quickly, with personality conflicts and problems of communication contributing to the split. The monogamous marriages contracted before the establishment of the group marriage generally endure.

## ALTERNATIVE LIFE STYLES

Despite the popularity of the institution, not everyone marries (Figure 13.2), and not everyone who marries remains wed. Some people incorporate sex into a single life, some choose celibacy, and some divorce and remarry or return to a single life style.

## *The single life*

The single life has become increasingly attractive. In only ten years, the number of singles more than doubled; by 1980, nearly 18 million American adults were living alone (Wolfe, 1982). At one time it was difficult to stay single. Since American society revolved around marriage and the family, the unwed were seen as deviants who threatened the natural order. Today, however, it is easier. In 1957, 80 percent of Americans believed that women who remained unmarried must be "sick," "neurotic," or "immoral"; by 1978, only 25 percent felt that way (Yankelovich, 1981).

Society has made it easier to be single in other ways as well. Frozen foods, clothes that don't need ironing, and improved transportation have made survival simpler for the lone adult. Jobs have made women financially independent, freeing them from the need to depend on a husband or family. As one woman said:

> Living alone is the only way for me. After fourteen years of living my life for everyone else, I finally discovered the joy and freedom of being single. There's no way in the world I'd think of getting married again. (Authors' files)

People who have chosen the single life point out its advantages: personal freedom, career opportunities, sexual availability and diversity, and a chance for self-improvement. These qualities, they feel, outweigh the economic, emotional, and sexual security of marriage (Stein, 1975).

Living alone does not mean being lonely. Many single individuals have one or more intimate relationships. Studies have found no difference in the physical or mental health of people who live alone and those who live with others (Rubenstein, Shaver, and Peplau, 1979). As a long-term option, however, being single seems to agree better with women than with men. Single women have more education, higher incomes, and better mental health than single men (Macklin, 1980). One single man who *was* lonely said:

> I don't much care for being single. You have all the privacy you could want and not many ties and responsibilities but it's very lonely, no one to share sadness and joys with. I would like to be married eventually. (Hite, 1981, p. 256)

Although single women may be better off than single men, they are likely to have a more difficult time finding sexual partners. Women have been socialized to expect sex in a context of love and to be "courted" by men. The aggressive pursuit of sexual partners is often difficult for them, and as the bloom of youth fades, they cannot compete in the singles bars, where physical attractiveness is usually the only criterion (Laws and Schwartz, 1977).

Perhaps for these reasons, most single women live with another person at some time in their lives, either cohabiting in a heterosexual or homosexual relationship or simply sharing a residence. As single life has become more popular, the number of heterosexual cohabiting couples has increased sharply. One estimate puts the number of unmarried people sharing living quarters with someone of the other sex at 2.7 million. In most cases cohabitation does not seem to be replacing marriage, merely delaying it, for more than 90 percent of young adult cohabitants say they plan to marry some day (Macklin, 1980).

# Celibacy

A possible choice for men and women who don't choose to marry is **celibacy**, or the abstention from sexual activity, a broad term that applies to a number of situations. Sometimes the abstinence lasts for a lifetime; for others, it is limited to a particular period of life. Celibacy can be voluntary or involuntary. The abstinence may be total, as when masturbation and fantasy as well as interpersonal activity are foregone, or partial, as in the case of a man or woman who masturbates but does not have any sexual partners.

**celibacy** abstention from sexual activity

Lifelong celibacy is typically chosen on the basis of strong moral or religious conviction. Admission to the Roman Catholic priesthood, for instance, entails a commitment to celibacy. Other religious groups consider physical purity to be necessary if one is ever to attain spiritual purity. One practicing nun described her celibacy as:

> A grace enabling me more easily to devote my entire being to God with an undivided heart, viewing life from a sacred perspective, as a means of growing in love and perceiving truth. (DeLora and Warren, 1977, pp. 300–301)

In recent years, celibacy has also become a fad. According to one psychologist (Brown, 1980), in a new form of celibacy practiced by some people, abstinence from sex is used to achieve higher levels of interpersonal or spiritual functioning. There is as yet no evidence as to the number of people who voluntarily choose such celibacy for nonreligious reasons. For some, lifelong celibacy is involuntary. Men and women who cannot find sexual partners or those who are limited by physical or mental disability may be forced to live celibate lives.

Temporary abstinence may be chosen for any of several reasons. Three common motivations today are health, feminist politics, and necessity (Laws and Schwartz, 1977). Health can be seen as the motive among individuals who have suffered from sexually transmitted diseases or who fear that they may contract one. In such cases, sexual abstinence may cover a brief period or several years.

Feminist politics can be a motive, for some radical and politically committed feminists believe that all male-female relationships are intrinsically oppressive and demeaning to women. Although a lesbian life style permits women with these beliefs to remain sexually active, many radical feminists are not able to accept same-sex relationships and become celibate.

At times poor physical health or the demands of work or family may require sexual abstinence. A woman whose pregnancy might be threatened by sexual activity may temporarily abstain from sexual activity. A person who is going through a difficult period of life may find abstention easier than coping with sexual relationships. A period of intense emotional or career stress may also cause a person temporarily to lose interest in sex and to become either partially or totally celibate.

Sexual appetite is very different from other appetites, such as hunger and thirst, for human beings can do without sex for most or all of their lives without endangering their survival. Celibacy presents no physical risks, although it may be linked to social or emotional problems. The contention of some spiritual authorities that abstinence enhances physical health and vitality has so far not been substantiated by scientific support.

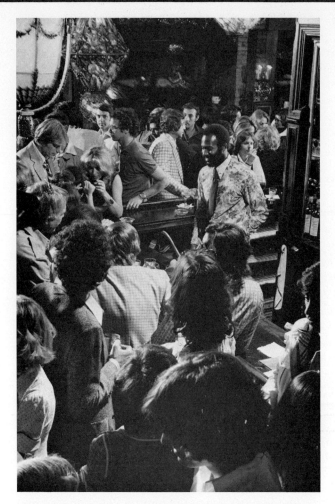

As the number of single adults has increased, places like singles bars, where unattached men and women can meet, have opened in every city. (© Burt Glinn/Magnum)

## Divorce and remarriage

Divorce has become so common that 60 percent of Americans believe people who get married today do not expect the marriage to last the rest of their lives (Yankelovich, 1981). The belief is grounded in experience; 44 percent of all American marriages wind up in the divorce court (Glick, 1980).

The process of divorce has effects far greater than simply the dissolution of an unworkable marriage. Even when the marriage breaks up because one of the partners has fallen in love with someone else, there can be deep pain in the partner who asks for the divorce. One man recalled:

> I cried often when I went through my affair and divorce. The conflict was overwhelming . . . married to one woman, loving my four children deeply, and being so much in love with another woman. It was a gut-wrenching experience. (Hite, 1981, p. 248)

Divorced men and women undergo a radical change in social role, from "wife" or "husband" (and thus part of a couple) to an unattached person for whom society has established no role or expectations. For this reason, recently divorced people often feel anxious and rootless. They often find that they have less money than they're accustomed to, and they may watch helplessly as the friends who saw them as half of a couple drift away. Many divorced people feel the broken marriage is evidence of personal failure. The stress of divorce shows in many ways. Compared with married (or remarried) people, divorced men and women get drunk more often, smoke more marijuana, are lonelier and more despondent, and are more likely to feel anxious or guilty (Cargan and Melko, 1982).

Divorced people have the same sexual options as other singles, but their sex lives are generally more active than those of men and women who have never married. About a third of the divorced have had more than ten sexual partners, compared with a sixth of the women and men who have never married (Cargan and Melko, 1982).

A count of the sexual partners of divorced people may not accurately reflect their sexual activity. Many divorced people go through a variety of partners during the first year after their divorce. This stage of sexual experimentation may be motivated by the feeling of escape from a sexually restrictive marriage, by a search for intimacy with someone new, or, as we saw in Chapter 2, by a wish to avoid commitment in another intimate relationship. Recently divorced people may also have a need to prove their sexual desirability with a new partner or partners. As one woman said:

> In the months after my divorce, I became a real "swinger." I was feeling very insecure at the time, and I needed to know that I was still attractive to men. (Authors' files)

The divorced person's new freedom may quickly pall. Before long, most men are looking for "meaningful relationships" and most women are complaining that casual sex lowers their self-esteem and leads to feelings of depression and even desperation (Hetherington, Cox, and Cox, 1979). Despite their flurry of post-divorce sexual activity, the divorced have sex less often on the average than most married people. They are also more dissatisfied with their sex lives than the married, the never-married, or the remarried (Cargan and Melko, 1982).

Many divorced people remarry. About a third of all marriages involve people who have been married before (Glick, 1980). The practice of entering a series of legal monogamous relationships can be considered a new form of marriage: **serial polygamy**. In most remarriages, the gap in age between partners widens. Two forces may be responsible. When men remarry, they tend to look for a younger,

**serial polygamy**
series of legal monogamous relationships

attractive woman; when women remarry, they tend to look for financial security, which is likely to be found with an older man. Women with college educations—especially those with graduate training—are the least likely to remarry (Glick, 1980).

When women or men do remarry, they generally marry for love, and many seem to be more successful on their second try (Schell and Hall, 1983). Remarriages seem about as happy as first marriages that endure. So despite the problems that divorce invariably brings—whether sexual, financial, social, or matters of child care and custody—once divorced people work through them, the picture seems to brighten.

## SEX AND AGING

The traditional image of sexuality in older men and women is as mythical and as wrong-headed as the Victorian idea that women cannot experience sexual pleasure. It's only reasonable that a society which limited sexual feeling to men would reject the idea that great-grandparents in their seventies and eighties not only think a good deal about sex, but also behave in bed much as they had when in their prime. But many do, and more would probably be sexually active if their health were better or if they had not come to believe the destructive myths about the elderly that pervade American society.

### *Myths about aging*

The major myths about aging lead to a view of old people as sexless and unattractive, and they often make the elderly self-conscious and embarrassed about their sexual needs (Kay and Neeley, 1982). The first myth, that "sex doesn't matter in old age," may spring from a religious tradition that condones sex only when procreation is possible. In such a view, the sexual needs of women who have passed menopause are unjustified. And since the responsiveness of older men may have slowed or changed somewhat, their sexuality is unimportant. Thus society believes that men and women will gracefully give up their sexual activities with increasing age.

The second myth, that interest in sex is abnormal for old people, results in the application of negative labels to individuals whose sexual interest continues throughout the life span. The sexually interested old man is often called a "dirty old man" or "lecher," while the sexually interested woman may be called "vain" or "silly."

These two myths lie at the basis of other sexual beliefs and practices. Because we don't expect a continued need for sexual contact in old age, the marriage of elderly people is seen as asexual companionship. When an older husband or wife loses a marital partner, we generally don't expect them to remarry. In fact, remarriage is often discouraged—especially by adult children with personal insecurities. If the remarriage is accepted, it is seen as "cute," as if the couple were children playing a game instead of adults committing themselves to intimacy and sexual contact. An eighty-two-year-old man who remarried complained because everyone who approved of the match said he needed companionship:

> It gets me mad. Sure I want companionship, but I also got married for sex. I always had an active sex life and still do. (Starr and Weiner, 1981, p. 5)

Another harmful practice is the custom of separating older women and men in nursing homes and other institutions. Sometimes even wives and husbands are separated (Kay and Neeley, 1982). Nursing home residents are often treated as children who cannot be trusted to make their own sexual decisions. In addition, the right to privacy is often denied them. At a time when older men and women may have an increased need for the intimacy of personal contact, they find themselves in institutions that do not recognize these needs.

After looking at nursing home practices, Alex Comfort (1976) suggested that the homes were run by people with sexual problems—the only reasonable explanation for their organization as mixed-sex nunneries. When homes for the aged follow the sexual customs of the rest of society, the residents are generally happier, healthier, and require fewer tranquilizers than do residents of conventional homes.

The sexual needs of elderly women tend to be even more suppressed than those of men. Not only is their sexuality denied, but society seems to believe that something is "wrong" when a younger man finds an older woman attractive. It is accepted that older men—especially if they are rich, powerful, or famous—will seek younger sexual partners. But an older woman who is involved with a younger man is generally ridiculed (Kuhn, 1976).

As we have seen, myths about aging and sexuality tend to suppress sexual activity among the elderly. However, a look at the physiology of aging shows no reason why sexual activity shouldn't continue into later years.

## Physiological changes with aging

The process of aging certainly produces changes in sexual structure and functioning, but sexual functioning doesn't suddenly disappear when a person reaches some biological marker. Instead, sexual physiology changes continuously throughout the life cycle. In fact, the general process of aging actually begins during youth. For example, the refractory period generally begins to lengthen when men are in their twenties. But because sex is mostly psychological, physiology has little to do with sexual satisfaction compared with such factors as sexual interest and a lifetime of patterns and habits.

**Women** A major factor in the lives of older women is menopause, which was discussed in Chapter 3. Menopause is the medical marker of middle age and occurs at about age fifty. Common myths about menopause warn that women may go insane, that they will lose their interest in sex, and that their femininity will be destroyed. Since psychology and physiology are so intertwined, women who believe these predictions may have a difficult time. Women who reject them are likely to find menopause no more than a slight discomfort. Although few women today accept the myths, a majority of those who have not been through the process regard it as "mysterious" (LaRocco and Polit, 1980).

Women who fear menopause are generally those who have not yet encountered it; those who have gone through it tend to be matter-of-fact and somewhat positive about the experience (Boston Women's Health Book Collective, 1977). Most women feel that menopause has no effect on sexual relations, and some find intercourse more important and enjoyable afterward (Neugarten et al., 1963).

Many of the psychological symptoms considered typical of menopause, such as irritability, headaches, tiredness, and depression, are not found among all women or all societies. Married women with high incomes and children in the home have the fewest menopausal symptoms, and a woman's reaction to menopause closely parallels that of her mother (Dosey and Dosey, 1980).

When studying the sexual response of women between the ages of forty-one and seventy-eight years old, Masters and Johnson (1966) found that some responses, such as nipple erection and clitoral response, were like those in younger women. Other responses either slowed or lessened in intensity. The sex flush was less prevalent, and vaginal response differed somewhat. In most women who reach menopause, lower levels of hormones lead to a shortening and narrowing of the vagina and cause the tissues of the vaginal walls to become thinner and less expansive (Hammond and Maxson, 1982). For some women, such changes may cause discomfort during and after intercourse, although as we'll see, intercourse may help to slow some of these changes. In fact, other researchers have found that few women report such discomfort (Starr and Weiner, 1981).

In addition, vaginal lubrication tends to be slower and less intense among older women. But this is not always true. Three of the women studied by Masters and Johnson, including one seventy-three-year-old, lubricated as quickly and as profusely as young women. These three women had maintained active sex lives, and had had intercourse once or twice a week throughout adulthood.

Although older women's vaginal contractions during orgasm were like those of younger women, their number tended to decline. Younger women generally have between five and ten contractions, but older women averaged three to five contractions. Once again, the same three sexually active women showed as many contractions as did the younger group. Finally, resolution was generally quicker among the older women.

Masters and Johnson concluded that although the intensity and duration of sexual response was reduced with age, older women were fully capable of sexual performance and orgasm, especially when their sexual stimulation was regular and effective. A regular sex life seems vital to sexual functioning in the aging woman. When older women who were regularly engaging in masturbation and coitus were compared with older women who had become sexually inactive, the genitals of those who were still sexually active showed fewer physiological signs of aging. Although estrogen levels in both groups of women were about the same, the sexually  active women had significantly higher levels of gonadotropic hormones (especially LH) and of androgens (Leiblum et al., in press). It appears that sexual activity—both coitus and masturbation—may even help to slow the aging process.

Among women who have always led an active sexual life, the hormonal decreases of menopause may be little more than an inconvenience that may require a slight adjustment in the sexual script. For example, if lubrication becomes a problem, artificial lubricants, such as K-Y Jelly, are often helpful. For women whose sexual interaction has been infrequent or unsatisfying, menopause may provide an excuse to give up sexual activity. Hormone replacement therapy may ease possible physical discomforts of intercourse for the aging woman by slowing physiological changes caused by decreased estrogen levels (Hammond and Maxon, 1982), but it will not directly increase her sexual interest.

**Men** The major effect of aging on male sexuality is a lengthening of each stage of the sexual response cycle. When Masters and Johnson (1966) studied sexual response in men between the ages of fifty-one and eighty-nine years, they found that penile erection takes considerably longer in older men, even when sexual stimulation is experienced as extremely arousing. The older man can maintain an erection for much longer periods without ejaculating than a younger man. It's not clear whether this prolonged erection is due to a less intense sexual response in older men, or whether they simply are more experienced at controlling ejaculation.

Like the aging woman, the aging man has orgasmic contractions that are essentially like those of his younger counterpart except that they tend to be fewer. The seminal fluid is typically expelled with less force. In addition, the feeling of "ejaculatory inevitability" commonly reported by younger men tends to be much shorter in older men, or to disappear. Resolution usually occurs much more rapidly with increasing age, sometimes within a few seconds. The refractory period, when a man cannot have another erection, lengthens considerably, especially in men past the age of sixty. Finally, most aging men say they are satisfied with one or two ejaculations a week.

Despite the absence of any ejaculatory urge, many older men can still enjoy sexual activity or provide pleasure to their partners. None of the physiological changes appear to lessen the pleasure older men find in sexual activity, and they have the positive effect of making intercourse last longer.

## Sexual behavior and aging

Biological aging does place some limits on sexual functioning, but as long as health remains good, sex remains possible. Ever since Alfred Kinsey (Kinsey, Pomeroy, and Martin, 1948; Kinsey et al., 1953) interviewed men and women, authorities have accepted the idea of a steady decline in sexual activity, beginning in the teens. An examination of most sex surveys would support this notion.

Kinsey found that married men in their teens had intercourse an average 4.8

times a week, dropping to 1.8 per week in their fifties and 0.9 per week in their seventies. However, Kinsey also found great individual differences in the way men responded to the aging process. Among men over the age of sixty, sexual activity occurred 1.0 times a week for sixty-five-year-olds, 0.3 times for seventy-five-year-olds, and less than 0.1 times for eighty-year-olds.

But there were exceptions to this picture of general decline. One seventy-year-old man said he averaged more than seven ejaculations per week, and an eighty-eight-year-old man was having intercourse at least once a week. It seems likely that group averages of sexual activity distort the activity of individuals within a group.

It may be that with increasing age more and more people become sexually inactive, but those who remain active show no decrease in levels of activity. Several studies support this suggestion. Among one group of men, the pattern of sexual activity that developed fairly early in life generally continued throughout the life cycle (Martin, 1977). Men who reported a good deal of sexual activity in the early years of marriage tended to maintain this pattern into old age. In contrast, men who were comfortable with low levels of sexual activity in their youth—say, once or twice a month—were likely to be content with even lower activities during old age.

When 800 adults between the ages of 60 and 91 were asked about their sexual activity, the year of their birth seemed to affect the frequency of their sexual relations (Starr and Weiner, 1981). The seventy- and eighty-year-olds in this study reported rates of intercourse similar to those found by Kinsey among forty-year-olds more than a quarter of a century earlier, perhaps indicating that a changing sexual climate encourages sexual activity.

Among these older people, eight out of ten were still sexually active. Many were still having intercourse three times a week. Most of those who were no longer sexually active said they simply lacked a partner or were too ill for sex. Asked how often she'd *like* to have sex, a seventy-year-old widow replied, "Morning, noon, and night" (Starr and Weiner, 1981, p. 47).

Up to this point, the focus has been on the effects of biological aging and previous sexual patterns. Other factors, such as physical, psychological, and social status, are also important.

Among men, the man who is physically healthy in his later years is likely to have more interest in sex than the man who is suffering from some disease. The availability of a compatible sex partner also plays an important role in maintaining sexual interest. Finally, the attitude that sexual activity is normal and appropriate for the elderly helps to maintain a man's interest.

The psychological factors that can lessen a man's activity and interest have been spelled out by Masters and Johnson (1966). The monotony that can develop from having a single sexual partner for thirty or forty years may cause a loss of interest. This factor may be particularly important if the female partner has lost her interest in intercourse, or if the couple is unwilling or unable to vary their sexual script. A man may also lose interest if he becomes deeply involved in vocational or economic pursuits. Someone who is preoccupied with work may simply be too

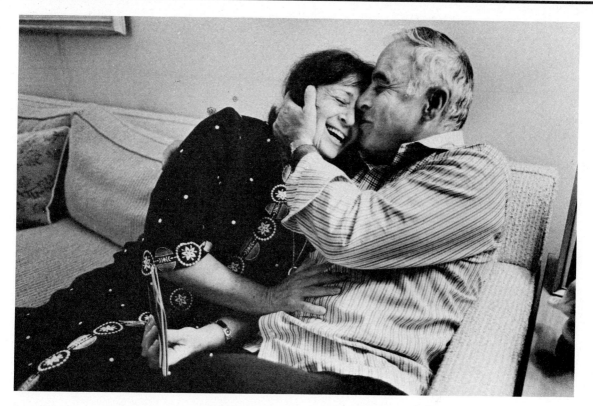

Sex can be a source of pleasure throughout life. Some women find sexual activity more enjoyable after menopause, and men generally find that their increased ability to maintain an erection makes longer intercourse possible. (© Joel Gordon 1979)

physically and mentally tired to devote any energy to sex. Fatigue and lack of energy can also result from bad health habits, such as overindulgence in alcohol or food.

Finally, aging men may be especially susceptible to the "fear of failure" that plays such an important role in the ability to have an erection. If monotony, fatigue, and alcohol combine to prevent an erection on one occasion, the older man may be reluctant to risk another failure. Combined with the cultural expectation that older men cannot and should not be sexually active, his failure may lead a man to conclude that he's too old to "get it up," and he quits trying. As we'll see in Chapter 14, many of these psychological problems can be reversed with sex therapy and sex education.

The sexuality of the aging woman has many parallels with sexuality in the aging man. The gradual decline in intercourse among women has an additional cause not reflected in the previous discussion. Since intercourse depends on the availability of a cooperative partner, intercourse rates are largely determined by male interest and not by female desire. The decline over the years in female intercourse rates does not necessarily reflect the level of a woman's sexual interest. Because there are so many older women without partners, or with partners who are no longer interested in sex, a better measure is a solo sexual activity, such as masturbation (Kinsey et al., 1953). Indeed, female masturbation rates gradually rise to a maximum level that is maintained until women are about sixty years old. Many older women in Kinsey's survey expressed a desire for higher rates of intercourse and blamed any decline on their husbands' lack of interest. The problem may be intensified by the tendency of American women to marry men who are older than themselves.

Although there seem to be few physiological limits on female sexuality, a number of other factors contribute to the overall decline with age. In addition to the lack of a willing partner, women are also subject to the same factors—monotony, fatigue, ill health—that limit the sexuality of the aging male.

When older adults were asked to reflect on their sex lives, about a third regretted lost opportunities. Not many were as exuberant as the sixty-three-year-old woman who said, "I wish I'd laid half the town (the male half)" (Starr and Weiner, 1981, p. 187), but regrets at lack of experience, ignorance, failure to communicate, and inhibitions were common. However, about half of these men and women said they were satisfied with their sex lives and would change nothing in their pasts. Clearly, many people born long before the sexual revolution are warm and responsive, and have full, rewarding sex lives.

# *Summary*

**1** Traditional marriage has four basic functions: economic security, reproduction of a family line, psychological security and a place in society, and the socialization of children. The American demand that it also provide romantic love, personal growth, and self-fulfillment has placed new strains on the institution. Americans have been marrying later, and when they choose a mate, they generally choose people who are like themselves in education, intelligence, attractiveness, age, socioeconomic level, ethnic background, and religion, and who live near them. Marriage requires adjustment to reduced freedom, changed financial situation, personality characteristics of the partner, and children. How decisions are handled has an important influence on marital satisfaction.

**2** The frequency of marital coitus declines with age, although not all individuals show similar declines. The rate of marital intercourse may be affected by boredom, pregnancy, childrearing, home care, career concerns, financial pressures, and the experience of aging in a youth-oriented culture. People who view intercourse as primarily procreative may lose sexual interest in a partner who can no longer have children. Marital satisfaction may depend more on the emotional tone of the marriage than on an absence of sexual problems.

**3** Although an overwhelming majority of Americans disapprove of extramarital sex, it is widespread. The Victorian double standard, which allowed only men to have affairs, is no longer so rigid. Today people are having affairs at a younger age, and middle-class, educated women are about as likely as men to have an affair. Among the reasons for extramarital sex are marital dissatisfaction, an interest in varied sexual experience, pressure from a friend or spouse, status seeking, a need for independence, and a desire to punish a spouse. In **open marriages**, extramarital affairs are allowed as long as each partner places the other first. Such affairs are known as **comarital relationships**, and they are successful when both partners have interpersonal skills and can handle stressful relationships. Extramarital affairs can stimulate jealousy and possessiveness and end marital trust and intimacy.

**4** **Swinging** incorporates extramarital sex into the marriage in the form of group sex. The majority of swingers are conventional, middle-class men and women. The positive effects of swinging are increased sexual excitement, the shedding of sexual inhibitions, and shared interests. The negative effects are the inability to live up to sexual illusions, sexual jealousy, and jealousy of the partner's popularity. Couples who stop swinging generally do so because of the impersonal nature of the practice. In **group marriages**, partners tend to be young, highly educated, and liberal. Jealousy is a problem in group marriages, and most break up quickly.

**5** As the single life has become increasingly attractive, society has come to accept it. People who choose to remain single say they do so because the personal freedom, career opportunities, sexual opportunities, and the chance for self-improvement outweigh the absence of the economic, emotional, and sexual security found in marriage. Single women may have a more difficult time than single men in finding sexual partners, especially as they grow older. Some women and men who remain single choose to be celibate. **Celibacy** can involve total abstinence, in which masturbation and sexual fantasy are foregone, or partial abstinence. Lifelong celibacy is usually based on moral or religious conviction, and temporary celibacy on health, feminist politics, or necessity.

**6** Divorce has far-reaching effects on social roles, financial situations, and the divorced person's image of him- or herself. Recently divorced people often feel anxious or rootless. Divorced people generally have a more active sex life than people who have never married, and the first year after divorce may be a period of sexual experimentation. Later, both men and women tend to look for intimate relationships. Divorced people often remarry, entering a series of legal monogamous relationships known as **serial polygamy**.

**7** Two myths about aging—that "sex doesn't matter in old age" and that an interest in sex is abnormal—have led to a view of old people as sexless and unattractive. These myths tend needlessly to suppress sexual activity in the elderly. Menopause is generally a less uncomfortable and negative experience than most younger women expect. After menopause, sexual responses such as nipple erection and clitoral response are like those in younger women, although other responses tend to diminish in intensity and duration. A regular sex life appears to slow the process of sexual aging in women. The major effect of aging on male sexuality is a lengthening of each stage of the sexual arousal cycle, although resolution is much more rapid. The physiological changes of aging do not appear to lessen the pleasure of sexual activity and they have the effect of lengthening intercourse.

**8** With increasing age, more and more people become sexually inactive.

Although the group average of sexual activity declines steadily throughout old age, that of individuals who remain active may not decline much. Among men, physical health, the availability of a compatible sex partner, and the attitude that sexual activity is normal help to maintain sexual interest. Boredom, an unwillingness to vary the sexual script, a preoccupation with work, bad health habits, and fear of failure can decrease sexual interest. Among women, the availability of a cooperative partner is the major determinant of sexual activity, since so many older women lack partners or are married to older men who may have lost interest in sex. Women are also subject to many of the factors that affect sexual activity and interest in men. But many people continue to have full, rewarding sex lives as long as they remain healthy.

# 14 Sexual Problems and Solutions

*Chapter 14*

The new cultural openness toward sexuality has uncovered hidden frustrations and anxieties and shifted the goals of sex therapy. A woman of the Victorian era who was unable to have an orgasm would not have sought professional help. She had little expectation of pleasure from sex, and her interest in it would have labeled her as a woman of doubtful morals. What's more, no one was available to provide counseling. Whatever "sex therapy" existed was aimed at controlling sexual expressiveness, not freeing it. Physicians believed that the less that was known about sex, the better (Leiblum and Pervin, 1980).

Today most men and women, whether homosexual or heterosexual, expect sexual activity to be satisfying, and many health professionals are ready to help solve their sexual problems. Sex therapists find that most of the people who consult them are unable to enjoy sexuality because they approach sex with ignorance, anxiety, and guilt. They are generally men and women who have thoroughly absorbed the old cultural message that sex is an evil, sinful, and dirty thing practiced with the person one loves best. To their ranks, however, have been added those who have rejected the old prohibitions but expect too much from the new freedom. Although there is nothing wrong with the sexual functioning of these people, they believe they are failing to meet the cultural standards for sexual performance set by the media and some sex manuals.

Many couples with sexual problems say their sexual satisfaction is high and their relationship happy (Frank et al., 1978), but others suffer a major loss of self-esteem. Self-esteem depends on how well we cope with our life roles, and a sexual problem can make us feel incompetent and convince us that we have failed as a spouse or sexual partner. This general sense of failure can produce shame and anxiety that intensify our original problem.

**LACK OF SEXUAL DESIRE**     *Causes of low sexual desire*     *Overcoming desire problems*
**SEXUAL COUNSELING AND THERAPY**     *Does sex therapy work?*
FOCUS: HOW TO BE YOUR OWN SEX THERAPIST

# Sexual Problems and Solutions

Almost every woman and man has some sexual problem at some stage of the life cycle. Any of the common sexual problems can become a **sexual dysfunction**, an incapacity that interferes with sexual functioning. Because sexual activity is interwoven with so many facets of everyday life, pressures from other areas can lead to sexual dysfunction. In many cases, after a period of sexual inadequacy, normal functioning returns. In other cases, however, the dysfunction becomes chronic and debilitating.

**sexual dysfunction** an incapacity that interferes with sexual functioning

In this chapter, we'll begin by looking at the ways sexual problems are labeled. Next we'll discuss common sexual problems—difficulties with orgasm and penetration on the part of women and with erection and ejaculation on the part of men, as well as a lack of sexual desire by both sexes. After investigating the effectiveness of sex therapy, we'll end the chapter by examining instances in which people can become their own sex therapists— and how to go about solving problems in personal sexuality.

## DESCRIBING SEXUAL PROBLEMS

Sexual problems have many sources. They can arise when we are unable to express our sexuality in satisfying and creative ways; when sexual activity becomes associated with anger, jealousy, fear, or guilt; or when we express our sexuality selfishly, without regard for the feelings of others (Calderone and Johnson, 1981).

The existence of a sexual problem is affected by how society defines sexual function-

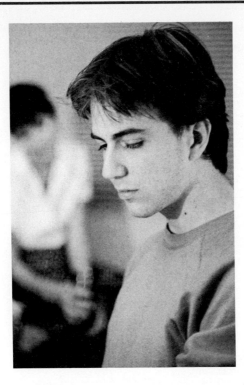

The feelings of incompetence and failure that often accompany sexual problems may lead to a major loss of self-esteem, which spills over into other areas of life. (© Paul Waldman)

ing, and the extent of any individual problem depends on physical health, beliefs, attitudes, childhood experiences, and the expectations of the culture. But the person's reaction to a sexual problem depends largely on how it is labeled.

Sexual problems can be labeled in either general or specific terms. The more specific the label, the more valuable it generally is. Traditional labels, such as frigidity or impotence, are vague terms that convey almost nothing about the sexual dysfunction. In addition, the negative connotations of such labels are destructive. Saying that a woman is frigid implies that she is cold and unresponsive, when in truth she may be warm and accepting. Saying that a man is impotent implies that he has no power, strength, or masculinity. Both terms have been criticized by professionals.

**situational orgasmic dysfunction** a condition in which a woman is unable to have an orgasm from certain kinds of stimulation

**erectile dysfunction** a condition in which a man cannot achieve or maintain an erection

**ejaculatory dysfunction** a condition in which a man either cannot ejaculate or ejaculates prematurely

The current practice is to label sexual dysfunctions with terms that are specific and carry no evaluative comment. For example, **situational orgasmic dysfunction** refers to the inability to have orgasms under certain conditions, **erectile dysfunction** means the inability to achieve or maintain an erection, and **ejaculatory dysfunction** denotes inability to ejaculate. Defining sexual dysfunctions in this way has important advantages: Once defined, the dysfunctions become easier for people to understand; counselors and therapists can communicate more easily about their work; scientific study of a dysfunction's causes and treatment is easier; and much of the shame and stigma associated with negative labels are removed.

Describing a sexual dysfunction is different from diagnosing a physical disease. In diagnosing disease, a physician thinks in such categories as healthy or sick,
normal or abnormal. But we have no absolute standard for sexual functioning,
only a range of possible capacities or incapacities. A particular dysfunction may
have meaning only for a given individual in a given context. Some people have
severe problems that affect all areas of sexual activity; other people have relatively
minor problems that interfere with (or are confined to) only a small part of sexual
behavior.

Exactly what is considered a sexual problem and how it is treated changes
with time. In the first half of the twentieth century, sexuality was viewed as a dangerous force (the raging libido), but Freud gave men permission to enjoy it. Men
were supposed to need sex frequently, although sexual pleasure was to be restrained. Women were expected to have only a limited interest in sex, and since
Freud had labeled clitoral orgasms and masturbation "immature," any therapy a
woman might receive would be aimed at switching her from clitoral to vaginal orgasms. But that therapy would not be direct. Professionals were reluctant to approach sexual dysfunctions directly, for they believed the problems reflected
broader emotional problems and were simply one aspect of a deep personality disturbance.

After Kinsey had prepared the way, William Masters and Virginia Johnson radically shifted the premises of therapy. The publication of *Human Sexual Inadequacy* in 1970 marked a new era in the understanding and approach to sexual
problems. This book challenged previous concepts of sexual dysfunction, particularly the concept that a sexual problem is always a symptom of some deeper problem. As a result, a wide variety of professionals now provide information and direct
counseling for sexual difficulties (Rosen and Gendel, 1981). Although the origins
of a specific dysfunction may lie in the remote past, the therapist focuses on present factors that affect current behavior.

## COMMON SEXUAL PROBLEMS: WOMEN

Our concepts of female sexuality have changed radically in the past century, and
particularly in the past twenty years. The work of sex researchers has liberated us
from the Victorian denial of female sexual potential, but general acceptance of their
right to sexual gratification has pushed women into a new set of dilemmas. Can a
woman be both "feminine" and sexually assertive? Is it "normal" for a woman to
want sex more often than her male partner? Should every woman have multiple
orgasms? Is something wrong with a woman who never reaches orgasm?

Such questions can create self-doubts that may become the source of sexual
problems. Women today are as susceptible as men to the demands of sexual performance. As a result, a considerable number are dissatisfied with some aspect of
their sexual lives. Common complaints center on the inability to have orgasms and
problems with penetration.

## *Lack of orgasm*

**primary orgasmic dysfunction** a condition in which a woman has never experienced orgasm from any kind of stimulation

**preorgasmic** a woman with primary orgasmic dysfunction

Although a sizable minority of women seem unable to have an orgasm, those with **primary orgasmic dysfunction,** who have never experienced orgasm from any kind of stimulation, remain a small group. The finding that about one woman in ten has never reached orgasm has turned up repeatedly in studies for thirty years (Kinsey et al., 1953; Hite, 1976; de Bruijn, 1982). Because most of these women can learn to have orgasms in at least some situations, they have also been called **preorgasmic** (Barbach, 1975).

A much larger group of women have situational orgasmic dysfunction; they have orgasms in some, but not all, situations. Typically, these women have difficulty reaching orgasm during intercourse, but not in response to manual or oral stimulation. As we saw in Chapter 8, up to three-fourths of married women but only about half of single women have orgasm during intercourse, and many of these women say that coitus must be accompanied by clitoral stimulation. The proportion of orgasmic women tends to increase with length of marriage and with age, with orgasmic ability apparently peaking between the ages of thirty and forty-five (Kinsey et al., 1953; Hunt, 1974).

Orgasmic dysfunctions are not necessarily a sign of disinterest in sex or of lack of sexual arousal. Women with this dysfunction often feel aroused, lubricate copiously, and show genital swelling in response to stimulation (Kaplan, 1974). A failure to reach orgasm during intercourse may not be dysfunctional at all, since so many otherwise responsive women never have coital orgasms. The condition may be a normal variation of female sexuality. For certain women, the thrusting of coitus is an inefficient method of stimulation that is not intense enough to trigger the orgasm reflex (Hite, 1976).

Some women may not find coital orgasm important. For them, love, intimacy, sensuality, and physical closeness may be the major source of sexual satisfaction. One such woman indicated that orgasm seemed somehow aggressive—an explosion that blotted out the warmth and trust of lovemaking, while another said:

> I prefer to experience orgasm while I'm on my own. My sexual relationship is for satisfying my need for warmth and love and friendship. (de Bruijn, 1982, p. 159)

In fact, two-thirds of the women in this group who did have regular orgasms during intercourse said that it contributed little to their general sexual satisfaction.

Women for whom orgasm is not an important goal probably feel contented without it. But some preorgasmic women are so frustrated and disappointed by their "failure" that they have major problems with self-esteem (Barbach, 1975).

**Causes of orgasmic dysfunction** Underlying most orgasmic dysfunction are learning factors, psychological inhibition, or some aspect of a woman's relationship. Margaret's case is an example of the simplest kind of orgasmic dysfunction, which can be traced to a learning deficit—she never learned how to experience orgasm.

*Case* Margaret D. grew up in a conservative middle-class home in which sex was a forbidden subject. A virgin at the time of her marriage, she enjoyed sex with her husband, despite a nagging feeling that "something was missing." Although Margaret was proud of her roles as teacher and mother, her sex life was disappointing and frustrating. Her husband ejaculated after a few minutes of intercourse without her ever experiencing orgasm. He blamed himself for being an inadequate lover, and in their discussions of the problem, he became increasingly defensive. At the suggestion of Margaret's gynecologist, the couple decided to seek sexual counseling. (Authors' files)

Although learning to ejaculate seems to happen naturally for the vast majority of men, not all women inevitably learn how to reach orgasm. Perhaps the difference stems from the fact that male ejaculation is required if conception is to occur. If orgasm did not develop "naturally" for men, the species would die out.

Among women, there may be a spectrum of orgasmic ability, ranging from orgasm with sexual fantasy alone to orgasm only after intense and prolonged clitoral stimulation (Kaplan, 1974). Discovering the level and type of stimulation required to trigger an orgasm is often a matter of trial and error. Most women discover masturbation accidentally while exploring their genitals, and women who masturbate to orgasm before marriage are more likely than other women to be orgasmic within the marital relationship (Kinsey et al., 1953). The experience of masturbation may not itself cause the ability to reach orgasm during intercourse, but it probably teaches women how to achieve orgasm. In one group of women, for example, orgasmic dysfunction was five times higher among those who had never masturbated (Hite, 1976).

Although orgasm is a physiological reflex, it can easily be inhibited by psychological factors. A strict religious upbringing may sometimes be responsible, although not all women with a religious background fail to reach orgasm (Morokoff, 1978).

The fear of losing control is another source of inhibition. This fear may take a specific form. Some women believe that in the throes of orgasm, they will faint, scream, or otherwise lose control (Barbach, 1975). Other women simply want to remain in emotional control throughout a sexual interaction. Although a momentary loss of consciousness during orgasm is common, some women fear losing touch so strongly that they simply cannot let go.

The relationship between a woman and her sexual partner may affect her ability to have orgasms in two ways. Nonsexual problems in the relationship—such as lack of trust or poor communication—can lead to a pattern of sexual withholding. A woman may take part in intercourse, but her negative feelings toward her partner may prevent an emotional involvement intense enough to achieve orgasm. Her partner's level of sexual functioning is also an important influence. Obvious difficulties exist if the man has serious erectile or ejaculatory control problems. If he loses his erection before or during intercourse, the woman will naturally find it difficult to reach orgasm. In cases of extremely rapid ejaculation, the woman may not be aroused enough before her partner ejaculates.

Time is extremely important if a woman is to reach orgasm. In one group of women, those who never had orgasms averaged about five minutes of manual stimulation, three minutes of oral stimulation, or six minutes of coital thrusting from their partners. But those who consistently had orgasms received ten minutes of manual stimulation, seven minutes of oral stimulation, or ten minutes of coital thrusting (de Bruijn, 1982).

A man who does not use proper techniques can keep his partner from reaching orgasm by failing to provide the necessary stimulation. But a man cannot use proper techniques if he does not know what they are, so it is up to such women to train their partners to be effective lovers (LoPiccolo, 1977). Some women who never reach orgasm during coitus admit that they fail to request or initiate the kind of sex play they find exciting (de Bruijn, 1982). Some women are too timid to ask for such stimulation; some say their partners either refuse their requests or get angry. A woman may believe that any stimulation which involves her own active movements either puts her in charge of the proceedings or interrupts her partner's actions—both violations of the traditional female sexual role (Gagnon, Rosen, and Leiblum, 1982).

**Becoming orgasmic**   One of the most significant developments in the field of sex therapy has been programs designed specifically to help women become orgasmic. The first important advance came when Masters and Johnson (1970) reported that most women—about 80 percent—could learn to become orgasmic without extensive psychotherapy or major personality change. Simply removing performance demands and providing direct instruction in techniques of genital stimulation was enough.

The next major advance came when psychologists Joseph LoPiccolo and Charles Lobitz (1973) augmented the Masters and Johnson approach with a guided masturbation training program for women who had never experienced orgasm. The LoPiccolo program for becoming orgasmic consists of nine sequential steps, beginning with the "looking phase," in which women explore their genitals with the aid of a hand mirror. The "touching phase" begins with clitoral stimulation, and moves on to intensive masturbation with the aid of lubricants to minimize discomfort. If orgasm does not occur, additional fantasy or the use of an electric vibrator is sometimes introduced.

Women who have trouble letting go are encouraged to role play an orgasmic reaction in order to get over their fears. Once orgasm has been reached in private, the woman masturbates to orgasm in the presence of her partner. He then attempts to do for her what she has been doing for herself, using either manual stimulation or a vibrator. Not until this last step is successful does the couple attempt intercourse—and in a position in which the woman can get manual or vibrator stimulation during coitus.

Preorgasmic women tend to be more successful at learning to have orgasm during intercourse than women who are situationally dysfunctional. Perhaps a woman who has never had an orgasm finds it easier to transfer her newly learned response to intercourse. Or perhaps a woman who is orgasmic during masturbation may rely on a pattern of stimulation that is difficult to transfer to intercourse. Among a group of Dutch women, those whose masturbation techniques were similar to the techniques used during intercourse were most likely to have regular orgasms (de Bruijn, 1982).

Many women with situational dysfunction find it difficult or impossible to reach orgasm during intercourse without additional clitoral stimulation. Nearly a third of the women in one study required this sort of stimulation to reach orgasm (de Bruijn, 1982). Yet many women are distressed by their persistent inability to reach orgasm without it. One woman expressed her shyness about asking for clitoral stimulation during coitus, saying:

> I have a fear of making the man feel shut down about the effectiveness of his penis. Equally, or more important, I have felt I ought to be able to do without it. (Hite, 1976, p. 256)

## Penetration problems

Two rare but distressing sexual problems that plague some women are vaginismus and dyspareunia. **Vaginismus** is a condition in which penetration is difficult or impossible because muscles around the vagina involuntarily contract. When the man attempts to insert his penis, a muscular spasm closes the entrance to the vagina so tightly that penetration is impossible. The woman has no voluntary control over this response.

**vaginismus** a condition in which intercourse is difficult or impossible because muscles around the vagina involuntarily contract

The other major problem, **dyspareunia**, consists of pain or discomfort during intercourse, and sometimes leads to vaginismus. Vaginismus is usually psychogenic in origin, but dyspareunia is often caused by physical factors.

**dyspareunia** pain or discomfort during intercourse

**Causes of penetration problems** In evaluating a penetration problem, the first step is a physical examination by a gynecologist. When a woman complains of dyspareunia, the physician usually looks for vaginal infections, endometriosis and infections of the cervix or uterus, or scar tissue in the vagina due to infection or surgery.

The most common cause of dyspareunia among the women treated by Masters and Johnson (1970) was inadequate vaginal lubrication, which can lead to intense burning, itching, or aching during intercourse. Since lubrication slackens in women who have passed menopause, they tend to be more susceptible to this problem. When dyspareunia can be traced to this cause, the use of an artificial lubricant, such as K-Y Jelly, is usually effective.

Vaginismus is usually associated with specific fears about intercourse or with negative sexual experiences in the past. Strong religious taboos are found in some cases. Women who have been raped occasionally develop vaginismus. Exaggerated fears of pregnancy or injury from intercourse are also important (Kaplan, 1974). Sometimes vaginismus is associated with serious erectile problems in the male partner (Masters and Johnson, 1970). In some cases, the man's repeated failure to penetrate his partner's closed vagina causes his erectile problem to develop. In other cases, the problem with erection develops first, and the woman's repeated frustration during intercourse leads to her vaginismus.

Whatever the original cause, therapists agree that if left uncorrected, vaginismus can completely disrupt a sexual relationship. It is often found in marriages that remain unconsummated for many years (Leiblum, Pervin, and Campbell, 1980).

*Case* Robert and Joyce had been married for four years without having intercourse. Although they had masturbated, and they enjoyed manual and oral stimulation together, each time they tried intercourse Joyce would become anxious, and her vagina tightened until penetration was impossible. She had been brought up as a strict Catholic and had received no formal sex education. When she was seven years old, the uncle of a neighborhood friend had molested her, and Joyce recalls this experience as extremely upsetting. When at the age of fourteen she first inserted a tampon, she became so anxious that her vagina tightened and she had to go to a physician to have the tampon removed. Although Joyce was physically attracted to her husband, she was afraid of his penis and felt that her vagina was not big enough to contain it. (Adapted from Leiblum, Pervin, and Campbell, 1980)

Since a woman with vaginismus may be capable of sexual arousal and orgasm, some women adjust by relying on manual or oral stimulation for sexual satisfaction. But the difficulty and frustration surrounding intercourse can also lead a woman to lose interest in sex or to avoid it. The response of a woman's partner to a large extent determines her adjustment to the problem.

**Treating vaginismus** Therapy for vaginismus always begins by teaching a woman to learn to relax in the presence of sexual stimulation. This can be accomplished in a number of ways, such as through sensual massage as described in Chapter 10. Behavior therapists may use deep muscle relaxation techniques as a first step. Muscle relaxant drugs, deep breathing, and relaxing imagery are also used for this purpose (Leiblum, Pervin, and Campbell, 1980).

Once the woman is able to relax, the second step is gradually to reduce her sensitivity to vaginal penetration. The therapist might begin by asking her to imagine inserting a tampon or her finger into her vagina, then slowly progress until she can imagine intercourse without discomfort. She is now ready to begin a carefully structured program of actual insertion. For instance, vaginal dilators of increasing thickness may be inserted (usually in a gynecologist's office), or the couple may practice insertion at home, relying on the woman's or man's fingers.

Several repetitions of each step may be necessary before the woman is relaxed enough to proceed to the next. The treatment often requires considerable patience from both partners. In the final step, the woman sits astride her partner and slowly inserts his penis into her vagina. Most women need several weeks—or even months—of practice before they are ready to attempt this step.

Some therapists also suggest the use of Kegel exercises, which were described in Chapter 7, to improve control over vaginal muscles. Although many women report increased confidence from these exercises, no research has yet documented their effectiveness in cases of vaginismus (Leiblum, Pervin, and Campbell, 1980).

When the therapy programs are carefully followed, vaginismus is usually

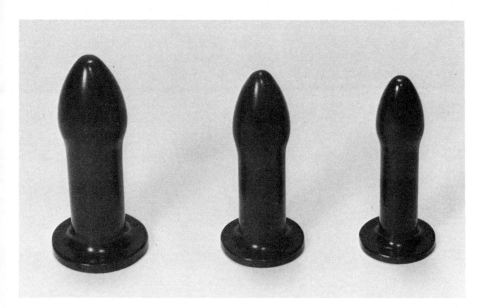

These vaginal dilators are used to treat women whose vaginal muscles contract so tightly that they cannot have intercourse, a condition known as vaginismus. (Courtesy, R. Rosen)

eliminated (Kaplan, 1974; Masters and Johnson, 1970). But many women with vaginismus either do not seek counseling or else drop out of therapy before the problem is solved. In some cases, the vaginismus is overcome only to have other sexual or interpersonal problems (which had been masked by the absence of intercourse) appear (Kaplan, 1974). However, most women who are successful in overcoming their vaginismus find that their future sexual relationships progress smoothly.

## COMMON SEXUAL PROBLEMS: MEN

Few men go through their lives without experiencing some form of sexual difficulty. An infrequent sexual problem is simply a normal part of life, as most men have discovered. When a problem persists and a man cannot cope with it, it becomes a sexual dysfunction. The common male sexual problems involve erection and ejaculation.

### Erectile problems

Several kinds of erectile dysfunction, which used to be called impotence, exist. In **primary erectile dysfunction,** a man has never been able to keep an erection long enough to have either heterosexual or homosexual intercourse. In **secondary erectile dysfunction,** the man fails in at least a quarter of his attempts. Some therapists (O'Connor, 1976) use the terms total and partial to distinguish between the man

**primary erectile dysfunction** a condition in which a man has never been able to keep an erection long enough to have intercourse

**secondary erectile dysfunction** a condition in which a man fails to keep an erection in at least 25 percent of his attempts at intercourse

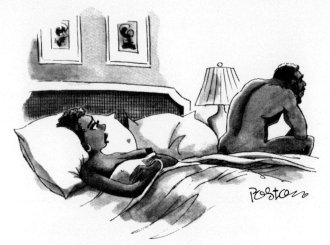

*"I thought with athletes, the legs were the first
thing to go."*

Reproduced by special permission of PLAYBOY Magazine;
copyright © 1983 by Playboy.

who is never able to become erect (whether or not he once had the ability) and
the man whose erection fails only part of the time. Clear-cut cases of total erectile
dysfunction include those in which a physical injury or disease has permanently
blocked the erection response. Within the category of partial erectile dysfunction
are men who cannot achieve an erection during foreplay, or men whose erection
wilts when genital intercourse is attempted or when their clothes come off, or who
can have erections only when they know that intercourse is impossible, or when
their partner dominates the sexual situation, or when their partner is passive (Kaplan, 1974).

Such problems can cause great personal distress. Because the ability to perform sexually is often linked to feelings of masculinity, and because erectile problems are obvious at a glance, the dysfunction usually threatens a man's self-esteem.
One man said of his intermittent problem:

> It makes me feel like I am a little helpless boy, guilty usually. I feel ashamed.
> (Hite, 1981, p. 340)

Men with erectile difficulties often compound their problem by withdrawing from
all forms of sexual interaction, as the case of Max demonstrates.

*Case*   Max T. had been married for 28 years when his wife
died of cancer. Several months after her death, he began to date again.
But he found himself unable to maintain an erection long enough for
intercourse. The harder he tried, the worse the problem became. Assured
by his physician that he was physically healthy, Max developed an intense
fear of sexual failure. He avoided sexual relations and stopped dating. His

sexual withdrawal was finally reversed when Max masturbated for the first time in more than twenty years. Upon his discovery that he could maintain an erection and reach orgasm, his confidence improved. He began dating again and gradually overcame his erectile problems. (Authors' files)

**Causes of erectile failure** Erectile problems are usually considered to have either an organic or a psychogenic cause, meaning that the problem has either a physical or a psychological basis. In some cases, the dysfunction has strong components of both (Rosen, in press). At one time researchers believed that 90 percent of all erectile dysfunctions were psychogenic (Magee, 1980); this is no longer the case. One study found organic disease in 73 percent of the men with erectile problems, as compared with only 12 percent of men without such problems (Schumacher and Lloyd, 1981).

Among the organic causes are any disease or disorder that affects the male hormone balance, nerve pathways, or blood supply to the penis (Figure 14.1). One list contains nearly a hundred possible organic causes of erectile dysfunction (Fracher, Leiblum, and Rosen, 1981). Some of these causes are rare, others are relatively common.

The long-term use of some drugs can cause erectile problems. As we'll see in Chapter 18 certain medications routinely prescribed for hypertension can, if taken for an extended period, lead to erectile dysfunction, as can high doses of alcohol or chronic alcoholism. A disease such as emphysema may not directly cause the erectile dysfunction. Instead, the body, under threat from the physical or psychological stress of the disease, may sacrifice sexual function in order to support systems that are vital to health (Schumacher and Lloyd, 1981).

The majority of erectile failures, however, are due to psychogenic factors, which may be either immediate or remote (Kaplan, 1974). Among the immediate causes are **performance anxiety,** or the fear of failure; the demands of the sexual partner; disagreements with the sexual partner; fear of premature ejaculation; an inability to relax; and emotional stress from nonsexual activities. The remote causes of erectile failure include childhood conditioning, the early learning of negative attitudes toward sex, religious indoctrination, the effects of paternal or maternal dominance on feelings of masculinity, and repressed or conflicting homosexual feelings.

**performance anxiety** the fear of failing at sexual performance

Psychogenic factors can also interact to produce erectile dysfunction. For example, when a man who is achievement-oriented and believes he should be able to get an erection on demand fails, he works even harder to force an erection. He begins "spectatoring"—that is, he remains somewhat detached from his sexual activity, watching himself in the act and monitoring the progress of his erection instead of enjoying sexual stimulation. Now less receptive to sexual pleasure, he finds that his erectile failures are even more frequent.

**Overcoming erectile problems** Several courses of action are open to a man with an erectile problem. If he has experienced the difficulty only once or twice, the obvious remedy is to try again, but under less demanding circumstances.

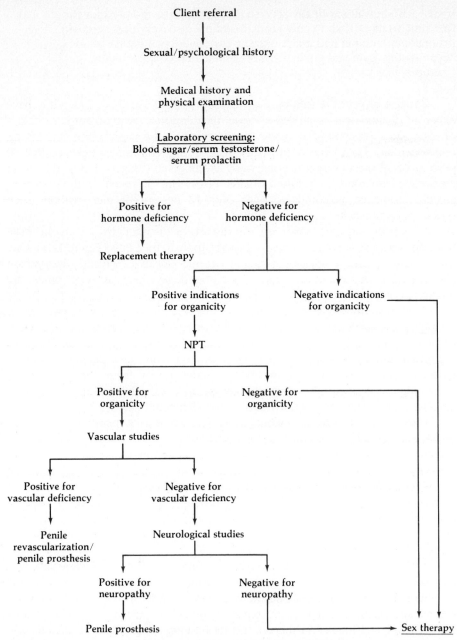

*Figure 14.1   A Flow Chart Model for Comprehensive Assessment of Erectile Dysfunction.*

This model was developed to show the steps involved in evaluating the possible medical factors in impotence. Most sex therapy clinics now employ a screening system like this for evaluating patients with chronic erectile dysfunction. (Adapted from Fracher, Leibium, and Rosen, 1981)

If he avoids all sexual activity, the problem is likely to worsen. Open communication with his partner concerning feelings about sex can help to overcome short-term erectile problems, but many men are reluctant to discuss their "failure" with anyone.

When the problem is persistent and grows progressively worse, professional help may be necessary. The first step is to consult a physician (usually a urologist) to rule out possible organic causes. Physical examination and laboratory tests can check for endocrine deficiency and interruption of nerve pathways or blood supply to the penis.

When laboratory tests indicate a deficiency of male hormones, testosterone injections or pills sometimes help to restore function. In one study, nearly a third of the men with erectile problems had a previously undetected disorder in hormone function (Spark, White, and Connolly, 1980). Most of them showed improved sexual functioning after hormone treatment.

It's probable, however, that hormonal imbalance is the culprit in many fewer cases than this study indicates. These cases were all referred by a physician, so many men with psychogenic dysfunctions may have been screened out. In addition, some of the men may have been so relieved to be given a physical reason for their dysfunction that they relaxed, lessening whatever psychological stress they were under. Other researchers have found a much smaller proportion of hormonal imbalance among their clients (Rosen, in press).

If hormone levels are within the normal range, a sleep erection test can indicate whether other organic factors may be involved. As noted in Chapter 4, men go through a nightly cycle of erections during sleep, which can be measured by placing a gauge around the penis. If nocturnal erections are absent, organic disease—either in the cardiovascular or nervous systems—may be involved.

When the blood supply is disrupted or the nerve pathways cease to function, whether from disease or injury, erection is permanently lost. But the outlook is hopeful for men willing to undergo surgery, in which a **penile prosthesis**—an inflatable or semirigid device—is implanted inside the penis (see Figure 14.2). Such a device produces an erection that is firm enough for intercourse but does not interfere with tactile stimulation or ejaculation. The implant is an important and justifiable last resort for regaining sexual capacity. As one man said:

**penile prosthesis** an inflatable or semirigid device surgically implanted inside the penis to provide an erection

> It took a lot of getting used to, but I have no regrets about my prosthesis. My major problem now is dealing with the reactions of a new partner. (Authors' files)

Since most men with erectile dysfunction think about their problem in unreasonable and self-defeating ways, the therapist generally discusses the patient's attitudes, beliefs, and expectations regarding sexual interaction (Gagnon, Rosen, and Leiblum, 1982). The goal is to encourage a more flexible, pleasure-oriented approach to sexual encounters. Relationship factors are also explored, because such seemingly minor elements as conflicts over childrearing or family finances can make therapy useless.

The next step is to overcome the man's fear of failure, for most men believe that even if they get erections during touching exercises, the erection will not last

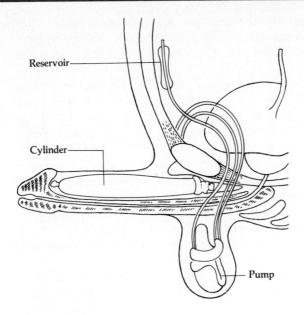

Reservoir

Cylinder

Pump

*Figure 14.2*

Penile Prosthesis with Pump for Inflations (American
Medical Systems, Minneapolis)

through intercourse. To overcome this fear, exercises are used in which the man
and his partner practice his getting erections and then deliberately losing them by
the withdrawal of stimulation (Zilbergeld, 1978). By developing a relaxed and
playful attitude, the man learns that a lost erection can be regained with further
stimulation.

Once confidence has been established, the man is given specific instructions
for intercourse, usually in the face-to-face, woman-above position. Some counselors suggest that at first the couple content themselves with merely experiencing the
sensations of the penis within the vagina. No thrusting or orgasm is allowed. Gradually, the man is permitted to attempt various positions and active thrusting to orgasm.

Among men who follow this program, 50 to 75 percent show improvement.
One reason that more men do not improve is the demand for a quick cure. Some
erectile problems take months, or even years, of counseling to overcome—particularly if the problem is related to underlying psychological difficulties. Many men
become impatient when treatment is not immediately successful and abruptly end
therapy.

The outcome appears most favorable when the man has a history of successful
sexual intercourse, has developed the problem suddenly, has had the problem
only a short time, is motivated to follow the therapist's recommendations, has an
affectionate and cooperative partner, and has no deep psychological problems
(Reynolds, 1977). In such cases, counseling is often effective in a few weeks.

# Premature ejaculation

**Premature** or **rapid ejaculation** is often considered the most common male sexual dysfunction. The prevalence of the problem depends on how "premature" is defined. The label certainly applies to men who ejaculate so rapidly that they do not penetrate their partner. But by Masters and Johnson's (1970) definition, in which prematurity is the inability to delay ejaculation until the female partner reaches orgasm at least 50 percent of the time, cases of premature ejaculation are widespread. They would include a man who ejaculates after 20 minutes of intercourse if his partner can reach orgasm only after 40 minutes of thrusting.

    In his study of male sexuality, Kinsey (Kinsey, Pomeroy, and Martin, 1948) argued that rapid ejaculation might be normal or even preferable for most men. Indeed, a highly aroused young man who ejaculates quickly is almost always in good sexual health and not at all dysfunctional. Such men generally have a short refractory period, so they can attempt more than one ejaculation during a session of lovemaking instead of focusing their attention on slowing their response.

    Yet a rapid response, although it may have some advantage for reproduction, can be a major drawback when considering the pleasurable aspects of intercourse. The man who feels he cannot control his own ejaculation may find that the pleasure of intercourse is lost. One man complained:

> It makes me feel very inadequate, unmanly, makes me feel like a wasted
> sexual experience, not satisfying to myself or my wife. (Hite, 1981, p. 354)

    For our purposes, premature ejaculation might be defined primarily in terms of lack of control (Kaplan, 1974). In this view, a man might have an ejaculation problem whether intercourse lasts for ten seconds or ten minutes if he lacks control over the reflex. As one man put it:

> Regardless of the time (one minute or fifteen minutes), if it is not when I
> want it, most of the normal bodily sensations are lost. (Hite, 1981, p. 358)

    Most men gain increased control as they age, but the problem sometimes becomes worse instead of better. In these chronic cases, feelings of anxiety and guilt usually play a major role, and the problem may require sex therapy. Certainly, the man who cannot enjoy intercourse because of persistent and uncontrollable rapid ejaculation has a sexual dysfunction.

    **Causes of premature ejaculation** The sexual response patterns that lead to premature ejaculation are often established during adolescence. Among youths, masturbation or intercourse is often accompanied by guilt or the fear of being caught, so a young man learns to reach orgasm as quickly as possible. When a man ejaculates within minutes of intromission, following rapid thrusting, the problem may have more to do with a limited view of sexual interaction than with any physical or psychological difficulty (Gagnon, Rosen, and Leiblum, 1982).

    Rapid ejaculation is rarely caused by physical or medical factors. Prostatic or urethral infections can lead to uncontrolled ejaculation, as can drugs that stimulate the central nervous system. But almost all cases of premature ejaculation are due to psychogenic factors. Because ejaculation is controlled by the sympathetic branch

**premature ejaculation** lack of control over the ejaculatory reflex so that a man ejaculates rapidly and involuntarily

of the autonomic nervous system, emotional factors can affect it. Fear or anxiety can cause the sympathetic nervous system to overreact, triggering ejaculation. As with erectile dysfunction, rapid ejaculation is often accompanied by performance anxiety, which compounds the problem. The more a man thinks about it, the more anxious he becomes, and the faster he ejaculates.

When premature ejaculation is associated with marital discord, it may be an expression of the husband's hostility. By ejaculating rapidly, he deprives his wife of sexual satisfaction. However, the problem also occurs in relationships where there is no hostility between the partners. Sometimes premature ejaculation *causes* hostility in the woman when she is repeatedly frustrated and disappointed by her sexual experience. Thus, a serious and long-standing ejaculation problem is often accompanied by an orgasmic problem in the female partner. For this reason, the problem is generally viewed as a dysfunction of the sexual relationship (Masters and Johnson, 1970).

*Case* Maxwell C. (age 34), who had been married for six years, consulted a psychologist after losing his erection for the second time during intercourse. His wife had been complaining a great deal about his rapid ejaculation, which seemed to occur more and more quickly as Maxwell became increasingly anxious about his problem. Finally, his anxiety became so intense the he lost his erection before penetration could take place. (Authors' files)

**Overcoming premature ejaculation** Sexual folklore offers many home remedies for rapid ejaculation. Some men attempt to distract themselves from the excitement of intercourse with mental gymnastics—reviewing the stock market, counting sheep, or remembering an unpleasant incident. Others use creams or lotions that numb penile sensation. Still other believe that cold showers or strenuous exercise will slow their response. Any of these techniques may have some success, but all have a major limitation—they distract the man from the experience he seeks to enhance.

The most effective technique for dealing with premature ejaculation was developed by urologist James Semans (1956). The **Semans technique** is based on the idea that the man reaches orgasm after very low levels of sexual stimulation. To increase the required level of stimulation, the man masturbates until he feels that he is about to ejaculate, stops the stimulation until the sensation decreases, then resumes stimulation of his penis. The procedure is repeated until he can experience high levels of arousal without feeling a need to ejaculate. As he learns to tolerate high levels of stimulation, he will need to stop the stimulation less often.

This basic procedure was modified by Masters and Johnson (1970) to include the female partner. In the **squeeze technique**, the woman stimulates her partner, and whenever he feels the urge to ejaculate, she squeezes firmly around the frenulum of his penis. This squeezing eliminates the urge to ejaculate and may cause a partial loss of erection. After the urge passes, the woman restimulates her partner until the next squeeze becomes necessary. For this technique to be successful, the man must be able to tell his partner that ejaculation is imminent.

**Semans technique** a method of treating premature ejaculation in which a man masturbates until he is about to ejaculate, stops, then resumes stimulation, repeating the procedure until he can experience intense arousal without ejaculating

**squeeze technique** a variation of the Semans technique for treating premature ejaculation, in which a woman stimulates her partner, then squeezes the frenulum of his penis each time he feels the urge to ejaculate

Both the Semans technique and the squeeze technique are effective, but there are advantages in using the Semans technique before involving the partner. When a man stimulates himself, he can focus exclusively on his own sensations and learn to recognize the point at which orgasm cannot be forestalled. By practicing alone, when he does not have to worry about communicating this urgent information, he may build up confidence and reduce his anxiety. When he feels confident with his ejaculatory control, he can teach his partner to apply the technique (Zilbergeld, 1978).

Once a man has gained control of ejaculation with his partner applying manual or oral stimulation, the therapist may suggest that they attempt intercourse—but in a limited way, as with erectile dysfunction. Gradually, the couple may begin active thrusting. Should the man feel he cannot control his response, the couple moves back to a less demanding sexual interaction. Although intermittent failure may occur, this program successfully solves a large majority of ejaculatory problems.

## Delayed ejaculation

Just as some men cannot delay ejaculation for a reasonable period, others are over-controlled and cannot ejaculate when they would like. To describe the condition of a man who is unable to ejaculate, Masters and Johnson (1970) used the term ejaculatory incompetence, but some men find this label humiliating. Most therapists call the condition either **delayed ejaculation** or **retarded ejaculation**.

**delayed ejaculation** the inability to ejaculate

Delayed ejaculation can be either primary (present from the first sexual experience) or secondary (developing after a period of satisfactory sexual functioning). There is also "partial retarded ejaculation," which describes cases in which ejaculation occurs but is accompanied by little sensation or muscular contraction (Kaplan, 1974). In all these forms of delayed ejaculation, the man feels unable to ejaculate in the right way or at the right time despite a firm erection and a willing partner.

**Causes of delayed ejaculation** Delayed ejaculation has been a rare form of male sexual dysfunction, although there is some indication that its frequency is increasing. The pressures on men to hold off ejaculation for longer and longer periods may be responsible. In attempting to delay ejaculation, some men lose ejaculatory ability altogether, as in the following case.

*Case* John S. (38 years old) had been married for nine years. The couple sought counseling because he could not ejaculate during intercourse. During the early years of their marriage, he had used mental distraction techniques and regularly smoked marijuana before making love in order to delay his ejaculation until his wife could reach orgasm. But after their only child was born, John began to lose his erection before he ejaculated. The harder he tried, the more difficulty he had in reaching orgasm. With each successive failure to ejaculate, John experienced increased performance anxiety and an increasing sense of helplessness. His frustration at last led the couple to avoid sex altogether. (Authors' files)

Many psychogenic factors can play a role in delayed ejaculation. For example, religious fears or strong sexual taboos can be involved, as can fear of making a partner pregnant. In addition, men who are emotionally overcontrolled may find it difficult to "let go" and allow ejaculation to take place. Such men may develop great skill in satisfying their sexual partners, but be unable to reach orgasm themselves. In other cases, relationship conflicts can lead a man to withhold ejaculation as an expression of hostility, anger, fear, or distrust of his partner (Kaplan, 1974).

Maladaptive sexual learning patterns can also play a role. Unusual methods of masturbation may be responsible for some cases of delayed ejaculation (Mann, 1976). For these men, the pattern of stimulation provided by intercourse is too different from the stimulation provided by such masturbation techniques as striking the shaft of the penis forcefully with the heel of the hand, stroking the urethral meatus lightly with a cotton swab, or stimulating a spot on the shaft with rotary movements of the index finger. Men who have unusual masturbatory fantasies—especially those involving masochism—may also find it difficult to ejaculate inside the vagina.

It has also been proposed that some delayed ejaculators feel no desire at all, and that they are either disgusted by intercourse or feel it an unpleasant duty (Apfelbaum, 1980). These men find only their own touch arousing and easily enjoy orgasm when masturbating. They feel compelled to satisfy a partner, however, and despite their own lack of desire, they can maintain an erection for an hour if necessary, so that their partners often have several orgasms. In this view, the man regards sex as a continuous demand for performance. As one man said:

> Sometimes I feel like a sex machine. I can go on and on, but there's nothing in it for me. (Authors' files)

Although physical factors are rarely the direct cause of delayed ejaculation, in a few cases certain drugs and diseases may be involved. For instance, major tranquilizers, such as Mellaril, inhibit the sympathetic nervous system, leading to retrograde ejaculations or delayed ejaculation. Any disease, injury, or drug that affects the sympathetic nervous system or the nerves that control ejaculation can also cause delayed ejaculation, as we'll see in Chapter 18.

**Overcoming delayed ejaculation**  As with other male sexual problems, the first aim of therapy is to confront and relieve any performance anxieties. Structured tasks, such as exercises involving sensual massage, can divert a man's attention away from his problem and to the pleasurable sensations experienced in various parts of his body.

Men with this problem are characteristically preoccupied with thoughts about ejaculation during intercourse. This preoccupation reduces their physical pleasure and thus the likelihood of reaching orgasm. For these men, establishing a relaxed attitude is the first step toward overcoming retarded ejaculation.

As we've seen, some men with this problem ejaculate when masturbating or when a partner stimulates them manually or orally. With such men, **behavior shap-**

**behavior shaping** a procedure in which behavior is encouraged that comes closer and closer to an ultimate goal, a step at a time

**ing** may be effective. In behavior shaping, behavior is encouraged that comes closer and closer to an ultimate goal, so that a man is led, a step at a time, toward ejaculation during intercourse. The steps begin at the point at which the man can already function, and progress from private masturbation to ejaculation through various interactions with the partner until at last the man is able to ejaculate within the vagina.

If the man actually finds coitus unpleasant, as has been suggested, a program of behavior shaping, which is aimed at "forcing" an orgasm, would be impractical. Since the person already feels a heavy demand, treatment should be aimed at lessening pressure. The emphasis would be on expressing feelings. The man may be encouraged to complain, to express the notion that because he gets little out of coitus, he may well feel left out or used. In short, treatment follows the course generally taken with women who do not reach orgasm during intercourse (Apfelbaum, 1980).

Treatment of delayed ejaculation has had varying degrees of success. The chances of overcoming the problem depend on its duration, the health of the partner relationship, and the overall psychological health of the individual. Among seventeen couples treated by Masters and Johnson (1970), only three cases were unresolved at the end of therapy. However, among another group of cases, therapy failed with about 40 percent of the men (Mann, 1976). Some cases of delayed ejaculation are related to deeply engrained interpersonal problems, but with extended counseling, significant progress can often be made.

## LACK OF SEXUAL DESIRE

Dysfunctions of sexual desire are difficult to define and the most difficult of all sexual problems to overcome. Part of the difficulty in definition comes from the wide individual range in sexual desire. Since we have no standards of "normal" or "healthy" desire, there is no objective basis for saying that a person's sexual interest is "too high" or "too low" (Zilbergeld and Ellison, 1980). Often, the individual who has little interest in sex may not perceive herself (or himself) as having a problem at all.

It is important to distinguish between lack of desire and lack of arousal. Lack of sexual desire refers to how often a person wants sex, whereas lack of arousal refers to how excited or turned on a person gets during sex (Zilbergeld and Ellison, 1980). Men and women with low levels of sexual desire may have little urge to initiate or participate in sexual activities, yet may get turned on during sexual activity. Those with a lack of arousal may not respond to sexual situations or may respond physiologically—the woman may lubricate and the man get an erection—but experience little sexual pleasure. Some people find the experience so unpleasant that they avoid sex. Others enjoy sexual interaction, but simply do not want it as often as most people.

There are important gender differences in the way people deal with low sexual interest or lack of responsiveness. A man with no desire for sex typically avoids it for fear that he won't be able to get an erection. Some men with low levels of desire may eventually develop delayed ejaculation. In contrast, since a woman can have intercourse without desire or arousal, women with low levels of sexual interest often continue to engage in sex. For many women, closeness and intimacy, not orgasms, are the major benefit of sexual activity.

Low sexual interest may be a chronic condition that characterizes the entire sexual life cycle, or it may develop after some specific event. For example, some women complain that their sexual interest decreases dramatically after the birth of a child. Often these acute lapses in sexual interest disappear once the external environment changes. When the lack of desire becomes chronic, however, therapy may be helpful.

### Causes of low sexual desire

A loss of interest in sex can be caused by physiology, emotions, learning, a specific situation, or a combination of causes. Illness or any physical condition that places an unusual strain on the nervous system may be followed by a loss of desire. Certain drugs, especially sedatives and narcotics, can lead to central nervous system depression and consequently to reduced sexual desire. In addition, illness or certain surgical procedures, such as mastectomy, can be accompanied by psychological stress that in turn produces sexual unresponsiveness.

Lack of interest or unresponsiveness may also be related to another, more specific, form of sexual dysfunction. For example, a woman who does not reach orgasm or a man who cannot get an erection might gradually lose interest in sex because of repeated frustration and disappointment.

Unpleasant early sexual experiences, such as incest, rape, or molestation, can sometimes result in chronic sexual disinterest, as can thoroughly learning the lesson that sex is evil. Learning can also lead to low levels of sexual desire in other ways. Some people may not have learned to perceive their arousal as sexual or to label erotic sensations and situations as sexual (L. LoPiccolo, 1980).

Men with unusual sexual preferences, ranging from exhibiting the genitals through strong sadomasochistic fantasies, may also show low levels of sexual desire or arousal with a partner. Placed in a conventional sexual setting, they become unresponsive and disinterested (Kaplan, 1977).

Sometimes the loss of sexual desire is due to a relationship problem. Painful sexual rejection by a partner can lead to a defensive denial of sexuality (Kaplan, 1977). For example, a woman whose mate consistently rejects her sexual advances may decide that sex simply is not important. When lack of sexual interest in a partner follows a general loss of interest in the relationship, the causes are likely to be complex. A range of factors, from simple boredom with the relationship to deep-seated hostility toward the partner, can lead to emotional detachment and loss of sexual desire (Barbach, 1982).

*Case* Max and Carol, a couple in their mid-twenties, had been living together for three years. Max, a third-year medical student, felt very frustrated by Carol's growing lack of interest in sex. Carol, who worked as a laboratory assistant, felt equally frustrated by Max's preoccupation with his medical-school training. His school pressures had become so great that the couple spent little time together. Carol also complained that when they had sex, Max was usually impatient and rushed through foreplay. Although Carol was able to become aroused and have orgasms, she was seldom in the mood for sex and rarely initiated it. Max agreed that during the week they saw too little of each other but usually planned to make it up on the weekends. By the time the weekend began, he said, he'd been bottling up his desire all week and generally felt very horny. When Carol showed no interest in his advances, he would become angry and the couple often found themselves arguing about something. Max saw Carol's low level of sexual desire as a major problem for them. (Authors' files)

In this case, Carol's lack of desire deepened as Max's medical training increasingly interfered with their general relationship.

Under the best of circumstances, however, Max and Carol may each have a different level of sexual desire. When couples complain that one partner lacks interest in sex, the problem is often due to a **desire discrepancy,** in which the partners' general level of sexual interest differs. When the relationship is going well, the partners may adjust to each other's wishes with only minor friction. But when the relationship is having other problems, the discrepancy may become the battleground, with resentments, hurts, and hostilities transferred to the issue of sexual frequency (Barbach, 1982).

**desire discrepancy** a difference in the general level of sexual interest between sexual partners

## *Overcoming desire problems*

Because problems of desire encompass a broad range of difficulties and are primarily subjective in nature, there is no generally agreed-upon course of treatment. Some therapists (Kaplan, 1977) report that sexual desire problems account for a significant number of failures in therapy programs and recommend psychotherapy as a way of gaining insight into the underlying cause. Although this might be valuable for some individuals, it would probably not help someone with a constitutionally low desire level or cases in which the lack of desire is primarily a relationship problem.

If a specific sexual problem, such as orgasmic or erectile dysfunction, exists, working on that problem is often helpful. Once the dysfunction is overcome, sexual desire often increases.

If sexual boredom is the problem, changing the script to make sexual activity more interesting to one or more partners may be the answer (Gagnon, Rose, and Leiblum, 1982). In such cases, techniques like those suggested in Chapter 13 would be helpful.

If the problem is a discrepancy in desire, a counseling approach based on compromise may work best (Rosen and Leiblum, 1976). Since low sexual interest may be more of a problem for the rejected partner than for the individual who is experiencing it, frank communication can sometimes lead to options acceptable to both partners. For example, mutual masturbation, oral sex, or massage might be included as substitute sexual activities, and the couple might compromise on their rate of sexual activity. At times, simply cuddling and being close might be enough. A mature recognition and acceptance of the differences in sexual need between partners is a great advantage in coping with this problem.

Not all cases of low sexual desire respond to counseling or therapy. Sometimes increasing dissatisfaction leads a couple to separate. In other circumstances, the couple may settle for a relationship without sex.

## SEXUAL COUNSELING AND THERAPY

When sexual problems arise, they don't always require intensive therapy or referral to a specialist. Short-term sexual difficulties that are accepted as a normal part of life often disappear with the passage of time. In other cases, a physician, a nurse, a minister, or even a sympathetic friend or family member can be of great help. As we'll see, sometimes we can solve our own sexual problems. When the problems become long-standing or complicated sexual dysfunctions, however, they usually require help from a qualified professional.

The first modern sex therapy was carried out in the late 1950s by behavior therapists, who stressed the role of learning and conditioning. Using these principles, they helped people overcome such common problems as lack of orgasm or erectile dysfunction.

It was the work of Masters and Johnson (1979) that provided the first detailed description of procedures for overcoming sexual dysfunction. They stressed the psychological basis of most sexual problems and the role of reeducation in solving them. Some of the earlier behavioral work was integrated into their approach. A little later, Helen Singer Kaplan (1974) combined the Masters and Johnson focus on specific problems with a psychoanalytic awareness of deeper conflicts. Yet she maintained that working on current anxieties instead of childhood problems was the most practical solution.

As we've seen in this chapter, sex therapists now use a combination of techniques aimed at eliminating sexual myths and misinformation, changing attitudes, enhancing communication, and altering specific behavior. Their strategies include masturbation, fantasy, behavioral rehearsal, ways to reduce anxiety, and explicit homework assignments (Figure 14.3) that range from massage and self-stimulation to exercises in communication. Programs are tailored specifically to the needs and goals of each person (Leiblum and Pervin, 1980).

Many large universities and medical schools have established sexual counseling services that provide treatment for a range of sexual problems. In addition to

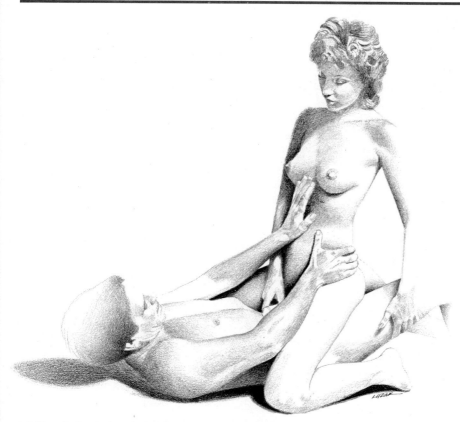

Additional stimulation during intercourse can be obtained by means of a vibrator. This method is sometimes recommended in sex therapy for women who wish to achieve orgasm with a partner.

offering basic therapy services, these programs generally provide educational and consultation services as well.

Most sexual counseling programs include certain basic elements. When either or both partners have negative attitudes toward sex, attitude change is necessary. In such cases, the development of positive attitudes is an essential aspect of counseling.

To eliminate performance anxiety, couples are usually instructed to refrain from intercourse during the first stage of counseling. Instead, they are instructed in techniques of nondemanding touching and caressing, so that they learn to relax in a sexual situation.

With the aim of improving communication as sexual technique, therapists encourage partners to use verbal and nonverbal methods to indicate the type of stimulation each finds most effective. They are also encouraged to invent new, mutually acceptable, patterns of sexual interaction and to share their fantasies (Gagnon, Rose, and Leiblum, 1982).

Sexual counseling, either individual, with couples, or in groups, can be of great help in teaching people to handle stressful situations. (© Bohdan Hrynewych/ Stock, Boston)

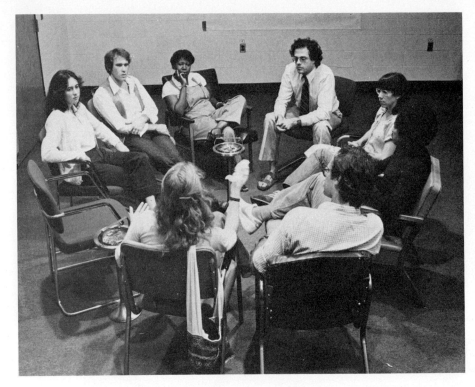

The dominant male and submissive female roles often inhibit progress in a sex therapy program. For this reason, counselors encourage couples to ease their rigid sex roles during the course of therapy and to share responsibility for initiating sexual experiences.

*Case* When Steve and Elaine M. (age 24 and 22) sought therapy, they were having sex less than once a month. Their problem appeared to be Steve's inability to maintain an erection long enough for intercourse. But questioning revealed that Elaine had never been able to have an orgasm during intercourse, although she easily reached orgasm with manual or oral stimulation. Elaine was not upset about her "problem," but Steve seemed to feel that her lack of orgasm during intercourse was due to his own incompetence as a lover. He felt guilty about sex and tried to perform in ways that would bring Elaine to orgasm, becoming so anxious about Elaine's orgasm that he could not maintain an erection. Steve's problem was directly related to Elaine's lack of orgasm during intercourse, and it was the couple—not either individual—that was sexually dysfunctional. The problem was overcome when both partners accepted their mutual responsibility, relaxing the traditional sexual script that required Steve to initiate and direct activities and limited Elaine to responding. (Authors' files)

In addition to a general therapy program, directive counseling is used from time to time. The therapist recommends specific techniques for dealing with the couple's particular problem.

A controversial innovation in treatment involves the techniques of nude encounter and sexual contact with the therapist. As yet these methods have been used in sex therapy programs in only a few isolated centers (Hartman and Fithian, 1974). During a "sexological examination," therapists touch and stimulate the breasts or genitals of patients to determine responses to stimulation and areas of maximum sensitivity. Such techniques are easily abused, and they have been rejected by most therapists. Similarly, the use of surrogate partners or "body therapists"—individuals who are paid to provide sexual instruction and participate in sex with the dysfunctional person—has been abandoned by most therapists because of the potential for abuse.

The first popular articles about sex therapy made it sound as if every dysfunction responds immediately to treatment. But the passing of time has made it clear that those articles were far too optimistic, and today a reevaluation of sex therapy has begun.

## Does sex therapy work?

The news that Masters and Johnson (1970) had treated nearly 800 cases of sexual dysfunction with two weeks of therapy and a reported failure rate of only 20 percent revolutionized the treatment of sexual problems. Their method was brief, but intensive. Couples had to spend two weeks in St. Louis, where they had physical examination, daily therapy sessions that lasted an hour or more, and extensive homework assignments. The therapy was aimed at dispelling sexual ignorance, changing attitudes, improving communication, and enabling the couple to enjoy physically pleasurable sexual interaction. A central technique was **sensate focus**, exercises in which the couples experimented with gently stroking and caressing each other's bodies free from the performance demands of intercourse.

**sensate focus** exercises in which couples experiment by gently stroking and caressing each other's bodies free from the performance demands of intercourse

Across the country, therapists began applying the Masters and Johnson technique—or some version of it—to the sexual problems of their clients. At first, reports were rosy. Men said their erections were firm or that they could delay ejaculation; women said that intercourse was no longer painful or that they were beginning to have orgasms. A sexual paradise appeared to be within the grasp of every human being.

Then came the disquieting news that the quick fix for sexual problems was not so successful. The "easy" cases seemed to have disappeared, and more and more therapists began wondering what had gone wrong. Some (Zilbergeld and Evans, 1980) charged that it was impossible to evaluate Masters and Johnson's research and that their published reports were vague, misleading, and riddled with statistical error. Other therapists (Levine and Agle, 1978), who began following clients closely after therapy was over, reported varied results. By the time a year had passed, success rates were down to only 6 percent (if the criterion was the elimination of all sexual problems in both partners) or 63 percent (if the criterion was

*Focus*

BEING
YOUR OWN
SEX
THERAPIST

When sexual problems are simple, many of them can be alleviated without the aid of a counselor. Therapists have tested the idea of simply giving written information to people with sexual problems and found that it often works. Married women with primary orgasmic dysfunction who followed a six-week program described in a booklet were about as successful in reaching orgasm as women who had been treated by Masters and Johnson in their intensive therapy program (McMullen and Rosen, 1979). Eighty percent of the women reached orgasm through masturbation, and more than half were able to transfer the response to intercourse.

As both this chapter and Chapter 10 have shown, sexual functioning is often disrupted by misinformation, unrealistic expectations, sexual anxiety, and faulty communication. By following this general guide, you may be able to tackle a problem that plagues your own sexual relationship and improve your own sex life.

First, inform yourself. The ignorance and misinformation that are the basis of many problems can be dispelled by reading one or more of the excellent self-help books that are available. These books, most of them in paperback, build on the information in this text and provide specific exercises and helpful examples.

FOR WOMEN
Lonnie G. Barbach. *For Yourself: The Fulfillment of Female Sexuality.* Anchor Books, 1976.
Lonnie G. Barbach. *For Each Other: Sharing Sexual Intimacy.* Doubleday, 1982.
Julia Heiman, Leslie LoPiccolo, and Joseph LoPiccolo. *Becoming Orgasmic: A Sexual Growth Program for Women.* Prentice-Hall, 1976.
FOR MEN
Joseph Nowinski. *Becoming Satisfied: A Man's Guide to Sexual Fulfillment.* Prentice-Hall, 1980.
Bernie Zilbergeld. *Male Sexuality.* Bantam Books, 1978.
FOR EVERYONE
Harvey L. Gochros and Joe Fischer. *Treat Yourself to a Better Sex Life.* Prentice-Hall, 1980.
Debora Phillips and Robert Judd. *Sexual Confidence.* Bantam Books, 1982.

If you've been unable to find a self-help book, try to develop a relaxed attitude toward sexual encounters. Anxiety over sex can lead to mechanistic, unfeeling sex or can totally disrupt interaction. For this reason, many therapists recommend a series of relaxation exercises to provide practice in reducing tension throughout the body. Simply taking deep, slow breaths can give you a start. Before engaging in sex, take a relaxing bath or practice body massage. Some of the suggestions in Chapter 6 may be helpful.

Slow down. Sexual performance is not the only

"some improvement"). One psychiatrist (Szasz, 1980) rejected the entire concept of sex therapy, saying that telling someone how to behave sexually was inconsistent with allowing people to discover and develop their own style of sexuality.

Robert Kolodny (1981), one of Masters and Johnson's collaborators, maintains that most therapists who have low success rates fail to adhere to the Masters and Johnson methods. (See Table 14.1.) Few require couples to leave their homes

criterion of enjoyment. Forget about erections, ejaculations, or orgasms and focus on the pleasure of sexual interaction. Above all, avoid watching yourself perform. Any self-monitoring of your sexual activities should be banished from the bedroom.

Talk to your partner about your concerns and express your feelings about the problem as fully as you can. Reread Chapter 10 and try some of the suggestions for communicating more effectively. Listen to your partner and try to see the problem from his (or her) point of view.

If you are thinking that sex would be wonderful if only your partner would change, you are almost certain to be on the wrong track. You are unlikely to change your partner's behavior as long as your own words and actions remain the same because much of your partner's behavior may be a response to something you are doing. Most sexual problems involve the relationship and require both partners to change. If there are major differences between you, try negotiation. Compromise is often the best course.

Apply the suggested methods for preventing sexual boredom that were suggested in Chapter 13. Sometimes these switches in sexual patterns and the devotion of special time to each other help to alleviate problems. For example, changing the time, the place, or the circumstances of sex may ease your situation. The old line about the frequency of intercourse—twice a week at home and every day on vacation—has a good deal of truth in it.

Try new methods of foreplay. Who ever said the sexual script had to progress in the same way in every encounter? Try new positions. If premature ejaculation is a problem, simply switching to a woman-above position may delay the response. Indeed, the woman-above position is the position most frequently prescribed by sex therapists for most dysfunctions. But don't let that recommendation confine you to a single position, either.

If you've tried all these steps and the problem persists, seek professional help. It may be that an undetected relationship problem is spilling over into your sexual life or that your dysfunction has some organic base.

The best course is to contact a university or medical school in your area. Many of them have sex therapy clinics. If there is no clinic near you, contact the American Association of Sex Educators, Counselors, and Therapists (AASECT), 600 Maryland Avenue SW, Washington, D.C. 20024 for a list of qualified sex therapists near you.

and to focus exclusively for two weeks on their sexual interaction. Many therapists have added new twists (such as the "sexological" exam) to the program or changed some of the practices. Kolodny admits, however, that the overall failure rate should have been reported as 23 percent, not 20 percent. He also agrees that therapy for these couples did not end in two weeks, but continued with lengthy telephone sessions over the next year or so—whenever a couple felt the need to

*Table 14.1   Success of sex therapy at the Masters & Johnson Institute (1959–1977)*

| TYPE OF PROBLEM | NO. OF CASES | OVERALL SUCCESS RATE |
| --- | --- | --- |
| Primary erectile dysfunction | 51 | 66.7% |
| Secondary erectile dysfunction | 501 | 78.4% |
| Premature ejaculation | 432 | 96.1% |
| Retarded ejaculation | 75 | 76.0% |
| MALE TOTAL: | 1,059 | 84.9% |
| | | |
| Primary anorgasmia | 399 | 79.0% |
| Situational anorgasmia | 331 | 71.0% |
| Vaginismus | 83 | 98.8% |
| FEMALE TOTAL: | 813 | 77.7% |

*Source:* R. C. Kolodny, "Evaluating Sex Therapy: Process and Outcome at the Masters & Johnson Institute," *Journal of Sex Research,* 17 (1981), 301–318, table from 312.

consult a therapist. Finally, he points out that the reversal of a sexual symptom does not always translate into marital satisfaction.

The argument is not over. Some therapists have concluded that the idea of a quick cure is foolish, but that the promise of improved sexual functioning can be made to most people with a clear conscience. When sexual problems are due to superficial causes and the couple's relationship is basically sound, therapy can clear up the dysfunction in short order. But when emotional conflicts or power struggles underlie a sexual problem, it may fail to respond to treatment or its solution may disrupt the relationship in other ways. Sexual paradise is still out of reach.

# *Summary*

**1** Almost every woman and man has some sexual problem at some stage of the life cycle, but to become a **sexual dysfunction**, the problem must develop into an incapacity that interferes with sexual functioning.

**2** The existence of sexual problems is influenced by the way a society defines sexual functioning and their extent depends on physical health, beliefs, attitudes, childhood experiences, and cultural expectations. There is no absolute standard for sexual functioning, so that what is considered a sexual problem and how it is treated change with time.

**3** About 10 percent of women have **primary orgasmic dysfunction**; they have never experienced orgasm from any kind of stimulation. Such women are called **preorgasmic** because most can learn to have orgasms in at least some situations. A larger group of women with secondary orgasmic dysfunction generally have trouble reaching orgasm during intercourse but often are orgasmic with manual or oral stimulation. The condition may be a normal variation of female sexuality, in which coital thrusting does not provide enough stimulation to trigger the orgasm reflex. Most orgasmic dysfunctions are caused by learning, psychological inhibitions, or some aspect of a woman's relationship. Orgasmic dysfunction has been successfully treated with a guided masturbation training program. A woman with secondary orgasmic dysfunction may require additional clitoral stimulation in order to reach orgasm during intercourse.

**4** Penetration problems include **vaginismus**, in which muscles around the vagina contract so tightly that intercourse is difficult or impossible, and **dyspareunia**, pain and discomfort during intercourse. **Dyspareunia** may be due to a vaginal, cervical, or uterine infection, endometriosis, scar tissue in the vagina, or inadequate vaginal lubrication. Dyspareunia can be treated by clearing up the physical causes or using an artificial lubricant. Vaginismus is usually due to fears about intercourse or negative sexual experiences in the past. Treatment for vaginismus begins with muscle relaxation and continues with the reduction of sensitivity to vaginal penetration.

**5** In **primary erectile dysfunction**, a man has never been able to keep an erection long enough to have intercourse; in **secondary erectile dysfunction**, he fails in at least 25 percent of his attempts. Erectile problems may have an organic or a psychogenic basis; sometimes both factors are implicated. Organic causes include drugs and medication and diseases or disorders that affect hormone balance, nerve pathways, or blood supply to the penis. Immediate psychogenic factors include **performance anxiety** (fear of failure), sexual demands, relationship factors, inability to relax, and emotional stress. Remote psychogenic factors include childhood conditioning, negative attitudes toward sex, religious indoctrination, parental dominance, and repressed or conflicting homosexual feelings. Where blood supply or nerve pathways are permanently disrupted, a **penile prosthesis** can be surgically implanted to provide an erection. In cases of psychogenic erectile dysfunction, therapists encourage a flexible, pleasure-oriented approach to sexual encounters, while working on relationship problems and overcoming the man's fear of failure.

**6** In **premature ejaculation**, a man lacks control over the ejaculatory reflex and ejaculates rapidly and uncontrollably. Although drugs and infection can lead to uncontrolled ejaculation, premature ejaculation is almost always due to psychogenic factors. Fear, anxiety, or hostility toward a partner can lead to premature ejaculation. The most effective treatments for premature ejaculation are the **Semans technique** and the **squeeze technique**. In **delayed ejaculation**, a man is overcontrolled and cannot ejaculate. The major causes of delayed ejaculation are religious fears, sexual taboos, the inability to let go, continual attempts to delay ejaculation, relationship conflicts, and unusual methods of masturbation. Delayed ejaculation is treated by relieving performance anxiety and establishing a relaxed attitude. **Behavior shaping** is useful unless the man actually finds coitus unpleasant. In this case, treatment follows a course similar to that used with women who have orgasmic dysfunctions.

**7** Dysfunctions of sexual desire are difficult to define and to treat. Lack of sexual desire can develop from illness, stress, drugs, other sexual dysfunctions, unpleasant early sexual experiences, or relationship problems. Sometimes the problem is the result of **desire discrepancy**, in which the partners' general level of sexual interest differs. There is no single course of treatment for problems of desire. Treatment may involve psychotherapy, overcoming specific sexual dysfunctions, and changing the sexual script. If a discrepancy exists, compromise is generally the most effective approach.

**8** The first modern sex therapy was carried out in the late 1950s by behavior therapists, who stressed the role of learning and conditioning. Adopting some of their techniques, Masters and Johnson stressed the psychological basis of most sexual problems and the role of reeducation in solving them. Helen Kaplan combined the Masters and Johnson focus with a psychoanalytic awareness of deeper conflicts. Today sex therapists use a combination of education, attitude change, enhancement of communication, and change in specific behavior. In recent years, many sex therapists have found that sexual dysfunctions do not always respond to treatment as rapidly as Masters and Johnson's reports indicated. However, few therapists follow Masters and Johnson's intensive approach to treatment. It appears that problems with superficial causes can be cleared up rapidly, but problems due to emotional conflicts or power struggles may require lengthy treatment and may not always respond to therapy. When sexual difficulties are simple and can be treated with specific information, improved communication, and varying the sexual script, people can often solve their own problems.

# Part Five

# Sexual Variations and Complications

Despite a long search, anthropologists, archeologists, and historians have been unable to find a culture with unlimited sexual freedom. Throughout history, societies have always placed restrictions on the sexual behavior of members. Yet there is little agreement among cultures as to which behavior is socially acceptable and which unacceptable.

Perhaps the only sexual conduct that is prohibited in virtually every society is incest, and there are even exceptions to this taboo. Among the royal families of ancient Egypt and Peru, marriage between brothers and sisters was encouraged in order to preserve the purity of the ruling family. Cultures cannot even agree on a definition of incest: some groups limit it to sexual contact between immediate family members, and others extend the definition to include second or third cousins or all the members of one's tribe.

A culture may enforce its standards of sexual conduct by passing laws that make their violation a criminal offense. However, laws against many sexual acts between consenting adults are rarely enforced. The private nature of sodomy, adultery, cohabitation, or homosexuality makes their prosecution almost impossible, and many people believe that such acts are not the business of society. Other laws against sexual acts are enforced sporadically and inconsistently. For example, crackdowns on prostitution seem to alternate with legal indifference, and the streetwalker runs much greater risk of arrest than the woman who works in a massage parlor.

In general, the law intervenes when sexual conduct falls into any of three categories: when there is no legal consent—as in rape or child molestation; when a social nuisance is created or public standards of decency are offended—as in exhibitionism; or when sex is used for commercial purposes—as in prostitution.

In the first of this unit's two chapters, we discuss unusual sexual variations called paraphilias and look at transvestism and transsexualism. The second chapter will investigate the many forms of sexual coercion and abuse, including rape, child molestation, sexual harassment, and incest—as well as prostitution, which may involve exploitation or coercion.

## exhibitionism experience

When I was younger, a man exposed his penis to me in a shopping mall. I couldn't believe it—it seemed ridiculous and also disgusting. I looked the other way and kept walking, and I never told anyone about it. When I thought about it afterward, it seemed like a pathetic thing to do, but also a very aggressive act. (Authors' files)

## fetishism experience

It's really weird, you know, these guys put out a lot of green to do some of the damnedest things ... like dressing up like a cheerleader and letting them feel me up under my sweater while they jerk off. Another guy pays me $50 every other Friday to sit on the john and take a leak while he stands in front of me and jerks off. Another kinky wants me to dress in this leather outfit I wear to ride my cycle and let him rub his joint all over me. (Tollison and Adams, 1979, p. 265)

# 15 Unconventional Sexual Behavior

# *Chapter 15*

As we grow up, most of us adopt the conventional sexual standards of our society. But some people become sexually attracted to odd objects, unusual partners, or unconventional acts. Their sexual standards are different from those of the community, and their sexual activities sometimes conflict with the laws of that community.

Implicit in the concept of sexual standards is the notion that some patterns of sexual behavior are "normal" and that any behavior falling outside this standard is "deviant" or "abnormal." However, the dividing line between the normal and the abnormal is not so clear as most people believe. A number of prominent sexologists have said that we have no absolute standards for sexual normality (Ellis, 1956).

In this chapter, we consider the various attempts people have made to distinguish normal sexual behavior from abnormal. Next we will discuss the unusual sexual acts that are called paraphilias, examining the motivations and characteristics connected with such behavior. We will then compare transvestism, which is considered a paraphilia, with transsexualism, a problem in gender identity. Finally, we will explore some of the methods that have been used to treat sexual variations.

## WHAT IS NORMAL?

There are several ways to define normality, and although each separates the normal from the abnormal in a fairly straightforward manner, none can by itself include all human sexual behavior. The approaches commonly used are moral, statistical, and psychological.

# Unconventional Sexual Behavior

Perhaps the most restrictive way of determining normality is the moral approach. The Judeo-Christian religious tradition maintains that only sexual behavior which can lead to conception within marriage is moral. All other sexual acts are immoral: they are perverted, debauched, aberrant, unnatural, abnormal, and so on. But there are problems with the moral approach. As noted earlier, what is considered moral in one culture may be immoral—or at least disapproved—in another. Among some groups, premarital intercourse is considered both moral and necessary. In other cultures, no man will take a bride who has not already demonstrated her fertility by producing a child.

In addition, standards of morality change, as we all know from the changing attitudes in our own culture. Today most of us see no conflict between morality and practices like oral sex and contraception.

Another way of defining normality is with the statistical approach. In this view, normal sexuality is average behavior—whatever many people in a society do. Normal in terms of this approach are masturbation, premarital and extramarital intercourse, oral sex, homosexual behavior, and prostitution. But normality in the statistical sense would also include child molestation, since it occurs with high frequency in the United States (Sanford, 1980).

Again, what is statistically normal in one culture may be extremely rare in another—because by a statistical standard, normal behavior receives this label whenever cultural attitudes approve of an act and it becomes widely practiced. If attitudes and habits change, so does the standard of normality. An act may be statistically abnormal at one period, but normal a decade or so later.

A third approach to defining sexual normality uses a psychological definition of acceptable behavior. Psychologically healthy sexuality is assumed to be mature, well-adjusted, and

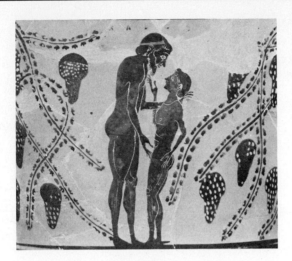

What is considered ''normal'' sexual behavior varies from culture to culture. A relationship between an older man and a youth was considered desirable in ancient Greece. (Cup, *Man and Boy,* Attic Black Figured. Gift of E. P. and Fiske Warren. Courtesy, Museum of Fine Arts, Boston)

personally and interpersonally fulfilling. It should not lead to such negative emotional states as anxiety or guilt. But many people who engage in coitus feel anxious or guilty about it, and some people who practice unconventional sexual acts are personally satisfied and feel little guilt or anxiety. The extent to which a person is upset about sexual behavior often has more to do with social training than with a specific practice.

The psychological definition of normality leads to the assumption that abnormal sexuality has its roots in psychological disturbance and that bizarre sexual behavior is the direct result of an underlying psychological "disease" or maladjustment. In this view, a man who is sexually aroused by, say, rubbing against a woman in a crowded subway car and regularly reaches orgasm that way would be considered "sick."

Many attempts have been made to classify sexual variations within a psychiatric framework, beginning with Richard von Krafft-Ebing, who compiled an impressive, if somewhat horrifying, compendium of all known forms of sexual deviance. Krafft-Ebing's work, and the psychiatric classification systems developed after him, were based on the notion that abnormal sexual behavior is directly linked to some form of mental illness. But "deviant" behavior takes place in a social context. In many cases, it is the process of being labeled as deviant by society rather than the specific sexual behavior that causes psychological problems. When a sexual act is labeled "deviant," the person who commits it is an outsider, because he or she has broken one of society's rules (Gagnon and Simon, 1973). Society typically responds to the "deviant" with ostracism, imprisonment, or some form of therapy.

The most practical and least harmful approach might be to consider as abnormal only those acts that a person feels compelled to perform, that make the person unhappy, or that bring physical harm or psychological distress to another person. Such a definition would take context into consideration and admit that what is normal in one situation might well be abnormal in another.

# THE CONCEPT OF PARAPHILIAS

Therapists no longer use the terms "sexual perversion" or "sexual deviance." Instead, they refer to unusual or bizarre sexual patterns as **paraphilias**. Paraphilia comes from the Greek word *para,* which means "beside," "beyond," or "amiss," and *philia,* which means "love." A person with a paraphilia is sexually aroused by behavior, objects, or partners that are forbidden or statistically abnormal in his or her society. For example, exhibitionism, which involves exposing the genitals to a stranger, does not exist in a society in which clothing is not worn. The American Psychiatric Association (Webb et al., 1981) takes the view that paraphilias can be considered disorders only if a person prefers the unusual sexual pattern or finds it necessary to achieve arousal or orgasm.

**paraphilia** preference for or dependence on unusual or bizarre objects, partners, or acts for sexual arousal and gratification

Because paraphilia is a medical diagnosis, inferring illness, some people object to its use when the unusual behavior takes place between two consenting adults. In such cases, the term "sexual variation," which is less judgmental, is generally used.

According to John Money (1981), all paraphilias involve some forbidden or unusual image that is enacted again and again, either in fantasy or in reality, for the purpose of becoming aroused and reaching orgasm. Thus, the action of a man who exposes himself to a passing woman might be based on his image of her shocked reaction to the sight of his genitals.

Money proposes that paraphilias belong to either the proceptive or acceptive phases of pair bonding (Chapter 2). That is, a paraphilia distorts a courtship ritual or the phase of mutual body contact. Sometimes the distortion displaces a typical element of the sexual relation from its normal sequence. For example, the fondling of an intimate partner may be displaced onto a stranger, as in the case of the man who becomes excited by rubbing against a clothed stranger. At other times, the distortion incorporates some element into the sexual script that is not typically part of it. For example, some people can achieve sexual gratification only if the partner gives them an enema.

Most paraphilias are restricted to males, and no one is certain just why this sex difference should occur. The major explanations focus on either biology or learning. A biological basis has been suggested by Money (1981). He believes that males' susceptibility to these disorders is related to the male vulnerability discussed in Chapter 2. Males lack the protection of the extra X chromosome and succumb more easily than females to disease and death at all stages of development. In this line of reasoning, the development of sexuality is more complicated and vulnerable in males than in females and so is more likely to go awry.

Not all authorities agree with this explanation. John Gagnon and William Simon (1973) emphasize learning and the importance of the male sex role in the development of paraphilias. Sexual patterns among males show wide variation; men are more likely than women to use sexual fantasy, to have variety, and to have impersonal sex. Men are also taught to initiate sexual encounters and thus have more opportunities to fail. These elements make men more likely than women to develop unconventional sexual patterns.

The most common paraphilias are voyeurism, exhibitionism, fetishism, sadism, masochism, and pedophilia. In many cases paraphilias are harmless, but taken to an extreme some can lead to injury, or even death.

## *Voyeurism*

Most men are sexually aroused by the sight of a nude—or nearly nude—woman. Beauty contests, topless bars, strippers, and men's magazines provide ample testimony to the appeal. But the businessman who ogles the topless dancer and the youth who masturbates while gazing at the centerfold in *Playboy* are not demonstrating a paraphilia. Neither is the pedestrian who stops to watch when his attention is caught by the sight of a woman disrobing in front of an open window.

**voyeurism** a preference for or dependence on the illicit observation of a woman or couple undressing or engaging in sexual activity for sexual arousal and gratification

**Voyeurism** becomes a sexual disorder when the watcher prefers his spying to intercourse, when the woman (or the couple) he is watching does not consent to his observations, and when he persists in his habit at considerable risk to himself. A voyeur will climb fences, perch on window ledges, or hide in bushes, sitting patiently for hours as he waits for a woman to disrobe (Tollison and Adams, 1979). Typically, he wants only to look and does not attempt contact with his victim. His

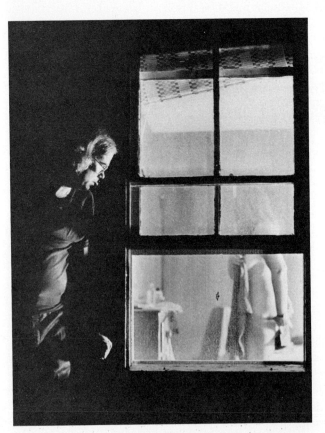

The voyeur's primary source of sexual satisfaction lies in watching an unsuspecting woman disrobe or a couple making love. (© Laine Whitcomb)

sexual excitement depends on viewing a forbidden scene—he must see without being seen. For this reason, the voyeur is not satisfied with watching women at nudist camps or in topless bars (Sagarin, 1974; Gebhard et al., 1965).

Many voyeurs masturbate while peering at their victims. Others achieve gratification later, recalling the scene from memory while masturbating or having intercourse with their wives. Some voyeurs cannot maintain an erection during intercourse unless they focus on images of their exploits.

Voyeurs are also called "Peeping Toms," after the thirteenth-century peeper who watched Lady Godiva ride naked through the market of Coventry, England, to protest against unreasonable taxation. Out of respect for her, the citizens of the town remained behind locked doors and barred shutters. However, one young man, named Tom, could not resist temptation. He peered out from behind the shutters and, it is said, was struck blind for his curiosity (Bullough, 1976).

Voyeurism is a disorder of the proceptive phase of sexuality, in which visual attraction to a partner is displaced from a preliminary to intercourse to the focus of sexual activity. Voyeurs seem invariably to be heterosexual men. No genuine case of compulsive voyeurism has ever been found among women, and therapists have reported no cases of homosexual voyeurs (Money, 1981).

The person who becomes a voyeur often has significant problems in his relations with others, as the following case indicates.

*Case* William V. (age 28) is a computer programmer who was arrested as a Peeping Tom. He lives alone and grew up in a rural area within a conservative, highly religious family. When he was fifteen, he masturbated for the first time while watching his older sister urinate in an outdoor toilet. Despite considerable guilt, he continued to masturbate two or three times a week while having voyeuristic fantasies.

On the summer evening when he was arrested, William had climbed a ladder and was peeping into the bedroom of a suburban home. Just before this incident he had been drinking heavily at a cocktail lounge featuring a topless dancer. When he left the lounge, he had intended to go home, but feeling lonely and depressed, he instead drove slowly through a nearby neighborhood, where he noticed a lighted upstairs window. With little premeditation, he parked his car and used a ladder he found nearby to climb up where he could look inside. The noise he made alerted the residents, who called the police. This was William's first arrest.

Although he was able to perform sexually with a female partner, William was beset with guilt over his sexual behavior, particularly his masturbation. Six months before his arrest, he had been rejected by a woman with whom he had had a lengthy relationship. He had not yet recovered from this experience. William was unassertive and timid, and so had responded to his rejection by withdrawing from social relationships and drinking heavily. As his self-esteem deteriorated, his voyeuristic fantasies became increasingly urgent. (Authors' files)

Research with convicted peepers indicates that the majority of voyeurs have little heterosexual experience, are shy with women, and have strong feelings of inferiority (Gebhard et al., 1965). Although some voyeurs are married, many say they are anxious and fearful at the prospect of forming a heterosexual relationship (Tollison and Adams, 1979).

How does voyeurism develop? Some psychologists say that shy, inadequate youths peep to satisfy their sexual curiosity and to meet their sexual needs without actually approaching a woman. In this way, they avoid whatever failure and low self-esteem might follow an unhappy heterosexual encounter. Peeping also gives voyeurs a feeling of power and allows them to feel superior to the women they watch (Coleman, 1972).

In the behavioral view, voyeurism is the result of learning and conditioning, in which orgasm reinforces the act of peeping. If the sight is sexually arousing and the watcher masturbates at the scene or while recalling the act, the association is strengthened. Inadequate social skills, a fear of women, or sexual guilt from a puritanical upbringing make it more likely that the association will become strong, because peeping provides enjoyable sexual satisfaction without the threat of heterosexual interaction (Tollison and Adams, 1979).

## *Exhibitionism*

**exhibitionism** the deliberate exposure of the genitals in a public place with the intent of obtaining sexual stimulation; also called "flashing"

Public display of the genitals is not always exhibitionism. For example, the drunk urinating on a streetcorner or the man whose zipper inadvertently slips open has no sexual intent. As a paraphilia, **exhibitionism** involves the deliberate exposure of the genitals in a public place with the intent of obtaining sexual stimulation. The exhibitionist feels compelled to repeat the performance and usually seeks no further contact with his victim, although he may be aroused by shock or surprise. Exhibitionism, also called "flashing," is extremely common and accounts for more than a third of all arrests for sexual offenses.

Like voyeurism, exhibitionism is a disorder of the proceptive phase of sexual activity, in which display of the genitals, part of the preliminary sexual activity, becomes the primary means of sexual stimulation. Again, nearly all exhibitionists are heterosexual men. Differences in sex roles may help to explain why there are almost no female exhibitionists. As girls grow up, they learn to place greater emphasis on modesty and the privacy of sexual contacts than boys do. In addition, women rarely see the exposure of their genitals as an affirmation of self-worth or identity, as some authorities believe men do.

There is no single kind of exhibitionist. Some expose a flaccid penis and make no attempt to approach the victim. Others masturbate while they expose themselves, fantasizing sexual intercourse with an aroused victim. Still others have aggressive fantasies and hope that the victim will be shocked or terrified (Hackett, 1971). This variety of patterns has made it difficult to establish the "average" flasher's motives or a typical family background.

Some researchers (Forgac and Michaels, 1982) have proposed that there are two major types of exhibitionists, the "pure" exhibitionist, who does no more than expose his genitals, and the "criminal" exhibitionist, who commits other acts besides exposure. In this view, the pure exhibitionist is a timid, inhibited, conscientious conformist; the criminal exhibitionist is an impulsive, aggressive, antisocial nonconformist.

In trying to explain this paraphilia, psychoanalysts propose that the urge to expose one's genitals develops in the family situation, and that most exhibitionists (60 percent in one study) have strong emotional ties to possessive or dominating mothers (Witzig, 1970). The shocked reaction of women to the exposed penis assures the flasher that his genitals are intact and that women fear him.

In the behavioral view, a man learns to associate the exposure of his penis with sexual satisfaction. It may begin when he is surprised by a woman while urinating or masturbating in an inappropriate place. The original embarrassment turns to arousal when he later thinks about the incident, and he begins masturbating regularly to fantasies of self-exposure. Eventually sexual arousal and genital exposure become closely linked (Tollison and Adams, 1979). But neither explanation accounts for all cases of exhibitionism.

Most exhibitionists are studied without comparing them to "normal" groups. When researchers did compare two groups of exhibitionists to "normal" men, they discovered fewer differences than they had expected (Langevin et al., 1979). Like "normal" men, exhibitionists responded with greatest arousal to sexually mature women, and their sexual responses to young girls and to other men were also alike. They were somewhat aroused by the children and not at all by the men. A sizable minority of exhibitionists expose themselves to children, but the researchers believe that this choice is often made because young girls are more likely to be impressed with the size of the exposed penis and less likely to report the exposure. When exposing himself to a young girl, said one flasher, "You can take your time and go all the way" (Langevin et al., 1979, p. 328).

What about the woman suddenly accosted by a stranger waving his penis at her? When twenty-five young women who had found themselves confronted by a flasher were interviewed, few seemed outraged or offended. Most said they had been afraid or surprised. Some thought the incident was funny. According to one woman:

> I was in the parking lot at [State College] coming out of the library. I see this really odd-looking man standing beside his car. He looks just like Yul Brynner; shaved head, sun glasses, a really funny shirt on. I thought, "Oh oh, he's really funny looking." All of a sudden he comes out from the car and flashes. It just struck me funny and I burst out laughing. I thought it was really comical. (Davis and Davis, 1977, p. 130)

Another woman didn't think her experience was at all funny. She had just finished taking an examination in a night class and was walking across the campus when she heard a rustling in the bushes. A man called her over, exposed himself, and propositioned her. She said she screamed and ran, and added: "I was really scared" (Davis and Davis, 1977, p. 126).

In retrospect, most of these women felt that the incident had not been dangerous, but rather annoying and weird. Some simply ignored the flasher; others left the scene. Those who reported the incident to the police tended to do so because someone else insisted.

## Fetishism

**fetishism**
dependence on some inanimate object or particular part of a partner's body for sexual arousal or gratification

**Fetishism** is a paraphilia in which a person must have contact with an inanimate object (such as a glove) or a particular part of a partner's body (such as a foot) in order to achieve sexual gratification. Often the person fondles, kisses, or smells the object while masturbating.

Mild degrees of fetishism are common and are encouraged by the underwear industry. For example, many men are more aroused by the sight of a woman in sexy lingerie than by a nude woman. Such a sexual preference becomes a paraphilia only when the man cannot function sexually without it, as when a man can get an erection only when his partner wears a garter belt and net stockings. Rubber, fur, and silk are said to be prevalent fetishes in the United States, and glove or shoe fetishes are often seen. One man, for example, was dysfunctional unless his wife wore elbow-length white kid gloves during their sexual activity (Chesser, 1971). A foot fetishist who was arrested in Texas was known as the "phantom female foot fondler." He grabbed women in public, slipped off their shoes, then caressed and kissed their toes (Tollison and Adams, 1979).

Fetishists who have come to the attention of the law or of therapists tend to be socially withdrawn, isolated, and lonely. They lack heterosexual social skills and are preoccupied with their fetish. Again, most fetishists are men, but fetishism comes to light primarily from arrest records, when a man commits burglary, theft, or assault to obtain a fetish such as women's underwear or locks of hair. Since fetishism is primarily a private activity, the extent of its occurrence among women is not known.

In fetishism, some outside element is incorporated into sexual activity and becomes its focus. The texture of an object is generally more important than its shape, and the smell may also be vital, as in the case of hair, shoes, or underwear (Money, 1981). As one fetishist said:

> When I rub them (panties) on my penis and over my stomach I feel an incredible sensation and I totally lose track of everything around me. It's very intense and goes on for about an hour, usually, until I have an orgasm. (Author's files)

**transvestism** a compulsion to dress in the clothing of the other sex in order to obtain sexual arousal or gratification

Psychoanalysts see the fetish as a substitute for the penis. In the behavioral view a fetish develops through conditioning, when sexual arousal and orgasm become associated with some object or part of a body. In fact, one researcher (Rachman, 1966) was able to condition young men to respond to the sight of a boot with an erection. He accomplished this by repeatedly showing the men photographs of women's boots immediately followed by photographs of nude women.

**Transvestism,** in which a person achieves sexual gratification by dressing in

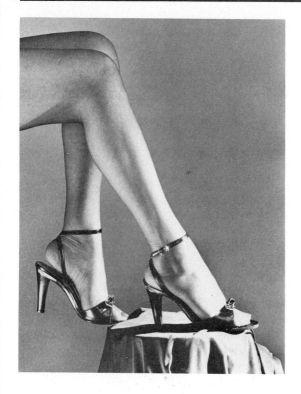

A person with a sexual fetish is aroused by some unusual object, such as a shoe. (© Joel Gordon 1980)

the clothing of the other sex, is classified as a form of fetishism by the American Psychiatric Association (Webb et al., 1981). But because it often includes components of gender identity, we will discuss it along with transsexualism.

## *Sadism and masochism*

As paraphilias, sadism and masochism are opposite sides of the same coin. In **sadism,** a person derives sexual gratification from dominating or inflicting physical or psychological pain on a partner; in **masochism,** a person derives sexual gratification from submission or pain. A sadist and a masochist may form a smoothly working relationship, or one person may respond to both kinds of stimulation. For this reason, these paraphilias are often referred to as sado-masochism.

Sado-masochism includes a wide variety of activities: verbal abuse or humiliation; smearing or soiling; binding, whipping, biting, pinching, burning, cutting, and piercing. The cruelty may be restricted to fantasy, or it may be acted out.

For many sadists, the motive is not the infliction of pain, but the need to dominate another person in order to get sexual gratification. Similarly, the masochist may derive pleasure not from the pain he or she receives, but from the act of submission.

**sadism** dependence on dominance or the inflicting of physical or psychological pain for sexual arousal or gratification

**masochism** dependence on submission or the reception of pain for sexual arousal or gratification

The pain involved may be extremely mild and primarily imaginative, as in the bondage "games" recommended in *The Joy of Sex* (Comfort, 1972), in which one partner ties up the other and stimulates him or her to orgasm. In this case, no one is injured, for the game is only mock sado-masochism.

Sometimes what starts out as a game with a consenting partner can become violent:

> It started out just as a game. I trusted him and thought he was just playing. He wanted to tie me down to the bed during sex. I thought it might be kinda fun so I agreed. I had no idea what would happen. After a while he started talking mean to me and slapping me on the face and breasts. I was getting scared and begged him to untie me. He went to the dresser and got a hairbrush and shoved it up my vagina over and over again. I screamed and thought he was going to kill me. I told him I was going to call the police. He seemed to lose control, slapping me and pushing the hairbrush up my vagina. I nearly passed out from the pain. (Tollison and Adams, 1979, p. 288)

Vicious sadism without the consent of the unsuspecting partner—who may be a stranger—can lead to serious injury or even death. The sadist who maims or murders may not have any genital contact with the victim at all. Instead, the sadist replays the scene from memory while masturbating or having "normal" intercourse with a partner. When the power of the image is no longer stimulating, the sadist strikes again (Money, 1981).

*Case* Donald (age 29) was confined as criminally insane after he attacked a woman with an axe. Since he was fifteen years old, Donald had masturbated frequently to fantasies of sexual violence, including bondage, whipping, spanking, torture, and forcible oral and vaginal intercourse. From time to time, he enacted these fantasies on women. He said that when he was his "normal" self, his sexual activity was confined to intercourse with willing female partners, but that when his "sadistic" self took over, only sexual violence excited him. (Adapted from Laws, Meyer, and Holmen, 1978)

Just as extreme sadism can lead to murder, extreme masochism can lead to suicide. Some individuals arrange to hang themselves until they are semi-conscious, but occasionally the "game" goes too far and they die of strangulation. A death by hanging may be revealed as a masochistic accident if the cord around the neck is padded with cloth to prevent rope burns. One man had a habit of torturing himself with jolts of electric current, which he delivered to his genitals and rectum through pads of aluminum foil. By using a rheostat, he could reduce the current below a fatal dosage. Finally, however, he turned up the rheostat too far and electrocuted himself (Morneau and Rockwell, 1980).

Sadism and masochism are varieties of paraphilias that are found in both heterosexuals and homosexuals, in women as well as in men. During sexual activity, men are more likely to inflict pain and women to receive it. Masochism appears to be the one paraphilia more common in women than in men; 10 percent

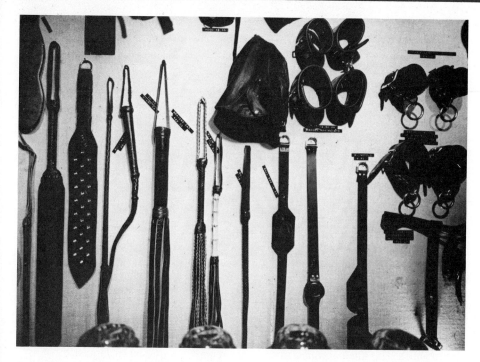

Sex shops that cater to sado-masochists sell a variety of whips, chains, handcuffs, masks, and leather-studded belts. (© Sepp Seitz 1983/Woodfin Camp & Assoc.)

of the unmarried women and 6 percent of the unmarried men in one national survey said that receiving pain gave them sexual pleasure (Hunt, 1974).

The general appeal of sado-masochism is apparent in the number of S-M clubs, bars, and newspapers that serve such inclinations. In sex shops, whips, chains, masks, handcuffs, and metal-studded belts are popular items. The clubs, such as the Eulenspiegel Society, which was founded in 1972 in New York, say that only consenting adults are involved, that all activities are planned in advance, and that each couple has a signal that stops the action when things get too rough for either partner. Whether their members engage in mock sado-masochism or actually injure one another is uncertain.

## *Other paraphilias*

In addition to the paraphilias described so far, there are a host of others. Pedophilia, in which the primary source of sexual gratification is the act or fantasy of sexual activity with prepubertal children, is a common paraphilia that will be discussed in Chapter 16. Some of the remaining paraphilias may be relatively normal among

**pedophilia** dependence on sexual activity with prepubertal children as a primary source of sexual arousal or gratification

people who grow up in a particular environment. Others are extremely rare, and their appearance usually indicates a major psychological disorder.

The number of these paraphilias is so great that we cannot describe them all. They include:

**apotemnophilia** dependence on fantasies about becoming an amputee for sexual arousal or gratification

**acrotomophilia** dependence on having an amputee as a partner for sexual arousal or gratification

**coprophilia** dependence on the smell, taste, or sight of feces for sexual arousal or gratification

**frotteurism** dependence on rubbing against a stranger, especially in a crowd, for sexual arousal or gratification

**klismaphilia** dependence upon receiving an enema for sexual arousal or gratification

**necrophilia** dependence on seeing, fondling, or having intercourse with the dead for sexual arousal or gratification

**telephone scatophilia** dependence on making obscene telephone calls for sexual arousal or gratification

**urophilia** dependence on the sight, smell, or taste of urine for sexual arousal or gratification

**zoophilia** dependence on sexual activity with an animal for sexual arousal or gratification

**Apotemnophilia.** In **apotemnophilia**, a person is aroused and reaches orgasm by fantasizing about becoming an amputee. Sexual gratification is so dependent upon being an amputee that the person tries to arrange things so that an arm or leg will be amputated (Money, 1980). (In **acrotomophilia**, it is the partner who must be missing a limb.)

**Coprophilia.** A person with **coprophilia** is sexually aroused by the smell, taste, or sight of feces and often is unable to reach orgasm without it. Coprophiliacs are often aroused by watching another person defecate.

**Frotteurism.** In **frotteurism**, a person depends upon rubbing against a stranger, especially in a crowd, for sexual arousal and gratification. A packed subway car often has a frotteur aboard, who rubs against the clothed breasts, buttocks, or legs of a woman (if heterosexual) or a man (if homosexual). The "partner" in this sexual activity is often unaware of his or her participation. Some frotteurs are also fetishists and will only rub against a person dressed in a particular fabric, such as corduroy, velvet, or leather.

**Klismaphilia.** The **klismaphiliac** must either receive an enema or fantasize about getting one in order to become sexually aroused or to reach orgasm.

**Necrophilia.** In **necrophilia**, a person obtains sexual gratification from the dead—from viewing a corpse, fondling it, or actually having intercourse with it. Some necrophiliacs get jobs in funeral homes, others resort to grave robbing. A few necrophiliacs can have intercourse with a living woman if she remains absolutely motionless (Tollison and Adams, 1979).

**Telephone scatophilia.** The **telephone scatophiliac** derives sexual gratification by making obscene phone calls. He phones a woman who is a stranger and makes sexual statements or propositions that are intended to offend or shock her.

**Urophilia.** Just as the coprophiliac depends upon feces for gratification, so the **urophiliac** depends upon urine. The smell or taste of urine or the sight or sound of a person urinating is necessary for arousal or orgasm.

**Zoophilia.** In **zoophilia**, a person depends upon sexual activity with an animal for arousal and orgasm. The contact may consist of masturbating the animal, oral sex, or actual intercourse. Zoophilia is relatively common among adolescents who grow up in isolated farming communities and usually disappears as human partners become available.

For the most part, these paraphilias are very rare. Although such paraphiliacs occasionally ask therapists for help or are arrested when some illegal activity comes to the attention of police, we really don't know a great deal about them. Often they escape public notice. People with these rare forms of parpahilia make up such a negligible part of the population that they have been neither surveyed nor studied.

# VARIATIONS OF GENDER IDENTITY: TRANSVESTISM AND TRANSSEXUALISM

The terms "transvestism" and "transsexualism" are sometimes confused. As we've seen, however, in most cases transvestism is a paraphilia in which dressing in the clothes of the other sex is arousing, but there is no wish to change one's sex. A male transvestite thinks and feels in predominantly masculine ways. In contrast, transsexualism is a conflict in gender identity, in which the person wants to change his or her body. A male transsexual thinks and feels in predominantly feminine ways. Yet the split is not as neat as it seems, because some male transvestites request surgery to change their sex so that they may live as women.

## *Transvestism*

Most authorities believe that all true transvestites are men (Levine and Lothstein, 1981). Women who dress in men's clothing tend to do so for practical reasons. The few women who are obviously cross-dressing are either lesbians or female-to-male transsexuals who feel at ease only when wearing men's clothes. Such women apparently get no sexual arousal from wearing male attire (Money, 1981).

Transvestites are not all alike. For some, sexual arousal comes from wearing one or two articles of female clothing, say a bra and lacy panties. At times, they wear these garments under their regular clothing. At other times, they wear them during masturbation or intercourse. These men have a fetish for women's clothing. But the majority of transvestites have moved beyond the fetish stage. They wear completely feminine garb—underclothes, outer garments, makeup, and wig. They may masturbate as they gaze at their mirror image, work their cross-dressing into sexual encounters with a partner, or go out in public, where they pass as women (Feinbloom, 1976).

The thrill of passing—which is always accompanied by the possibility of detection—and the attention they get from men combine to arouse them. Afterward they may masturbate or have intercourse while recalling the situation. In one study, nearly half of a group of transvestites said they never engaged in sexual activity of any kind while they were cross-dressed (Croughan et al., 1981). For some transvestites, the sexual feelings associated with cross-dressing diminish with time and are replaced by a sense of having another personality, or a "female self," which they seek to express.

Transvestism often begins with a fetish for women's undergarments and gradually progresses to cross-dressing. The case of John W., whose sexual pattern followed this course, distinguishes transvestism from transsexualism and shows the close relationship between sexual adjustment within a marriage and the expression of paraphilias.

*Case* John W. (age 45) is a school superintendent. He has been married for 22 years and has two teenaged children. John's mother died when he was twelve years old. Before her death he used to wear her underclothing, and the feel of silk gave him an erection, which led him to masturbate. By puberty, John wore his mother's clothes whenever he had a chance and developed a fetish for women's garments, which he used in masturbation. When he was a college freshman his father died, and John joined the service.

When he married, his wife was unaware of his sexual patterns. She was never able to reach orgasm during sexual activity. Although they had intercourse regularly, neither partner received much sexual satisfaction from their marriage. John began to masturbate to transvestite fantasies and periodically cross-dressed. After nineteen years of marriage, his wife learned of his cross-dressing and was outraged. She demanded that he never again wear female clothing in their house.

John began cross-dressing in the back seat of his car. At first he restricted himself to deserted parking lots, but as his relationship with his wife deteriorated, he progressed to a public exhibitionistic phase and began exposing himself to passing men. He never intended to have sexual contact with these men; instead, he was sexually stimulated by the act of exposure in female clothing. Although his cross-dressing was always accompanied by masturbation, the specific sexual stimulus that triggered it changed considerably as time passed. Three years after his wife forbade him to cross-dress at home, John was arrested for exposing himself in a public parking lot while wearing women's clothes. (Adapted from Rosen and Kopel, 1977)

John is not a typical transvestite. Many lead model, even conservative, lives. Their cross-dressing is limited to particular times and places, and their appearance, jobs, and hobbies are quite masculine (Feinbloom, 1976).

Most transvestites are heterosexuals, although some are bisexual or homosexual. Often their wives know about the practice, and some cooperate with their husbands, helping them with dress and makeup and incorporating the husband's paraphilia into their joint sexual activities.

Transvestites can be distinguished from homosexual "drag queens" by dress, movements, and eye contact. Transvestites dress conservatively, and their gestures are not effeminate. Drag queens dress in stylish, eye-catching costumes, and their clothes, gestures, and eyes all send sexual signals. The transvestite blends into a crowd; his cross-dressing is meant to fulfill his own erotic or personality needs. The drag queen always stands out; his cross-dressing is meant to attract other men.

Transvestism appears to be a deeply ingrained pattern of sexual behavior that originates in childhood or early in puberty. Psychoanalysts say it is connected with the Oedipal conflict and represents an attempt to overcome castration fears. Cross-dressing protects males from castration and, by creating a woman with a penis, assures them that they are no different from girls (Fenichel, 1945). Barred from having sex with their mothers, they have it with her clothes. Some psychoanalysts regard cross-dressing as a sign of homosexual conflict.

In the behavioral view, the gradual development of transvestism—from masturbation with an article of women's clothing to the inability to achieve sexual gratification without cross-dressing or fantasizing about it—shows the process of conditioning at work. The connection between sexual satisfaction and cross-

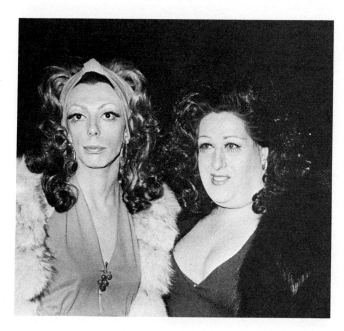

In recent years, many transvestites have "come out," and transvestite bars and clubs are increasingly common in large cities. (© Charles Gatewood)

dressing is strengthened each time sexual arousal or orgasm occurs when a man is cross-dressed or is imagining the practice.

Transvestism apparently allows some men to cope effectively with life. Their compartmentalization of the practice keeps it from interfering with work, family, friends, and intimate relationships (Feinbloom, 1976). When transvestites come to terms with the practice, some gain social support for the activity by joining transvestite groups—much like the homosexual person who joins a gay community group. Such subcultures tend to stabilize the activities of the "deviant" group, aid members in accepting their own behavior, and work to remove the stigma placed on them by society (Plummer, 1975).

The attempt to come to terms with transvestism is not always successful. When it is not, the transvestite is filled with anxiety and discomfort. Without a sympathetic listener in whom he can confide, a transvestite may experience intense guilt and shame, and low self-esteem. Among seventy middle-aged men who belonged to transvestite groups, all but two had tried at some time in their lives to give up the practice (Croughan et al., 1981).

## Transsexualism

Transsexuals may be either male or female, although as we saw in Chapter 1, men are believed to outnumber women about six or eight to one (Levine and Lothstein, 1981). The feeling of each transsexual—that he or she is trapped in the body of the opposite sex—almost always is present during childhood, but no one knows what causes the development of discordant gender identity.

By taking androgens and undergoing sex change surgery, Annie M., the young woman on the left, was transformed into the young man on the right. (© Associated Press Photo)

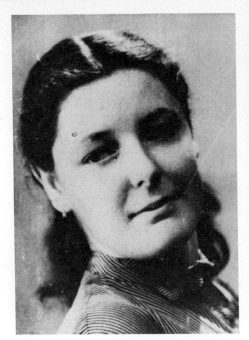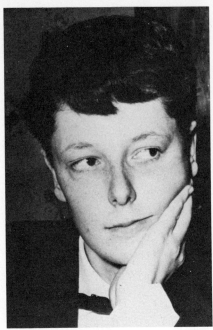

Some authorities believe prenatal hormones may have something to do with it, yet girls who are known to have been exposed to androgens before birth develop normal female gender identities. Since the hormone level of adult transsexuals tests within the normal range for their own biological gender, there seems to be no obvious disturbance of the endocrine system. And because it is impossible to reconstruct the prenatal history of an adult transsexual, there is no way to identify any hormonal involvement (Ehrhardt, Grisanti, and McCauley, 1979).

It is agreed that some aspects of the behavior of a child who will become a transsexual usually resemble the behavior of the other sex. Boys prefer feminine activities; girls, masculine activities. But there is no way to tell whether a very feminine boy, for example, will develop into a heterosexual, transsexual, transvestite, or homosexual adult (Green, 1980).

In one study (Ehrhardt, Grisanti, and McCauley, 1979) that compared fifteen female-to-male transsexuals with fifteen lesbians of the same age, race, educational level, and socioeconomic background, a few differences did turn up. As girls, the transsexuals dressed as boys and wanted badly to become one; the lesbians did neither. Any wish to become a boy felt by the lesbians was temporary; with the transsexuals, it was a painful experience that left them unhappy and confused. Both groups had been seen as tomboys, but transsexuals were more likely than lesbians to prefer boys as friends during childhood. Neither group had cared much for dolls or infant care, and both had preferred to play with trucks, cars, and guns.

The most striking difference between the two groups appeared at puberty. Transsexuals were disgusted at their menstruation and breast development, and several began binding their breasts tightly in early adolescence. Only one of the lesbians had a negative reaction to the physical signs of puberty.

Both psychoanalytic and behavioral views of transsexualism hold that childhood experiences are important in the development of gender identity. But no unusual pattern of family interaction appeared in either group. In most cases, both parents were present throughout childhood and adolescence. Some of the women in both groups had developed close attachments with their mothers, some with their fathers, and some were equally attached to both parents.

One problem with all studies that ask adults about their childhood is that memories are continually being reshaped. People generally remember their childhoods in ways that fit into their adult lives. However, the finding that family background seems to have little influence on gender identity was supported in a different way by another researcher (Green, 1978). In this case, the continuing study focuses on children between the ages of three and twenty years old who are being reared by or have grown up with transsexual parents. All but four of the children are aware of the mother's or father's sex change and know that such switches are not typical.

As yet, all sixteen children are heterosexually oriented and none has developed gender identity problems. Two of the girls are considered tomboys; one is a thirteen-year-old who wants to be a veterinarian and the other a three-year-old who wants to be a "mommy."

As noted in Chapter 11, psychoanalysts believe that a child must identify successfully with the parent of the same sex in order to develop normally, and social learning theorists stress the importance of appropriate role models for growing children. But some of these children watched as Daddy grew breasts and became their mother or Mommy lost her breasts and became their father. Others were children of women who divorced and married a female-to-male transsexual. In one family, the biological parents remained together, but the father is a male-to-female transsexual who lives as a woman and has undergone treatment with female hormones. Yet in every instance, the children's development appears to be "normal."

*Case* The biological mother of a two-year-old daughter and a three-year-old son began to receive androgen injections, to live as a man, and told the children she was now their "father." This mother then married a woman who assumed the role of the children's mother. The children, who are now seven and eight years old, have no conscious recall of their "father" ever being their mother. Both children are contentedly female or male. The girl's favorite toy is a set of dishes, and she prefers girls as playmates. The boy's favorite toy is a walkie-talkie, and he prefers to play with boys. (Adapted from Green, 1978)

If the cause of transsexualism is uncertain, so is its remedy. Psychotherapy has not been successful in solving the identity problems of transsexuals. Only a few cases of successful identity change are known, and when identity is changed, a homosexual orientation often remains (Barlow, Abel, and Blanchard, 1977).

Many transsexuals attempt to cope with their conflicting identity by living in

*Focus*

DOES
SEX-CHANGE
SURGERY
HELP?

During the 1960s and 1970s, surgery became the accepted treatment for transsexuals, and some universities set up special gender identity clinics to carry out this treatment. Surgery as a treatment for transsexualism became so well known that a major character in a best-selling novel and movie, *The World According to Garp* (Irving, 1978), was a male-to-female transsexual, Roberta Muldoon, who before her surgery was a tight end for the Philadelphia Eagles.

In 1979, however, investigators at Johns Hopkins University followed up a number of patients and discovered that those without surgery seemed to do as well as those who had received the extensive and costly procedure (Meyer and Reter, 1979). As a result, Johns Hopkins ended its surgery program. Other investigators criticized this study, pointing out that the results on men and women were mixed together and that success was defined by such standards as the sex of a transsexual's roommate, the socioeconomic rating of the transsexual's job, and whether there had been any arrests or psychiatric treatment after surgery. Completely ignored were the patients' personality and emotional reactions—the reasons for surgery in the first place (Fleming, Steinman, and Bocknek, 1980).

Sex reassignment surgery does not end a person's social and emotional problems. Most people who request the surgery also have psychological disorders that need treatment. For example, at one gender identity clinic, only 7 percent of the men and 40 percent of the women who requested surgery had no significant psychological problems apart from gender identity (Levine and Lothstein, 1981).

In addition, not all patients who request surgery are "primary" transsexuals, men and women who have known from early childhood that their biological sex did not match their gender. No more than 25 percent of the

accordance with their gender instead of their biology. Making this decision is often painful, and one transsexual described the conflict involved:

> The one flaming truth is that Martha is a real being, not a fun and games figment of Mark's imagination. To repress her too much longer could mean disaster. To bring her out in the wrong way could bring harm to many people. So the dilemma is as real as Martha. . . . I think it is all going to boil down to the inner strength of Mark, and if it isn't there, it has to be built up. Martha has come out of the closet of Mark's mind—now she has to come out of the closet of the world. (Authors' files)

If the switch is limited to cross-dressing, there is always the risk of detection. Besides, the conflict between biology and life style remains. As a result, some transsexuals have their bodies altered to conform to their gender identity. This is a lengthy, expensive process.

Biological men who want to become women take estrogens, which enlarge the breasts and redistribute body fat in a feminine pattern. Electrolysis removes facial and body hair, and plastic surgery can make noses look feminine and Adam's

men who asked for surgery fit this description. The rest were "secondary" transsexuals, men whose feelings that they were meant to be women had developed after years as a transvestite, an effeminate homosexual, or a bisexual with a low sex drive. These men seemed pushed into the decision for sex change by some personal stress, as the following case shows.

Case: Henry (age 30) was a chronically depressed, bearded, twice-married, responsible childcare worker. He was also a transvestite who cross-dressed for intercourse or masturbation. His father died suddenly, and at about the same time Henry discovered he was infertile. He began to drink heavily, and his depression deepened. He became unable to get an erection, and his job performance deteriorated. Henry decided he was meant to be female and that his life as a male was a charade. He seriously considered jumping off a bridge. But he rejected suicide and instead asked his wife for a divorce, announcing that he was going to have sex-reassignment surgery. While awaiting surgery he began living as a female, but found that the feminine sex role did not lift his depression. Temporary psychiatric hospitalization was followed by a year of psychotherapy, during which he returned to his male role, remarried his wife, and found himself once again able to have an erection. (Adapted from Levine and Lothstein, 1981)

It may be that there are many secondary transsexuals among the people who have had surgery, and perhaps these people are later more likely to have serious psychological problems or to decide that the surgery was a mistake.

Studies have found that when patients are carefully selected, their life generally improves and most are glad they chose surgery (Lothstein, 1980; Walinder and Thuwe, 1975). Surgery does not seem to eradicate all discomfort over gender, but it does appear to lessen the transsexuals' preoccupation with gender and allows them to turn their attention to other aspects of life.

apples less prominent. Nothing can be done to alter the voice except to practice speaking within the female register. Genital surgery begins with castration. The penis is removed and a vagina constructed, using skin from the penis in the lining. Scrotal skin is used to build the vaginal lips, and a cosmetic clitoris is made. Since all this skin is sensitive, orgasm can be reached through vaginal stimulation. The urethra is shortened and redirected to make urine flow downward instead of outward into an arc.

Biological women who want to become men take androgens, which make facial hair grow, shrink the breasts slightly, suppress menstruation, redistribute body fat in a masculine pattern, and thicken the vocal cords, lowering the voice. Surgery removes the uterus and remaining breast tissue. Building external genitals for women is the least satisfying part of the reconstruction. A penis and scrotum can be built, using skin and bone grafts, but the new penis—although adequate for urination and realistic enough to allow the transsexual to pass—is not satisfactory for intercourse. It cannot change back and forth from a flaccid to an erect state, and the skin is not sensitive. Orgasm must still be based in the clitoris, which is kept and which has become larger in response to androgens.

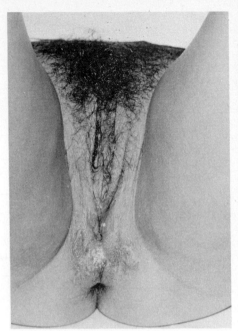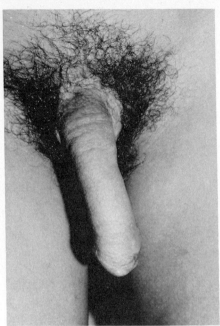

Transsexuals sometimes undergo surgery to transform their genitals. The construction of female genitals for a biological male (a) is usually more satisfactory than the construction of male genitals for a biological female (b).

Surgery does not always bring transsexuals the happiness they envisioned when they began the complicated procedure. Because many transsexuals are still dissatisfied after surgery, there has been controversy about its use.

## TREATMENT OF PARAPHILIAS AND SEXUAL DISORDERS

If a paraphilia is harmless and does not interfere with other aspects of a person's life, there is probably no need for treatment. A person who is turned on by fur or enemas and who has a cooperative partner may live a reasonably contented life. A paraphilia requires treatment when it has led to arrest; when the person's life situation is in jeopardy (a wife threatens to leave her husband, a man fears that his employer will find out); or when the person is so embarrassed, anxious, or guilty about the practice that he or she seeks professional help.

Although psychotherapy has sometimes been used to treat paraphiliacs, it is a lengthy, expensive, and time-consuming way of approaching the problem. Most paraphiliacs who apply for therapy are treated either pharmacologically or with behavior therapy.

## Pharmacological treatment

Since 1966, Provera, an androgen-depleting hormone, has been used on an experimental basis with masochists, sadists, voyeurs, exhibitionists, and pedophiliacs who were either in trouble with the law or feared they might be arrested. Provera drastically reduces a man's testosterone level, causing it to drop to levels normally found in a prepubertal boy. It is believed that this anti-androgen also has a direct effect on brain pathways that govern sexual behavior (Money and Bennett, 1981). Provera decreases frequency of erection and ejaculation, lowers sexual desire, and leads to diminished sexual fantasies. In effect, it gives the paraphiliac a "vacation" from his sex drive (Money, 1981).

The effect of Provera has been called "chemical castration." When the drug is withdrawn, sexual interest and potency gradually return, with erections appearing in about ten days. The erotic apathy caused by the drug may be welcome relief to a paraphiliac who has felt driven by his sexual urges. While he is taking the drug, the patient is given psychological counseling to help him establish a new life style.

Although the immediate effects of Provera are striking, the risks of relapse after the drug has been withdrawn are high. The long-term effectiveness of this treatment depends on a number of factors. Among twenty paraphiliacs who had been treated with the anti-androgen, those who were most successful in overcoming their paraphilia had stayed off alcohol or drugs, regularly attended the counseling sessions, followed the therapist's recommendations, and established a pair bond. The pair bond seemed especially important, for many paraphiliacs have never known this sort of intimacy (Money and Bennett, 1981).

Anti-androgens are fairly effective while they are taken, but the approach is so drastic that their use is controversial. Provera is usually given only to people whose paraphilia is dangerous or so overpowering that they cannot control it by any other means.

## Behavioral treatment

Most paraphilias are also treated with behavioral methods; behavior therapy is used in hospitals, prisons, clinics, and in private practice. Unlike psychoanalytic treatment, which explores early childhood, searching for the causes of a paraphilia, behavior therapy focuses on the unwanted sexual behavior itself, using methods that attempt to change the person's response to sexual situations. Since behavior therapists believe that sexual responses to unusual objects, partners, or acts are developed through learned associations, they use similar associations to eliminate unwanted thoughts and behavior and to establish desirable thoughts and behavior. Both aspects of therapy are important, because the elimination of an unacceptable sexual pattern can be successful only if an acceptable and satisfying means of fulfillment is substituted.

Unless sexual response can be measured, a therapist has no way of knowing whether treatment is effective (Abel and Blanchard, 1976). A variety of techniques has been developed to meet this need, including physiological tests of arousal (Rosen and Keefe, 1978) and questionnaires that ask a person about his or her sexual responses. For example, the penile plethysmograph, which monitors erections, is commonly used to measure arousal (see Chapter 5). These devices are used at every stage of therapy. They assess the person's initial sexual preferences, aid in the modification of the preferences, and evaluate the success of therapy.

**aversion therapy** elimination of unwanted responses by punishing them with electric shock or other painful stimuli

One method of eliminating unwanted responses is through **aversion therapy**, in which a person's unacceptable sexual responses are punished with electric shock. A sadist, for example, might look at slides of multilated women. Each time he becomes aroused, he receives an electric shock that he can stop by flipping a switch that changes the slide to one of heterosexual intercourse (Bancroft, 1974).

**covert sensitization** elimination of unwanted responses by imagining unpleasant consequences following them

Another, more common, method is **covert sensitization**, in which a person simply imagines the unpleasant consequence. Sometimes covert sensitization is supplemented by an unpleasant stimulus, such as a foul odor. For instance, after an exhibitionist relaxes, he is encouraged to imagine a scene in detail. He drives down a street, sees a young woman, stops his car, and exposes his erect penis to her. As he visualizes exposing himself, he imagines being struck by nausea, losing his erection, vomiting all over himself, and being seen in that condition by the woman and a gathering crowd. As he imagines the nausea, a vial of valeric acid, which has a noxious odor, is thrust under his nose. Among ten exhibitionists who were treated by this method, nine stopped exposing themselves after a series of treatments (Tollison and Adams, 1979).

As we have seen, paraphiliacs are often unassertive and uncomfortable in heterosexual situations, and find it difficult to make friends with women. Thus, while the covert sensitization is going on, the paraphiliac also learns social skills, perhaps learning how to approach a woman and talk with her, and how to ask a woman for a date. If he is married, he may be taught some of the communication skills discussed in Chapter 10.

**orgasmic reconditioning** the transfer of sexual responses from unacceptable objects or acts to acceptable objects or acts by masturbating to thoughts or representations of the acceptable stimuli

Another technique commonly used by behavior therapists is **orgasmic reconditioning**, in which the fantasies a paraphiliac has while masturbating are gradually shifted from unacceptable to acceptable sexual images. If the shift is successful, arousal and orgasm may become associated with acceptable fantasies, strengthening their appeal and weakening the power of the undesired fantasies. A voyeur is told that whenever he feels the urge to peep, he should masturbate while looking at a series of pornographic pictures. Over several months, the pornographic photographs are gradually replaced by photographs of his nude wife (Tollison and Adams, 1979).

Despite the obvious appeal of the behavioral approach—it is both pragmatic and efficient—some aspects of it remain controversial. The use of aversive conditioning, even if the paraphiliac agrees, is unacceptable to some people. In most instances, behavior therapy quickly decreases the power of unacceptable sexual stimuli, but there are few studies of its long-term effects. In addition, most studies focus on individual cases. But the treatment that is effective with one person will not always be effective with another, even if they share the same paraphilia. Relapse is always a danger and is likely to occur unless treatment continues for months or even years (Rosen and Kopel, 1977).

Behavior therapy is probably more successful for some paraphiliacs than for others. Those who are unmotivated, mentally retarded, or psychotic are unlikely to be helped by these methods (Bancroft, 1974). But if the person who is being treated participates wholeheartedly, the therapy may be extremely successful.

# Summary

**1** There are several ways to define "normal" sexual behavior—moral, statistical, and psychological—but none is completely satisfactory. The moral approach, based on the Judeo-Christian tradition, maintains that only sexual behavior which can lead to conception within marriage is acceptable. The statistical approach sees normal sexual behavior as whatever many people in a society do. The psychological approach sees normal sexual behavior as mature, well-adjusted, fulfilling, and without guilt or anxiety. The most practical approach might be to consider all behavior as normal except for those acts a person feels compelled to perform, that make the person unhappy, or that bring physical harm or psychological distress to another person.

**2** A **paraphilia** is a sexual pattern in which a person is sexually aroused by behavior, objects, or partners that are forbidden or statistically abnormal in the society. A paraphilia is not considered a disorder unless the person prefers the unusual pattern or finds it necessary to achieve arousal or sexual gratification. Paraphilias are also called "sexual variations." Most paraphilias are restricted to males, perhaps because they lack the protection of an extra X chromosome, making the development of sexuality more vulnerable in males, or perhaps because of socialization into the male sex role.

**3** In **voyeurism,** a person prefers or is dependent on the illicit observation of a woman or couple undressing or engaging in sexual activity for sexual arousal or gratification. **Exhibitionism** involves public display of the genitals with the intent of obtaining sexual gratification. In **fetishism,** a person must have contact with an inanimate object or a particular part of a partner's body for sexual gratification. In **sadism,** a person derives sexual gratification from dominating or inflicting physical or psychological pain on a partner; in **masochism,** a person derives sexual gratification from submission or pain. Masochism may be the only paraphilia more prevalent among women than men. Other paraphilias include **pedophilia, apotemnophilia, acrotomophilia, coprophilia, frotteurism, klismaphilia, necrophilia, telephone scatophilia, urophilia,** and **zoophilia.**

**4** **Transvestism** is a paraphilia in which men become sexually aroused by dressing in women's clothing. A male transvestite thinks and feels in predominantly masculine ways. Transsexualism is a conflict in gender identity, in which a person thinks and feels predominantly as a member of the other biological gender. As a child, a transsexual's behavior usually resembles the behavior of the other sex. Although childhood experiences are believed to be important in the development of transsexualism, studies have found no unusual patterns of family interaction, and children who are reared by transsexuals appear to have normal gender identity. Through hormone treatment and surgery, some transsexual men and women have their bodies changed to fit their gender identity. There is considerable controversy over surgical treatment for transsexuals, and some universities have stopped their sex-reassignment surgery programs.

**5** A paraphilia requires treatment only when it leads to arrest, when the person's life situation is in jeopardy, or when the person is so embarrassed, anxious, or guilty about the practice that he or she seeks professional help. Pharmacological treatment, which uses an androgen-depleting hormone that greatly reduces sexual interest and potency, is effective but highly controversial. Behavior treatment attempts to eliminate unwanted thoughts and behavior and to establish wanted thoughts and behavior. Behavior therapists use **aversion therapy**, in which unwanted sexual responses are punished; **covert sensitization**, in which a person imagines unpleasant consequences of the unwanted behavior; and **orgasmic reconditioning**, in which masturbatory fantasies are gradually shifted from unwanted to wanted sexual images. As behavioral treatment goes on, paraphiliacs are often taught social skills to ease their sexual adjustment. Behavior therapy is most successful when the paraphiliac participates wholeheartedly in the treatment.

## the victim's view

I always thought of rape as something that happened to somebody else. When it happened to me, I couldn't believe it. I knew that it wasn't my fault, but I still had the feeling that somehow I was the guilty one. It's left me with a terrible mistrust of most men. (Authors' files)

## the rapist's view

They was all asking for it. They'd flaunt themselves. And if I wasn't in the position to do it, somebody else would. I got my satisfaction not out of raping them but by sodomizing them. That was my satisfaction—to take them in the back. . . . I won't say I'll never tie a woman down [again]. I might do it. I might do it again. There's no tellin'. (Sussman and Bordwell, 1981, pp. 40–41)

# 16 Sexual Coercion and Exploitation

*Chapter 16*

Rape, the sexual abuse of children, raids on houses of prostitution, and the arrest of people who produce child pornography are everyday events in the news media. As small children, we are taught to be wary of strangers who offer us rides and candy. When we become adults, we learn more about a dark and disquieting aspect of human sexuality—coercive and exploitative sex.

How do some people, most often men, come to associate sex with aggression or power? Why is the most tender connection between a man and a woman turned into brutal violence? Under what conditions do people use this connection to exploit others? And why is society unable to control sexual abuse and exploitation?

Many researchers and scholars have attempted to answer these questions, with varying degrees of success. The primary focus has been on the link between sex and aggression. Some see sexual coercion and abuse as the inevitable expression of a human instinct for violence. Others see it as being built into the culture and an inevitable outgrowth of the male sex role.

In this chapter, we'll look at some theories about the association of sex and aggression before we take up the various kinds of abuse and exploitation. First, we'll investigate rape, especially the myths that have grown up around this act of violence, the characteristics of rapists, and the effects of rape on the victim. A survey of the nature and scope of child molestation will lead us into a consideration of incest, which often involves the exploitation and molestation of children. Then we'll examine the question of pornography, and search for a link between this sort of exploitation and violence. Next we will explore the problem

# Sexual Coercion and Exploitation

of sexual harassment, a type of coercion that has only recently become a public concern. Finally, we will look at the problem of prostitution and the ways in which both prostitutes and their clients can be abused or coerced.

## SEX AND AGGRESSION

One explanation for the frequency of sexual violence puts the blame on human nature. Human aggression is said to be instinctive, an element that will always be part of human life. Some people learn to express their aggression in nonphysical ways; others go through life using fists, guns, or knives on anyone who gets in their way.

Another explanation proposes that a predisposition toward violence is part of being male. As we saw in Chapter 1, a tendency toward aggression seems to be linked to male hormones. But whether or not the predisposition exists, not everyone accepts the inevitability of its expression.

Still others see violence as part of the culture, as behavior acquired through personal experience and observation (Bandura, 1973). By the time they are three or four years old, American boys have developed aggressive ways because they are encouraged—by attention or success—each time they are aggressive. On television and in films, they see violent men glorified, held up as heroes when they use fists, guns, or automobiles to impose their wish-

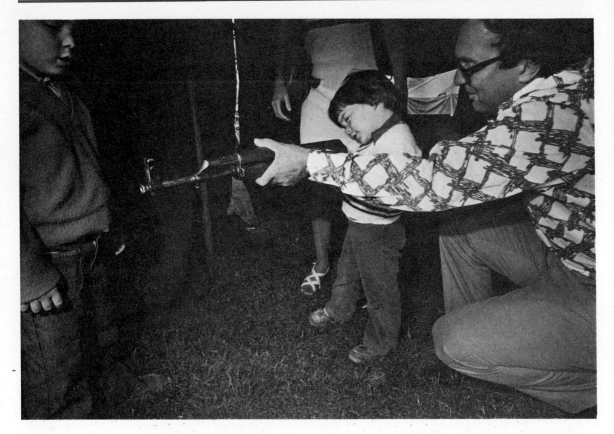

In many ways the culture encourages boys to be aggressive; the combination of male aggression and an inferior social role for women may encourage violent sexuality.
(© George W. Gardner)

es on others. Long before boys reach manhood, they discover that raping or batter-ing a woman is both safe and rewarding, because women are weaker and less like-ly to strike back than most men. Finally, some believe that women's inferior social position is the primary cause of sexual coercion and abuse (Gates, 1978). In this view, the stereotypical male sex role, not just the encouragement of male aggres-sion, fosters abuse and coercion.

There is some indication that the encouragement of male aggression and an inferior role for women are both linked with violent sexuality. Among 156 tribal societies, rape was either unknown or extremely rare in 47 percent. In these "rape-free" societies women were treated with considerable respect, and their reproduc-tive, social, and economic roles carried prestige. There was little violence of any kind in these cultures; the people generally regarded the natural environment with reverence. In 18 percent of the tribal societies, rape was prevalent. A "rape-prone" society was characterized by high levels of violence throughout the culture, the view of women as property, and the separation of the sexes into social groups (Sanday, 1981).

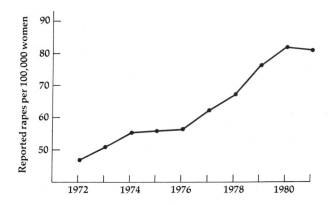

**Figure 16.1  Number of Reported Rapes per 100,000 Women in the U.S. (1972–1981).**

(Statistical Abstract of the United States, 1982–1983. U.S. Bureau of the Census [1982])

# RAPE

Rape is the fastest-growing violent crime in the United States (see Figure 16.1). In 1979, more than 76,000 attempted or completed rapes were reported to the police (FBI, 1980). These figures represent only those cases the police considered valid— the cases in which they believed the victim. Approximately 15 percent of rape complaints are considered "unfounded" and receive little or no official attention.

**rape** sexual relations with another person obtained by using force, threat, or intimidation

Rape is also believed to be the most underreported major crime. It is generally believed that only 20 percent of all rapes are reported, indicating that more than half a million women are assaulted each year. A careful analysis of rape statistics led one researcher to propose that between 20 and 30 percent of all American girls who are now twelve years old will experience a sexual assault some time in their lifetimes (Johnson, 1980).

In recent years the definition of rape has been changing, and a number of cultural myths about it have been exposed. Researchers have come to a better understanding of the rapist and have begun to explore the physical, psychological, and sexual aftereffects of rape on the victim.

## *What is rape?*

Rape is generally defined as sexual relations with another person obtained by using force, threat, or intimidation. But this simple and straightforward definition is only a starting point in understanding the act. Rape can take many forms. It includes stranger rape, gang rape, date rape, marital rape, statutory rape, homosexual rape, and rape by women.

Rape by a stranger conforms to the common image. It accounts for at least half of all reported rapes, can take place on a dark street or within the victim's home, and sometimes occurs during a burglary or robbery (Katz and Mazur, 1979).

In gang rape, two or more people sexually assault another person or persons. Often the rapists are strangers to the victim, and they may stalk a solitary woman who is walking or driving. Sometimes a gang rape is a required part of a new member's initiation into a street gang.

Many are date rapes, which occur during a prearranged date or shortly after a woman has met a man at some social occasion. The victim of a date rape may know the rapist only casually, be his steady date, or even be engaged to him. Among a large group of college students, nearly a quarter of the men admitted having become so aroused that they could not stop themselves from having intercourse—even though the woman they were with begged them to stop (Koss and Oros, 1980).

Marital rape, in which a husband forcibly has intercourse with his wife, is undoubtedly much more common than most people believe. Among more than 600 San Francisco women, 14 percent had been raped by their husbands or ex-husbands; in every case the man used physical force (Russell, 1982). Until recently, laws specifically excluded forcible sex with a spouse from the definition of rape. Since 1978 when the first case of marital rape reached the Oregon court, at least forty-seven American husbands have been charged with the crime; twenty-three of them were convicted (Russell, 1982). Cases concerning marital rape are rarely brought to court for several reasons: some states still allow husbands to rape their wives, courts are reluctant to interfere in "family matters," and many women are even more reluctant to bring charges against their husbands.

The first case of marital rape to reach American courts occurred in 1978, when Greta Rideout charged her husband, John, with raping her. The jury found John innocent, but by 1982, at least twenty-three American husbands had been found guilty of the crime. (UPI)

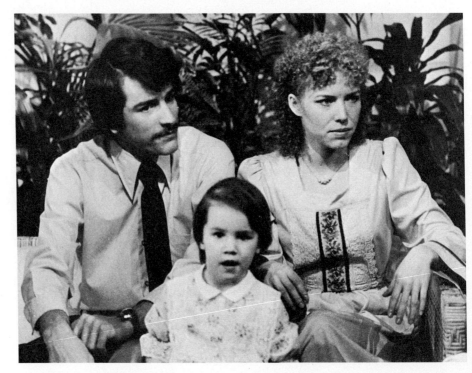

Statutory rape refers to sexual intercourse with a female who has willingly agreed to the act, but who is under the legal age of consent. Statutory rape laws are intended to protect girls from sexual exploitation, but they are often inconsistent. The legal age of consent, for example, varies from state to state, and ranges from fourteen to twenty-one years of age. In addition, a woman may have the legal right to a marriage license before she is legally old enough to consent to sexual intercourse. Some authorities have suggested lowering the age of consent to twelve, on the grounds that many young teenage girls lead active sex lives, but the legal system regards such girls as incompetent to make sexual choices.

Homosexual rape is relatively common in prison, but it occurs in some segments of the homosexual community and among male gangs as well. Most men who rape men do not consider themselves homosexuals. Instead, the very act of rape establishes the rapist's power and degrades the victim (Groth and Birnbaum, 1979).

Although cases in which women have raped men are on record, the act is extremely rare. Most women who are charged with rape have assisted men who were raping another woman.

Perhaps because of women's social and sexual role, the rape victim is often disbelieved or scorned. Rape may be the only major crime in which the victim has borne the burden of guilt and responsibility. This attitude appears to pervade the criminal justice system. Among judges, prosecutors, and police officers, most tended to place a good deal of the blame for rape on the woman and believed that only about half the women who reported a rape to the police had actually been raped and could correctly identify their assailant (Feldman-Summers and Palmer, 1980). As we've seen, police fail to believe at all about 15 percent of the women who report they have been raped.

When a rape is reported to the police, they decide whether it is "founded" before they search for and arrest the accused man. Police are most likely to believe a rape has been committed if victim and rapist were strangers, if the rapist used physical violence, if the victim bears signs of resistance, if the victim has a "good reputation" or is seen as respectable. The police are more likely to investigate the rape of a woman who is married, badly bruised, and assaulted by a stranger. Since the victim's reputation for sexual promiscuity is often considered by legal authorities, a prostitute finds it extremely difficult to make a successful charge of rape.

Few men who are accused of rape are actually charged with the crime. Prosecutors will not bring charges unless they feel relatively confident of conviction, and conviction is almost impossible when there is no physical evidence to support the accusation.

The legal treatment of rape has been changing, with police relying more on establishing the force or threat of force by the rapist and less on the victim's resistance or reputation. This change has not increased the number of prosecutions for rape, nor has it decreased the number of acquittals. It has, however, made it possible to convict men for rape who would formerly have been convicted for assault or indecent liberties. The new laws might be called "truth-in-labeling" laws (Loh, 1981).

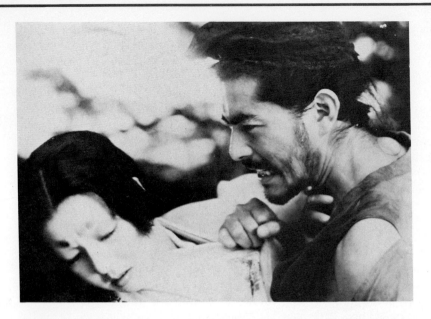

In the film, *Rashomon,* from which this scene was taken, Japanese director Kurosawa shows the complex meanings and motives that surround an act of rape. (The Museum of Modern Art/Film Still Archive)

## Facts and fallacies

In Western society, until recently, rape was not seen as a crime against a victim. The view of woman as first the property of her father and after marriage the property of her husband made rape a violation of a man's property.

Traditional punishment for rape reflected this view. In the Bible, the rape of a virgin required the rapist only to reimburse her male guardian for the decrease in her value on the marriage market. In medieval England, only forcible intercourse with a virgin was considered rape. The punishment was death, but the rapist could escape by marrying the victim. Not until the thirteenth century was the legal concept of rape expanded to include the violation of wives, widows, and nuns. But always the burden of responsibility to prove rape was placed on the victim. Traces of these attitudes remain. The concept of the wife as her husband's property implies that he has the right to do with her as he wishes and has led to the view that marital rape is not a crime. The recognition that rape is a crime against a woman is fairly recent.

In addition to bearing the burden of this history, women who are raped must overcome the cultural myths that encourage rape by blaming the victim. The continual exposure of women to these myths may foster the development of a "victim mentality" in women, which further contributes to the incidence of rape (Brownmiller, 1975). Four common and destructive myths permeate American society.

   **Myth number one:** *All women want to be raped* The idea that women secretly desire rape is a popular theme in movies, books, and pornography. It also plays a prominent role in the work of psychoanalyst Helene Deutsch (1944), who believed that women's psychological preparation for sexuality was primarily masochistic. As girls grew up, sexual intercourse became connected with rape, painful penetration, and the act of deflowering the virgin. As proof, Deutsch pointed to the frequency of rape in women's dreams and fantasies. Although many women do include rape in their sexual fantasies (Chapter 7), most of them have no wish to see their fantasies become reality. The notion that all women yearn to be sexually assaulted has no basis in fact.

   **Myth number two:** *No woman can be raped against her will* The prevalence of this myth makes rape impossible in the minds of many people, and it absolves the rapist of responsibility. Its supporters quote Honoré de Balzac, a nineteenth-century French novelist, who said: "You can't thread a moving needle." A moving needle suddenly becomes still, however, when it is held by a person who knows that she will be shot, stabbed, or choked if she moves. Most rapists hold a weapon on their victim or threaten them with violence or death (Gardiner and Torge, 1979; Schram, 1978).

   In addition, not all rapes involve penile-vaginal penetration. Some rapists insert objects into the vagina, some have oral or anal sex, and some masturbate while abusing a woman (Holstrom and Burgess, 1980). Some rapists are dysfunctional and cannot penetrate their victims. Sadistic rapists may find their sexual gratification in the infliction of pain.

   **Myth number three:** *All women who are raped ask for it* According to this pervasive myth, a victim causes her own rape by hitchhiking, walking in unsafe places, leaving her door unlocked, wearing "seductive" clothing, or acting in a "provocative" manner. This myth also transfers responsibility for the rape to the victim. The act becomes victim-precipitated—that is, the victim has caused the crime. The National Commission on the Causes and Prevention of Violence describes victim-precipitated rape as occurring "when the victim agreed to sexual relations but retracted before the actual act or when she clearly invited sexual relations through language, gestures, etc." (1969, p. 226). Using this definition, the commission reported that only 4.4 percent of rapes were victim-precipitated. The notion that victims cause their own rape is probably an outcome of sex-role socialization: women are taught to be attractive and seductive by a culture that values these qualities, while men are encouraged to believe that any attractive woman is "fair game" for aggressive sexual advances.

   The "she asked for it" myth has led to suggested restrictions on women's actions. They are advised to dress decorously, told never to hitchhike or walk alone at night, and instructed to be extremely cautious in social situations. However, such precautions would not end rape: About half of all rapes occur in the victim's home.

Restrictions on women's behavior also place the responsibility on the potential victim. When Golda Meir was prime minister of Israel, she was asked to place a curfew on women in the hope of ending a series of rapes. She refused to do so, saying: "But it is the men who are attacking the women. If there is to be a curfew, let the men stay home" (Gardiner and Torge, 1979).

**Myth number four: *if you're going to be raped, you might as well relax and enjoy it*** This myth picks up the theme of popular movies like *Straw Dogs* or *Gone with the Wind,* in which the victim is at last swept away by passion, perhaps reaching orgasm for the first time in her life. It is closely linked to Myth Number One, and it completely misinterprets the victim's emotional reaction to a sexual assault. Victims perceive rape as a threat to their lives, not as a sexual intrusion (Schram, 1978).

If these myths bear no resemblance to reality, a new explanation for rape is needed. Many researchers have come to believe that rape is not a sexual crime at all, but an act of aggression. Sexual gratification does not seem to be the primary motive for rape; instead, most rapists seem motivated by anger or a need for power. They appear to use sexuality as a way of expressing their aggressive feelings (Groth and Birnbaum, 1979). Perhaps rape should be treated as an act of violent assault rather than as a sexual crime.

## Men who rape

The mingling of sexuality with aggressive needs and feelings seems to produce three distinct patterns: the anger rape, the power rape, and the sadistic rape (Groth and Birnbaum, 1979).

In an anger rape, the rapist's aim is to hurt the victim; he uses sex as an instrument of revenge. The anger rapist uses far more force than he needs to overpower his victim, and he is not sexually aroused when he begins the attack.

Anger rapes usually do not last very long. They are not planned, and the rape is often a response to some stressful event in the rapist's life, such as the loss of a job. For whatever reason, the rapist feels he has been wronged or in some way treated unjustly. He reacts by taking revenge on a victim. The anger rapist strikes infrequently and sporadically; and at the time of the assault, he is "blind with rage." He rarely finds any sexual gratification in his rape. As one convicted rapist described it:

> I was enraged when I started out. I lost control and struck out with violence. After the assault I felt relieved. I felt I had gotten even. There was no sexual satisfaction; in fact, I felt a little disgusted. I felt relieved of the tension and anger for a while, but then it would start to build up again, little things, but I couldn't shake them off. (Groth and Brinbaum, 1979, p. 15)

In a power rape, the aim is conquest; the rapist uses sex to compensate for feelings of inadequacy and to establish his mastery, identity, and capability. Rape demonstrates the rapist's heterosexuality and preserves his sense of manhood. As one convicted power rapist put it:

> In my rapes, the important part was not the sexual part, but putting someone
> else in the position in which they were totally helpless. I bound and gagged
> and tied up my victims and made them do something they didn't want to do,
> which was exactly the way I felt in my life. I felt helpless, very helpless in that
> I couldn't do anything about the satisfaction I wanted. Well, I decided, I'm
> going to put them in a position where they can't do anything about what I
> want to do. They can't refuse me. They can't reject me. They're going to have
> no say in the matter. I'm in charge now. (Groth and Birnbaum, 1979, p. 30)

The power rapist often strikes in response to some incident that has undermined his sense of masculinity, and commits a series of assaults in a relatively short
period. He uses only enough force to overpower his victim. He may deny that he
forced her and insist that she enjoyed the experience.

In a sadistic rape, the aim is to abuse and torture the victim; the rapist uses sex
to punish and destroy. Some bizarre form of bondage or torture often characterizes
these rapes, and sometimes the rapist uses a stick or bottle instead of his penis to
penetrate the victim. For some rapists, inflicting pain brings sexual gratification; for
others, it serves to arouse them. The violence often escalates over time.

The sadistic rape is deliberate and planned, and the rapist often stalks his victim. Sadistic rapes tend to be repetitive, but they are not the rapist's only form of
sexual gratification. He often has consenting sexual activity with other partners.
One convicted rapist who murdered his victims reported that his sexual relations
with his wife were "satisfactory" and that he had never struck her. But of his rapes,
he says:

> Murder was always a part of all these plans. Murder is sadistic, and there's no
> doubt that I planned to be sadistic. The very thought of murder was
> appealing, even though I don't consider murder as evil as rape. In the first
> killing, I had an erection up to the point I fired the gun. I have no memory of
> ever having a legitimate, consenting sexual fantasy. Originally, the fantasy
> associated with my offenses was that sexual intercourse itself would be painful
> to the victim. (Groth and Birnbaum, 1979, p. 56)

Although the anger rape is usually spontaneous, many others seem planned.
About 71 percent of the rapes in a Philadelphia study were planned in advance
(Amir, 1971). In some cases, the rapist selected a particular victim; in others he decided that any victim would do. In 43 percent of these rapes, two or more rapists
were involved with a single victim. Often a group of male friends planned a rape in
advance, but left the selection of the victim to chance. The men studied tended to
belong to a generally violent subculture, and rape was only one way in which they
showed generally aggressive and antisocial behavior.

No two rapists are alike. In fact, along with all the other myths about rape is
the rape of the "typical rapist." There appears to be no such thing. Although some
studies have found rapists to be below average in intelligence, others have found
their intelligence to be average or above average (Schram, 1978). Although the majority of rapists are less than thirty years old, one rapist in four is older than that
(see Figure 16.2). Although the majority of rapists are single, about one in three is
married (Katz and Mazur, 1979). Although rapists have often been drinking heavily, one out of two rapes is committed by a sober man (Rada, 1978).

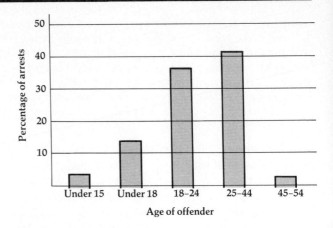

**Figure 16.2 Rape Arrests by Age of Offender: 1981**

Rapes are committed by men of all ages. This figure shows the percentage of rapists arrested in each age group. it is important to note, however, that statistics from police records do not include the large majority of rapes, which are never reported. (Statistical Abstract of the United States, 1982–1983. U.S. Bureau of the Census [1982])

Whatever common background has been discovered is undermined by the fact that most studies are based on convicted rapists. Men accused of rape but not convicted are likely to have more personal, social, and economic resources than those who wind up in prison. Further, since rape is such an underreported crime, perhaps 80 percent of rapists are never charged with an offense. There is no way to find out about the background of these men.

In an attempt to discover whether rape might have some link with male hormones, investigators (Rada et al., 1976) measured the level of testosterone in the blood of rapists and child molesters. Rapists who had inflicted physical injury on their victims had significantly higher levels of testosterone than did child molesters and rapists who did not injure their victims. Since other studies have found elevated testosterone levels in young men with a history of violent criminal activities, it would appear that male hormones are not linked to the act of rape as such, but may be related to the tendency toward violence.

The suggestion that because of the male sex role "any man" might become a rapist was explored with a group of college men (Malamuth, 1981). These men were asked how likely they would be to rape if they thought they would never be caught. About 20 percent said they would be quite likely to rape under such circumstances, and another 15 percent said they might. When these men listened to tapes that described rape scenes in explicit terms, men who said they'd rape if they could get away with it responded just as convicted rapists did to such scenes: They found them highly arousing. Men who said they'd never rape were much more aroused by scenes of consenting sexual activity.

Men who said they'd rape if they could get away with it differed from men who said they wouldn't in two other ways: They were more aggressive toward women during an experiment, and they believed strongly in the cultural myths about rape. In this belief they again resembled convicted rapists, who generally hold callous attitudes about rape and believe strongly in the myths (Malamuth, 1981). Indeed, some researchers (Burt, 1980) believe that myths play an important role in causing rape by permitting the rapist to justify his behavior.

## The female victim

Although women between the ages of fifteen and twenty-five seem to be at greatest risk of rape, age is no protection. Women as old as ninety-one have been victims. The risk increases for women who live in poorer areas of a city. Since the majority of rapes occur within the rapist's neighborhood, the typical victim belongs to the same race and socioeconomic group as her attacker.

When a woman is assaulted, her first reaction is generally disbelief. As the rape proceeds and she feels her life is in danger, shock turns to near panic. Whether she resists may depend in part on her background: women who have never encountered violence tend to confine their resistance to words; women who have been exposed to violence tend to use physical resistance. If the rapist threatens a victim with a weapon, she is likely to submit without a struggle. No one is certain just how many women do resist: Reports of physical resistance range from 17 to 90 percent, depending on the study (Katz and Mazur, 1979).

Being raped is a devastating experience that can affect the victim's life for years. Women's reactions appear to go through two stages: an acute phase lasting from a few days to several weeks, and a long-term phase, during which they learn to cope with the experience (Burgess and Holstrom, 1974).

During the acute phase, victims seem disorganized. Their lives are disrupted. In the first few hours after the attack, some women are agitated and seem frightened, angry, restless, or tense. The rest maintain a façade of composure and calm but admit they are numb or in a state of shock. In the weeks following the attack, physical reactions include headaches, disturbed sleep, edginess, appetite changes, and vaginal itching, burning, or pain. Emotional responses range from fear and humiliation to anger and thoughts of revenge. Some women blame themselves for the attack and search their memories for ways in which they might have avoided it.

In the long-term reorganization phase, victims often move, change telephone numbers, visit family or friends for emotional support, or take long trips. They may have upsetting dreams or nightmares. Some develop intense fears that affect their life styles. For example, women assaulted while at home may be afraid to stay at home, and women attacked outdoors may feel safe only at home. Most women are afraid to be alone.

Such fears seem to be centered on stimuli associated with the rape: being alone, darkness, a man who resembles the rapist. Because the victim often rearranges her life to avoid such stimuli—making sure she is not alone, leaving lights on at night, refusing to interact with men she does not know—their power remains strong. Her fears persist in part because she avoids harmless situations that would destroy the association with her rape (Kilpatrick, Resick, and Veronen, 1981).

During the first two months after the rape, victims generally face financial difficulties and problems at work. Moving, taking time off, and involvement with the criminal justice system can lead to docked pay or loss of a job. Some women quit their jobs because their work takes them into situations where they feel vulnerable (Resick et al., 1981).

The effects on the victim's sexual life may persist for years (Feldman-Summers, Gordon, and Meagher, 1979). The majority of women in one study (Becker et al., 1982) reported a fear of sex, a lack of sexual desire, and difficulty in responding to a partner that lasted for at least two months after the rape. In another study (Ellis, Calhoun, and Atheson, 1980), about one out of ten victims who had been active sexually before the rape still refused all sexual activity a year later. Among women who had resumed sexual activity, some had flashbacks during sexual encounters. A partner's gestures, actions, words, the weight of his body, or sexual activity in the dark made them recall the rape so vividly that they experienced attacks of anxiety.

Most rapes are reported to the police by someone other than the victim—witnesses, friends, or family members (Katz and Mazur, 1979). From the victim's point of view, telling the police may only add to her problems. She may feel that reporting the crime will do little good, that she will only be embarrassed, that the police will not believe her, or that the rapist will seek revenge. In search of the factors that influence a woman to report a rape, researchers (Feldman-Summers and Ashworth, 1981) interviewed more than 400 women. White women were more likely than black, Hispanic, or Asian women to say they would report a rape to authorities, and a woman's perception of the result of her report was the best predictor of her in-

Rape crisis centers, like this, provide emotional support and guidance immediately after the rape—when sympathetic, enlightened intervention is needed. At most centers, follow-up counseling to help women handle possible psychological problems is also available.
(© Bettye Lane)

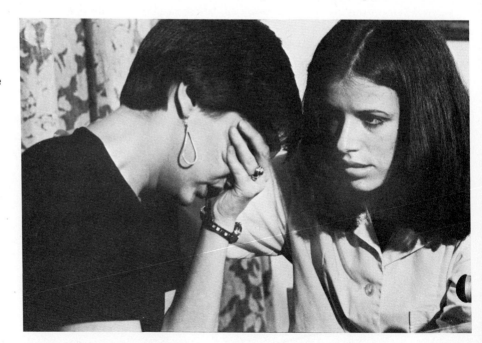

tentions. Many women believed that their family, friends, and sexual partners would provide little social support if they did report a rape.

Nearly half the victims in one study feared the reaction of their sexual partner to the news (Burgess and Holstrom, 1979). They worried that he might think the rape had been their fault, that he would not believe them, that he would suspect they'd enjoyed it, or that he would see them as soiled or undesirable. Over half the women who did tell their partners found them helpful, and partners provided most support when they were gentle and put no sexual pressure on the victims.

To help victims deal with their experience, rape crisis centers have been established across the country. Most centers regard the rape victim as a healthy, normally functioning person who merely needs assistance to deal with a temporary crisis. Counseling is generally directed at speeding recovery by helping the woman to cope with what has taken place.

## *The male victim*

Most male rape victims are attacked by other men. The information we have on homosexual rape comes from male prison populations. As with heterosexual rape, the question often arises as to whether force or coercion has actually been used. Young prisoners may be "seduced" by older inmates who offer various goods and services—cigarettes, food, the promise of special privileges, or protection from other inmates. The provider of these services expects sexual favors in return. If the young prisoner refuses, rape may follow. Homosexual rape, like heterosexual date rape, may often result from a seduction that has gone wrong (Gagnon and Simon, 1973).

Like heterosexual rape, homosexual rape is an extremely underreported crime. One study of sexual assault in the Philadelphia prison system estimates that of 2,000 assaults that occurred, only 96 were reported to the prison authorities (Davis, 1970). Victims hesitated to report rapes because they were afraid of retaliation. Prison authorities discouraged complaints and were slow to act on them.

Sexual aggressors tended to be older, taller, and heavier than their victims; however, both victims and aggressors were younger than the average inmate. Victims tended to look young for their age and to be less athletic and more attractive than their aggressors. Aggressors tended to be serving time for more violent and more serious crimes than their victims. Finally, in many of the rapes several aggressors attacked a single victim (Davis, 1970).

One young prisoner, who was sentenced for assault while drinking, reported that prison guards sometimes made possible the gang rape of inmates:

> I have seen the guards set someone up . . . unlocking an inmate's cell door and letting other inmates go in and, actually what you call rape. Maybe the inmate gave the guard a hard way to go and he gets back at him. . . . I seen it three times. And you know, it's unbelievable. You can hear a guy hollering and no one doing nothing about it. And you know it could have been you as well as anybody else. (Money and Bohmer, 1980)

# *Focus*

PREVENTING
OR DEALING
WITH RAPE

Since no woman is safe from rape, it is important to take precautions that decrease vulnerability and prepare you to deal with a rape should it occur.

**How to avoid rape** The more difficult it is for a rapist to gain access to you, the less likely you are to be raped. At home, keep doors and windows locked, never open the door to a stranger, and never list your first name on a mailbox or in a phone book. If you are at home alone, close the curtains at night and turn on more than one light so it looks as though you are not alone. If someone rings the bell, pretend that a man is in the house, calling out, "I'll answer the door, Jim!" before you go to the door. If you are frightened, buy a dog.

When you go out, avoid solitary walks on dark streets. If you have to be out alone, carry a police whistle on a key chain or some practical weapon such as a lighted cigarette, a hat pin, a plastic lemon, or an umbrella. If you think you're being followed, zigzag across the street. If you find you're right, seek help quickly. Don't ride in an elevator when the only other occupant is a male stranger. If you are driving, keep gas in your tank, the doors locked, and check the front and back seats before you get in (Katz and Mazur, 1979).

In social situations, make sure your date knows the sexual limits early in the evening. Be careful about picking up men, especially if you've been drinking heavily or using drugs. If a man keeps bothering you in a disco or a bar, tell the bartender or the waiter. If the situation gets too bad, go to the women's room and ask some woman if you can sit at her table. When you leave, if you think someone is following you, take a cab and go to a friend's house or ask the driver not to pull away until you are inside your house (Gardiner and Torge, 1979).

**Dealing with a rapist** When it becomes clear that you are about to be assaulted, try to escape if possible. If you decide to scream, yell "Fire!"—not "Rape!"—you'll get a much quicker response.

Authorities disagree on whether or not physical resistance is a good idea, and it may depend on the situation. Some believe that screaming, crying out, or fighting (kicking or biting) at the very beginning of the attack is the best way to avoid a rape (Selkin, 1975). The women's movement recommends that women learn the martial arts so they can defend themselves. Such techniques may work best when the rapist is a stranger and if the resistance is initiated before the rapist is caught up in the assault. But a sadistic rapist may be further aroused by the struggle, and an untrained woman who carries a gun or a knife may find that the rapist takes it away and uses it on her.

Some authorities advise delayed resistance. The victim plays along with the rapist, treating him as a human being, gaining his confidence, and helping him sexually (Storaska, 1975). Delayed resistance may work best when the rapist is an acquaintance or a "friend." When using delayed resistance, the woman is gentle, perhaps caressing the rapist's face until her thumbs are over his eyes, then pressing hard, or caressing his testes, then suddenly squeezing them so hard that he is disabled. Some women simply cannot bring themselves to use such techniques, and when used with the wrong rapist, they have been

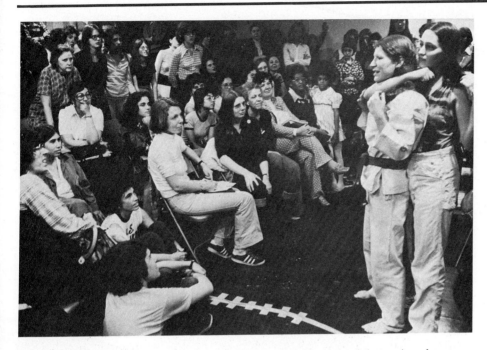

By learning the martial arts, women are better equipped to defend themselves from a rapist. Self-defense works best when the rapist is a stranger, if the resistance starts immediately, and if the rapist is not a sadist. (© Bettye Lane)

called an "invitation to murder" (Selkin, 1975).

Most rapists are *not* murderers. If there is no way to escape, the experience may be less devastating if you try to escape mentally, going off somewhere in your head. But first memorize the man's features so you can identify him later.

**After the rape** If you are raped, the first thing to do is get medical help for any injuries. The next step is to get emotional support and guidance. A person you can confide in, who will not be judgmental, and who can help you decide on the best course of action is essential. The staff at a rape crisis center can provide this sort of help.

The decision on whether to report the assault to the police must be made fairly quickly, and if the crime is reported, medical evidence will be needed. For your own well-being, you should have a medi-cal examination to make certain there are no internal injuries, and you should be checked for sexually transmitted diseases and discuss the possibility of taking a drug to prevent pregnancy (see Chapter 20). Rape often has long-term effects on the victim. If any adjustment problems are apparent, some sort of counseling may be needed.

This prisoner reported that two men who had been raped in this way committed suicide.

The majority of prison rapists do not view their behavior as homosexual—as long as they assume the active, aggressive male role, they define themselves as heterosexual. The primary motive for homosexual rape appears to be the need to conquer and degrade the victim. Sexual assault provides men who have failed to succeed in traditional paths a way to assert their masculinity and power in a prison environment that denies them all other opportunities to succeed (Davis, 1970).

Men who are sexually assaulted or abused by women have a hard time persuading attorneys or legal authorities that the attack has taken place. Most people assume that a frightened or angry man will be unable to maintain an erection. Yet men interviewed by Kinsey and his associates (1948) reported boyhood erections and ejaculation when they were scared, feared punishment, were angry, or were yelled at, and other research has described genital arousal as part of the body's reaction to emotional turmoil (Bancroft, 1980).

When women forcibly assault a man, the victim is generally tied up or threatened with a weapon. Despite his embarrassment, fear, or anxiety, the victim functions sexually. In one case, a woman threatened a medical student with a scalpel until he had intercourse with her; in another, a truck driver who fell asleep after accompanying a woman to a motel was gagged, blindfolded, and tied to the bedposts, then forced to have sex repeatedly with several women over a twenty-four-hour period. Whenever his erection flagged, the women threatened to castrate him and held a knife to his scrotum (Sarrel and Masters, 1982). At times, women simply dominate the man, reversing traditional sex roles. The woman's forcefulness completely overpowers the man, and he submits (Sarrel and Masters, 1982).

There is no way to discover how often women assault men sexually. The truck driver who was assaulted told no one of his experience until a sexual dysfunction that developed after the attack sent him to a sex therapist. He felt disgraced by the episode and believed his friends would think him "less than a man" if they found out about it (Sarrel and Masters, 1982). If this male reticence afflicts most victims of female sexual assault, the practice, although undoubtedly rare, happens oftener than people believe.

## SEXUAL ABUSE OF CHILDREN

**child molestation**
sexual contact between an adult and a child

Children—both boys and girls—are more vulnerable to sexual abuse than women. **Child molestation** includes a wide range of behavior, from obscene language, innocuous staring, and casual touching to coitus with a young girl or anal intercourse with a young boy. Almost all child molesters are men, and they are known as pedophiles. Pedophilia, as we saw in Chapter 15, is a paraphilia in which sexual arousal or gratification is focused on children.

**hebephilia**
contact between an adult and a young adolescent

When the victim of a child molester is past puberty, say between the ages of twelve or thirteen and fifteen, the act is called **hebephilia**. In some societies, girls of this age are married. Among the ancient Greeks, homosexual hebephilia—sexual contact between a man and a boy in his early teens—was incorporated into social institutions. The young boy's lover was morally—and sometimes legally—responsible for the boy's education and development, and the relationship was closer than that between parent and child (Bullough, 1976). In contrast, American society severely condemns such behavior.

The sexual abuse of children so often goes unreported that the actual incidence is unknown, but it's been estimated that from 200,000 to 500,000 sexual assaults on girls between the ages of 4 and 13 occur each year in the United States. Boys are abused less often. The number of boys between 4 and 13 who are molested each year may be as few as 20,000 or as many as 200,000. Add to those figures the molestation of infants and toddlers, and the total becomes disturbingly large (Sanford, 1980).

Child molestation is likely to go unreported for several reasons. A child's perception of sexual activity is so different from the adult view that the child may not know that anything wrong has happened. A child is more likely to report a stranger's improper behavior than the advances of others, since most children are taught to be suspicious of unknown adults. Sexual advances from friends or family members are especially confusing to the child. Yet about three child molesters out of every four are known to the victim—family member, relative, neighbor, baby sitter, or someone connected with church, school, or recreational programs (Sanford, 1980). The most common child molester is a relative of the child.

Once a child informs parents about a sexual advance, the information is not always reported to the police. Several considerations enter into this decision. Parents have a well-founded hesitancy about exposing a child to the stress of legal proceedings. Many authorities believe that the emotional damage caused by the system's handling of these cases is at least as harmful to the child as the molestation (MacFarlane, 1978). Even when the case is handled sensitively, the parents must consider that the chances of catching and imprisoning the offender are slight. If the molestation has not involved physical injury, many parents decide that protecting their child from courtroom procedures is more important than imprisoning the offender.

## The child molester

Just as there is no typical rapist, so there is no typical child molester. A child molester is not a dirty old man in a raincoat who offers candy to passing children. In age, intelligence, education, income, occupation, race, religion, and family background, child molesters resemble the general population (Mohr, Turner, and Jerry, 1964). Neither alcohol nor drugs is involved in the majority of offenses, and pedophiles are not psychotic.

Convicted child molesters tend to be psychological children with adult bodies. They find it difficult to delay gratification or to control impulses; they suffer from low self-esteem; they seem concerned only with their own needs and feelings. Most tend to feel isolated from others, to feel inadequate, and to be inept in social relationships (Groth, 1978).

Less than 10 percent of child molesters use force (Sanford, 1980). Instead, they persuade children to have sexual activity with them or else they place a child under some obligation. If the child refuses, they will not use force. Most child molesters use sex to get physical contact and affection (Groth, 1978).

### The young victim

Any child can become the victim of a child molester. The incident often takes place in the child's home or in other familiar places, but in a sizable minority of cases the child and the molester make contact in a public place, such as a park, a playground, or a street. Boys—perhaps because of their greater freedom—are more likely than girls to meet their molester in a public place (Ellenstein and Cavanaugh, 1980).

Because molestation covers such a wide range of activity, it is often difficult to draw firm conclusions about its effect on the young victim. Most connections between child molestation and later psychological disturbance are based on studies of adults in therapy, but there is no indication that such adults are typical of men

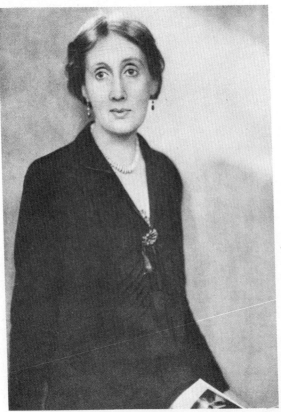

A child who is sexually abused may have sexual problems as an adult. As a child, the writer Virginia Woolf was molested by her half-brother. Throughout her marriage, she had no interest in sexual relations with her husband. (Culver Pictures)

and women who were molested as children. In a search for the factors connected with childhood sexual abuse that increase the likelihood of lasting damage, researchers (Tsai, Feldman-Summers, and Edgar, 1979) compared women whose molestation had led them to seek therapy with women who had been molested as children but felt no need of therapy. Lasting damage appeared to be connected with sexual abuse that lasted nearly five years, that occurred frequently during that period, that continued until the girl had passed her twelfth birthday, and that included attempts at genital intercourse.

As this study indicates, the child's age and developmental level at the time of the abuse may be particularly important. A young child who does not understand what has happened is less likely to be harmed than an older child who believes that the incident is wrong, that he or she has been violated, or that he or she is responsible for the incident. Similarly, a child who is fondled in the park by a stranger is less likely to show lasting effects than a child who is repeatedly molested in a relationship that lasts for several years.

The reaction of parents and other adults to knowledge of the offense is also likely to have a powerful effect on the child. A child who is not believed, whose parents react with strong emotions, or whose life is significantly disrupted by the incident may have a difficult time coping with the abuse. A child who is made to feel that disobeying a parent led to the incident ("I told you never to go to the park alone") may have similar difficulty. And when parents cut off spontaneous hugs and kisses on the assumption that physical demonstrations of affection will bring back memories of the incident, a child may feel no longer worthy of affection, that all normal displays of affection are connected with sexual abuse, or that she or he is being punished (Sanford, 1980).

When the child molester is a family member, the act becomes incest, and additional problems arise.

# INCEST

Incest refers to any intimate, sexually arousing, physical contact between members of a family who are not married to each other (Justice and Justice, 1979). Human beings seem to have a horror of incest, and sexual activity between parents and children has been prohibited in every known society (Murdock, 1949). Sexual activity between brothers and sisters has also been forbidden with only a few exceptions, such as ancient Egypt and Persia. Incest inspires such revulsion that in many cultures offenders are put to death.

**incest** intimate, sexually arousing physical contact between members of a family who are not married to each other

No one is certain exactly how the incest taboo developed, but it appears to serve humanity well. From a biological viewpoint, inbreeding appears to reduce size, fertility, longevity, and resistance to disease in a species, as well as allowing certain abnormalities, such as dwarfism, to emerge. When more than a 150 children of incestuous matings in Czechoslovakia were compared with their half-sisters and brothers of nonincestuous matings, 25 percent of the incest group but none of the nonincest group were retarded, and 20 percent of the incest group but only 5 percent of the nonincest group had some abnormality (Seemanova, 1971). From a psychological viewpoint, incest stirs up jealousies and stresses within the family, confusing family roles and keeping the child's needs from being met (Justice and Justice, 1979). From an anthropological viewpoint, incest prevents families from using marriage to form cooperative networks for trade and mutual protection (Cohen, 1978).

Beyond the bounds of the nuclear family, the definition of incest varies from culture to culture. Most societies forbid marriages between uncle and niece, aunt and nephew, or first cousins, and some restrict marriage among very distant relatives, or even their in-laws. But a few societies define incest quite narrowly and allow half-brothers and sisters to marry.

Although incest was once believed to be extremely rare, with the rate set at one person per million in English-speaking countries, authorities now believe it is much more common. Earlier estimates were based on reported cases of incest, but research made clear that most cases never come to the attention of courts, social workers, or therapists.

The concept of the "typical incest family" has undergone a sharp change, and it has become apparent that incest occurs at all levels of society. Early studies showed a high proportion of cases among poor families in rural areas (Gebhard et al., 1965), leading to the stereotype of the uneducated, backwoods family. However, the bulk of cases in a California incest treatment program come from middle-class suburban neighborhoods.

When sexual surveys of the general population were made, about one in every hundred women reported a sexual experience with her father or stepfather (Justice and Justice, 1979). Brother-sister incest is believed to be even more common, but mother-son incest is so extraordinary that only twenty-two cases have ever been documented. In every reported case, one or both partners was severely disturbed before the incest began.

Incest is hardly ever a single, isolated event. In most cases, the relationship lasts for more than a year, and sexual activity occurs anywhere from once a week to every day (Katz and Mazur, 1979).

## Father-daughter incest

The father who begins an incestuous relationship with his daughter is rarely retarded, psychotic, or pedophilic. Instead, he is a man with some sort of personality disturbance that makes him unable to control his impulses. He is likely to be under considerable stress, engrossed in his family, and with no outside social contacts. When his marital relationship does not meet his sexual needs, he turns to a daughter for sexual and emotional fulfillment (Meiselman, 1978). In most cases, his wife is either emotionally distant or physically absent, and she is often extremely passive and dependent.

Women who as girls were incestuously involved with their fathers describe them as patriarchs whose authority was absolute, leading some therapists to blame father-daughter incest on male and female sex roles (Herman and Hirschman,

1981). Family sex roles in incestuous families are generally highly traditional, and mothers are often ill or absent. In this view, the powerful father—who regards his powerless daughter as property—forces her to pay with her body for affection and care.

Some incestuous fathers do regard their children as their property and feel they may do what they please with them. In initiating sexual activity, such a father may tell his daughter that all fathers behave this way with their daughters. Other fathers may say that they are providing sex education, protecting the daughter from corrupt men in the outside world, or expressing their love. If the daughter is young, she may believe her father:

> As a child I thought, why would someone that I love and who loves me do anything wrong to me. There seemed to be no answer but . . . this is natural, and this is the way it is. I thought maybe, just maybe, this was my personal indoctrination into womanhood. (Herman and Hirschman, 1981, p. 85)

Father-daughter incest may be increasing as divorce and remarriage weaken the barriers against it in remarried families (Perlmutter, Engel, and Sager, 1982). Stepdaughters who are victims of incest are less likely to feel the same affection for the offending parent that biological daughters often continue to show. Most simply want to get away, and many girls who leave feel a mixture of guilt for deserting their mothers and anger toward them for not preventing the abuse:

> I feel bad about leaving my mother because she needs me, but I know we have to split eventually anyway. When I have my own children I'll never allow her and John to visit me because I'd be afraid of having him near my children. (Perlmutter, Engel, and Sager, 1982, p. 92)

Like child molestation, incest when reported brings the child into the legal system. Once the case comes to the attention of the authorities, the result may be a lengthy jail term for the father or destruction of the family through divorce. When this happens, the child is likely to blame herself for the situation. One nine-year-old girl who was ready to testify against her father was devastated to see him brought into the courtroom in handcuffs and with chains around his waist. She said, "I did *that* to my Daddy?" and collapsed (MacFarlane, 1978).

The long-term effects of father-daughter incest appear to include difficulty in relationships with men and various sexual problems, such as lack of orgasm and lack of sexual desire. Some researchers believe an incestuous relationship may sometimes set up a chain of events that leads the victim into prostitution (Katz and Mazur, 1979).

## Other forms of incest

Although father-daughter incest is the most common form in court records and the files of therapists, many researchers believe incest between brothers and sisters is much more prevalent. The scarcity of records on sibling incest may be explained by the fact that society is less upset by it, so cases are less likely to be reported, and that it is less likely to have lasting repercussions.

Sexual activity among siblings is certainly not rare. Among nearly 800 college and university students in New England, 15 percent of the women and 10 percent of the men reported some kind of sexual activity with a sibling (Finkelhor, 1980). Those who had engaged in sexual activity as young children tended to report the sort of behavior that sounds at first like typical childish sex play—showing, exploring, and fondling the genitals. However, many of the cases were closer to child molestation, because the young child was usually involved with a much older sibling. In a third of the cases, the older sibling was a teenager. As children grew older fondling continued to be common, and it progressed to intercourse in a number of cases. Not one child who was involved with an older sibling had ever told about the experience.

Reactions to this childhood sexuality varied. When the relationship had been exploitative, as when an older brother coerced a younger sister, the experience was generally recalled as negative and was related to later problems in sexual adjustment. But when the experience was a mutual activity between siblings born only a few years apart, it tended to be remembered positively. Among women, such incidents were related to a belief in their sexual desirability. Among men, perhaps because of their cultural role as initiator of sexual activity, sexual experience with siblings seemed related to doubts about their own sexual desirability.

Little is known about homosexual incest between siblings, but a number of cases of incest between father and son are on record. In such cases, the father generally has strong homosexual desires but lives an apparently conventional heterosexual life. The affair usually stops when the son becomes upset about it, and the son's turmoil produces guilt and depression in the father (Meiselman, 1978).

We know so little about these other forms of incest that we can't be certain as to their prevalence or long-term consequences. Except for cases of incest among brothers and sisters who are close in age, however, incest can be regarded as coercive sex and a special form of child molestation.

Whether the incidence of coercive sex is actually rising or whether a greater proportion of cases is now being reported, statistics of violent sex have been climbing. As concerned people look for causes, attention has turned to the effects of pornography.

## PORNOGRAPHY AND SEXUAL VIOLENCE

For many people, the key issue in debates over pornography is whether its use leads to antisocial behavior and violence. Does pornography lead men to rape or encourage violence and hostility toward women? Does it promote sadism and child molestation?

Before considering those questions, we need to know the status and recent history of pornography in the United States. According to the Random House dictionary, **erotica** is literature or art dealing with sexual love, but **pornography**, derived from a Greek word meaning "writing about prostitutes," is defined as

**erotica** literature or art dealing with sexual love

**pornography** obscene literature, art, or photography, especially that having no artistic merit

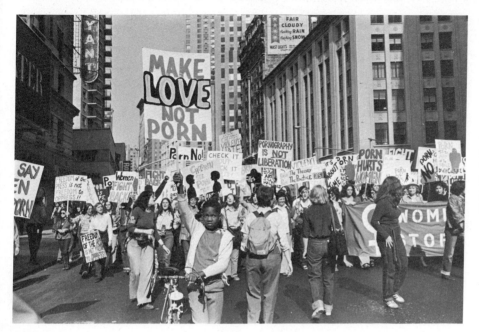

This anti-pornography march is directed against pornography that uses children or that portrays women as victims or passive sex toys, on the grounds that such material encourages violence and hostility toward women. (© Barbara Alper/ Stoch, Boston)

"obscene literature, art, or photography, especially that having no artistic merit." An object that is **obscene** causes sexual excitement or lust, but is offensive, disgusting, or repulsive. Thus the difference between erotica and pornography appears to be in the realm of emotion and artistic merit. Pornography does not recognize the complicated emotions involved in a sexual relationship, and lacks artistic intent and quality. These definitions have evolved gradually, in response to court decisions; however, in many cases it is still difficult to draw the line between erotica and pornography. Since the judgment is subjective, a work that is erotic to one person may be obscene to another.

**obscene** an object that causes sexual excitement or lust but is offensive, disgusting, or repulsive

## The legal issues

Attempts to separate the erotic from the obscene began in 1933, when James Joyce's *Ulysses,* which has been considered pornographic and was not allowed to be sold in the United States, was ruled not obscene. The federal judge who heard the case wrote that "in its entirety," *Ulysses* "did not tend to excite sexual impulses or lustful thoughts" (Woolsey, 1934). This line of reasoning was upheld by the Supreme Court in 1957, when it ruled that obscenity was not protected by the First Amendment, but that material could be deemed obscene only if the average person, using community standards, would regard the dominant theme of the entire work as "appealing to prurient interests."

But the definition of obscenity was still unclear. In 1966 the Court tried again, this time adding that a work was obscene only if it was "utterly without redeeming social value." This last phrase gave pornographers a technical loophole. By including a single quotation from Shakespeare or providing medical captions for blatantly sexual photographs, they could redeem a pornographic book in the eyes of the law. The Court went even further in 1969, when it decided that a person could possess and use obscene materials in his or her home. Producers and distributors of pornography claimed the same right until in 1973 the Court retreated. It ruled that local community standards—not those of the national community—could be used to define obscenity. With this ruling, a movie that was acceptable in a major city could be prosecuted in a rural area, and a book forbidden in one part of the country could be sold freely in another.

This confusing situation continues today. Although Supreme Court Justice Potter Stewart said of pornography, "I know it when I see it," personal standards vary as much as local standards. Two people, armed with the same definition of pornography, are likely to come up with radically different judgments of sexual materials.

## The Commission on Obscenity and Pornography

Behind attempts to ban pornography is the assumption that it is dangerous. But at the time of many important Court decisions, no one really knew much about its effects. In 1968, the country decided to find out. The Commission on Obscenity and Pornography, which included clergy, educators, health care professionals, researchers, and lawyers, was formed to investigate the effects of pornography on American society.

In 1970 the Commission's findings filled eight volumes with information from fieldwork and experimental research. Some of the studies focused on public attitudes toward pornography; others evaluated the effects of pornography and the kinds of individuals likely to buy or use it. Researchers found, for example, that the typical patron of an adult bookstore was a white, middle-class, middle-aged, married man, dressed in a business suit or neat casual attire (Winick, 1970), and that 93 percent of the audience at an X-rated movie had a regular sex partner who was aware of their interest in pornography (Nawy, 1970). After studying the voluminous data, the commission decided there was no evidence to show that looking at, reading, or listening to explicit sexual material led to delinquent or criminal behavior. It saw no reason to ban pornography and instead advised massive sex education programs.

### Pornography and sexual aggression

The commission also studied the relationship between sex and aggression by checking the experience of convicted sex offenders with pornographic materials. A study conducted by the Kinsey Institute (Gebhard et al., 1965) found that sex offenders were more likely to say that pornography did not arouse them and less likely to report strong arousal than were offenders with no history of sex crimes or "normal" men. The researchers who conducted this study believe that arousal to pornography depends on the user's imagination and sensitivity—qualities found most frequently among young, well-educated people. Since most convicted sex offenders are neither young nor well-educated, they were less likely than others to be aroused by pornography. In another study with convicted sex offenders, rapists and pedophiles reported having seen much less pornography—either during their adolescence or in their last year of freedom—than had a group of "normal" men (Goldstein et al., 1971).

However, there are problems with such studies. When people answer questions about their responses to pornography, few say that it arouses them. Yet when response is measured in the laboratory, the proportion who are sexually aroused is much higher. It seems likely that pornography arouses a majority of people but that they hesitate to report this arousal, particularly if they—or the people they are with—disapprove of sexual material.

Researchers who have continued to study the connection between pornography and sexual violence have found that under certain circumstances, erotic materials may indeed be associated with increased aggression. In most studies that investigate this relationship, researchers bring men into the laboratory, make them very angry, and then show them some type of erotic material. Afterward, they are asked to take part in an experiment that provides them with an opportunity to give electric shocks to another person.

In one study (Donnerstein and Berkowitz, 1981), angry men who watched aggressive pornography gave women, but not men, increased electric shocks. And when the erotic film depicted a woman who was raped but seemed to enjoy it, even men who were not angry gave increased shocks to women. Such movies apparently justify aggression, for they indicate that the attacker is repaid for his aggression with pleasure. In view of the widespread belief that women really want to be raped, these films are more likely than depictions of consenting sexual activity to have serious consequences. A diet of such films might stimulate already aggressive men with weak inhibitions to assault available women.

It appears, then, that hard-core pornography as such may not be the issue; it may be the *type* of pornography. Some people have noted that the amount of aggression in pornography has increased in recent years. Films that show rape instead of consenting intercourse and some "snuff" films, in which women appear to be murdered, have become more prevalent, and a few video games that require a player to overcome obstacles in order to rape a woman have been introduced.

Although pornography may not lead directly to rape or child molestation, it does appear to encourage a view of sexuality that equates pleasure with power. Most users of pornography recognize that it is fantasy. However, if images of women as passive sexual objects who enjoy being dominated become part of the fantasy lives of men and women, men will think that they should dominate and women that they should be dominated.

Perhaps the best solution to the problem is that offered by the Commission on Obscenity and Pornography: better and more widespread sex education. By providing information that is accurate, honest, and emotionally meaningful, sex education may change how people think about sexuality, and thus alter or replace the use of pornography.

# SEXUAL HARASSMENT

Unlike most forms of sexual coercion, sexual harassment aroused little concern until a few years ago. It has always existed, but until recently sexual harassment was simply a subject for jokes. We are all familiar with cartoons that show the lustful boss chasing his secretary around the desk. In life, sexual harassment is not funny. As defined by the Equal Employment Opportunity Commission (1980), **sexual harassment** consists of unwelcome sexual advances that are a condition of employment or that affect personnel decisions, or sexual conduct that interferes with job performance or makes the work environment offensive.

**sexual harassment**
unwelcome sexual advances that are a condition of employment, that affect personnel decisions, that interfere with job performance, or that make the work environment offensive

Most working women have encountered some form of this coercive treatment, which can range from continual ogling or leering at a woman's body, or "accidentally" brushing up against her, to rape. In various surveys, from 49 to 88 percent of women say they have been sexually harassed on the job. When it happened, they felt upset, angry, guilty, or frightened, and they found the unwanted advances embarrassing, demeaning, or intimidating (Evans, 1978). About two-thirds of the harassment is verbal—off-color remarks, propositions, or outright demands for sex—and the other third is physical.

Sometimes men's behavior becomes so offensive that a woman quits her job:

> A vice president of the company where I worked made overt advances following a company banquet. This included stroking my buttocks and continually rubbing himself against me. At one point he got me alone—away from the group—and put his hand down my dress. I finally managed to get rid of him. For several weeks afterward he kept calling me at work. When I talked to my supervisor about it, his only reaction was amusement. A few months later, my supervisor started making advances. When I found another job, I left. It's much better where I am now. (Collins and Blodgett, 1981, p. 77)

One black woman said the advances began on the first day of her new job, when her employer asked if she'd make love with a white man. When she repeatedly refused, she was fired. Her employer's parting words were, "If you would have intercourse with me seven days a week, I might give you your job back" (Mackinnon, 1979).

Sexual harassment has flourished because men believe that it is fun, that its consequences are trivial, that it affects only women in low-status jobs, and that any woman can handle unwelcome advances (Evans, 1978). But women find no fun at all in these advances, and the consequences are major. A woman who rejects them without losing her job may find herself demoted.

As for the belief that only waitresses, clerks, and secretaries are sexually harassed, that is a myth. University professors and executives also face this kind of treatment. A forty-year-old bank vice president discovered:

> I was hit from all directions at once with several important bank clients offering me their business on the condition that I go out with them. I was responsible for keeping and building up these large accounts. If they pulled out, my career was finished. (Bralove, 1976)

In most cases, sexual harassment is not easy for a woman to handle. Reports from women who have been harassed indicate that direct confrontation with the man is ineffective, that ignoring advances leads to their increase, and that refusals are often followed by reprimands for job performance, sabotage of the woman's work, and other sorts of retaliation (Working Women United Institute, 1975).

Like rape, sexual harassment is not just a sex game. Some believe that power is the real issue, and that sex is used to remind women of their "proper place" (Evans, 1978). Economic power is used in sexual harassment in the same way that physical power is used in rape (MacKinnon, 1979).

Since sexual harassment appears to be part of the working world, what can a woman do? For generations, women had only three choices: submit, quit, or be fired. It is now possible to fight back with legal action against the employer, the harasser, or both. In 1981, the U.S. Court of Appeals ruled that sexual harassment is a violation of Title VII of the Civil Rights Act and that it constitutes discrimination on the basis of sex (Mastalli, 1981). Courts have found the employer responsible if the employer knew or should have known of the offensive conduct and did nothing to stop it. By complaining to her employer about persistent, unwelcome advances, a woman can establish the employer's knowledge and simplify any legal action.

Court action is lengthy, slow, and often requires appeals. As long as women hold generally subordinate positions in the working world, sexual harassment will be with us. Some men say they do not realize when they have been offensive, and that they expect women to let them know when they've gone too far. That puts women in a double bind: If they don't speak up, the harasser assumes his attention is welcome; if they do speak up, they may face other forms of retaliation. Unless companies establish and enforce policies against harassment, many women will continue to be silent (Collins and Blodgett, 1981).

If the relationship between men and women becomes more nearly equal, will men become victims of sexual harassment? Some may. One case has already surfaced in Wisconsin, where a male employee of the State Bureau of Social Security Disability Insurance was awarded damages, back pay, and attorneys' fees when his female supervisor demoted him after he had rejected her sexual advances (*New York Times*, 1982).

# PROSTITUTION

In other forms of sexual coercion, the woman is forced to participate. **Prostitution** is an emotionally indifferent but voluntary commercial transaction, in which money is exchanged for sexual services. Although prostitution has been called a "victimless crime," prostitutes or their clients may be subjected to various forms of abuse or coercion. This is especially true when children or young adolescents are involved. Because prostitution is governed by social values, the treatment of the prostitute differs from one society to the next.

**prostitution** the emotionally indifferent but voluntary sale of sexual services

## *Cultural views of prostitution*

The career and status of the prostitute have been very different in different societies and at different times in history. The courtesans of the Renaissance and the *hetaerae* of ancient Greece were often freer and more independent than married women of their cultures. In many societies, prostitution has a religious function. Young girls often acted as prostitutes in the temples of ancient Greece, and the proceeds from their work maintained the religious establishment. In ancient Babylon, women were expected to prostitute themselves once and donate the earnings from this act to the temple. After this single occasion, they resumed a chaste home life. Religious prostitutes in Egypt and India often had high status and provided entertainment as well as sexual services.

In each society, a prostitute's status depends on her social background, personal skills, and professional success. The Greek *hetaerae* served upper-class men and were regarded as personal companions, but Greek prostitutes who worked in lower-class brothels had little status or independence.

A prostitute's status in the United States varies in a similar way. At the top of the hierarchy is the call girl, who works only for a select group of clients, is highly paid, and is relatively safe from the police. In the middle is the prostitute who works in a brothel or massage parlor and who serves a diverse clientele. At the bottom of the hierarchy is the streetwalker, who actively solicits unknown customers or is available to their invitation, receives less money than other prostitutes, and may have to cope with repeated arrests.

## *The world of the prostitute*

As the object of social stigma and police scrutiny, the prostitute is ripe for victimization. She is victimized by society, in the discriminatory enforcement of laws against prostitution. Although both are equally guilty under the law, it is almost always the prostitute and not the customer, or "john," who is arrested.

The prostitute may also be victimized by people connected with her work— the pimp, who "protects" her; the brothel or hotel owner; the bartender or cabdriver who sends her customers. Because her employment is illegal, the prostitute has little recourse against thefts or physical abuse from these groups. Sometimes a prostitute dies at the hands of a pimp or a client; in one three-year period, 200 New York City prostitutes were murdered (Sanford, 1980).

In the past, the "stereotypical" prostitute seemed to be recruited from the poor, minority groups, or was a woman already labeled delinquent by police and social agencies. However, in some ways the prostitute's image has changed. Among more than a hundred streetwalkers, 64 percent were from middle- or upper-middle-class families (James, 1978), and among women employed in massage parlors, most were middle class and had some college education (Rasmussen and Kuhn, 1977).

A woman may enter prostitution for any number of reasons: money, independence, or excitement (James, 1978). The major appeal of prostitution as a profession is economic. It pays far more than most women can earn without extensive education. A call girl may earn $50,000 a year; a woman in a massage parlor may earn half that. One masseuse was frank:

> If I could find a straight job that paid as well, I'd take it in a minute. But where can anyone just out of college find a job that pays twenty-four thousand dollars a year? Where could anyone find a job like that? It's good money and I enjoy it. (Rasmussen and Kuhn, 1977, p. 16)

Housewives and college students often turn to prostitution for extra income.

However, not all women who want money, excitement, and independence become prostitutes. Those who choose prostitution instead of a "straight" career tend to have some common experiences (James, 1978). Most become sexually active at an early age, but have no intimate relationship with their first partner. This pattern of superficial sex is not typical of American women, as we saw in Chapter 12. Many prostitutes have been abused or neglected as children, and the proportion who have been victims of rape or incest is much higher than in the rest of the population.

Perhaps the heaviest toll for the prostitute is emotional. The woman who has learned to view sex as a commercial transaction may have a difficult time breaking this connection in her personal life. Personal accounts by prostitutes reveal that, in order to protect themselves from their work situation, some develop an emotional numbness or a disdain or dislike for their customers.

The prostitute apparently serves a variety of symbolic and fantasy functions for her clients. New York City call girls describe the encounter between prostitute and

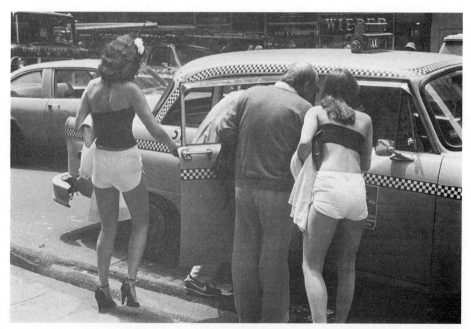

Prostitution in large cities takes many forms. Contact can be made in bars, over the telephone, or on the streets, and either prostitute or client may find themselves subjected to abuse or coercion. (© Michael Weisbrot & family/Stock, Boston)

*Focus*

ROBERTA
VICTOR—
PROFILE OF A
PROSTITUTE

Roberta was an overweight child but precociously intelligent and sensitive. She learned early to seek appreciation and attention from men by offering her body as a sexual reward. Accustomed to using sex as a form of manipulation, she found it easy to adjust to prostitution. Roberta tells her story in her own words.

"The favors I granted were not always sexual. When I was a call girl, men were not paying for sex. They were paying for something else. They were either paying to act out a fantasy or they were paying for companionship or they were paying to be seen with a well-dressed young woman. Or they were paying for somebody to listen to them. They were paying for a *lot* of things. Some men were paying for sex that *they* felt was deviant. They were paying so that nobody would accuse them of being perverted or dirty or nasty. A large proportion of these guys asked things that were not at all deviant. Many of them wanted oral sex. They felt they couldn't ask their wives or girlfriends because they'd be repulsed. Many of them wanted somebody to talk dirty to them.

"I was about fifteen, going on sixteen [when I got into prostitution]. I was sitting in a coffee shop in the Village, and a friend of mine came by. She said, 'I've got a cab waiting. Hurry up. You can make fifty dollars in twenty minutes.' Looking back, I wonder why I was so willing to run out of the coffee shop, get in a cab, and turn a trick. It wasn't traumatic because my training had been in how to be a hustler anyway.

"I learned it from the society around me, just as a woman. We're taught how to hustle, how to attract, hold a man, and give sexual favors in return. The language that you hear all the time—'Don't sell yourself cheap.' 'Hold out for the highest bidder.' . . . It's a marketplace transaction. . . . What I did was no different from what ninety-nine percent of American women are taught to do.

. . .

"It was a tremendous kick. Here I was doing absolutely nothing, *feeling* nothing, and in twenty minutes I was going to walk out with fifty dollars for twenty minutes' work? Folks work for eight dollars for take-home pay. . . .

"At the beginning I was very excited. But in order to continue I had to turn myself off. I had to disassociate who I was from what I was doing.

"It's a process of numbing yourself. I couldn't as-

client as a "scene" in which both participants play certain roles: opportunist/ hooker, adventurer/playmate, lover/romantic partner, slave/master, friend/confidante. The prostitute seems to provide far more than a simple sexual service. Some men demand a form of emotional relationship; others require sexual education or "therapy"; and most customers expect sexual imaginativeness, variety, and enthusiasm. The men tend to be middle-aged, professional or in business, and many have no other sexual outlet. The researcher who studied these call girls (Stein, 1977) concluded that prostitution may often operate as an "underground sexual health service" that aids men with various sexual and emotional needs. However, these women were relatively elite call girls; the streetwalker may provide a less complex set of services. Some men who hire prostitutes may have physical handicaps or deformities or be unable to establish intimate relationships with women.

sociate with people who were not in the life—either the drug life or the hustling life. I found I couldn't turn myself back on when I finished working. When I turned myself off, I was numb—emotionally, sexually numb.

"Almost all the call girls I knew were involved in drugs. The fast life, the night hours. At after-hours clubs, if you're not a big drinker, you usually find somebody who has cocaine, 'cause that's the big drug in those places. You wake up at noon, there's not very much to do till nine or ten that night. Everybody else is at work, so you shoot heroin. After a while the work becomes a way of supplying drugs, rather than the drugs being something we took when we were bored."

[The process of deterioration began for Roberta with her increasing dependence on drugs. As her physical attractiveness declined, she began to work off the street, where she ran into the dangers that face all streetwalkers.]

"For the first time I ran the risk of being busted. I was never arrested as a call girl. Every once in a while a cop would get hold of somebody's book. They would call one of the girls and say, 'I'm a friend of so-and-so's.' They would try to trap them. I never took calls from people I didn't know. But on the streets, how do you know who you're gonna pick up? . . .

"I once really got trapped. It was about midnight and a guy came down the street. He said he was a postal worker who just got off the shift. He told me how much money he had and what he wanted. I took him to my room. The cop isn't supposed to undress. If you can describe the color of his shorts, it's an invalid arrest. Not only did he show me the color of his shorts, he went to bed with me. Then he pulled a badge and a gun and busted me."

[As a result of her arrest and subsequent conviction, Roberta served a prison sentence of almost four years. After her release, she went back to the world of heroin and prostitution.]

"You become your job. I became what I did. I became a hustler. I became cold. I became hard. I became turned off. I became numb. Even when I wasn't hustling, I was a hustler. I don't think it's terribly different from somebody who works on the assembly line forty hours a week and comes home cut off, numb, dehumanized. People aren't built to switch on and off like a water faucet" (Terkel, 1972, pp. 91–103).

Clients can also be victimized, especially if they hire streetwalkers. The victimization usually takes the form of theft, in which the prostitute or her accomplice steals a watch, wallet, or other valuables. On occasion, johns are beaten by a pimp, and in rare instances they are arrested.

Men also work as prostitutes, but few male prostitutes serve a female clientele. When such contacts exist, they tend to parallel the relationship of a man who supports a mistress—the woman pays a man who provides her with both sexual service and some form of companionship. But the majority of male prostitutes work for male customers.

Although some male prostitutes are homosexual, most are not. In fact, the male prostitute's success as a "hustler" often depends on his ability to present himself as exclusively heterosexual (Gagnon and Simon, 1973). Most male prostitutes do not consider themselves homosexual, and the etiquette of the contact between male prostitute and male customer is carefully structured to maintain this perception (Hoffman, 1979).

The contact is usually brief and restricted to fellatio or manual masturbation. To maintain his self-image as heterosexual, the male prostitute forbids any form of intimacy with the client and may use heterosexual fantasy in order to reach orgasm—as did the hustler played by Jon Voight in *Midnight Cowboy.*

## Child prostitution

The use of children as prostitutes has become a matter of public concern. Even people who do not regard adult prostitution as coercive are usually shocked and dismayed at the growing number of reports concerning child prostitution in large cities.

Most girls and boys who become prostitutes are runaways who leave home to escape sexual or physical abuse, school problems, or family dissension. On their own in a big city, with no friends, no money, nowhere to turn, they are extremely vulnerable. Many get no farther than the bus station before they are contacted by a pimp's representative, who buys them a meal and gives them a place to stay. Before long, they are into the life:

> At first I thought this guy just liked to help kids. I felt lucky that he saw me in
> the bus station and came over to help me. I don't know what I would have
> done otherwise—later I learned he worked for the pimp I got mixed up with.
> Some friend! (Sanford, 1980, pp. 128–129)

Some youngsters begin by posing for child pornographers. In most cases, however, pornographic models cannot make enough to live on, especially after they've been introduced to drugs. If they don't want to steal or push drugs, their only option is prostitution.

In line with traditional sex roles, boy prostitutes usually strike out on their own. Taught to be independent, they do not feel the need of a "loving" protector, and they don't want to turn their earnings over to someone else. But girl prostitutes, taught to be dependent, feel the need of protection from customers and police. To the girls, the pimp becomes a father figure; many pimps have names such as Cotton Candy, Sugar Daddy, Poppa Bear, and Sweet Honey. One West Coast pimp explained:

> Boys just aren't worth the trouble. They can move on easily and they don't
> follow orders as well as girls. Too much of a mind of their own—my
> investment is much better with girls. (Sanford, 1980, p. 135)

Although pimps insist they are providing an important service to these girls, they—and the customers of boy and girl prostitutes—are sexually exploiting children.

The theme of this chapter has been the exploitation of women and children by men. Again and again, what appears to be a misdirection of sexuality in individuals is shaped by the sex roles of society. As we've seen, there's no reason to believe that men's sexual needs are greater than those of women. But when sexuality takes an unusual turn in women, it is rarely coupled with violence or the exploitation of others. A social structure that makes men dominant and women submissive encourages men to coerce those they see as weaker than themselves.

# Summary

**1** The existence of rape and other forms of sexual coercion has been explained as the inevitable expression of a human instinct for violence, as an expression of the male predisposition for violence, as the result of social learning, or as the result of woman's inferior social position. The encouragement of male aggression and woman's inferior position may both be linked with violent sexuality.

**2** **Rape** refers to sexual relations with another person obtained by force, threat, or intimidation. It includes stranger rape, gang rape, date rape, marital rape, statutory rape, homosexual rape, and rape by women. Rape may be the only major crime in which the victim has borne the burden of guilt and responsibility. Until recently, rape was not seen as a crime against a woman but as a violation of male property rights. By blaming the victim, cultural myths encourage rape. Many researchers believe that rape is not a sexual crime at all, but an act of aggression directed at women.

**3** Three distinct motives lead men to rape: anger, power, and sadism. In an anger rape, the aim is revenge; in a power rape, the aim is sexual conquest; in a sadistic rape, the aim is abuse and torture. Although anger rapes are usually spontaneous, most other rapes are planned. There appears to be no "typical rapist." Women's reactions to rape go through an acute phase and a long-term reorganization phase. Being raped often has long-term sexual consequences. Most male victims are attacked by other men, especially in prisons; however, women occasionally sexually assault or abuse men.

**4** **Child molestation** refers to any sexual contact between an adult and a child; sexual contact between an adult and a young adolescent is known as **hebephilia**. Child molestation often goes unreported, since the child may not be aware that improper behavior has occurred, the child molester may be a relative, or parents may wish to protect the child from the stress of legal proceedings. The child molester, who is almost always a man, resembles the general male population. Molesters rarely use force; instead they persuade the child to have sexual contact or else place the youngster under some obligation. A molested child is most likely to be emotionally damaged if the abuse lasts over a long period, if it occurs frequently, if it lasts past the twelfth birthday, and if it includes attempts at genital intercourse. Parents' reactions to the discovery that their child has been molested also have a powerful influence on the incident's effects.

**5** **Incest** refers to intimate, sexually arousing, physical contact between members of a family who are not married to each other. Incest is much more common than was once believed, and surveys indicate that about one woman in every hundred has a sexual experience with her father or stepfather. The incestuous father is likely to be a man with no outside social contacts who is under considerable stress and is unable to control his impulses. The long-term effects of incest on the daughter appear to include difficulty in relating to men and various sexual problems. We know little about other forms of incest, but incest between brothers and sisters appears to be more prevalent than father-daughter incest.

**6**   The legal status of **pornography** in the United States is uncertain, in part because judgments of pornography are subjective and vary among individuals and in part because of confusing court decisions. After commissioning many studies, the National Commission on Obscenity and Pornography decided there was no evidence to show that pornography led to delinquency or criminal behavior. Studies have shown that some types of pornography may be associated with increased aggression. Although pornography may not lead directly to rape or child molestation, if it encourages a view of sexuality that equates pleasure with power and portrays women as enjoying sexual domination by men, it may shape views of sexuality.

**7**   **Sexual harassment** consists of unwelcome sexual advances that are either a condition of employment or that affect personnel decisions, or sexual conduct that interferes with job performance or makes the work environment offensive. Most working women have encountered some form of sexual harassment. It flourishes because men believe that it's fun, that its consequences are trivial, that it affects only women in low-status jobs, and that any woman can handle unwelcome advances. In fact, the consequences are major (firing or demotion); it affects women at all levels; and it is extremely difficult to handle. Now that sexual harassment has been ruled a violation of Title VII of the Civil Rights Act, a woman who is harassed may take legal action against both the harasser and the employer.

**8**   **Prostitution** is an emotionally indifferent but voluntary sale of sexual services. The status of the prostitute varies from one society to the next. Prostitutes may be robbed, physically abused, or killed by people connected with their work. Prostitutes come from all social classes, and they tend to enter the life for money, independence, or excitement. Most women who become prostitutes are sexually active at an early age but have no intimate relationship with their first partner. They may also have been abused or neglected as children, and there may be a background of rape or incest. The prostitute's clients are infrequently arrested. Most male prostitutes serve male customers, and the contact is usually a brief episode of fellatio or manual masturbation. The number of child prostitutes in large cities has been growing; most are runaways who find themselves in a large city without money or friends. Although boy prostitutes often strike out on their own, most girls are "protected" by a pimp.

**9**   Most coercive sex seems linked in some way to the male sex role, for unusual variations of sexuality in women rarely take a violent or exploitative form. The dominant role given men by society may encourage them to coerce those they see as weaker than themselves.

# Part Six

# Sexual Health and Reproduction

Books on health regularly appear on best-seller lists, health food stores seem to sprout on every corner, and those of us who aren't dieting are jogging. Health has become big business in the United States, and for good reason. The state of your health affects the way you look, how you feel, and what you do at work and at play. If you are in good physical health, you probably take your body and its workings for granted. But if you became seriously ill or were severely injured, nothing would seem more important to you than your health. A recent survey of 25,000 Americans discovered that nearly half thought about their health more often than they thought about work, money, or love (Rubinstein, 1982).

Health problems can have both direct and indirect influences on sexuality. Disease, disability, and drugs can directly alter the body's capacity for sexual response, or they can act indirectly by affecting mood and self-image. Despite diseases and disabilities, few people are too sick or too disabled to enjoy some form of sexual expression.

Just as health affects sexual expression, so sexual expression can affect health. Various diseases can be passed from one person to another by sexual contact; some forms of contraception appear to have widespread effects on the body; and a tardy decision to end a pregnancy can carry physical risk. Of course, the reproductive process has major effects on women. Bearing a child not only leads to temporary changes in the way a woman feels and acts, but can affect her sexual activity as well.

In the four chapters of this unit, we'll cover the interrelationship between sexuality and physical functioning. The first chapter will be devoted to sexually transmitted disease. In the second, we'll investigate some health problems of the reproductive system as well as the influence of disease, injury, and drugs on sexual expression. In the third chapter, we'll explore the issues of contraception, sterilization, and abortion. We close this section with a chapter on pregnancy and childbirth.

Even though I think of myself as a sexually liberated person, it came as a tremendous blow when a guy I had been seeing called me up to tell me he had the clap. At first I just couldn't believe it, and afterwards I found myself getting really mad at him for not being more careful. We had a real blowup and that more or less ended the relationship. (Authors' files)

I never thought much about VD until recently when I read a newspaper article about herpes. Since then I think twice about who I go to bed with. The whole idea of catching something that you'll have for the rest of your life is pretty frightening. I must say it's put quite a damper on sex for me. (Authors' files)

# 17 Sexually Transmitted Diseases

# Chapter 17

**sexually transmitted disease (STD)** any disease that *can* be passed by sexual contact

None of us likes to talk about **sexually transmitted disease (STD)**, which refers to any disease that can be passed by sexual contact. When the topic comes up in any personal way, we usually feel embarrassed, guilty, ashamed, distressed, or confused. Many people who inadvertently contract an STD feel as did this young woman:

> I was brought up to believe that "nice" people don't get VD, so how do you think I felt when I got gonorrhea? . . . I felt dirty. Like I was crawling with bugs. (Bell, 1980, p. 217)

Indeed, our attitudes toward STD, which make it a moral or social rather than a medical problem, are perhaps the single most important reason for the current epidemic in the United States. These attitudes can be traced to traditional views of sexuality and illness.

Before it was possible to identify the microorganisms that cause disease, many people thought illness was a punishment for bad or immoral behavior. In fact, before the connection between sexual activity and syphilis was known, this sexually transmitted disease was believed to be God's punishment on the human race for the sin of blasphemy (Rosebury, 1971). Once it was understood that STD was passed by sexual activity, the diseases were considered punishment for promiscuity.

Attitudes change slowly, and although the precise organisms that cause most STD are known, people persist in regarding an STD as a badge of shame. Such attitudes seem strongly related to cultural standards of acceptable sexual behavior. In a culture that sets up premarital chastity and marital fidelity as the standard, the acquisition of an STD is often seen as proof of sexual misconduct.

# Sexually Transmitted Disease

Making the diseases a moral instead of a medical issue can be harmful. The stigma often keeps people who believe they have an infection from seeking medical treatment. If they do consult a physician, it ensures that they are too embarrassed to identify their sexual contacts, who might also have the disease. The stigma also makes the prevention of STD difficult by creating a barrier against the flow of information about it. The result is that, despite the existence of effective cures for most STDs, they continue to be a worldwide health problem.

Although many people believe syphilis, gonorrhea, and herpes exhaust the category of sexually transmitted disease, there are at least a dozen different STDs, and they range from the annoying to the dangerous. Some varieties used to be referred to as **venereal disease** (VD). The word "venereal" comes from Venus, the goddess of love, and it was applied to diseases such as syphilis and gonorrhea that are nearly always passed from one adult to another by sexual contact. However, a number of diseases or infections that are often transmitted by sexual contact, such as pubic lice ("crabs") or scabies, can also be picked up in other ways. Calling them venereal diseases usually embarrasses people who might have acquired them in some nonsexual way, and it's not accurate because these diseases are not so closely linked to sexual activity as are the traditional venereal diseases. So most authorities have dropped the term "venereal disease" in favor of the broader term "sexually transmitted disease," which also lacks the cultural stigma associated with VD.

In this chapter, we investigate the most common diseases that can be passed through sexual activity. We also explore myths and misconceptions about STD and close by discussing ways of preventing STD.

**venereal disease** any disease that is *primarily* passed by sexual contact

# GONORRHEA

Gonorrhea, which is often called "clap," "drip," or "a dose," is a bacterial infection that has afflicted humanity all through recorded history. References to it appear in ancient Egyptian, Assyrian, Chinese, Japanese, and Indian sources. But gonorrhea had to wait until about A.D. 200 before it got the name by which we know it. Gonorrhea means "flow of seed," an apparent reference to the penile discharge resembling semen that accompanies the disease in men (Lasagna, 1975).

The erroneous belief that gonorrhea is spread by public toilet seats may have its origin in the Bible, which in Leviticus says: "Everything, whereon he sitteth shall be unclean. . . . And what saddle soever he rideth upon that hath the issue shall be unclean." "The issue" in this case is the penile discharge.

Perhaps because some people contracted both gonorrhea and syphilis, by the sixteenth century medical authorities believed gonorrhea was not a separate disease, but merely a symptom of syphilis. Not until 1879 was the specific organism that causes gonorrhea identified: a tiny bacterium, christened *gonococcus,* that looks like a pair of coffee beans lying side by side.

This bacterium cannot penetrate the human skin; it can enter the body only through warm, moist surfaces, such as the genitals, the anus, and the upper throat. Gonorrhea spreads through genital, oral, or anal sexual activity. The germs thrive in the upper throat—not the mouth—of a person who has contracted the disease through oral intercourse (Lasagna, 1975). Because the germs die very quickly when outside the human body, there is no danger of picking up gonorrhea from toilet seats, clothing, or other objects.

## *Symptoms*

The symptoms of gonorrhea appear between two days and two weeks after exposure. In men, the symptoms tend to take the form of pain during urination and a penile discharge. The discharge is at first clear or milky, but later may become white, yellow, or yellowish-green. In women, a green or yellow-green vaginal discharge is the primary early symptom, although some women may also find urination painful. (In both sexes, an anal infection may show itself in mild irritation or a discharge from the rectum, and an oral infection may lead to slight hoarseness, a sore throat, or swollen glands.)

Although 80 to 90 percent of men develop warning symptoms of a genital infection, only about 10 percent of women show any symptoms. Since women may not know they have contracted the disease, they often develop secondary infections. The most common complication among women is an infection of the pelvic area, called pelvic inflammatory disease, which may cause severe pain, fever, vomiting, and menstrual irregularities. When the inflammation is extensive, the woman may become sterile.

Untreated gonorrhea can also cause sterility in men. In rare instances, an untreated gonococcal infection spreads to the heart, nervous system, or joints. When gonorrhea invades the joints, a form of arthritis develops. Some women develop

painful adhesions between the liver and surrounding tissue that can be misdiag-
nosed as gall bladder disease (Keith and Brittain, 1978).

Although a woman does not pass gonorrhea to her unborn baby in the uterus,
during the birth process the bacteria may enter the infant's eyes. If left untreated,
the baby will become blind. For this reason, the eyes of newborn infants are routinely treated with erythromycin, tetracycline, or silver nitrate, which protects
against this threat.

In men, gonorrhea is usually diagnosed by examining a few drops of the urethral discharge under a microscope. In women, a culture is made by taking a swab
from one of the affected sites, placing it on a special culture medium, and waiting
for the germs to grow. It may be necessary to make cultures from several areas—
the cervix, anus, urethra, and so on—in order to find the bacteria. The culture is
necessary, because without it other vaginal infections cannot be distinguished from
gonorrhea.

## Treatment

Once a positive diagnosis is made, treatment is relatively simple and straightforward. Penicillin is the usual choice, although other antibiotics, such as tetracycline,
can be used with people who are allergic to penicillin or for penicillin-resistant
gonorrhea. Gonococcal bacteria have become increasingly resistant to penicillin,
but they still succumb to the drug if it is given in large enough doses. The required
dose for gonococcal bacteria is now more than thirty times as large as it was during
the 1940s, but the antibiotic is still effective (Cooke and Dworkin, 1981).

Some gonorrhea bacteria have mutated to produce beta gonorrhea, a strain
that breaks down penicillin, making it ineffective against them. Beta gonorrhea was
first reported in the Philippines in 1976, and has since been found in eighteen
countries. Many of the cases discovered in the United States have been brought in
from Southeast Asia or the West Coast of Africa, where the strain is more prevalent
(U.S. Public Health Service, 1980). Beta gonorrhea is curable, however, and suc-
cumbs to another antibiotic, spectinomycin.

## The gonorrhea epidemic

In the army of common infectious diseases, gonorrhea may rank second only to
the common cold. In 1979, more than a million cases of gonorrhea were reported
to government health authorities, and the best guess is that another 600,000 to one
million cases went unreported (U.S. Public Health Service, 1980). The incidence of
gonorrhea began skyrocketing in the late 1960s. In the past few years, however, the
increase has slowed down and the rate has remained relatively steady. But gonorrhea is twice as prevalent as it was less than ten years ago (see Figure 17.1).

The young run the greatest risk of contracting the disease, with 38 percent of
all cases among twenty- to twenty-four-year-olds and another 25 percent among
teenagers between fifteen and nineteen years old. If you live in a large city, your

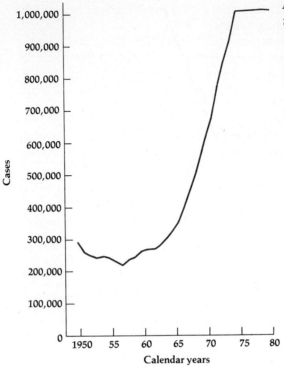

**Figure 17.1   The Gonor-
rhea Epidemic.**

After an alarming rise since
1960, the number of cases
of gonorrhea reported to the
U.S. Public Health Service has
leveled off in the past few years—
but a decline is not yet in sight.
(U.S. Public Health Service. STD
Fact Sheet, 35th ed. Atlanta: Center
for Disease Control, 1980)

chances of picking up gonorrhea are increased, but the incidence fluctuates widely
from state to state. Alaska has the highest rate in the nation, with 1,275 cases per
100,000, and New Hampshire the lowest, with only 105 cases per 100,000 (U.S.
Public Health Service, 1980). As we'll discover, there are ways to protect yourself
from contracting gonorrhea.

## NONGONOCOCCAL URETHRITIS

**nongonococcal ure-
thritis (NGU)**  any
urethral infection that is
not caused by gono-
coccal bacteria

It's been estimated that about half of all men who visit a physician's office complaining of urethral discharge do not have gonorrhea at all. Once the possibility of
gonorrhea has been eliminated, the infection is usually diagnosed as **nongonococcal** or **nonspecific urethritis** (NGU)—a catch-all term that simply means a urethral
infection not caused by gonococcal bacteria.

### Symptoms

Among men, the symptoms of nongonococcal urethritis may be similar to those
produced by gonorrhea—a burning sensation during urination and a penile discharge—or they may be mild and barely noticeable. The discharge may be thin and

clear or thick, white, and creamy like the discharge of gonorrhea. A woman may also develop NGU, but in most cases she has no symptoms at all.

Authorities agree that nongonococcal urethritis has more than one cause, but can't agree on exactly what the causes are. Some cases may be caused by a fungus, others by a bacterium, yet others by chlamydia, an organism that has been described as "somewhere between a virus and a bacterium" (Secondi, 1975). Some specialists suggest that mechanical irritation of the genitals, perhaps by vaginal sprays, soap, or contraceptive creams or jellies, may stir up a latent infection. When NGU is passed through anal intercourse, both men and women may complain of an inflamed rectum.

## *Treatment*

Left untreated, nongonococcal urethritis can produce complications; men may develop an inflamed prostate, and women may develop pelvic inflammatory disease. For many infected individuals, however, the only consequences of this disease seem to be mild discomfort. It is usually treated with the antibiotics tetracycline or doxycycline. Unlike gonorrhea, which is quickly eliminated with adequate doses of penicillin, nongonococcal urethritis must be treated for several weeks. If the treatment is not thorough, some of the organisms may survive, multiply, and cause the condition to flare up again. Since NGU often has no symptoms, a man's sexual partners—whether male or female—should be treated at the same time in order to avoid passing the infection back and forth between them (Felman and Nikitas, 1981). In some men, NGU may become a chronic condition—episodes may sporadically recur without any new exposure to the infection.

Cases of NGU are usually not reported to American public health officials, so there is no solid information as to its prevalence. However, in Great Britain and Sweden, where the infection is reported, it is twice as prevalent as gonorrhea among men (Felman and Nikitas, 1981). According to the National Center for Disease Control, between 25 and 30 percent of men reporting to U.S. clinics for treatment of STD had nongonococcal urethritis (U.S. Public Health Service, 1979). However, NGU is believed to be more common than gonorrhea among university students and upper socioeconomic groups who are not generally treated at public clinics (Felman and Nikitas, 1981). In any event, the incidence of nongonococcal urethritis seems to be on the rise, and it may become a major health problem.

## SYPHILIS

Syphilis, a chronic bacterial infection that is transmitted by sexual activity, also seems to have been humanity's constant companion. At one time, people believed that the crew of Christopher Columbus's expeditions to the New World were the first Europeans to encounter the disease.

Many authorities no longer accept this explanation. They point to descriptions

**syphilis** a chronic disease caused by a spirochete, which is transmitted by sexual activity

of "leprosy" in the Bible and other ancient writings that, from their symptoms, appear to be cases of syphilis. Some believe that David's lament in the Thirty-eighth Psalm indicates that this Old Testament king had syphilis, which he apparently contracted from Bathsheba (Rosebury, 1971). Other references establish the presence of syphilis in ancient China, Japan, and India, and in the pre-Columbian European civilizations of Greece and Rome.

Even more ancient evidence has connected syphilis with prehistoric human beings. The skeletons of Neanderthal men and women bear all the signs of congenital syphilis, a form of the disease passed from mother to child before birth (Lasagna, 1975). If these skeletal abnormalities are the result of syphilis, the disease may be older than gonorrhea.

Syphilis was always regarded as a foreign disease: the English called it the French disease, the Dutch called it the Spanish pox, and the French blamed it on the Italians. No matter what its ancestry, syphilis was rampant in sixteenth-century Europe. Ten percent of the population was probably infected. Among its royal victims was Henry VIII of England. His daughter Mary, who later became queen, appears to have had congenital syphilis (Lasagna, 1975).

Syphilis is caused by a spirochete, a thin, corkscrew-shaped bacterium that can penetrate the human skin and enter the body through the mouth, anus, or genitals, or through any slight break in the skin. From there it travels by way of the bloodstream to every part of the body. Syphilis can be spread through genital, oral, or anal sexual activity. Like the gonococcus, the spirochete dies quickly outside the body and can be killed by soap and water.

### Symptoms

**chancre** a hard, painless sore that is the first visible sign of syphilis

Syphilis, which develops slowly, passes through four stages. During the *primary stage,* the only sign of infection is a hard, painless sore called a **chancre.** Typically, this chancre appears near the place where the bacteria have entered the body—

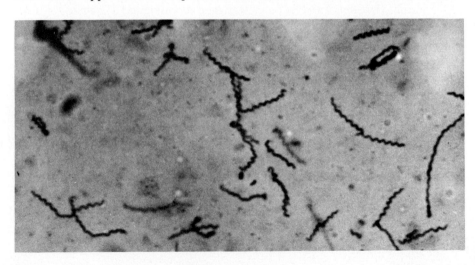

The spirochete that causes syphilis is a thin, cork-screw shaped bacterium that can enter through the mouth, anus, genitals, or any break in the skin. (© Rotker/ Taurus Photos)

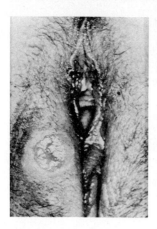 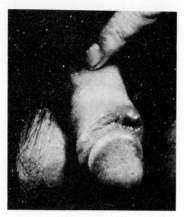

The only symptom of primary syphilis is a hard, painless chancre, such as in these chancres on the vaginal outer lip (a) and the shaft of the penis (b). (From: *Color Atlas of Venerelogy* by Anthony Wisdom)

usually the genitals—about ten to ninety days after exposure. The sore, which grows from the size of a small pimple to that of a marble, has a ring of hard, rubbery tissue around its base, but is soft and generally open at the top. Because the chancre is filled with bacteria, the disease is highly contagious during the first stage. Since the chancre is painless, the infected individual may not notice it or consider it a sign of disease. In women, the chancre may develop internally. Regardless of whether the infection is treated, the chancre disappears within one to eight weeks.

From two to ten weeks during the *second stage,* the effect of the syphilis bacteria spreads from the genital area to other parts of the body. At this time, the disease is still highly contagious. A common symptom of this stage is a rash or blisters that may appear anywhere on the skin. Like the chancre, the rash disappears without treatment. Other symptoms of second-stage syphilis may include headache, fever, loss of appetite, or sore throat. These symptoms may be so mild that they are ignored, or they may be confused with other diseases, such as flu.

Now the disease enters the *latent stage,* and its signs may disappear for ten, twenty, or even thirty years. The disease is usually not contagious at this time, except for a pregnant woman, who may infect her unborn baby. During the latent stage, the syphilis bacteria may attack and destroy various parts of the body, including the circulatory and nervous systems.

Finally, in *late* syphilis, the internal damage becomes apparent. Among a third of the untreated cases, it takes the form of cardiovascular disease, paralysis, mental incapacity, blindness, or other serious health problems.

When a woman with syphilis becomes pregnant, the spirochetes may travel into the body of the unborn child, causing congenital syphilis. An infected fetus may miscarry, be stillborn, or die shortly after birth. If the infant lives, it may appear healthy but later become crippled, blind, or deaf, or develop characteristic facial, dental, or bone abnormalities.

## Treatment

Before the advent of penicillin, there was no reliable cure for syphilis, and the standard treatment, which dates back to the seventeenth century, was mercury or other heavy metals. There is little evidence that the mercury treatment worked, and many patients suffered serious side effects or even death from it.

Since the early 1940s, when penicillin came into use, syphilis has been completely curable. The disease may be halted at any stage by adequate doses of penicillin or other antibiotics, such as tetracycline. In fact, syphilis that is treated before it reaches the late stage can be cured with little or no permanent damage. In cases that have reached the late stage, damage cannot be reversed, but any further damage can be prevented.

## The waning of syphilis

Although syphilis has been, with good reason, the most feared STD, it is becoming increasingly less common in the United States (see Figure 17.2). There are still nearly a half million cases of untreated syphilis, but its incidence has dropped dramatically in this century.

However, the incidence of syphilis rises and falls. In 1979, about 25,000 cases of primary and secondary syphilis were reported to public health authorities, an increase of nearly 15 percent from the previous year. Since the mid-1970s, syphilis has become increasingly a male disease, perhaps because its rate is rising among the gay male population. For whatever reason, more than three cases of syphilis among men are reported for every case among women (U.S. Public Health Service, 1980).

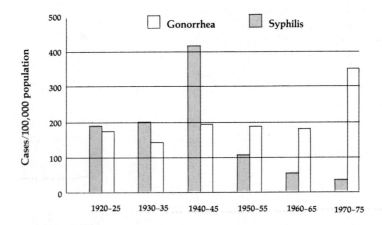

**Figure 17.2**

The Incidence of Reported Cases of Gonorrhea and Syphillis, 1920–1975.

# HERPES

The sexually transmitted disease that has received the most public attention in recent years is **herpes,** a virus infection of the mucous membranes or skin surface. Herpes has a history that runs back at least as far as ancient Greece. It was the Greeks who called it herpes, which comes from the Greek word meaning "to creep." The name describes the disease's primary symptom: sores that creep across the skin's surface (Hamilton, 1980).

**herpes** an infection of the mucous membranes or skin surface, caused by herpes type 1 or herpes type 2 virus, and often transmitted by sexual contact

Herpes is actually a family of more than fifty different viruses, but two familiar types are connected with sexual activity. Herpes type 1 causes cold sores on the mouth; herpes type 2 produces genital infection. It was once believed that herpes type 1 could not infect the genitals and that herpes type 2 could not infect the mouth. It now appears that some herpes infections are "crossovers"—that is, genital herpes can be caused by type 1, and a cold sore by type 2. Some authorities believe that the increase in oral sexual activity is partly responsible for the increased number of crossover infections, which have risen from 5 percent of herpes infections in the mid-1960s to between 10 and 15 percent today (Hamilton, 1980). Although herpes is passed by direct physical contact, the virus may live for a brief time outside the body, making it possible (but highly unlikely) to contract herpes from damp towels or other objects.

## *Symptoms*

The first attack of herpes tends to produce the most severe symptoms. Before any trace of the infection is visible, most people notice a tingling, itching, or burning sensation near the place the infection will appear. A few hours or perhaps a couple of days later, a small patch of measlelike rash appears, which quickly develops into blisters. These blisters itch or burn and often feel tender to the touch.

In women, groups of blisters tend to appear on the cervix, vulva, and sometimes the thighs or buttocks. In men, similar blisters tend to appear on the penis, although they may also develop on the thighs or buttocks or in the urethra. In severe cases, both men and women complain of fever, swollen glands, headache, and other flulike symptoms. However, the symptoms are often so mild as to escape notice. For instance, a woman who develops a herpes infection that is limited to the cervix may be unaware that she has contracted the disease.

As the infection progresses, the blisters form scabs and begin to dry up. They disappear spontaneously within one to three weeks. Herpes is contagious as long as any symptoms are present, from the initial tingling through the healing of the sores.

Although the recovered patient feels and looks well, the herpes virus remains in the body, having retreated to nerve cells where it cannot be reached by protective antibodies in the bloodstream. About two-thirds of those who contract herpes apparently build up an immunity to the virus and never experience another attack, but the other third have recurrences at sporadic intervals. These recurrences are of-

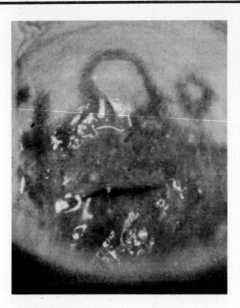 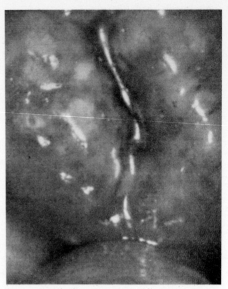

After a week or so, the herpes blisters that cover this woman's cervix (a) begin to dry and heal by themselves (b). When blisters are limited to the cervix, a woman may be unaware that she has contracted the disease. (From: *Color Atlas of Venerelogy* by Anthony Wisdom)

ten linked with emotional or physical stress. In women, they may occur during certain phases of the menstrual cycle. Recurrences are usually less severe than the primary infection and tend to disappear more quickly

Aside from the discomfort that accompanies an outbreak of herpes, additional complications can occur. If the virus is transferred to the eyes, the cornea can become infected, a condition known as keratitis. Since the herpes virus is killed by soap and water, keratitis can be prevented by two simple precautions: always wash the hands before rubbing the eyes, and never use saliva to lubricate contact lenses.

Far more serious is the association of herpes type 2 with cervical cancer. Research indicates that women with cervical cancer are more likely to have been exposed to herpes type 2 than women who do not develop this cancer. Not all women who have had herpes type 2 develop cervical cancer, but such women should have Pap smears each year to monitor the health of the cervix (U.S. Public Health Service, 1982a). When cervical cancer is caught in its early stages, cure rates are extremely high.

Another serious consequence of herpes type 2 is the possibility of passing the infection to an infant during the birth process. Until recently, up to 70 percent of the newborns who contracted the virus died, and many who survived had brain damage (Babson et al., 1980). The outlook may not be as bleak for these babies as it once was, however, because a new drug now being tested, vidarabine, appears to cut the death rate in half (Leary, 1980). A baby can contract herpes only if the infection is active at the time of delivery, when the infant is exposed to the virus during the trip through the cervix and vagina. If a woman has a case of active herpes, most physicians recommend a Caesarean section so that the infant is not exposed to infection in the vaginal canal.

Contracting a herpes type 2 infection seems to have widespread psychological effects on some people. Physicians report that some of their male patients develop erectile dysfunction after contracting the disease. Since the virus has no direct effect on sexual function, it appears that the fear of spreading herpes and the fear of being rejected as a sexual partner can combine to make erection virtually impossible. The fear of passing herpes to others can be so deep that people who contract it sometimes withdraw from social contacts and seem to lose all interest in sex (Hamilton, 1980).

## Treatment

For thousands of years, all that could be done for people with genital infections of herpes was to make them as comfortable as possible. Even today there is no cure for the disease, in the sense that all the virus is eliminated from the body. However,

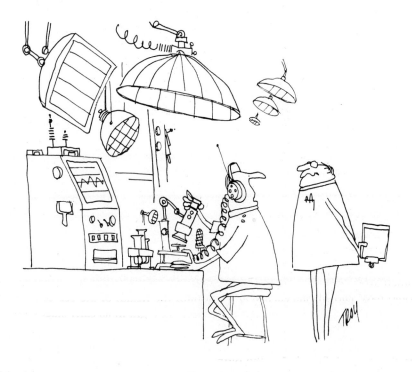

"I'm in touch with the herpes virus. They say they have a right to life, too."

(Reprinted courtesy *Omni Magazine*, © 1983)

a new drug, acyclovir, does speed the recovery from an initial outbreak, even though it does not eradicate the virus and is not effective against recurrences (Saral et al., 1981). Acyclovir works by causing the herpes virus to commit suicide. Because the drug resembles an enzyme the virus needs to reproduce, it mistakenly uses the drug, producing an incomplete virus that cannot survive. And since the drug is ignored by normal body cells, it seems safe as well as effective (Hamilton, 1980).

Most creams and ointments simply delay healing and may spread the virus, creating new blisters. Although the open blisters are susceptible to bacterial infection, most specialists believe that antibacterial, corticosteroid creams, antiseptics, or lemon juice may do more harm than good. The recommended procedure is to keep the sores dry and clean, using only water unless soap can be used without too much pain. Epsom salts and Burow's solution may be applied to the sore and allowed to dry in the air, since these compounds speed the drying of the blisters (Hamilton, 1980). To avoid infecting others, it is necessary to abstain from sexual activity until all symptoms disappear.

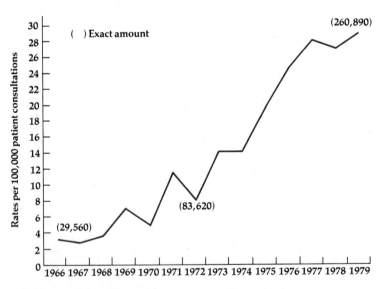

*Figure 17.3 Herpes—The New Epidemic.*

This graph of patients' consultations with private physicians for genital herpes infections shows the rapid rise in herpes infections over a thirteen-year period. (U.S. Public Health Service. *MMWR: Morbidity and Mortality Weekly Report,* March 26, 1982, vol. 31, no. 11, p. 138)

## *The new epidemic*

The U.S. Public Health Service (1982a) believes there is a national epidemic of herpes type 2 and points out that in just over a decade, voluntary reports from private physicians indicated that they had seen nearly a tenfold increase in cases of herpes type 2 in the past thirteen years (see Figure 17.3). More than a quarter of a million cases were seen by private physicians in 1979, but since there is no record of cases seen at public health clinics and hospitals, the actual incidence is unknown.

We do know that both type 1 and type 2 are extremely common. When the herpes virus enters the body, the immune system goes to work, producing antibodies that fight the virus and help to guard against new outbreaks of infection. So the presence of antibodies in the bloodstream indicates a previous infection. Tests have shown that about 90 percent of adults in the United States have been infected by herpes type 1, and about 60 percent have been infected by herpes type 2—usually without any symptoms.

The sensational treatment of sexually transmitted herpes in the media has made many people afraid of sexual activity and led to warnings that the disease could end the sexual revolution. Our fear is reflected in a common joke: "What's the difference between true love and herpes? Herpes is forever." As we've seen, the joke is only partly right: The herpes virus does live forever in the body, but only a third of the people who contact it ever have another infection, and it appears to be transmitted only when the infection is active.

## ACQUIRED IMMUNE DEFICIENCY SYNDROME (AIDS)

Among the newest diseases associated with sexual contact is **acquired immune deficiency syndrome (AIDS)**, a disease that involves a breakdown of the body's natural immune system, leaving a person susceptible to a host of serious infections and diseases. Since the first case was reported in 1979, the number has increased dramatically to about 600 by mid-1982, with one to two new cases being diagnosed every day (U.S. Public Health Service, 1982c). AIDS is a serious disorder, with death occurring in 41 percent of the diagnosed cases.

AIDS is concentrated among homosexual and bisexual men, who make up 75 percent of the cases, and it seems to be associated with a large number of sexual partners. One study found that gay men with AIDS had had an average of 1,160 sexual partners, compared with an average of 524 for gay men without AIDS (Levine, 1982). For this reason we are considering AIDS as an STD, although the disease can be acquired in other ways. It is believed that AIDS can also be spread by contaminated needles or blood transfusions; most heterosexual patients with AIDS use intravenous drugs and some are hemophiliacs (who receive frequent transfusions). The appearance of a few cases among heterosexual, non-drug-using Hai-

**acquired immune deficiency syndrome (AIDS)** a disease that involves a breakdown of the body's natural immune system

*Focus*

MYTHS AND MISCON-
CEPTIONS
ABOUT STD

Myths and misconceptions about sexually transmitted diseases pervade American society. Most of these myths promote the spread of STDs or interfere with their treatment, so it would seem that as long as people believe them, the epidemic is likely to continue.

### Myth number 1. Nice people don't get STD

Many nice people *do* get STD. Sexually transmitted diseases are democratic; they pay no attention to social class, race, religion, educational level, marital status, or sexual orientation. Since "nice" people have sexual contact, we all need to be aware of the signs and symptoms of STD. Although multiple sexual partners increase a person's chances of contracting some sexually transmitted disease, these infections can be acquired by people whose sex life is relatively conventional. A man on a business trip who visits a prostitute may become infected and pass the disease to his wife. Or a woman can infect her new husband, unwittingly passing to him an STD she received from her former spouse.

The myth that nice people don't get STD may be encouraged by information from the U.S. Public Health Service, which reports data on the number and types of some STDs, basing its figures on information from public health clinics, private clinics, and physicians. Although these reports are legally required of all health practitioners, not all physicians report cases among their regular patients. A private physician is often reluctant to expose a long-time patient to the tracing of his or her sexual contacts that follows an official report of STD. But public health clinics—which generally treat the economically disadvantaged—tend to be conscientious in fulfilling this requirement. It has been estimated that less than half the cases of syphilis and gonorrhea are reported to public authorities, and that the uncounted cases are concentrated among older middle- or upper-class men and women.

### Myth number 2. You can get an STD only once

There is no limit to the number of times an individual can be reinfected with the same STD. Unlike many infectious diseases—measles, mumps, and so on— STDs do not provide immunity to later infections. Except for herpes, a person who contracts a particular STD does not develop antibodies that will protect him or her against later exposure.

### Myth number 3. STDs are acquired only through genital intercourse

STDs may be acquired through a variety of sexual activities. Both oral

tians suggests that crowded living conditions and poor sanitation may also help to spread the disorder.

Researchers have been puzzled by the concentration of AIDS in the gay community, and it has been suggested that changes in the gay life style during the past fifteen years may be responsible, including an increase in the number of sexual partners and the widespread use of amyl and butyl nitrite as recreational drugs (Friedman-Klein et al., 1982).

and anal sex can transmit an infection, as can skin contact with an area infected by syphilis. However, few cases of serious STDs are acquired through contact with inanimate objects, such as sheets or the notorious public toilet seat. The microorganisms that cause most STDs can survive only on warm, moist skin—typically, the mouth and genital areas.

**Myth number 4. Sexual contact with an infected partner invariably results in STD** Exposure to the microorganisms that cause STD does not always lead to infection, just as not everyone who is exposed to influenza or tuberculosis contracts it. When public health officials trace the sexual contacts of someone infected with, say, gonorrhea, they often find that only about half the contacts have the disease. Some STDs are

more contagious than others, but even those that are highly contagious do not infect on every exposure.

**Myth number 5. Nothing can be done about the signs and symptoms of STD** Early treatment of most STDs, including gonorrhea and syphilis, will completely eliminate the infection. If treatment is delayed, however, the damage caused by these infections cannot be reversed. But even years after an infection has been acquired, treatment will halt its progress and no further damage can take place. The most important exception to this rule that treatment can eliminate STD is herpes; however, the disease apparently is not contagious unless symptoms are present.

**Myth number 6. The signs of STD are easy to recognize** Although most men develop warning

signs that lead them to seek treatment for STD, women are often completely unaware of their infection. Yet without such recognition, prompt and effective treatment is impossible.

When the internal male organs become infected, a man generally has a penile discharge or finds urinating painful. But because the female urinary tract is separate from the genitals, it may not be involved in the infection. Women often develop symptoms in the vagina or cervix, where they cannot be detected without an internal examination. Unless a woman develops pain or vaginal discharge—and most infected women do not—she may not realize she is infected until the disease progresses to a later, more severe stage. It seems that women are forced to depend on the honesty and responsibility of their male sexual partners for protection.

Although the disorder remains mysterious, one researcher (Levine, 1982) has proposed that AIDS begins when the immune system malfunctions—perhaps due to the use of nitrites—but no symptoms appear. Whether the disease progresses further may depend in part on genetic factors. The individual may eventually develop symptoms that resemble a chronic virus infection, including fever, diarrhea, weight loss, and general weakness. The lymph nodes may become enlarged. This condition can last for weeks or months. AIDS becomes life-threatening when the individual encounters a serious disease the body can no longer defend itself against. The most common complications of AIDS are Kaposi's sarcoma, a rare form of skin cancer that often invades the lymph nodes, and a type of pneumonia caused by a protozoan that rarely leads to disease in people with a normally functioning immune system. Both complications are frequently fatal.

Although the actual number of AIDS cases is small, its startling rise among homosexuals has led many gay men to reevaluate their life styles (Smith, 1982). There have been suggestions that gay men are changing their sexual practices by decreasing their impersonal, anonymous sexual encounters, and developing small circles of men who confine their sexual partners to members of the group or cultivating monogamous relationships.

## SEXUALLY TRANSMITTED HEPATITIS B

**hepatitis B** an inflammation of the liver caused by a virus (HBV) that can be passed by sexual contact

Another disease that has been linked to sexual activity in homosexual men is **hepatitis B**, an inflammation of the liver caused by a virus (HBV) that produces a serious infection. It has been estimated that 40 percent of all new HBV infections in the United States are sexually transmitted and that between 3 and 6 percent of gay men are carriers of the virus, infecting others without showing any symptoms themselves (Ostrow et al., 1982).

It has been known for some time that HBV was passed by contact or innoculation with products in human blood, but until recently researchers were at a loss to explain why homosexual men were at such risk for the disorder. It now appears that injury to the rectal tissues allows the virus to pass from one person to another. Among a group of nearly 4,000 homosexual men at STD clinics, HBV was strongly connected to anal-genital intercourse and oral-anal contact with large numbers of partners, as well as to the practice of rectal douches before or after sexual activity (Schreeder, 1982). There was no connection between HBV and oral-genital intercourse. The researchers speculate that injury to rectal tissue allows the virus to pass into the body from infected semen or to be acquired orally from injured rectal tissue.

Hepatitis B is a serious disease. There is no effective treatment, and it generally takes weeks or months to recover completely. Its first symptoms are generally tiredness, depression, fever, and loss of appetite. As with other liver infections, jaundice, a yellowing of the skin and the whites of the eyes, often develops. Most people recover from HBV infections, but in about 10 percent of cases it can become a chronic condition with such serious side effects as cirrhosis.

Although there are no drugs that effectively treat hepatitis B, a vaccine has recently been developed that could eventually eliminate the disease. Three injections of the new vaccine appear to immunize between 80 and 100 percent of recipients with no more serious side effects than a sore arm (Francis et al., 1982). At present the vaccine is both scarce and expensive, but a task force (Ostrow et al., 1982) has recommended that all homosexually active men be vaccinated as soon as possible.

# "MINOR" STDS

Along with syphilis and gonorrhea, three other sexually transmitted diseases must be reported to public health authorities. These three "minor" conditions are chancroid, granuloma inguinale, and lymphogranuloma venereum. Discovered about a hundred years ago, these diseases were thought to be found only among the economically disadvantaged people in tropical climates. They have now been reported in all social classes and, although they are still more prevalent in the tropics, they have been found in every sort of climate.

These three infections are minor in the sense that they are far less common than either gonorrhea or syphilis. They are not at all minor, however, in the discomfort they can cause. They often cause painful, itching skin lesions and growths in the genital area. A fourth minor STD, but one that is not reported to public health authorities, is venereal warts.

## Chancroid

Chancroid is caused by a bacterium that infects the genital area, producing a smooth, round sore that resembles the chancre of primary syphilis. Unlike the syphilis chancre, however, the chancroid is usually painful. There is another important difference between chancroid and syphilis: chancroid remains in the genital area, but syphilis spreads through the blood to infect many parts of the body.

In men, the sore usually appears at the head of the penis or on the shaft; in women, it commonly appears around the vulva. However, the infection may show up in other places. Men may find the sore around the anus, scrotum, or thighs, and women may find it in the vagina. Sores may also appear on the hands or mouth, since pus exuded by the chancroid is full of bacteria.

In fighting off this infection, the body sends out white blood cells, which drain the bacteria through the lymph nodes. Thus the lymph nodes in the groin may become infected and swell, causing abcesses. The skin lesions may persist and spread to cover the genitals, causing disfigurement and pain.

Treatment for chancroid is relatively simple and extremely effective. Erythromycin or sulfa drugs, given by mouth, usually clears up the infection within several weeks. This lengthy treatment can be cut in half with frequent applications of wet compresses, followed with a prescribed lotion (Keith and Brittain, 1978).

**chancroid** a sexually transmitted disease that is caused by a bacterium and characterized by a soft, painful sore resembling the syphilis chancre

## Granuloma Inguinale

Granuloma inguinale is also caused by a bacterium. "Granuloma" refers to scar tissue that develops in response to the invasion of microorganisms, and "inguinale" simply means the groin. When this bacterium invades the body, there is a continuous growth of scar tissue on or near the genitals or anus.

**granuloma inguinale** a sexually transmitted disease that is caused by bacteria and characterized by the continuous growth of scar tissue in the genital area

Early symptoms are painless sores, which may spread from the genitals to the thighs or buttocks. Since the body cannot fight off these bacteria, the sores continue to spread, causing weakness and discomfort. When granuloma is left untreated, anemia, arthritis, and distortions of the genitals sometimes develop. Because the sores are not painful, people often wait until the disease is firmly entrenched before seeking treatment. Various antibiotics are effective against granuloma inguinale, but the more advanced the case, the longer it takes and the more difficult it is to reverse its course.

## *Lymphogranuloma venereum*

**lymphogranuloma venereum (LGV)** a sexually transmitted disease caused by chlamydia, which is characterized by swollen, tender lymph nodes and grotesque swelling of the genitals

Lymphogranuloma venereum (LGV) is caused by an organism called chlamydia, which is also suspected of involvement in nongonococcal urethritis. Among the symptoms of LGV are fever, chills, abdominal pains, headaches, loss of appetite, and pains in the joints. If the disease has been acquired through anal intercourse, there may also be backaches. From five to twenty-one days after exposure, the first visible sign of infection appears: a small blister that usually escapes notice, especially in women, and soon vanishes. In the next stage, the organism causes the lymph nodes in the groin to swell and become tender or painful. If untreated, infection may cause enormous and grotesque swelling of the genitals. Once again, antibiotic treatment halts the progress of the disease, with early treatment being faster and more effective than delayed treatment.

## *Venereal warts*

**venereal warts** soft, pink, fleshy growths on the genitals, which are caused by a virus and transmitted by sexual activity

Far more common than the other "minor" STDs—and much less serious—is a condition called condyloma acuminata and commonly known as **venereal warts.** These warts, found on the genitals, are similar to warts that often develop on other parts of the body. They are caused by a virus that prefers the warm, moist environment of the genitals. The warts' first appearance is usually as small, soft, pink or fleshy growths. With time, they may spread until they cover much of the genital area. For most people, however, the warts tend to remain small, painless, and unnoticed.

If the warts do spread, they may cause itching and irritation, which makes sexual contact unpleasant or painful. If the person scratches the warts, they may become inflamed and infected. In many cases, the warts disappear spontaneously.

Since warts, like herpes, are caused by a virus, they cannot be cured by antibiotics. Treatment is local; usually a chemical ointment is applied directly to the warts to destroy them. One common form of treatment is podophyllin, a chemical that "burns" off the warts. In more severe cases, electricity or extreme cold may have to be used, and the treatment may require several sessions.

# PARASITIC INFECTIONS

Two uncomfortable conditions that are often sexually transmitted are infestations of tiny animals: pubic lice and scabies. Either one of these parasites can also be picked up from clothing, bedding, towels, or toilet seats that have come in contact with an infected person. Thus, a case of pubic lice or scabies does not necessarily indicate sexual activity.

## *Pubic lice*

**Pubic lice** are often called "crabs" and when magnified, they do look like miniature crabs. They are yellowish-gray creatures, about the size of a freckle, that have three pairs of claws in front and four pairs of legs in back. They live on blood, which they get by burrowing into human skin. Their home is human hair: pubic hair, armpit hair, eyelashes, and eyebrows. Since lice drop off the body and since they can live for twenty-four hours after leaving their host, they may be picked up from bedding or towels an infected person has used.

**pubic lice** parasites that infest human hair, primarily in the genital area, and are often transmitted by sexual activity

Most people are first aware of the infestation when an intense itching develops. The itching is an allergic reaction to the louse bite, so that some people, who are not allergic, have no symptoms (Keith and Brittain, 1978). The condition is easy to diagnose, because once it is suspected no microscope is needed to discover either the lice or their eggs, which are cemented onto human hairs.

Treatment is swift and effective, and it is available in shampoo, cream, or lotion form. Kwell is the trade name for a prescription shampoo, which is applied to the infested hair, left on for a time, and then rinsed off. If necessary, the shampoo can be repeated in twenty-four hours. Eurax, the prescription cream or lotion, is applied after bathing and left on for twenty-four hours; it can be repeated after four days (U.S. Public Health Service, 1982b). Treatments available over the counter are Triple-X and A-200. Because pubic lice are so easy to transmit, the sexual partner of an infected person should also be treated and all bedding and towels disinfected.

## *Scabies*

A tiny mite that burrows into the skin, where it lays its eggs, causes **scabies**, another parasitic infection that can be transmitted sexually or through contact with infested clothing or other objects. The scabies mite is much smaller than the pubic louse, and can set up its living quarters almost anywhere on the body—genitals, breasts, buttocks, armpits, wrists, and between the fingers are favorite places.

**scabies** parasites that burrow into human skin, causing intense itching; often transmitted by sexual activity

Again, itching is the first warning of an infestation. The itching is so intense that the infected person feels compelled to scratch, setting up a secondary inflammation. This condition often obscures the dark wavy lines that mark the mite's burrow, so diagnosis must sometimes be made from microscopic examination of skin scrapings. In fact, scratching is often so deep that it may be weeks after the mite has been eradicated before all signs of the infestation disappear.

Scabies is treated with daily applications of Eurax, the prescription lotion that is also effective against pubic lice. Eurax is applied following a long, hot bath. Two treatments are generally enough to eliminate the mite. Calamine lotion, starch baths, or—for small areas—a corticosteroid ointment can be used to relieve discomfort.

## VAGINAL INFECTIONS

Within the healthy vagina live a large number of microorganisms kept in delicate balance by one another and by the vaginal environment. Some of these microorganisms help keep the vagina acidic, so that potentially harmful organisms find it difficult to flourish there. The natural secretions of the healthy vagina and cervix lubricate the vagina and keep it moist; they also nourish the acid-producing bacteria, especially lactobacilli, which are related to the bacteria found in milk products.

If this balance is upset and the vagina's normal acidity decreases, acid-producing bacteria die and harmful microorganisms multiply, producing unpleasant symptoms. The hormonal changes that accompany pregnancy often encourage the development of vaginal infections. In the same way, some women are vulnerable to infection just before or during menstruation. Finally, commercial douches, sprays, and "feminine hygiene" products may cause an irritation that paves the way for infections. In fact, some authorities believe that such irritation may cause more women to seek medical treatment for vaginal infection than any other source (Keith and Brittain, 1978).

Vaginal infections are not always the result of sexual contact, and in cases where the infectious microorganisms are sexually transmitted, they may live in the genital tract for several years without producing any symptoms. Symptoms develop only when the vaginal environment permits the microorganisms to multiply. Men are as likely as women to harbor the microorganisms but rarely develop any unpleasant symptoms. The major vaginal infections are trichomoniasis and monilia.

### *Trichomoniasis*

**trichomoniasis** a protozoan, usually transmitted by sexual activity, that can cause vaginal infection

Trichomoniasis, commonly called "trich," is caused by a protozoan, a one-celled organism (Figure 17.4) that lives in the vagina, although, it may also inhabit the urinary tract. This extremely common parasite can be found in more than half of all women and is most prevalent during the childbearing years. The trich parasite, Trichomonas vaginalis, may inhabit the vagina peacefully, or it may cause acute or chronic discomfort. Trichomoniasis is usually passed through sexual contact, but

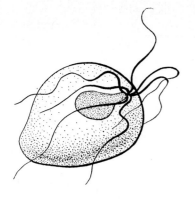

***Figure 17.4   The Trichomonas Vaginalis Parasite.***

because the protozoan can live for several hours after leaving the body, it is sometimes picked up from damp towels or toilet seats.

The major symptom of trichomoniasis is a foamy vaginal discharge, which may be greenish, yellowish, or gray, and which often has an unpleasant odor. This discharge, which may be slight or heavy, tends to irritate the vulva and vagina, often causing itching. The inflammation may make sexual intercourse painful or unpleasant. Trichomoniasis is usually diagnosed by examining a slide of the discharge under a microscope. In men, who tend to have no symptoms at all, the parasite may be diagnosed microscopically or by making a culture.

The most effective treatment for trichomoniasis is a drug called metronidazole, which kills the protozoan. However, this drug, marketed as Flagyl, may have harmful side effects, particularly when large doses are taken by mouth. It is not recommended for pregnant women. People who do take Flagyl should not drink alcohol while under treatment, because the combination sometimes causes abdominal pain. Less severe treatments, such as vaginal suppositories or creams containing sulfa, are effective for some women but do not work as well as Flagyl. Vinegar douches, which increase the acidity of the vagina, can be effective in the early stages of a trichomonal infection. To prevent recurrence, it is important to treat the male sexual partner at the same time.

## Monilia

Next to trichomoniasis, the most common vaginal infection is **monilia**, also called "thrush." Monilia is caused by a yeast fungus known as both Candida albicans and Monilia albicans. This fungus usually inhabits the vagina, but in quantities too small to be noticed. When the vaginal environment is disturbed, the yeast may multiply and cause physical distress.

Monilia may be passed by sexual activity, or it can be introduced into the vagina from the anal area. Monilia often inhabits the large intestine and can travel along a menstrual pad or be brought near the vaginal opening when a woman wipes from back to front after defecation (Keith and Brittain, 1978).

**monilia** a yeast fungus, usually transmitted by sexual activity, that can cause vaginal infection

The major symptom of a yeast infection is a thick white discharge with a yeasty odor and the texture of cottage cheese. This discharge may irritate and redden the vulva, causing intense itching. Diagnosis is usually made from slides or cultures.

Several treatments are helpful for monilia infections. A drug called nystatin may be taken by mouth or in a vaginal suppository. Or gentian violet may be applied to the affected areas. The direct application of plain, unsweetened yogurt to the vagina has been recommended as treatment for mild cases of monilia, since yogurt contains high levels of lactobacillus (Cooke and Dworkin, 1981). Effective creams or ointments can also be used with the male partner, who may harbor the yeast fungus under the foreskin or on the scrotum.

Yeast infections may be stubbornly persistent or respond easily to treatment, only to reappear during the next menstrual cycle. If the infection seems related to birth control pills, switching to a low-progesterone pill or using a different method of birth control may be necessary. Treatment is often complicated because several vaginal infections may occur together.

## Other infections

Vaginal infections that are not caused by either trichomonas vaginalis or Candida albicans are often classified as "nonspecific vaginitis"—a category that roughly corresponds to nonspecific urethritis in men. As with other infections, its symptoms usually include some kind of vaginal discharge and an irritation of the vulva. One type of vaginitis is now attributed to hemophilis vaginalis, a bacterium that can be identified through microscopic examination. Since this bacterium is passed by sexual activity, treatment—usually with antibiotics or sulfa creams—must be given to both male and female partners.

**cystitis** a bladder infection caused by microorganisms, allergic reactions, anxiety, excessive intake of coffee or tea, or irritation

Although not a vaginal infection, **cystitis**, or bladder infection, is related to vaginal infections, as it can be caused by organisms that normally inhabit the vagina or rectum or that lead to vaginitis when they infect the vagina. Not all cases of cystitis are caused by microorganisms: allergic reactions, anxiety, excessive intake of coffee or tea, and irritation can also lead to bladder infections. In fact, constant pressure on the urethral opening during prolonged intercourse can be followed by a bladder infection often called "honeymoon cystitis."

The symptoms of cystitis are a frequent urge to urinate, along with pain and burning on urination. Most cases of cystitis respond promptly to sulfa drugs, which end the symptoms within 36 hours and usually clear up the infection within two weeks. Drinking plenty of water, urinating before and after intercourse, and the application of K-Y Jelly before intercourse can help to prevent bladder infections.

## Prevention of vaginal infections

Probably there is no way to avoid acquiring the microorganisms that produce vaginal infections. But one practical approach is to attempt to maintain a vaginal environment that inhibits the growth of these microorganisms. There are several things you can do.

Most microorganisms flourish in warm, moist places. You can help keep the vulva dry by switching from nylon to cotton underwear and avoiding tight clothing, which builds up heat and moisture.

Wash or bathe daily.

Because sugar encourages the growth of many vaginal infections, try to avoid sweet foods.

Don't use "feminine hygiene" products, douches, and sprays that irritate the vaginal area.

Take antibiotics only if necessary, because they tend to destroy the lactobacilli that are the body's natural defense against vaginal infection. If you do have to take antibiotics, try eating yogurt to reestablish your own lactobacilli.

These precautions may help you to avoid vaginal infections—or at least minimize their severity. Making it difficult for hostile microorganisms to grow within the vagina helps to decrease the incidence of some infections that are often picked up through sexual contact. More important, however, is to stop the spread of all STDs, especially the ones that used to be called venereal disease.

## THE PREVENTION OF SEXUALLY TRANSMITTED DISEASE

Clearly, the best way to eliminate sexually transmitted diseases is to *prevent* them, rather than to treat them after infection has occurred. Unfortunately, most prevention efforts have been hampered by moralistic attitudes. Those who see STD as a just punishment for "promiscuity" and believe that fear of syphilis, gonorrhea, or herpes deters nonmarital sex are usually not eager to develop or publicize preventive measures. As a result, much of what passes for "education" about STDs takes the form of scaring people. Some may be so frightened they give up sex entirely, but many are likely to dismiss the information:

> Sure, we had that sex ed lecture they give you, but after you hear that, you'd have to be crazy to want to have sex. They make it sound like you'd end up crippled for life or blind or maybe even dead if you do anything. So of course nobody listens to them. I mean, you see plenty of people walking around the street and you figure at least some of them must have had sex without anything happening. (Bell, 1980, p. 217)

Yet measures that lessen a person's chances of contracting an STD do exist, and some of them are extremely simple. None of these precautions provides complete protection, and following them doesn't eliminate the need for personal caution and medical treatment (Table 17.1). But even if a preventive measure works only half the time, it can still do a great deal to halt the spread of sexually transmitted disease. The various preventive measures include visual inspection, condoms, vaginal protection, soap and water, urination, and antibiotics.

## Table 17–1  Common STDs

| DISEASE | TRANSMISSION | SYMPTOMS | TREATMENT |
| --- | --- | --- | --- |
| Gonorrhea | Bacterium passed through oral, genital, or anal intercourse. | Men: penile discharge; painful urination. Women: usually none; sometimes yellow-green vaginal discharge or painful urination; can cause sterility. | Penicillin; tetracycline in case of allergy; in beta gonorrhea, spectinomycin. |
| Nongonococcal urethritis (NGU) | Any of several microorganisms passed during sexual contact; irritation from sprays, soaps, etc. | Penile discharge; painful urination; can cause sterility. | Tetracycline, doxycycline, erythromycin in case of allergy. |
| Syphilis | Spirochete passed during sexual contact or skin contact with open sore. | Primary stage: hard chancre; secondary stage: rash, flulike symptoms; latent stage: none; late stage: severe organ damage or death. | Penicillin; tetracycline or erythromycin in case of allergy. |
| Herpes | Virus passed through sexual contact or contact with sores. | Blisters, which become open sores, then scab over. | Acyclovir (does not eliminate virus from body). |
| Acquired immune deficiency syndrome (AIDS) | Uncertain, but believed linked to multiple sex partners. | Fever, diarrhea, weight loss, weakness; may lead to Kaposi's sarcoma or other disease. | None. |
| Hepatitis B | Uncertain, but virus believed passed through anal intercourse or oral-anal contact. | Tiredness, depression, fever, loss of appetite, jaundice. | None (vaccine available). |

### Visual inspection

The first precaution is to examine your new partner's genitals—or the genitals of your regular partner if he or she may be seeing other people. The inspection can take place during sensual caressing or love play, which means, of course, that you're not making love in the dark.

Visual inspection of the male genitals, the "short-arm" method, can often reveal signs of venereal infection. If this short-arm inspection, in which the penis is "milked" by grasping the shaft and pulling the loose skin back and forth several

| DISEASE | TRANSMISSION | SYMPTOMS | TREATMENT |
|---------|--------------|----------|-----------|
| Chancroid | Bacterium passed during sexual contact. | Soft chancre. | Sulfa drugs, erythromycin. |
| Granuloma inguinale | Bacterium passed during sexual contact. | Scar tissue, gradually spreading to cover genitals. | Sulfa drugs. |
| Lymphogranuloma venereum (LGV) | Chlamydia passed during sexual contact. | Small blister, followed by swollen lymph nodes, then greatly swollen genitals. | Tetracycline or sulfa drugs. |
| Venereal warts | Virus passed during sexual activity. | Soft, pink, fleshy warts. | Podophyllin; electricity; freezing. |
| Pubic lice | Lice move into pubic or armpit hair, eyelashes, eyebrows during sexual activity or contact with contaminated objects. | Intense itching. | Shampoos, creams, lotions. |
| Scabies | Mite moves onto skin during sexual activity or contact with contaminated objects. | Intense itching; secondary skin inflammation. | Lotion. |
| Trichomoniasis | Protozoan passed through genital sexual activity or contact with contaminated objects. | No symptoms unless vaginal ecology is disturbed; frothy, foul-smelling vaginal discharge; inflamed vulva and vagina. | Flagyl; if pregnant, sulfa drugs. |
| Monilia | Yeast fungus passed through genital sexual activity; by careless wiping after defecation; along menstrual pad. | No symptoms unless vaginal ecology is disturbed; thick, white, cheesy vaginal discharge; inflamed vulva and vagina. | Nystatin; gentian violet; creams and ointments. |

times, produces a cloudy discharge, it's possible that your partner has NGU or gonorrhea. Prostitutes routinely inspect their customers this way in order to safeguard their own health. Visual inspection of the female genitals seldom reveals signs of infection, but should a white, yellow, or yellow-green discharge be evident, no intercourse should take place.

Recognizing other signs of STD takes some practice, but skin sores or eruptions in the genital area of either sex should be a warning signal. As we've seen, however, many infected people have no visible signs of disease. So even if your partner looks healthy, it's wise to follow the rest of these precautions.

## Condoms

**condom** a thin rubber sheath that covers the penis, worn to prevent conception or the transmission of disease

A properly used **condom**, a thin rubber sheath that covers the penis, is probably the best prevention against STD. It prevents the transmission of gonorrhea more than 90 percent of the time (Secondi, 1975), and will prevent most other STDs unless the source of infection is a nongenital area, such as the inner thighs. For this reason, it will not always protect against syphilis. Nor is a condom a certain protection against herpes; the herpes virus is so small it can pass through the wall of a condom. To be effective against gonorrhea and other STDs, the condom must be put on before contact between sexual partners and must remain on the penis until contact is over.

The protective function of the condom has been known for more than five hundred years. In some countries, such as Sweden, health authorities actively publicize the importance of condoms in preventing STD. During World War II, members of the U.S. armed forces were often supplied with condoms when given leave. In recent years, however, the condom's value as a health protection device has been obscured, and some authorities trace the sharp increase in gonorrhea during the 1970s to its declining popularity. As birth control pills replaced the condom, STD rates climbed. Both partners lost their protection against most STDs, and the hormonal changes caused by the pill in women seemed to decrease their resistance to the STDs they did encounter (Secondi, 1975).

## Vaginal protection

Contraceptive creams and jellies provide some protection against STDs. Women who use these products have lower rates of STD than women who use other forms of contraception. Although the primary purpose of contraceptive products is to kill sperm, they seem to kill other organisms as well.

Another form of vaginal protection, a gel called Progonasyl (from "*protection against gonorrhea and syphilis*"), has been developed but is not widely available. When this substance was used in Nevada's legal prostitution establishments, it decreased the incidence of gonorrhea and syphilis among the women who worked there. For the moment, Progonasyl is available to individuals only through a doctor's medical prescription.

## Soap and water

Washing the genitals with soap and water before and after sexual activity may sound too simple to be effective, but it does help. Although washing does not provide complete protection, it may decrease the chances that an infection will be transmitted. A romantic bath or shower together is one way to make sure this precaution is taken.

## Urination

Another relatively unknown protective technique is urinating after sexual intercourse. Germs may travel up the urethra in both sexes, and urine is a sterile but acid solution. Urinating washes out any germs that are in the urethra. It's important, however, that neither partner have intercourse with a full bladder, since pressure on a distended bladder can cause the kind of damage that increases a person's susceptibility to infection.

## Routine antibiotics

Because large doses of antibiotics such as penicillin can cure certain STDs, it's logical to suppose that smaller doses—taken before the infection can become established—will prevent these STDs. The technique sometimes works, but it is highly controversial and few people use it.

Taking antibiotics either just before or just after sexual contact will often prevent an infection, but it also carries some danger. First, without a doctor's advice, it is difficult to know exactly how large a dose must be taken. People who use the leftover antibiotics in their medicine cabinets may take an insufficient dose—high enough to eliminate the symptoms of disease but too low to kill off the infectious microorganisms. The development of penicillin-resistant strains of gonorrhea has been blamed on such insufficient dosages, because penicillin kills off the weaker germ strains but leaves the stronger strains free to multiply. This is also true of other antibiotics. Tests among a group of gay men indicated that routine doses of a tetracycline drug after sexual activity drastically reduced the incidence of gonorrhea, but the cases that did develop took longer to show up and were extremely resistant to treatment when they finally appeared (Keith and Brittain, 1978).

Antibiotics also have powerful effects on the body. An overuse may cause additional health problems, develop resistance to the drug's effects, or induce an allergy to the drug.

Finally, disease does not necessarily follow every sexual contact with an infected partner. There is usually a better than even chance that the "healthy" partner will not contract the disease, making routine treatment an unnecessary use of a potentially dangerous drug.

## Regular medical checkups

No matter how wary a person is, it's always possible to pick up an STD from someone who has no symptoms. Medical checkups won't prevent STD, but they can detect many silent infections that are not producing any signs of their presence. If you have more than one sexual partner, or if your partner has other partners, make a medical checkup a twice yearly routine. If asking your own doctor for this kind of examination embarrasses you, go to a public health clinic. And if you have *any*

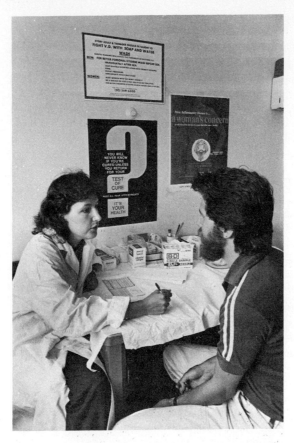

STD clinics serve many functions in society. They provide information to the public and private counseling to individuals. (© Hazel Hankin)

questions, suspicions, or fears about STD, call the National VD hotline. This twenty-four hour, toll-free number is 800-982-5883 in the western states and 800-227-8922 in the eastern states. The person who answers will give you the information you seek but won't ask your name.

# Summary

**1** **Sexually transmitted diseases** (STDs) are any disease that *can* be passed by sexual contact, whereas **venereal diseases** are any disease that is *primarily* passed by sexual contact. The public stigma attached to STD is probably the primary reason for the current epidemic in the United States.

**2** **Gonorrhea** is a bacterial infection that enters the body through warm, moist surfaces and is spread through sexual contact. Although men tend to have painful urination and penile discharge, most women show no symptoms. Untreated gonorrhea can cause secondary infections and sterility. Penicillin cures most cases of gonorrhea, although beta gonorrhea, caused by a mutated form of the bacterium, must be treated with spectinomycin.

**3** Nongonococcal urethritis (NGU) is any urethral infection not caused by gonococcal bacteria. Its symptoms resemble those of gonorrhea, and it can be treated with antibiotics. NGU is believed to be more common than gonorrhea among upper-income groups.

**4** **Syphilis**, a chronic bacterial infection transmitted by sexual activity, can enter the body through the mouth, anus, genitals, or any break in the skin. Syphilis goes through four stages: a primary stage, in which the only sign of infection is a hard, painless sore (**chancre**); a second stage, characterized by a rash and other mild symptoms; a latent stage, with no symptoms; and a late stage, in which damage to major organ systems becomes apparent. Syphilis can be cured at any stage by penicillin.

**5** **Herpes**, a virus infection of the mucous membranes or skin surface, is caused by either of two viruses: herpes 1, which primarily affects the mouth, and herpes 2, which primarily affects the genitals. Crossover infections, in which type 1 affects the genitals and type 2 the mouth, are becoming increasingly prevalent— perhaps due to the increase in oral sexual activity. The primary symptoms of herpes are itching, burning blisters, which disappear in a few weeks. Since the herpes virus cannot be eradicated from the body, new outbreaks are always possible. About one-third of the individuals who contract herpes have recurrences. Acyclovir can shorten an initial infection, but there is no known cure.

**6** **Acquired immune deficiency syndrome (AIDS)** is a disease that involves a breakdown of the body's natural immune system, leaving a person susceptible to serious infections and disease. AIDS is concentrated among homosexual and bisexual men and appears to be associated with a large number of sexual partners and perhaps with the use of amyl and butyl nitrate as recreational drugs. The most common complications of AIDS are Kaposi's sarcoma, a rare form of skin cancer that can invade the lymph nodes, and a sometimes fatal form of pneumonia caused by a protozoan.

**7** **Hepatitis B**, a liver inflammation caused by the HBV virus, has been linked to sexual activity in homosexual men. It may be spread through anal-genital intercourse or oral-anal contact with a large number of partners. There is no effective treatment for hepatitis B, from which recovery is slow. However, a vaccine that effectively protects against hepatitis B has been developed.

**8** Six myths about STDs pervade American society: (1) Nice people don't get STD. (2) You can get an STD only once. (3) STDs are acquired only through genital intercourse. (4) Sexual contact with an infected partner invariably results in STD. (5) Nothing can be done about the signs and symptoms of STD. (6) The signs of STD are easy to recognize. These myths, which are all wrong, promote the spread of STDs and interfere with their cure.

**9** **Chancroid** is caused by a sexually transmitted bacterium that produces a painful sore resembling the syphilis chancre. It can be effectively cured with erythromycin or sulfa drugs. **Granuloma inguinale**, which is caused by a bacterium, causes continual growth of scar tissue in the genital and anal areas. It can be cured by various antibiotics. **Lymphogranuloma venereum (LGV)** is caused by chlamydia, which are sexually transmitted. It leads to painful swelling of the genitals and may be cured by antibiotics. **Venereal warts** are caused by a sexually transmitted virus. They may be treated by chemicals or destroyed by electricity or extreme cold.

**10** **Pubic lice** are parasites that inhabit human hair and are often spread by sexual activity. They cause intense itching and can be eliminated by special shampoos, creams, or lotions. **Scabies,** a tiny mite that burrows into the skin, where it causes intense itching, can be eliminated by the same lotion that eradicates pubic lice.

**11** Vaginal infections develop when the natural ecology of the vagina is upset and harmful microorganisms are allowed to proliferate. **Trichomoniasis,** a protozoan infection, is usually passed by sexual contact. It causes an irritating vaginal discharge and may be killed by Flagyl. **Monilia,** or thrush, is an infection caused by a yeast fungus. It is usually passed by sexual activity and causes an irritating, cheesy discharge. Several drugs can eliminate it. **Cystitis,** or bladder infection, which is characterized by frequent, painful urination, may be caused by organisms that inhabit the vagina or rectum or by a number of other factors, including lengthy, protracted intercourse (honeymoon cystitis). Cystitis responds to sulfa drugs.

**12** The spread of STDs can be reduced by visually inspecting a partner's genitals for signs of STD, using a **condom** during intercourse, using contraceptive creams or jellies, washing the genitals with soap and water before and after intercourse, urinating after sexual intercourse, taking small doses of antibiotics (a controversial procedure), and having regular medical checkups to detect silent infections.

## a paraplegic's view

One thing I do know is that I'm a much better lover now than I ever was before (the accident). There are a lot of reasons for that, but one of the biggest is that I'm more relaxed. I don't have a list of "do's and don'ts," a timetable, a proper sequence of moves to follow, or the need to "give" my partner an orgasm every time we make love. Sex isn't just orgasm for me, it's pleasuring, playing, laughing, and sharing.
(Lenz and Chaves, 1981)

## a cancer patient's view

I found I needed to give directions to what areas were sensitive and arousable. My nerve sensation around my labia and clitoris was less than 50 percent of what it had been prior to my radical surgery. However, other parts of my body seemed to develop increasing sensitivity. I was orgasmic in new ways, such as through breast and neck stimulation and fantasy. Yes, these orgasms were different, but sexually satisfying.
(Burger, 1981, p. 53)

# 18 Sexuality and Health

# *Chapter 18*

Imagine you are just recovering from a heart attack and fear you may have to give up sexual activity to prevent a second attack. Or imagine you have been injured in a skiing accident and are confined to a wheelchair. You worry about how to manage sexual contact when you can't even move your hips or legs. Many Americans have faced these problems, but until recently they have done so mostly without professional help.

The attitude that illness is punishment lingers, and many people who suffer a stroke, a heart attack, or a major accident see it as some kind of personal judgment. Some make bargains with God, vowing to give up "all that" (sex) if they are allowed to recover (Renshaw, 1978). Whether or not patients see their physical misfortunes as punishment, a reluctance to speak of forbidden topics often rules out sex as a subject of conversation between doctors and most patients—unless, of course, the patient has been so unfortunate as to contract an STD.

Not many years ago, when a medical condition interfered with sexual functioning or desire, the patient and his or her partner nearly always accepted the complication in silence. Should the patient raise the question of sexual functioning at all, physicians often said that nothing could be done or else brushed the problem aside as inconsequential—especially if the patient was middle-aged or female.

In the past few years, there has been what amounts to a "patients' liberation." Physicians have been investigating the relationship between illness or accident and sexuality and discovering that disease or disability need not end a person's sexual life. A cardiac patient,

# *Sexuality and Health*

who once would have been forbidden sexual activity, is likely to be encouraged to try sex. And a paraplegic, who once would have been considered lacking either sexual desire or capacity, is likely to be shown ways of expressing sexual feelings.

In this chapter, we begin by exploring sexual functioning in chronic disease, such as heart disease, cancer, diabetes, and multiple sclerosis. Next, we examine sexual functioning in disability, such as spinal cord injuries, cerebral palsy, and mental retardation. We close by investigating the effects of drugs—both prescription and recreational—on sexuality.

## SEX AND ILLNESS

Chronic or debilitating disease can affect sexuality either directly or indirectly. Some diseases interfere with the nervous or endocrine systems, or with the supply of blood to the pelvis, so that the effect is direct. Sexual response is sluggish, diminished, or even eliminated. Other diseases affect sexual response indirectly by changing body image, lowering energy levels, or making movement painful.

Yet people suffering from chronic illness often feel a special need for the comfort and intimacy sex provides. For example, among a group of cancer patients, 70 percent said that sexual activity was more important to them now than before their cancer was discovered (Bullard, 1981).

Many patients who curtail or eliminate their sexual activities do so unnecessarily, or for reasons that are more psychological than physiological. The close relationship between physical health, emotional well-being, and sexual functioning can be seen in heart disease, cancer, diabetes, and multiple sclerosis.

## Heart disease

It has been estimated that more than 14 million Americans have some sort of heart or blood vessel ailment. Until recently, however, cardiac patients received little advice concerning sexuality. They were usually told to stop smoking and alter their diet, but no mention was made of sexual activity. Often, fear of a second heart attack led them to curtail sexual expression or to become abstinent, as it did this man:

> I was too anxious and afraid even to try sex. I thought I could die during it. It took six months before I finally tried it and it was no good. I had some chest pain and I panicked. I didn't try it for another two months and I was still fearful; it wasn't much, because my wife is just as afraid as I am. (Hellerstein et al., 1977)

Frustration and marital stress often follow such sexual avoidance. Within a year, these problems had sent this patient and his wife to a therapist.

Such experiences were common in the past. Studies consistently found that sexual activity diminished markedly among most male cardiac patients, and up to a fourth of them became abstinent. Little is known about the responses of women following heart attack, but among a small group of women patients, ten of the fourteen had decreased their sexual activity, although none had lost the ability to have an orgasm (Kolodny, Masters, and Johnson, 1979).

Even when illness interferes with sexual functioning or desire, it need not end a couple's sexual relationship. Adjustment may be required in the sexual script, but some sort of intimate contact is almost always possible. (Photo Unique)

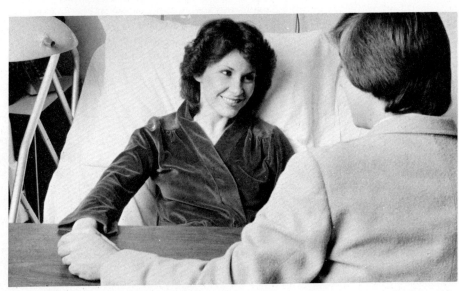

Now, however, research has resulted in a more realistic evaluation of the cardiac patient's sexual abilities. Medical authorities have developed guidelines for the safe resumption of sexual activity, and fewer patients are likely to be faced with unnecessary abstinence and troubled relationships. It appears that 80 percent of heart-attack patients can resume sexual activity at their pre-attack levels. Sexual intercourse with a regular partner is safe if the patient can comfortably climb two flights of stairs (Hellerstein et al., 1977).

Physicians and patients alike once believed that sexual activity placed a heavy stress on the cardiovascular system. The belief was apparently mistaken. Among a group of married, middle-aged men who suffered from heart disease, the peak heart rate at orgasm averaged about 117 beats per minute—less than these men's normal heart rate while working (Hellerstein and Friedman, 1970).

Sexual activity is a form of mild exercise. Most cardiac patients are given systematic physical exercise to improve their physical functioning, and the safety of sexual activity seems related to the ability to perform these exercises. One group of patients who followed a 16-week physical conditioning program found that their peak heart rate during intercourse dropped from 127 beats a minute to 120 beats a minute (Stein, 1977). A patient's ability to tolerate intercourse can be determined by an exercise stress test that evaluates cardiac response to mild exercise.

Sexual activity is usually permitted about six weeks after a heart attack. One way to reintroduce sexual activity is through masturbation (Wagner, 1975). A patient's urge to masturbate can be a sign of returning health. As a first step, masturbation has advantages over intercourse: sexual stimulation is completely under the patient's control, and there is no need to contend with any fears the partner might have about the resumption of sexual activity. Moreover, successful masturbation may increase a patient's confidence in the ability to perform with a partner.

After intercourse has resumed, following a few simple rules can minimize any risk to health (Mackey, 1978). Since extremes of temperature—either heat or cold—make the heart work harder, room temperature should be comfortable. And because digestion puts a strain on the heart, it is best to wait several hours after a large meal before starting sexual activity. Finally, large amounts of alcohol or excessive fatigue may cause additional and unnecessary strain on the heart. Contrary to popular opinion, sex in the man-above position does not place additional strain on the male heart, so any comfortable position may be selected for intercourse.

## Cancer

When a person develops cancer, medical attention is focused on halting the spread of the disease, not on the effects it might have on sexual functioning. Yet cancer patients often have many years of relatively normal life, and their sexual needs do not disappear. Men and women in one group of cancer patients said that although their interest in genital intercourse had lessened, their need for physical closeness had increased (Leiber et al., 1976).

Cancer can have direct effects on sexual functioning, as when a liver cancer radically shifts the body's balance of sexual hormones or when surgery constricts the vagina or damages the nerves that control erection. But the psychological effects of cancer are more common and often more profound.

The discovery of cancer produces a deep emotional shock, generally followed by fear, anger, and despair. A patient's body image deteriorates, a process that may be intensified if treatment leaves disfiguring scars or causes hair to fall out. In addition, the patient may feel guilty for developing cancer; self-esteem may plummet; and the fear that the cancer will recur may always be present (Kolodny, Masters, and Johnson, 1979).

The attitude of the patient's partner is critical in determining the level of sexual functioning. If he or she is repelled by the disease or mistakenly fears contracting it, problems intensify and the relationship may deteriorate. Because cancer takes many forms, it is impossible to discuss each one. We can see how it can affect sexuality, however, by exploring the relationship between sexual activity and four types of cancer.

**Breast cancer**  Because the female breast is a potent sexual symbol, breast cancer can have powerful effects on sexuality. Monthly self-examination, using procedures discussed in Chapter 6, may detect breast cancer so early that only the lump itself need be removed. When the cancer has begun to grow, a woman generally has a **mastectomy**, a removal of the cancerous breast, that often leaves her feeling she has been mutilated and her femininity destroyed. She may keep this feeling to herself:

**mastectomy**  the surgical removal of a breast

> After surgery my doctor said that I was doing beautifully. I smiled bravely and
> didn't show my horror, anger, and self-pity. (Kriss, 1981, p. 185)

It's been suggested that a woman who has lost a breast suffers a shock as deep as that felt by a man who has lost his penis (Kriss, 1981). Others propose that re-

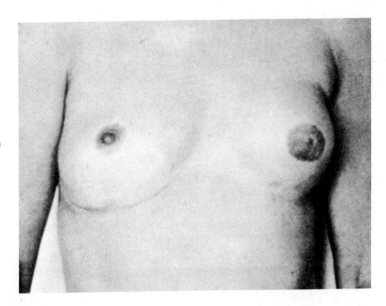

When a breast must be removed, it is often possible to reconstruct a new one, using a graft from the labia to form a sensitive nipple and inserting a prosthesis beneath the skin.

sponse to the loss of a breast is identical with the reaction that follows the death of a parent, child, or husband (Wabrek and Wabrek, 1976).

Running through these reactions is the woman's fear that her husband or sexual partner may reject her, that she will no longer be seen as sexually desirable. These fears may make her unable to abandon herself to sexual pleasure. Among a group of women with mastectomies, more than half said their sexual adjustment was "poor" or "very poor," and no more than half of the younger women and a quarter of the older women were having intercourse as often as once a week (Kriss, 1981).

The woman's perception that she is no longer desirable may lead her to erect subtle, unspoken barriers to sexual activity. Her response may help shape her partner's reaction to her mastectomy—and the partner's reaction is vital to the woman's sexual adjustment. Sometimes the partner does have difficulty in accepting the mastectomy, but often what the woman perceives as distaste or rejection is simply uncertainty or a concern about the woman's physical and emotional health (Green and Mantell, 1978).

Sexual partners seem more likely to take the mastectomy in stride if they are also partners in dealing with the physical problem. It has been recommended that a partner be drawn into the decision to have surgery and that afterward he help the woman change her dressing and massage her arm. Extremely important in her adjustment is his willingness to look at the scar.

The sexual adjustment is never easy, as one woman made clear five years after her mastectomy:

> My husband is and always has been my number one champion and supporter.
> He tells me that the fact I have only one breast makes no difference to him,
> that he is grateful to have me around, alive and well—and I believe him. But
> in our intimate moments, it is a hard thing for me to do to present him with
> this disfigurement. One breast by itself is rather obscene, I think. My husband
> says it doesn't look that way to him, but it looks that way to me. . . . Our
> lovemaking, so far as tenderness and wanting one another, has not been
> affected, but my enjoyment of it has, because my left breast was always
> extremely sensitive and was one of my most important erogenous zones. Now
> it isn't there anymore, and I miss it to this day. (Cope, 1978, pp. 146–147)

The difficult adjustment to mastectomy can be smoothed by participation in therapy groups composed of mastectomy patients. Through sharing their experiences, women can explore their own feelings and come to terms with them. By discussing the sexual aspects of mastectomy, they can learn to deal with whatever misapprehensions, fear, or guilt might be standing between them and their partners.

**Gynecological cancer** The effect of gynecological cancer on sexual functioning depends in part on the site of the cancer: vulva, vagina, cervix, uterus, tubes, or ovaries may be involved. No matter where the cancer is located, however, the fact that the sexual system is involved may lead women to withdraw from sexual activity almost as soon as the cancer is diagnosed. Among nearly a hundred women whose cancer had been diagnosed within six weeks, most had either ceased coitus or reduced the frequency (Harris, Good, and Pollack, 1982). In the majority of cases, the change was initiated by the woman, either because of actual physical symptoms (pain or bleeding), fear of such symptoms, or general anxiety.

Knowledge of the cancer sometimes reduces intimacy between a woman and her partner. Before their diagnosis, half the women in this study found it easy to talk to their partners about sex; afterward, only about a third found such conversation comfortable. Women with cancer of the reproductive system often require special counseling, especially if they see their cancer as a punishment for past sexual activity (Good and Capone, 1980), or if they immediately assume their sexual lives are ended.

At any stage of gynecological cancer, a woman can be encouraged to have intimate, but nongenital, contact with her partner. After treatment, fear of injury or of a recurrence of the cancer may interfere with the resumption of sexual activity. In some cases, a couple may have to alter their sexual script, especially if the extent of surgery in vulvar or vaginal cancer has made intercourse impossible. Even after radical surgery, however, some women have been able to develop natural functioning. One young woman with vaginal cancer who lost her uterus, an ovary, and the upper two-thirds of her vagina was able, after reconstructive surgery, to have genital intercourse. Three years after her initial surgery, she was married (Burger, 1981). In fact, researchers (McGregor, 1973) have reported that some younger women whose vulvas had been removed were able to conceive, carry, and deliver a baby normally.

**Testicular cancer** Although cancer of the testes is comparatively rare, causing less than two out of every hundred male cancer deaths, it has effects on sexual functioning similar to those produced in women by breast cancer: the man's sexual image is deeply involved. As we saw in Chapter 6, young men may develop testicular cancer, and it may be discovered early by self-examination, making the chances of complete recovery extremely good.

A man who develops testicular cancer generally has the diseased testis removed. Since the other testis remains, in most cases there is no physiological reason for impairment in sexual function or fertility. Sometimes, however, complications may lead to impaired functioning. If the lymph nodes are removed along with the testis, the ability to ejaculate generally disappears, although the patient still has erections and orgasms (Kedia, Markland, and Farley, 1977). And if the cancer is so far developed that both testes must be removed, sexual desire and the ability to have erections are usually lost.

The loss of a single testis can have psychological effects on sexual functioning. Some patients feel they have lost their masculinity. Such men tend to be anxious about their own sexual ability. After surgery, they begin observing their sexual performance to reassure themselves they are functioning properly. As we saw in Chapter 14, the habit of "spectatoring" can lead to various sexual dysfunctions. Other patients view the cancer as a punishment for their sexual "sins." Still others equate manhood with fathering children. If they lose the ability to ejaculate, they may also develop erectile failure (Kolodny, Masters, and Johnson, 1979).

**Prostate cancer** More common than testicular cancer is cancer of the prostate, a form of the disease that sometimes requires the removal of the prostate gland—a procedure called **prostatectomy**. The prostate rarely becomes cancerous in young men, but most men—if they live long enough—develop this cancer. In the majority of cases, the cancer is harmless: it remains small, has no symptoms, and has no perceptible effect (Silber, 1981). When a prostate cancer does begin to spread, however, the entire prostate is removed. In order to get all the tissue, the surgeon enters the body through the perineum—the area between the scrotum and the anus. In the process, nerve pathways are damaged, and erection is no longer possible. Thus, the man who has a prostatectomy for cancer may want to consider a penile prosthesis (discussed in Chapter 14).

**prostatectomy**
surgical removal of the prostate gland

Most prostatectomies are *not* performed to eradicate cancer, however, but to remove excess tissue from a greatly enlarged, noncancerous prostate. If the surgeon enters through the perineum, nerve pathways may be damaged, although not always. About half of the men who have surgery in this manner are no longer able to get an erection. In most cases of noncancerous enlargement, the surgeon enters the body in the pubic area, above the penis, or else inserts a tube into the penis without making an incision in the skin.

Men who undergo the latter procedures should have no problem with erections, for the nerve pathways that control erection are not touched. Yet about 20 percent of those with pubic incisions and about 5 percent of those with no incision at all develop erectile failure. This inability to have an erection may be primarily psychological, perhaps because the men believed that the surgery would affect their sexual functioning. When physicians carefully explained the operation to a group of men who were to have prostatectomies, none developed erectile problems. But among men who had no explanation, erectile problems were prevalent (Zohar et al., 1976). If such men continue to have nocturnal erections (discussed in Chapter 7), the psychological nature of the erectile failure is established. These men may find that sexual therapy can restore their potency.

The less radical prostatectomies often affect sexual functioning in another way, however. Afterward, most men develop retrograde ejaculation (see Chapter 4). Damage to the nerves or the tissue around the neck of the bladder keeps the bladder from closing as semen passes its entrance on the way from the body, and the fluid passes instead into the bladder. The sensation felt during orgasm undergoes a slight change, but is just as pleasurable (Silber, 1981). Since there is no sperm emission, the man becomes infertile. As in the case of testicular cancer, if the patient confuses manhood with fertility, secondary erectile failure may develop. Otherwise, the lack of ejaculate should not seriously affect the sexual relationship.

## Diabetes

Diabetes, a chronic disease in which an insulin deficiency impairs the body's ability to use sugar, can have a far-reaching effect on sexual function in both sexes. Because the effects are more dramatic in men, more is known about them.

Among male diabetics, approximately 50 percent have erectile dysfunction (Wagner, Hilsted, and Jensen, 1981). The ability to get erections is generally lost over a long period of time, and does not begin until several years after the disease is discovered. In a few cases, however, erectile failure is an early symptom that brings the diabetic to medical attention. Erectile dysfunction is not related to the severity or duration of diabetes, nor does the patient experience any decline in sexual desire. What's more, nearly all diabetics with erectile dysfunction are able to ejaculate.

The precise cause of this erectile problem is not clearly understood, and many different factors may play a role in its development. It was once believed that hormonal deficiencies were the cause of erectile failure, but this theory was rejected after tests showed that most diabetics have normal testosterone levels. Nerve and blood vessel damage are believed to be involved, and nerve damage has been found among some diabetic men who were unable to have erections (Wagner, Hilsted, and Jensen, 1981).

The male diabetic's erectile problems are not always physical by-products of the disease. Psychological pressure, such as the need to cope with a chronic debilitating disease, can lead to depression, and that in turn to sexual difficulties (Renshaw, 1975). Indeed, some of the same personality and marital problems that operate in nondiabetic men may sometimes be responsible for precipitating or worsening sexual dysfunction. If the patient who complains of erectile dysfunction has nocturnal erections or erections during masturbation, the problem is psychological, and sex therapy may be helpful. Even in patients with severe diabetes, sexual counseling and careful treatment can often restore a satisfying sexual relationship (Wagner, Hilsted, and Jensen, 1981).

Although less is known about sexual functioning in female diabetics, the primary effect of the disease in women appears to be lack of orgasm. Among sexually active women, 35 percent of the diabetic women had not had an orgasm in the past year, compared with only 6 percent of nondiabetic women. It appears that women with diabetes become less responsive, so that it takes longer, more intense stimulation to bring them to orgasm. Sensitivity diminishes gradually, and the condition is apparent in both coitus and masturbation. However, sexual desire may remain high for some women (Kolodny, Masters, and Johnson, 1979).

A troublesome sexual problem for some diabetic women is monilia, which was discussed in Chapter 17. Excess sugar in the body, which can be detected in blood and urine, apparently upsets the vaginal ecology, allowing the fungus to flourish.

## Multiple sclerosis

Multiple sclerosis is a disease of the nervous system in which degenerative changes affect the material covering nerve cells in the brain and spinal cord. Its victims are almost entirely young adults, and the disease's progress is slow, often taking more than twenty years to run its course. Although there is no cure, some patients have shown improvement after taking ACTH, a hormone produced by the pituitary gland.

The symptoms of multiple sclerosis include clumsiness, double or blurred vision, tingling, and patches of numbness in the limbs or body. In the early and middle stages of the disease the symptoms come and go, so that at times the patient seems completely recovered. Finally, however, the symptoms become more severe and permanent.

Since multiple sclerosis involves the nerves, it is not surprising that patients report a variety of sexual dysfunctions. In fact, sexual problems may be the first signs of the disorder, and because the symptoms of multiple sclerosis disappear for a time, only to return, physicians may erroneously assume that any sexual difficulty is psychological (Kolodny, Masters, and Johnson, 1979).

Men with multiple sclerosis tend to have erectile problems, and women may experience diminished sexual desire, orgasmic problems, pain during coitus, or a lack of vaginal lubrication. In a study of more than three hundred patients with advanced multiple sclerosis, 64 percent of the men and 39 percent of the women said that their sex life was unsatisfactory or that they had given up all sexual activity (Lilius, Valtonen, and Wikström, 1976). About half of both sexes reported a lessening or absence of interest in sexual activity. Most of the men had erectile problems, and about half of the women said their clitoris was losing its sensitivity.

Yet the prospect for sexual functioning is often hopeful, as this case shows.

*Case* Dan has had multiple sclerosis for twenty years. At the time of his diagnosis, he was told to expect a progression of symptoms, including tingling in the hands and feet, weakness, and erectile dysfunction. Shortly after the onset of the other symptoms, Dan became unable to have an erection. The condition persisted for ten years, and Dan assumed he would never have another erection. Then a woman who later became his sexual partner urged him to experiment. They found that a vibrator provided enough stimulation for an erection, and Dan also learned to enjoy a wide range of sexual pleasure, including body massage. Today he considers intercourse as only one of the available sexual options. (Adapted from Bullard, 1981)

Because so many of the patients are young and because the progress of the disease is so slow, therapists can generally be of help in suggesting sexual aids and alternatives to genital intercourse. Counseling also keeps patients aware that the frequent disappearance of symptoms will give them periods when sexual functioning returns to normal.

Although we've considered only a few of the illnesses that can affect sexual functioning, a similar thread seems to run through accounts of the relationship between physical illness and sexual functioning. Since the psychological component of human sexual function is so strong, some sort of satisfactory sexual adjustment can often be made, even in cases that involve extensive physical damage.

## SEX AND DISABILITY

Many adults suffer from a physical disability that seriously interferes with daily life. The disability may be paralysis, physical deformity or scars, sight or hearing impairment, or a developmental abnormality. According to popular ideas, these disabled people are not—and should not be—interested in sex, and the medical profession often pays little attention to their sexual needs. For many disabled people, however, sexual activity is a primary consideration in adjusting to their disability.

These individuals must often cope with a sudden and negative change in body image. For example, a man who has had a limb amputated may see himself as unattractive and feel ashamed and self-conscious about displaying his body. Disabled people may have to accept sudden limitations in their ability to control their bodies. Even when a disability does not directly affect the sexual organs, it is likely to produce sexual side effects.

Since disabled people may equate their individual worth with their sexual functioning, discouragement in the sexual area may lead them to lose the self-confidence and assertiveness they need if they are to form intimate relationships, develop work ability, and be generally productive citizens. Adequate sexual functioning is not a luxury for the physically disabled, but is probably a central element in their rehabilitation (Bullard, 1981).

The way in which a physical disability affects sexual functioning may depend on the age of the patient at the time the disability was acquired and whether the condition is stable. Disabilities that begin early in life often affect socialization. For example, a handicapped child may have limited contact with other children, less opportunity to date and learn about sex, and a limited choice of marriage partners. In the case of disabilities that are acquired after puberty, the maturation process is completed and the individual may have been sexually active before the injury. Many disabilities in this category, such as spinal cord injury, are conspicuous, and the individual may worry about his or her sexual and reproductive capabilities.

Regardless of the nature of the disability, the disabled man or woman is likely to need counseling, information, and reassurance. As Alex Comfort (1978) has pointed out, the disabled person has two types of disabilities: physical problems that limit activity or response and psychological problems that arise from misinformation and lack of social permission to be sexually active. The patient needs two kinds of assistance: up-to-date information about the sexual consequences of the disability and help in dispelling myths and stereotypes.

Both kinds of help can be provided by a physician who follows a systematic program with disabled patients. The program begins with a thorough evaluation of the physical problem—for example, using a sleep-erection test to discover whether a man's erectile physiology is intact. Next, patient and partner are encouraged to widen their sexual repertoire; for example, when erection is impossible, the couple might be educated in oral-genital techniques or the use of sexual aids. Finally, realistic sexual goals are set. A couple who cannot expect to reach the levels of sexual activity they enjoyed before the disability can learn ways of outwitting the limitations it imposes (Comfort, 1978).

Such help is essential if the patient is to develop a satisfying life. Efforts to pro-

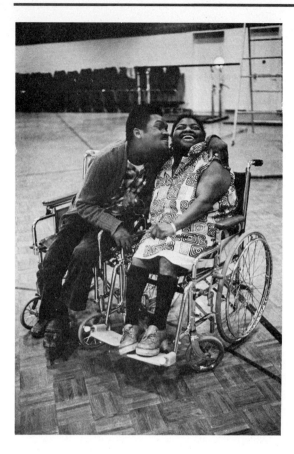

Individuals who are able to make a satisfactory adjustment to their disability need not sacrifice the rewards of sexuality. (© Abraham Menashe 1980)

tect disabled patients from sexual frustration by pretending there is no problem may be well-intentioned, but they are certain to fail.

## *Spinal cord injury*

As a result of advances in medical technology, most men and women with spinal cord injuries can expect a normal life span. However, the complications of such injuries may interfere with sexual activity in many ways. For instance, in addition to losing sensation in the lower body, the paraplegic, who is paralyzed on both sides of the body, loses control of the bowel and bladder.

Many of the typical responses to sexual arousal can be seen in men and women with spinal cord injuries. Respiration, heart rate, and blood pressure increase during arousal; nipples become erect; and often a sex flush breaks out on the skin of the trunk, neck, and face. The extent of the injured person's sexual disability depends on the exact location and amount of spinal cord damage. For example, when a man's spine is injured so that signals cannot travel down the spinal cord from the brain, he will not have an erection, no matter how exciting he finds sights, sounds, thoughts, or other psychogenic stimuli. But he may still be able to have reflexive erections in response to local stimulation. Ejaculation is less common than erection, but some men who have no sensations in their genitals may ejaculate. Orgasm is uncommon, but it may persist even though the nerve connections to the pelvis have been severed.

Some adults with spinal cord injuries say they can concentrate on sensation from an intact portion of their bodies, reassigning it to their genitals and using fantasy to reach orgasm (Cole, 1975). Throughout the book, we've stressed the sexual importance of learning, thoughts, and fantasy. Although the connection between brain and genitals may be severed, the fact that sex is mostly psychological enables injured adults to experience orgasm. One young man who was a quadriplegic (both arms and legs paralyzed) learned to reach orgasm when his partner licked, kissed, and stroked his neck, ears, face, and shoulders. He said that it took him a long time to learn that he could have orgasms without ejaculation (Lenz and Chaves, 1981).

The realization that sexual pleasure is not restricted to the genitals may take some time to discover, as another young man explained:

> I felt asexual for a long time because a man's sex was supposed to be in his penis, and I couldn't feel my penis. . . . It didn't occur to me that it felt good to have the back of my neck licked, or that it felt good to have my arms stroked lightly. Stroking the wrists, then to the arms, then up the arms, is a sequence that I've since learned can be very exciting. (Smith, 1981, p. 16)

Although most attention has been focused on men, women also have sexual problems following spinal cord injury. Since the injury rarely interferes with the menstrual cycle, most paraplegic women are able to conceive and have a relatively normal pregnancy and delivery. However, the absence of sensation in the genitals can interfere with arousal and orgasm in women just as it does in men. Like men, some women learn to reach orgasm through fantasy and other forms of stimulation.

Through masturbation, paraplegics can relearn the sensual potential of their bodies. Such self-exploration provides a pleasant experience and also enables them to tell a partner just what sort of stimulation feels best (Becker, 1981). This need to ask for specific stimulation or to reassure a new partner that stimulation is pleasurable, not painful, makes sexual assertiveness (see Chapter 10) extremely important for people with spinal cord injuries. Often, becoming sexually assertive enhances the injured adult's self-esteem, so that improvement in the sexual area spills over into the rest of life (Dunn, Lloyd, and Phelps, 1981).

## Cerebral palsy

Cerebral palsy is a catch-all term covering motor disturbances caused by a variety of prenatal brain defects or injuries during the birth process. A person with this disorder tends to make involuntary movements and to have difficulty controlling the voluntary muscles. Cerebral palsy can be thought of as a miscommunication between the brain and the muscles, so that movements tend to be uncoordinated. Walking may be difficult, and speech may be distorted. If the person becomes upset or anxious, muscle spasms may occur. Sometimes there is mental retardation, but many people with cerebral palsy have normal intelligence.

The reproductive system of people with cerebral palsy is not affected by the disorder, nor is there usually any effect on sexual functioning, including sexual desire. The problem faced by these people is a possible difficulty in establishing intimate relationships. Because the disorder is often conspicuous, opportunities for socialization and sexual learning in adolescence may be difficult. Victoria, a young woman with cerebral palsy, recalled her adolescence:

> The sexual feelings I had, I saw others having also, but they were not
> disabled. I thought, "I have these feelings, too, but I am ashamed because I
> realize I am not supposed to have them." So I walked around with a lot of
> emotional pain. (Thornton, 1981, p. 28)

As with spinal cord injuries, learning to talk comfortably about sex eases sexual adjustment for people with cerebral palsy. Because of spastic muscle movement, some intercourse positions may not be possible, and explicit communication with a partner may be necessary. As in the case of other disabilities or chronic disease, people with cerebral palsy often report that sexual relationships are extremely important to them. The acceptance and intimacy that characterize a sexual relationship appear to help them overcome basic problems of self-image and self-esteem.

## Mental retardation

Like the physically disabled, mentally retarded people have been subjected to sexual myths and repressive attitudes. After denying that retarded people have sexual feelings, society discourages them from becoming involved in any form of sexual activity. At one time, compulsory sterilization was routine, and retarded people were forbidden to marry. The vast majority of institutions for the retarded still prohibit any form of sexual expression, including masturbation, and refuse to provide sex education for residents. Recently, the increasing recognition that the retarded individual should be encouraged to live as much as possible within the mainstream of society has led to attempts to recognize and deal with their sexual needs.

The term "mental retardation" covers a large group of individuals with widely differing skills and abilities. Those who are considered "mildly retarded" have IQs between 52 and 67. Most of these people—and they are 90 percent of the mentally retarded—can hold jobs, marry, and become parents. Although they develop slowly, they can function independently but need assistance in such matters as budgeting and handling money. "Moderately retarded" people can learn to care for their personal needs and do simple work, but rarely marry or become parents. "Severely retarded" people, who can be trained to do simple tasks under considerable supervision, and "profoundly retarded" people, who require continual supervision and care, are likely to live in institutions (Bootzin and Acocella, 1980).

The sexual maturation of mentally retarded people reaches different levels of

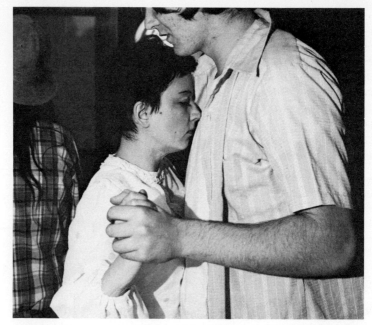

Society rarely considers the sexual feelings of mentally retarded individuals, whose sexual needs are no different from those of other men and women. (Mary Ellen Mark/Magnum)

competence and ability, with the retarded following the same developmental pattern of sexuality as the nonretarded. Research has shown that a relationship exists between IQ and sexual maturation—the lower the IQ, the slower the sexual development.

Typically, the first sexual behavior to appear is masturbation. Children are normally sensitive to cues that parents disapprove of masturbation and carry it out in private to avoid punishment. But retarded children often miss these cues, and most must be specifically taught that masturbation is a private activity. Because retarded children are watched closely, they are likely to be caught and punished for their sexual activity. Given society's attitudes toward masturbation, most parents simply try to eliminate this behavior instead of trying to teach the retarded child when and where the activity is appropriate.

Things become more complicated when retarded people become sexually mature and show interest in sexual activity with others. Most retarded girls and boys are cut off from the social interaction that would bring them to some level of social maturity. For example, they may be closely protected by parents who forbid such learning experiences as dating and interaction with the other sex. Parents may fear that a retarded daughter will be sexually exploited.

Another fear is that the retarded will produce retarded children or that, even if they have normal children, they will lack the resources to be effective and responsible parents. Although some retarded adults are unable to undertake the responsibility, most of the mildly retarded can learn to become at least adequate parents.

Even men and women who are so retarded that they clearly cannot rear children can be given the opportunity for sexual intimacy. If society recognizes that recreational sex is necessary for psychological well-being, then there seems to be no reason to forbid this experience to retarded people simply because they cannot accept procreational responsibility (Johnson, 1977). Of course, methods of contraception that are appropriate to the individuals involved would have to be used. Mildly retarded people may be able to use techniques such as birth control pills or intrauterine devices (discussed in Chapter 19).

Because retarded people have been seen as children in need of sexual protection, they are not considered mature enough to make sexual decisions. As a result, most retarded people have been denied the usual sex education or information about contraceptives. Since they lack both information and opportunity, it is not surprising that as yet they have been unable to demonstrate their sexual responsibility (Hall, 1975).

Illness and disability force individuals to confront problems and make adjustments to ensure satisfactory sexual experiences. Sexual problems may be compounded by the drugs taken to alleviate a physical or psychological difficulty. Most drugs can change sexual functioning in some way, even when taken for recreational purposes.

# SEX AND DRUGS

Whether a drug is prescribed for some ailment, taken to relax, or used to get high, it can have effects—physiological or psychological or both—on sexuality. A drug might increase the desire for sexual experience, but have no effect on performance. Or a drug might make it easier to engage in sex by removing self-consciousness or guilt. However, the same substance might also interfere with performance, perhaps by making it difficult to reach orgasm. Or a drug might not change a person's sexual activity, but alter the subjective experience. For example, marijuana may make an orgasm seem longer and more intense, although the time and the physiological reactions have not changed. To further complicate the picture, the same drug does not always have the same effects.

## *The effects of drugs*

Whatever effects a drug has on sexuality, they differ from person to person and from one occasion to another in the same person. Personality, mood, needs, expectations, physical condition, and setting all influence reaction to a drug.

Most drugs alter body chemistry in some way, although few directly affect the sexual organs. Most drugs work their influence indirectly, perhaps by changing arousal in the central nervous system, metabolism, coordination, or general health. By themselves, these physiological changes are unlikely to have a radical effect on sexual behavior.

The way a person expects a drug to act goes a long way toward determining its influence. Generally, if a drug is expected to heighten sexual arousal, it will. But if the drug is expected to interfere with sexual functioning, the user is likely to experience problems. For example, during the nineteenth century, marijuana was used in houses of prostitution as a sexual stimulant and by religious ascetics to destroy their sexual appetite. It appeared to be successful in both cases. Clearly, personal and cultural expectations play a major role in determining the sexual side effects of a drug.

Obviously, the effect of one glass of wine is very different from the effect of an entire bottle. This dosage relationship can be predicted for almost any drug, whether a prescription for high blood pressure or marijuana. In large quantity, most substances—even those that are relatively harmless—are likely to present sexual obstacles. Familiarity with a drug also alters its effects. A short-term user is sensitive to the novelty of a substance, but the long-term user may be immune to these effects or require higher dosages that impair sexual performance.

Our present knowledge about the effects of drugs—whether prescription or recreational—on sexual functioning is scanty and subject to change. The available information describes the possible effects a drug can have on sexuality, but cannot predict the effects on a particular person. And since most laboratory research has been done on men, more is known about most drugs' effects on male sexual response than on female arousal or orgasm.

## Prescription drugs

Dozens of drugs that are commonly prescribed by physicians and psychiatrists can affect sexual functioning. The effects are often positive. Any drug that successfully treats an incapacitating physical condition can indirectly improve sexual functioning. In the same way, psychiatric drugs that reduce anxiety or lift depression may improve sexual functioning. If these drugs enhance personal relationships, improved sexual performance is likely to follow.

Some drugs, however, can lead to sexual difficulties, and patients should be aware of the possibility when they begin taking the drug. The expectation that a sexual problem may arise can, of course, sometimes provoke it, but the patient's knowledge that such side effects are normal and that they can be controlled by changing medication will keep serious concern from developing.

**Antihypertensive drugs** Many drugs are used to treat high blood pressure, and most of them can impair sexual functioning in some people. The problem does not need to be permanent, however, for if a patient encounters difficulties, the dosage can be reduced or a new drug substituted. When the drug is stopped, the symptoms generally disappear. (These drugs are also taken by some cardiac patients.)

Drugs (such as spironolactone) that work by stepping up kidney function rarely cause problems at low dosages. When the dosage is increased, however, men may be plagued by erectile failure, diminished sexual desire, and enlarged breasts, while women may suffer from irregular menstrual periods and tender breasts. Drugs (such as reserpine) that reduce blood pressure through their effects on the nervous system have a variety of effects, depending on the drug that is taken. Decreased sexual desire is a common side effect, perhaps because some of these drugs tend to cause drowsiness or depression. These drugs sometimes cause erectile failure, retarded ejaculation, and enlarged breasts in men, and a lack of orgasm or the secretion of milk in women.

**Psychiatric drugs** Major tranquilizers, such as the phenothiazines, have revolutionized the treatment of serious mental disorders, especially schizophrenia. The phenothiazines have permitted patients who would formerly have been hospitalized to live at home. Because phenothiazines work on the endocrine system as well as on the brain, they can affect sexual functioning. Diminished sexual desire is reported by about 20 percent of women and men alike. A much smaller proportion of women experience a decrease in vaginal lubrication or have irregular menstrual periods—or none at all. At high doses, men occasionally have erectile failure and inability to ejaculate, and the size of their testes decreases (Kolodny, Masters, and Johnson, 1979).

Drugs used to treat depression have varied effects. Since depressed people tend to be apathetic toward sexual activity, any drug that lifts the depression should improve sexual functioning. And so it is with most patients who take antidepressants. However, among patients who continue to have sexual activity during a depression, about five in every hundred developed sexual difficulties as the drug lifted their depression (Simpson, Blair, and Auso, 1965).

**Hormones** The power of hormones to disrupt sexual function was made clear in the discussion of hormonal treatments of paraphiliacs (Chapter 15). However, people who take hormones for other reasons may also develop sexual problems. For example, male athletes who take large doses of anabolic steroids to improve muscle mass may become sterile, and men with prostatic cancer who are given female hormones may develop erectile problems (Kolodny, Masters, and Johnson, 1979).

## *Recreational drugs*

When drugs, such as alcohol, marijuana, or street drugs are taken for their effect on sensation or perception, they are called recreational drugs. Both legal and illegal drugs are widely used for recreational purposes. For some users, the sexual side effects are welcome and intended. For others, sexual side effects are unpleasant, unintentional, and unwelcome. The folklore surrounding the effects of drugs on sexuality is enormous, as the Focus on aphrodisiacs shows, but scientific research is relatively scarce.

# *Focus*

THE SEARCH
FOR THE
PERFECT
APHRODISIAC

**aphrodisiac**  a drug
that heightens sexual
desire, pleasure, or
performance

Myths and folklore about the effect of drugs on sexuality pervade almost every culture. The search for the perfect **aphrodisiac**—a drug that will heighten sexual desire, pleasure, and performance—has been a cultural theme since ancient times. Yet the search appears to have been in vain. Few drugs have a direct and positive effect on sexuality. In fact, it is far easier to find drugs that are *an*-aphrodisiac—substances that diminish desire and pleasure.

Nevertheless, the search for aphrodisiacs has never ceased. Natural substances such as datura, belladonna, and henbane were used in the sexual orgies of ancient fertility cults. Tribes that worshipped the Greek god Bacchus, also known as the "phallus god," used the poisonous psychedelic mushroom *Aminita muscaria* to create sexual frenzy. Marco Polo chronicled the sexual effects of hashish in the Eastern palaces of the eleventh century. In Africa, yohimbine was used to increase

sexual powers, and in medieval Europe, the aphrodisiac of choice was the mandrake plant.

Certain foods have acquired a reputation as aphrodisiacs. Oysters, celery, bananas, and tomatoes are among the delicacies that are supposed to have sexual powers. Some societies have placed their faith in animal parts—powdered rhinoceros horn or raw bull's testicles. Natural food advocates may believe in the powers of ginseng root or vitamin E. A sign in a popular New York seafood restaurant reads FISH IS FOOD FOR LOVE.

One of the best-known aphrodisiac drugs is cantharides, also called Spanish fly, made from a beetle that is dried and powdered. Taken by mouth, cantharides irritates and inflames the genitourinary tract, causing an unpleasant genital stimulation. It sometimes produces an erection that refuses to subside until the drug wears off. However, cantharides does not increase sexual desire

and may cause illness or even death.

The drugs with the most powerful reputations as aphrodisiacs today are alcohol and marijuana, although neither acts directly on sexual desire or performance. The effects of either drug seem to depend on the amount used, the setting in which they are consumed, and the personality of the user. Of critical importance in their effect is the strength of their reputation as sexually stimulating substances. If a person truly believes in the aphrodisiac powers of, say, a banana, then eating it may prove to be a sexual turn-on.

Why do we continue to search for that perfect aphrodisiac? Perhaps our search is for instant ecstasy. Sexuality is a complex and often troubled area of human behavior. Insecurity, confining sex roles, myths, and misinformation keep many of us from responding freely. If only we could find the perfect drug, we believe, the obstacles would disappear and we would find ourselves in sexual paradise.

## *Alcohol*

Many people believe that alcohol breaks down the barriers to sexual activity and acts as an aphrodisiac. The investigation of this question has long been hampered by moralistic attitudes toward both alcohol and sex, and only recently has research into alcohol's effects on sexuality become possible.

Perhaps Shakespeare was right when he wrote of alcohol: "Lechery, sir, it [alcohol] provokes and unprovokes; it provokes the desire, but it takes away the performance" (*Macbeth,* act 2, scene 1). In the past decade, research has uncovered a more complicated picture, one in which a person's expectations are extremely important.

In one experiment (Farkas and Rosen, 1976), sixteen young men drank various mixtures of orange juice and tasteless alcohol, and then their responses to erotic films were measured. As the alcohol level in the blood rose the men's heart rates increased, but their erections were slow to develop (as measured by a penile plethysmograph) and were weaker (see Figure 18.1). The men's subjective experience of arousal matched the physiological recordings: they felt most aroused when their alcohol level was lowest. This experiment was the first controlled demonstration of the direct effects of specific alcohol dosage on human sexual response to visual stimuli.

Further research indicated that alcohol's physiological effects are influenced by the person's beliefs about the drug's power as an aphrodisiac. In a second study (Briddell and Wilson, 1976), one group of young men was told that alcohol would increase their sexual arousal as they watched an erotic film. A second group was told that alcohol would decrease arousal. Varying amounts of alcohol were given

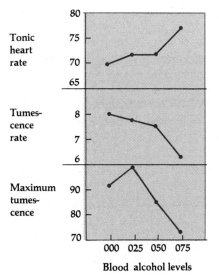

### *Figure 18.1*

The Relationship Between Blood Alcohol Level, Penile Tumescence, and Heart Rate. (Farkas and Rosen, 1976)

to the men, who were unaware of the drink's alcohol content. As they viewed the film, their erections were measured. Again, increased alcohol levels were associated with weaker erections. However, the sexual response was also affected by the men's expectations (through suggestion). Men who heard that alcohol increased arousal had larger erections than men who had heard that the drug decreased arousal.

Alcohol appears to affect ejaculation as well as erection. In a somewhat similar study (Malatesta et al., 1979b), men were given varying doses of alcohol and asked to masturbate to orgasm while watching sexually explicit videotapes. As levels of alcohol increased, the men felt less aroused, derived less pleasure from the films, took longer to reach orgasm, and said their orgasms were less intense than usual. What is more, at the two highest alcohol levels, nearly half the men failed to reach orgasm.

Alcohol appears to have similar effects on sexual arousal in women. In one study (Malatesta et al., 1979a), women who drank alcohol and then masturbated to orgasm while watching erotic films took much longer to reach orgasm, found it more difficult to climax, and had less intense orgasms when their alcohol level was high. These results paralleled the reactions of men. However, unlike men, the women in the study said they felt *more* aroused at high alcohol levels and enjoyed their orgasms more.

Taken together, these studies indicate that large amounts of alcohol suppress sexual response in both men and women. The studies also show that expectations about the effects of alcohol have considerable influence on the way people react. In American society, most people believe that alcohol and sex go together, and this belief was reflected in the subjects' reports. Small quantities of alcohol may help to set a sexual mood, without necessarily interfering with ability to perform, but as Shakespeare pointed out nearly four hundred years ago, too much alcohol "takes away the performance."

Alcohol is a powerful drug, and when abused it can have deleterious effects on sexual functioning. Alcoholic women report high levels of sexual dysfunction, including reduced responsiveness and inability to reach orgasm. Their reproductive function also seems to deteriorate. Studies have found a higher than expected level of menstrual disorders, early menopause, premenstrual tension, and reduced fertility among alcoholic women. Not all these problems may be the direct result of alcoholism. Perhaps sexual problems or gynecological or obstetric problems come first, with women drinking for relief. Then, as their alcohol consumption steadily increases, the problems worsen. When alcoholic women do become pregnant, they tend to miscarry and to have complications during pregnancy and delivery (Wilsnack, 1982). In addition, their babies often suffer permanent harm, as we'll see in Chapter 20.

Chronic alcoholism also causes sexual problems in men. Loss of sexual desire, erectile dysfunction, sterility, testicular atrophy, low testosrone levels, and enlarged breasts are all found in alcoholic men (Wilson, 1981). The steady intake of large quantities of alcohol seems almost invariably to lead to some kind of sexual dysfunction.

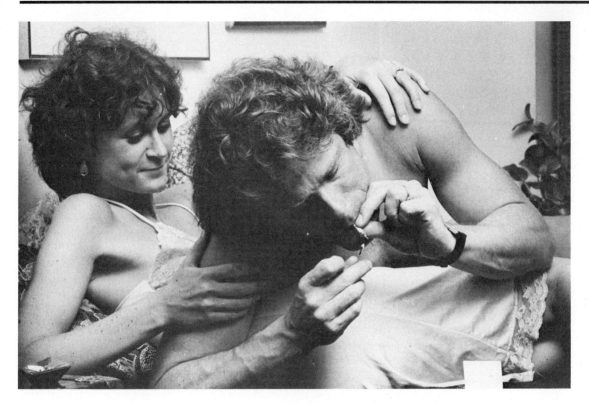

The user's expectations and the setting determine the sexual effects of any drug taken as an aphrodisiac. (© Joel Gordon 1980)

## Marijuana

In different parts of the world, marijuana is used to ward off fatigue, to treat diseases such as glaucoma, and as part of religious rituals. Within such settings, it has few sexual side effects. In the West, however, marijuana has acquired a reputation as an aphrodisiac. At the potency usually consumed in the West, both the physical and psychological effects of marijuana are relatively mild. Nevertheless, the belief that the drug enhances sexuality persists among users and nonusers alike, and the strong expectation of increased sexual pleasure is often borne out in experience.

Most users of marijuana describe their experience in pleasurable terms (Goode, 1972). Among 150 college students, for example, marijuana increased sexual desire—but only when the user was in the company of a likely sex partner. In such a situation, desire was intensified and sexual sensations enhanced. Users often felt greater contact, responsiveness, sharing, and empathy with a sexual partner (Tart, 1971). Most users said that marijuana was the ideal aphrodisiac and that the level of intoxication was related to feelings of sexual pleasure. But with very high levels of intoxication, some users reported that their involvement with their own fantasies and inner experiences detracted from their sexual involvement.

When another group of college students replied to a questionnaire, nearly half said that marijuana increased sexual desire, and just over half said that it increased sexual enjoyment. Once again, high doses of the drug were said to be associated with lessened desire and pleasure. Among these students, men and women reacted differently to marijuana: women were more likely to report increased sexual desire, and men were more likely to note increased enjoyment. The researcher (Koff, 1974) believes that traditional sex roles can explain the sex differences. Marijuana is powerful in releasing women's sexual inhibitions, probably because they have traditionally been taught to repress their sexual desires. It seems less likely to increase their enjoyment because most women are uncomfortable at the prospect of losing control during sexual encounters. The drug seems to affect enjoyment in men because they have been taught to value the intensity of physical sensation during sex.

Interviews with more than 1,300 men and women over a period of five years also produced testimony to marijuana's power to enhance sexual enjoyment. But when these adults were asked about marijuana's specific effects, their answers were surprising. No, said the men, marijuana did *not* increase sexual desire, firm or prolong erections, allow them to control ejaculation, or increase the intensity of orgasm. In a similar vein, the women said that marijuana did *not* increase their interest in sex, their arousability, their vaginal lubrication, or the intensity or frequency of their orgasms. Then how does marijuana increase sexual enjoyment? According to these men and women, it heightens sensory awareness, relaxes them physically and mentally, and puts them in tune with their partners (Kolodny, Masters, and Johnson, 1979).

These reports seem consistent with what is known about the effects of marijuana on the body and indicate that expectations, set, and setting—not the physiological effects of the drug—are responsible for the glowing reports of marijuana users. A candle-lit room, burning incense, music, a desirable partner, and the conviction that the drug will intensify sexual pleasure could account for most experiences described by users.

Although marijuana does seem to enhance sexual activity for many individuals, there has been concern that the drug may interfere with sexual function by altering hormone levels. Little is known about the effect of the drug on women's hormone levels. After evaluating a number of studies, the National Academy of Sciences (1982) reported that marijuana indeed suppressed testosterone production, decreased the size and weight of the prostate and testes, and reduced sperm production, but that the effects were rapidly reversed as soon as men stopped using the drug. The report concluded that marijuana did not cause sterility.

## *Other illicit drugs*

A variety of illicit drugs have acquired reputations as aphrodisiacs in the past fifteen years. Among them are amphetamines, cocaine, amyl nitrite, LSD and other hallucinogens, barbiturates, and Quaaludes. Their reputation as sexual enhancers generally comes from those who use them illicitly. However, the major illicit drug, heroin, has earned a reputation for diminishing sexual activity and desire.

**Heroin**   Heroin, like other narcotic drugs, seems to depress sexual function. Addicts of both sexes report that it reduces sexual desire and delays orgasm. Male addicts say heroin causes erectile problems. Not all users report these effects, and degree of sexual impairment is often associated with amount and duration of drug use.

As with other drugs, a distinction can be made between the effects of chronic and occasional use. Initial experimentation with heroin often produces desirable effects. Ejaculation is delayed, so intercourse can continue for long periods. Sexual difficulties usually emerge with continued use. In one study (DeLeon and Wexler, 1973), ex-addicts were interviewed about their sex lives. Almost all of them reported a decrease in the frequency of intercourse, masturbation, and nocturnal emission while on heroin. When a heroin user ejaculated, it took him an average of forty-four minutes to reach orgasm.

Many ex-addicts enroll in methadone maintenance programs. In these programs, the ex-addict receives a daily dose of methadone that is intended to block the craving for heroin without interfering with general functioning. Although some addicts on methadone maintenance continue to have sexual problems, most report improved or normal sexual functioning (Cushman, 1972).

**Amphetamines**   Various effects have been claimed for amphetamines—commonly called "speed" by their users—from heightened sexual interest but decreased ability to perform, to definitely increased powers, to decreased sexual interest, to no interest at all (Cox and Smart, 1972). There is simply no agreement among users as to how amphetamines affect sexuality. Differences in dosage, method of administration, and drug experience may be partly responsible for this disagreement, but it appears that there are large individual differences in reaction to the drug.

Amphetamines stimulate the central nervous system, increasing heart rate, blood pressure, and muscle tension. Speed has its most powerful effect when taken intravenously, for it provides an overwhelming orgasmic "rush" that involves the whole body. Men may get an erection as they inject the drug. Users frequently say they have an increased desire for sexual activity accompanied by aggressiveness during the sexual act. Although sexual activity is often prolonged, orgasm may become difficult or impossible (Gay and Sheppard, 1973). Other researchers report that chronic amphetamine use may prevent orgasm without interfering with erection; however, some users also report multiple orgasms.

**Cocaine**   In 1884 Sigmund Freud, who used cocaine to lift his own depression and fatigue, wrote about the power of cocaine as an aphrodisiac: "The natives of South America, who represented their goddess of love with coca leaves in her hand, did not doubt the stimulative effects of coca on the genitalia." For many drug users, cocaine remains the ultimate mood elevator and energizer. Like amphetamines, cocaine is a stimulant, and in its effects on sexuality, it tends to resemble amphetamines. It increases the ability to maintain an erection, prolongs sexual activity, and interferes with the attainment of orgasm. When large amounts of cocaine are used, its strongly stimulative nature may result in sexual frustration. Once again, dosage and the individual's level of sexual functioning before drug usage appear to play a major role in sexual reactions.

**Amyl nitrite** Amyl nitrite, commonly known as "poppers," is sometimes used with cardiac patients to treat the pain of angina. It expands the blood vessels, rapidly dropping the blood pressure. This drop is usually accompanied by faintness, skin flush, and a feeling of heat in the skin. The body's response to amyl nitrite is immediate, intense, and may be extremely dangerous.

Amyl nitrite first gained popularity as an aphrodisiac among homosexual groups, but its use has spread to some heterosexual circles. It appears to be more popular with men than with women. Generally, the drug is inhaled at the moment of orgasm, when it is reported to prolong and intensify the climax. The drug's effect is short-lived—usually a minute or two. As indicated in Chapter 17, heavy use of amyl nitrite may be associated with the development of AIDS.

**Psychedelics** During the 1960s, when psychedelic drugs burst onto the American scene, drugs such as mescaline and LSD were proclaimed as powerful aphrodisiacs. Testimony to their power in heightening sexual experience from prominent figures in the drug culture influenced the expectations of drug users for many years.

The limited research on psychedelics indicates that their effects depend entirely on the setting in which they are used and the empathy between sexual partners. Drug users at a San Francisco clinic reported that with a compatible partner, psychedelics increased sexual sensitivity, heightened awareness, and improved communication. But if the user was uncomfortable with either the setting or the partner, sexual experiences were generally unpleasant (Gay and Sheppard, 1973). Reactions to psychedelics are unpredictable, and the amount used seems to be critical. At high dosages, users are likely to find that sex is difficult or impossible.

**Barbiturates** Barbiturates, such as seconal, phenobarbital, nembutal, or tuinal, are depressants. They slow the action of the central nervous system, decreasing alertness, reaction time, and motor coordination. A small dose may make a person euphoric, but a large dose will produce unsteadiness or unconsciousness. If they make the user feel more relaxed, sexual activity may increase, but at higher dosages they slow or stop sexual activity. Although barbiturates may release inhibitions, they usually interfere with sexual performance. Chronic users report loss of desire, erectile problems, and inability to reach orgasm.

**Quaalude** Methaqualone, marketed in the United States under the trade name Quaalude, is a sedative-hypnotic drug that is chemically unrelated to barbiturates. Although it is also a depressant, it acts on different brain centers. Quaalude is generally prescribed to produce sleep or relaxation in agitated patients.

When it first became popular as an illegal drug, Quaalude was regarded as an aphrodisiac. However, its sexual effects appear to be unimpressive. At low dosages, it has been reported to increase desire and break down sexual resistance, but at the expense of erectile ability. At high dosages, Quaalude's relaxing qualities are likely to produce a lack of interest in sex and an inability to perform.

Drug use is certainly one of today's major health issues. It is almost impossible to find an American who has never used alcohol, an illegal drug, or one of thousands of prescription drugs. Although we know very little about how most drugs interact with sexuality, we do know that expectations and beliefs about the effects of any drug on sexuality play a major role in the way it is actually experienced.

# Summary

**1** Chronic or debilitating disease can affect sexuality directly (by interfering with the nervous or endocrine systems) or indirectly (by affecting body image, energy levels, or movement). Most reduction of sexual activity by patients with serious disease is unnecessary. Since sexual activity is only a mild form of exercise, 80 percent of heart attack patients can probably resume their regular levels of sexual activity. Cancer has deep psychological effects, and the attitude of the patient's partner plays a critical role in determining the level of sexual functioning. Diabetes can have far-reaching effects on sexual functioning. Although nerve and blood-vessel damage may be partly responsible, psychological factors can also be important. Since multiple sclerosis involves the nerves, it has a physical effect on sexual functioning. However, the intermittent nature of the disease and the youth of most patients enable the majority to make a satisfactory sexual adjustment.

**2** Sexual functioning is probably central to the rehabilitation of disabled patients. The disabled person has physical problems that limit activity or response and psychological problems that arise from misinformation and society's view that the disabled are not sexually active. In spinal cord injury, the connection between the brain and the genitals may be severed, but many patients can learn to reassign sensation from an intact portion of their bodies and reach orgasm through fantasy. Cerebral palsy does not affect the sexual system, so the major problem for people with this disorder is establishing intimate relationships. Although society restricts the sexual activities of mentally retarded people, 90 percent of them can marry and have children. Even those who cannot could enjoy recreational sex if appropriate methods of contraception are used.

**3** The effects of various drugs on sexuality are influenced by personality, mood, needs, expectations, physical condition, and the setting. Dosage and familiarity with the drug also influence its effects.

**4** Antihypertensive drugs can impair sexual functioning at high dosages, but so many drugs can be used to treat high blood pressure that a patient who has problems can easily be switched to a new drug. Major tranquilizers that are used to treat schizophrenia can directly reduce sexual functioning, while drugs used to treat depression generally improve functioning indirectly by lifting depression. Hormones can have a powerful effect on sexual functioning and may reduce or eliminate desire or performance.

**5** People have always looked for a perfect **aphrodisiac**, a drug that heightens sexual desire, pleasure, and performance, but few drugs have a direct, positive effect on sexuality. Large amounts of alcohol suppress sexual response in men and women. When abused, alcohol can lead to sexual dysfunction. Marijuana users generally report enhanced sexual desire or enjoyment, yet it appears that expectations, set, and setting are responsible for these effects. Among other illegal drugs, the effects on sexual functioning vary. Heroin seems to depress sexual functioning; amphetamines and cocaine have uncertain effects; amyl nitrite has momentary, intense positive effects, but can be quite dangerous. Psychedelics depend entirely on setting and empathy between sexual partners; high doses of barbiturates slow or stop sexual activity; and Quaaludes appear to depress sexual functioning. Expectations and beliefs about a drug's effects on sexuality appear to play a major role in its perceived effect.

*one couple's experience*

My old boyfriend felt that if I was on the pill or using a diaphragm I would become promiscuous. We fought about it a lot. We always said we would use the foam and condom method, but, actually, we rarely did. (Authors' files)

*another couple's experience*

When my husband and I started going out, we used foam and condoms. That worked okay for a while, until we had two rubbers break on us in one week. I ran off to a clinic and went on the pill. That worked fine for more than a year. Lovemaking became more spontaneous. No more "Are you ready now? Let's stop and get our stuff." Then I started getting really bad headaches. I went off the pill and we're back to foam and rubbers again! It's a nuisance, but okay. (Authors' files)

# 19 Birth Controls: Contraception, Sterilization, and Abortion

*Chapter 19*

---

Our bodies are designed to reproduce themselves. If we have sexual intercourse on a regular basis without interfering with the system, the expected outcome is conception, pregnancy, and childbirth. **Contraception**, or the intentional prevention of conception, is actually a process of redesign—an attempt to separate sexuality from its possible reproductive consequences.

**contraception** the intentional prevention of conception

The search for the perfect contraceptive began as early in human history as women and men became aware of the link between intercourse and pregnancy. Four thousand years ago, ancient Egyptian writings described various vaginal suppositories, including crocodile dung mixed with paste, that were meant to prevent conception. As for men, Egyptian wall paintings show men wearing sheaths over their penises—apparently forerunners of the modern condom. And one Greek writer suggested washing the penis in vinegar or very salty water before intercourse. Among women of ancient Rome, a "natural" method of birth control was popular: a woman held her breath, rose immediately from bed, squatted down, and tried to sneeze. When these early techniques failed, the ancients limited family size through abortion or infanticide.

Effective, widespread, and socially approved contraception is a relatively recent practice. Today's contraceptive freedom is a product of slowly changing social, sexual, economic, and political conditions. The view that contraception is a right, if not a duty, developed gradually. Not too long ago, any attempt to prevent conception was considered immoral, unhealthy, and socially destructive. As recently as twenty years ago, it was even illegal in some states.

# Birth Controls: Contraception, Sterilization, and Abortion

After tracing the contraceptive revolution, we'll look at the many methods of preventing conception, considering the effectiveness of each as well as its drawbacks. Because of the prevalence of contraceptive failures, other methods have also been used to prevent birth. We'll investigate **sterilization,** or the use of surgery to make a person incapable of conceiving a child. Then we'll look at **induced abortion,** or the intentional termination of a pregnancy. Although abortion is not a contraceptive, it is the most widely used means of birth control in the world. We'll close by exploring the decision to use birth control and the importance of fitting the method to the way we live.

**sterilization** the use of medical techniques to make a person incapable of conceiving a child

**induced abortion** The intentional termination of pregnancy

## THE CONTRACEPTIVE REVOLUTION

What seems like a revolution in contraception has taken place in two areas: technology and attitudes. Researchers have developed medically sophisticated contraceptives that are close to 100 percent effective. But more important, the vast majority of people have come to accept the use of contraceptives as a desirable way to limit fertility. This change in attitude occurred only in the second half of the twentieth century, and it represents a sharp break with the past. Before this century, contraceptive knowledge was the privilege of a restricted few—physicians, prostitutes, and the upper classes of certain cultures. In most societies, any limit on fertility was discouraged by legal, religious, and social codes.

We have become accustomed to the notion of birth control as a necessary part of life. But previous generations struggled over this issue. Because fertility has such important consequences for society, birth control has always been socially regulated (Gordon, 1976). Since population size is directly related to the use of contraceptives, a society that wants to expand is likely to prohibit contraceptive measures.

Our present concern with overpopulation is a relatively recent development. Most past societies have had the opposite concern—they needed to increase population levels. Before the twentieth century, many factors kept population levels low: high infant mortality, short life span, disease, famine, high maternal mortality during childbirth. From a political standpoint, most societies needed a high birth rate. Western religious tradition supported this need. For example, Christian churches generally condemned sexual activity that had no procreational intent.

In the second half of the nineteenth century, people had begun to accept the notion that motherhood should be voluntary, and the importance of choice in childbearing was stressed. But because most medical authorities believed that contraception was unhealthy, even dangerous, and because the moral ethic of the time called for restraint of sexuality, abstinence was advocated as the best technique for limiting family size. Contraceptive devices were considered obscene, and possessing them—or information about birth control—was illegal.

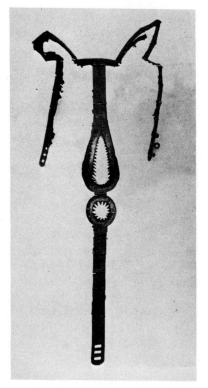

For centuries, contraception was seen as unneeded by "good and faithful" wives. During the Middle Ages, female faithfulness was ensured by the chastity belt, which the husband locked in place before he left on a journey. (© Eric John Dingwall/Clarion Press)

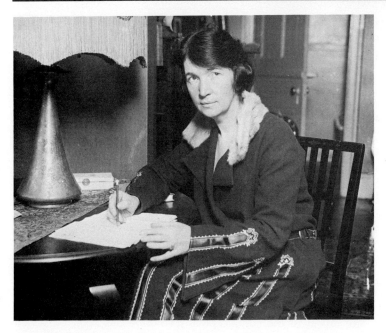

Margaret Sanger, a nurse among New York City's poor, was primarily responsible for the American acceptance of contraception. Early in this century, she defied law and custom in order to protect women from death by illegal and dangerous abortions. (© Culver)

With time, however, the view that birth control devices were unhealthy, unnatural, or obscene began to change. The change was primarily the work of two women: Margaret Sanger in the United States and Marie Stopes in England.

Just after the turn of the century, Margaret Sanger began work as a nurse in the poor neighborhoods of New York City's Lower East Side. Her interest in birth control developed as she discovered the lack of contraceptive knowledge among poor immigrant women, who begged her for advice on ways to limit their families. Again and again, she found these women resorting to illegal and dangerous abortions.

Her concern for these women led her to adopt birth control as a personal cause. Although not the first to speak out on the issue, Sanger attracted considerable public attention. In 1914, she began publishing a magazine called *Woman Rebel*. The magazine voiced her political ideals and printed articles on socialism, class division, and women's rights. Sanger was arrested and charged with violating the law forbidding the distribution of contraceptive information. The government subsequently dropped its case against her because of the publicity her arrest had received as a free speech issue. Sanger next opened a birth control clinic in a poor area of Brooklyn. Her activities led to another arrest, and she eventually served thirty days in prison.

Others, including Robert Latou Dickinson, the gynecologist who first studied women's sexual anatomy (see Chapter 3), became involved in the struggle, and contraception finally won public acceptance. The valiant efforts of Sanger and other advocates of birth control were not the only factors in the widespread support of contraception. Urbanization and industrialization probably played an equally important role in the change. Among a rural population, children are a source of labor and financial support; in an urban, industrial society, they are a financial drain. Children must be fed, clothed, and educated, yet there is no productive work for them. Even now, countries with large agricultural populations are slow to limit their family size, but the birth rate has dropped markedly in most industrialized nations (Figure 19.1).

A final factor in the public acceptance of contraception has been the changing role of women. The sexual double standard, in which women remained faithful to their marital partners while men indulged in sexual wandering, helped to keep contraception out of favor. The faithful wife who regarded sex as a route to motherhood had no need for birth control. Although motherhood is still a primary role for many women, few still regard sex as only a means of procreation. Women's legal right to control their own fertility has expanded their choices in many areas besides sexual behavior, including education, career, and family structure.

The most recent aspect of the contraceptive revolution has been the acceptance of birth control for the unmarried. Until the 1970s, contraceptives were considered proper only as a form of family planning within marriage, and many states had laws against providing birth control devices for single women.

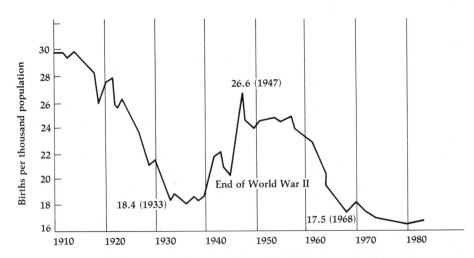

*Figure 19.1   Birth rates in the United States since 1910.*
The birth control movement has received widespread public accepance in the twentieth century.

The assumption that easy availability of contraceptives led to promiscuity and the breakdown of the family is still with us, but discriminatory laws no longer keep contraceptives out of the hands of unmarried women. Concern with the rising tide of pregnancies among unwed women has eliminated the last legal barrier to birth control information.

However, a new federal regulation would require family planning clinics to inform the parents of adolescents who request contraceptive devices. This rule has generated a storm of protest on both constitutional and practical grounds. Opponents point out that a survey of adolescents who now use the clinics indicates that about 16 percent would switch to less effective methods of conception and that 5 percent would continue to have sex, but without using any sort of contraception. Only 2 percent said they would stop having intercourse (Kenney, Forrest, and Torres, 1982). The courts have so far prevented the Department of Health and Human Services from putting the regulation into effect, with one judge declaring it "unlawful" (Pear, 1983a).

## METHODS OF CONTRACEPTION

At least ten different contraceptive techniques are commonly used today in the United States, and each has several variations (see Table 19.1). In order to make an intelligent selection, we need to be aware of what is available and what best suits our individual needs.

Most contraceptives are designed for women, a few are meant for men, and some require the cooperation of both. None of these methods is perfect. The ideal contraceptive would have at least four characteristics: (1) It would be completely effective, with no instances of unwanted pregnancy; (2) it would have no negative effects on physical or psychological health; (3) it would be easily reversible; and (4) it would fit well into the user's personal and sexual needs, being easy to get, inexpensive, and convenient.

Until a perfect contraceptive is developed, we're forced to choose on the basis of trade-offs. For instance, greater effectiveness often means an increased health risk, but less harmful methods tend to disrupt sexual spontaneity. Some compromise is necessary, and so we accept the disadvantages of a method in order to obtained its valued advantages.

### *The pill*

The development of the **pill**, which controls fertility with synthetic hormones, was at first hailed as the perfect solution to contraception. It apparently gave women safe and complete control over childbearing decisions. Then the pill's effects on general health brought all hormonal contraceptives under increasing scrutiny. A few years later, some varieties of the pill were found to have distinct health benefits

**pill** a synthetic hormone preparation that prevents conception

## Table 19.1   *Contraceptive effectiveness*

| METHOD | FAILURE RATE WHEN USED CORRECTLY (%) | ACTUAL FAILURE RATE (%) | PROBABLE REASON | AVAILABILITY |
|---|---|---|---|---|
| Combination pill | .34 | 4–10 | Forgetting to take pill | Requires prescription |
| Minipill | 1–1.5 | 5–10 | Forgetting to take pill | Requires prescription |
| IUD | 1–3 | 5 | Expulsion | Requires trained insertion |
| Diaphragm with spermicide | 3 | 17 | Incorrect placement Tears or pinholes Premature removal | Requires trained fitting |
| Cervical cap | 2 | 16 | Incorrect placement Dislodged by partner's penis Premature removal | Requires trained fitting |
| Condom | 3 | 10 | Break or tear | Over-the-counter |
| Foam | 3 | 22 | Insufficient amount | Over-the-counter |
| Sponge | said to be about same as diaphragm | | Premature removal | Over-the-counter |
| Rhythm (calendar) | 13 | 21 | Irregular ovulation | Chart from physician or church |
| Rhythm (temperature) | 7 | 20 | Unclear temperature pattern Temperature change from stress or infection | Thermometer over-the-counter |
| Rhythm (mucus) | 2 | 25 | Unclear pattern Changes from illness or diet | Mirror and speculum over-the-counter |
| Withdrawal | 9 | 25 | Sperm present in preejaculate Failure to withdraw in time | No preparation required |
| Vasectomy | .15 | .15 | Vas deferens reconnects | Surgery required |
| Tubal ligation | .04 | .04 | Tubes reconnect | Surgery required |

Failure rates are based on use by 100 women over the period of one year.
(Data from Hatcher et al., 1980; Koch 1982b; Pear, 1983)

for some women. Although the pill provides the most effective reversible protection from unwanted pregnancy, it is no longer viewed as the most suitable contraceptive for all women.

Hormonal contraceptives could be developed only after scientists had a clear idea of how the menstrual cycle works. By the 1930s, researchers understood the relationship between changing hormone levels and ovulation, which was discussed in Chapter 3. Now the task was to find ways to intervene in the cycle and prevent ovulation. This was accomplished in the 1940s, and by 1956 the first commercially marketed birth control pill, called Enovid, was tested, At present, from ten to fifteen million American women use some variety of the pill.

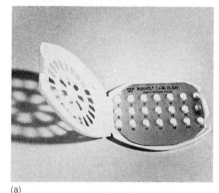

(a)

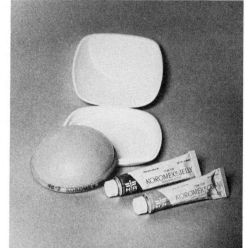

(b)

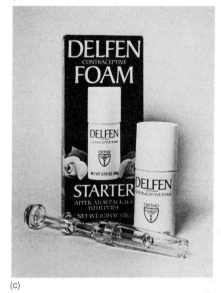

(c)

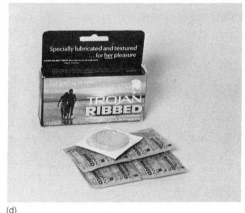

(d)

No contraceptive method is perfect, and before we select one, we need to know which technique best suits our needs. The pill (a) is extremely effective and keeps sexual activity spontaneous, but carries risks. Among other methods, the diaphragm (b), foam (c), and condoms (d) are without risk, but are less effective than the pill and may disrupt spontaneity. (© Leonard Speier 1983)

All hormonal contraceptives rely on the influence of estrogens or progestins— or both—to disrupt the normal processes of ovulation and pregnancy. Synthetic estrogens have two major effects on the menstrual cycle: They keep the plug of mucus that covers the cervix impenetrable to sperm, and they keep the uterus from developing the lining in which a fertilized egg can implant itself.

**Types of pills** The most widely used hormonal contraceptive is the *combination pill*. It contains constant amounts of estrogens and progestins and is taken for twenty-one consecutive days, stopped for seven days, and then resumed. Since the combination pill contains both hormones, it works by inhibiting ovulation, maintaining a thick cervical plug, and inhibiting the development of the uterine lining. Unlike the shifting levels that characterize the normal cycle, hormone levels in the pill user remain relatively stable throughout the month. Since pill users do not build up a normal uterine lining, they don't actually have a normal menstrual period. Instead, several days after they stop taking the pill, they have what is called "withdrawal bleeding." The absence of true menstruation explains why the pill user's bleeding tends to be shorter and scantier than nonuser's.

Another form of dual hormone contraceptive is the *once-a-month pill,* developed because it is more convenient than a daily pill. The combination of estrogen and progestin is rapidly absorbed by body tissues and then slowly released into the bloodstream. A monthly *injection* of combined hormones has been tested in Egypt, Cuba, Mexico, and Sweden, and trials showed that the injection effectively stops ovulation (Fotherby et al., 1982). Neither the pill nor the injection is yet available in the United States.

Women who experience negative side effects from the estrogen in the combination pill may be switched to the *mini-pill,* which contains only progestins. Although mini-pills produce fewer side effects, they are also slightly less effective than combined pills. The major side effects of the mini-pill are irregular bleeding and spotting in midcycle. The mini-pill is less effective because its primary action is to maintain a mucous barrier that keeps sperm from entering the uterus, not to inhibit ovulation. Unlike other pills, mini-pills are taken every day, with no breaks.

Another form of contraception based on progestins is the progestin *capsule* implanted under the skin of the forearm. The capsule can remain in place for several years, and in a five-year test with more than a hundred Chilean women, no pregnancies occurred. The major side effect is an irregular menstrual cycle (Diaz et al., 1982). The capsule is not generally available in the United States. A long-lasting progestin injection that is needed only four times a year is used in more than eighty countries. This injected drug, Depo-Provera, is considered an ideal contraceptive by some experts and regarded as dangerous by others, since it produces cancer in some laboratory animals (Boffey, 1983). In 1983, Depo-Provera was being considered for use in the United States. Long-term progestin effects can also be obtained by using a vaginal ring that contains the hormone, or by including progestins in certain types of intrauterine devices (IUDs), which we'll discuss later. In all these methods, the progestin is released slowly into the bloodstream.

A final type of hormonal contraceptive is the *morning-after pill,* designed for use when a woman has had unprotected intercourse in the middle of her menstrual cycle. Morning-after pills contain extremely high doses of estrogen and should be used with caution. If taken regularly, they can have severe side effects. Some morning-after pills contain diethylstilbestrol, commonly called DES, a drug that has been associated with increased risk of cancer in the children of women who took it while pregnant. Thus, if the morning-after pill fails to prevent pregnancy, the woman is strongly advised to have an abortion.

Morning-after pills, which work by preventing the fertilized egg from implanting itself in the uterine lining, must be taken within seventy-two hours of intercourse. Some pills are taken for five consecutive days, others for ten. They can have severe side effects, including nausea, vomiting, headaches, and breast tenderness. A safer morning-after pill containing only progestins is being tested by researchers.

Major efforts have gone into developing hormonal contraceptives for women, but little is heard about a "male pill." The aim of such a pill would be to interfere with sperm in some way, probably by halting sperm production. Most American researchers have used male or female hormones, and they have had only limited effectiveness. In China, researchers have been working on a male pill that contains gossypol, an ingredient of cottonseed oil. They report some success in suppressing sperm production without depressing sexual interest (Djerassi, 1979).

**The pill's effectiveness** Theoretically, the combination pill is nearly 100 percent effective. The effectiveness of progestin-only pills seems to be slightly lower. However, pills that must be taken every day may sometimes be forgotten, and it has been estimated that the actual failure rate of the pill is between 5 and 10 pregnancies for every 100 woman years of pill use (Hatcher et al., 1980).

There are two major types of error. If a woman forgets to take several pills, particularly in the first half of her cycle, she may be unprotected—an egg may develop. A woman who misses more than one pill can guard against this kind of failure by using a back-up method of contraception for the rest of that cycle. For the same reason, women who are just starting to take the pill should use a secondary means of protection during the first cycle. The second error that leads to pill failure occurs when women who dislike the side effects of the pill stop taking it but fail to use an additional means of contraception.

In rare cases, a woman who has taken her pills regularly becomes pregnant. If this happens, the increased chances of developing a malformed baby usually lead physicians to recommend a therapeutic abortion. Among babies conceived while women were taking the pill, the proportion of boys seems to increase (Shiono, Harlap, and Ramcharan, 1982).

**Reversibility—pregnancy after the pill** In the 1960s, authorities assumed that a woman would be especially fertile after she stopped taking the pill;, therefore conceiving a child presented no problem. This has not proved to be the case. Although most women who stop taking the pill resume their normal menstrual cycle and promptly become pregnant, a few women experience the **oversuppression syndrome**. The pill has suppressed ovulation for so long that the normal menstrual cycle does not begin immediately, and she is temporarily infertile. The oversuppression syndrome is most likely to occur in women whose menstrual cycle was irregular before they began using the pill, so most physicians do not prescribe the pill for women with irregular cycles. Even when the normal menstrual cycle resumes immediately, it's best to wait several months after stopping the pill before trying to become pregnant. The waiting period ensures that all synthetic hormones will leave the body before conception, reducing the risk of miscarriage.

**oversuppression syndrome** Temporary infertility in women who take the pill for so long that ovulation does not resume when they stop taking it

**Side effects** Because the pill's synthetic hormones reach all areas of the body, their effects are not restricted to the reproductive system. Unpleasant (or pleasant) effects of the pill are referred to as side effects, but potentially life-threatening changes are called complications. Side effects are relatively common among pill users; complications are much less frequent, but a far greater cause for concern.

About 40 percent of women who use the pill experience some side effects, and the actual rate may be even higher. Many women may fail to report symptoms because they simply don't connect their headaches or mood changes to the pill. This supposition is supported by the fact that as many as half of all women who start using the pill stop taking it before a year has passed. Many of these women are probably experiencing unpleasant side effects.

The most frequently reported side effects are nausea, weight gain, headaches, spotting (slight bleeding between periods), susceptibility to vaginal infections, depression, and mood changes. Some of these side effects, such as nausea, seem to lessen with continued use; others, such as headaches during the week the pill is not taken, tend to get worse with longer usage. Such symptoms as fatigue and mood change tend to remain constant. Some women also report decreased sexual interest and difficulty in reaching orgasm.

These symptoms are sometimes eliminated by switching a woman to another brand of pill, but when side effects persist it may be necessary to find a different type of contraceptive. For other women, nausea and weight gain seem a small price to pay for an effective and convenient contraceptive. In addition, many women report positive effects. Shortened, lighter withdrawal bleeding is often welcomed in preference to regular menstruation. As one woman said.

> I was suddenly set free. I knew exactly when my period would begin—almost to the hour, when it would end, and I stopped worrying about embarrassing accidents. (Authors' files)

Pills also seem to lessen premenstrual discomfort and cramping. Since they regularize hormone levels throughout the cycle, pills may eliminate the drastic mood swings and physical symptoms some women report as the premenstrual syndrome (see Chapter 3). Finally, some women say that the pill increases their sexual interest—an effect that may simply reflect the removal of any fear of pregnancy.

**Complications** When the pill first appeared on the market, it was greeted with enthusiasm. In recent years, however, researchers have realized that the pill can present serious health hazards to some women.

The pill is clearly associated with increased risk of heart attack, blood clots, stroke, high blood pressure, severe headaches, gall bladder disease, diabetes, liver tumors, and hepatitis. However, the overall risk for pill users is actually very small, and going by it is deceptive, because the risk is not shared equally by all users. For instance, women with blood type O seem to be less susceptible to clotting disorders than women with other blood types. Similarly, pill users with a history of hypertension are more likely to suffer heart attacks than those with normal blood pressure levels. Smoking also increases the risk. In fact, smokers in their forties who have stopped taking the pill, but who used it for at least five years, appear to run an added risk of heart attack until menopause (Layde, Ory, and Schlesselman,

1982). Risk of heart attack or hypertension may also depend on which pill is pre-scribed. Combination pills that are high in estrogen appear to increase the sort of blood cholesterol that protects against these disorders, while pills that are high in progestins appear to increase the kind of cholesterol that is associated with them (Wahl et al., 1983). For some women, then, the health risks of the pill are smaller than average; for other women, the risks of illness or death are much greater than the statistics indicate.

The relationship of the pill to cancer is under intense study. A connection has been found only in a variety of pill that has been removed from the American mar-ket, and there is no increase among women who take the combination or mini-pill (U.S. Public Health Service, 1982). As we'll see, these pills may even protect wom-en against some forms of cancer. However, since estrogen speeds up the growth of existing cancers, any woman who has ever had cancer or who is considered at high risk for cancer should not use the pill.

**Advantages** Even critics of the pill admit it has several advantages. When used correctly, it is the most effective form of reversible contraception. It does not intrude on the sexual experience. It is convenient, and some of its side effects are positive. With only these advantages, many women would continue to use the pill.

Now it appears that the pill may bring substantial health benefits to many women, for it seems to help prevent several diseases and common medical condi-tions (Ory, 1982). For example, women who take the pill have reduced rates of breast disorders and only half the rate of pelvic inflammatory disease of women who use no contraceptive at all. The pill also appears to prevent the development of iron deficiency anemia, probably because it usually reduces the quantity of men-strual flow.

One of the diseases that seems to be prevented by the pill is a disease physi-cians once suspected it caused: cancer. Women on the combined pill seem to have lower rates of endometrial and ovarian cancer than women who don't take it. The pill seems to prevent endometrial cancer only among women who use it for at least a year, and the effect is strongest in women who have never had children (U.S. Public Health Service, 1982). Protection against both forms of cancer may persist for as long as ten years after a woman stops taking the pill. Finally, the pill may help to prevent rheumatoid arthritis, a painful and crippling disease (Ory, 1982).

Before deciding to take the pill, a woman needs to know all about its benefits and risks. All too often the pill is dispensed automatically to any woman who en-ters a family planning clinic or physician's office. Once a woman and her physician decide that the pill is appropriate, they share a responsibility for monitoring her health for as long as she takes the pill.

## *Intrauterine devices (IUDs)*

The origin of the modern **intrauterine device** (IUD), a small piece of plastic or metal that is inserted into the uterus, is generally credited to Richard Richter, a Ger-man physician who in 1909 developed such a device from silkworm gut and

**intrauterine device (IUD)** a small piece of plastic or metal that, when inserted in the uterus, sets up an in-flammation that pre-vents implantation of a fertilized egg

bronze. Its inspiration may have been the mushroom-shaped stem *pessary,* which was used in the nineteenth century to prop up a sagging uterus. The stem of the pessary was inserted into the uterus and the cap covered the cervix. Although pessaries often led to infection, they also seemed to reduce fertility.

Richter's IUD also was associated with infections and was not much used. About a quarter of a century later, a silkworm gut and silver IUD was reintroduced in Germany, and a similar device was developed in Japan. Although the first modern IUDs were brought to the United States by German scientists at the time of World War II, they were not widely available until the early 1960s. About 15 million women around the world now use some type of IUD.

**Effectiveness and use** The majority of IUDs contain small amounts of copper. Copper IUDs seem to be more effective in preventing pregnancy than the plastic models, but the long-term effects of copper on the body are not completely understood. The body seems to absorb less copper from an IUD than it does from food. An increasingly popular form of IUD contains small amounts of progestins that are slowly released into the uterus. Unlike plastic models, which can be left in place as long as they produce no side effects, the copper IUD must be replaced every three years and the progestin-releasing IUD must be changed every year.

No one is certain exactly how the IUD prevents pregnancy. The most commonly accepted explanation is that since the IUD is a foreign object, it causes an inflammatory response within the uterus, which prevents a fertilized egg from implanting itself in the uterine wall. This means that the IUD does not prevent conception—the egg and sperm can still meet—but instead halts the development of

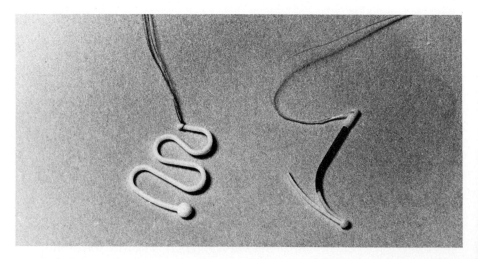

The intrauterine device (IUD) is an effective means of contraception that allows complete spontaneity, but can lead to serious complications. (© Leonard Speier 1983)

the egg. The copper-releasing IUDs seem to give added protection by altering the enzymes required for implantation and perhaps by killing sperm.

Because the effectiveness of an IUD depends upon its correct placement, it needs to be inserted by an experienced person, whether a physician or a paraprofessional at a family planning clinic. The physician first measures the depth and shape of the uterus and selects an appropriately sized device. Generally, the IUD is placed in an inserter (shaped like a thin plastic straw), which passes through the cervix and deposits the IUD within the uterus. Insertion is usually highly uncomfortable, and afterward there may be bleeding and severe cramps as the body tries to rid itself of the foreign object. If these symptoms persist, the physician will have to remove or adjust the device. Most IUDs have a string attached to them that is left hanging in the vagina so that the woman can be sure the IUD is still in place.

IUDs are highly effective. Their failure rate is usually estimated at between one and seven pregnancies for every 100 woman-years of use. Effectiveness varies with the type of IUD used, the ease of insertion, the physician's experience, and the likelihood of expulsion. Many women spontaneously expel an IUD; others request its removal because of pain or discomfort. The likelihood of expulsion is increased if the woman has just had a child or if she has recently had an abortion. The safest time to insert an IUD seems to be during a menstrual period, since the cervix is already somewhat dilated and there is almost no chance that the woman is pregnant at the time of insertion.

**Side effects and complications** The most frequently reported side effect of the IUD is dysmenorrhea, or painful menstrual periods. Menstruation is likely to be longer than normal, the menstrual flow much heavier, and the cramping more severe. Blood loss is especially heavy with the copper IUD; users of the progestin-filled IUD seem to have a much smaller increase in menstrual flow (Djerassi, 1979). Many women have their IUDs removed because of these problems; others simply take vitamin and iron supplements to make up for the loss of blood and to prevent anemia.

Women who have anemia or dysmenorrhea probably should not consider using an IUD. Physicians also advise against the IUD for women who have any uterine or cervical disorder, any STD, who have recently been pregnant, had genital surgery, have heart conditions or clotting problems, or who are allergic to copper (Holt and Weber, 1981).

Three serious, but less common, complications sometimes follow the insertion of an IUD. Pelvic inflammatory disease may signal its presence by a continual vaginal discharge, sometimes accompanied by pain and fever. Women with a history of pelvic infections may find that the IUD makes them more susceptible to infection and that it is more difficult to treat existing infections. One type of IUD, the Dalkon Shield, was withdrawn from the market in part because the type of string attached to it was believed to aid the passage of bacteria from the vagina into the uterus.

A second complication traced to the IUD is also linked with pelvic inflammatory disease: ectopic pregnancy, in which the fertilized egg implants itself in the Fallopian tube. About 5 percent of the women who become pregnant while wearing an IUD have ectopic pregnancies, and there is some indication that such pregnancies are connected with the progestin-filled IUDs (Cooke and Dworkin, 1981).

The final IUD-related complication is perforation of the uterus. The device can puncture the uterine walls and even enter the abdominal cavity. Perforation is usually the result of faulty insertion. A misplaced IUD is located by ultrasound (a device that produces a picture by bouncing sound waves off an object) and removed.

The long-term effects of the IUD are not clear. If the device is left in place for more than four or five years (as the older IUDs could be), it may cause permanent structural changes in the lining and muscles of the uterus. Since the IUD appears to work by causing a chronic inflammation of the uterus, such a change in cell structure would not be surprising.

Although the IUD is highly effective, on occasion a woman does become pregnant while the device is in place. About 50 percent of such pregnancies end in spontaneous abortion. Some physicians recommend ending these pregnancies by therapeutic abortion because the risk of serious infection during pregnancy is high. If a woman decides not to have an abortion, the physician will probably remove the IUD.

Not all women can tolerate the IUD, but for women who can, the device has several advantages. A college woman explained her reasons for using an IUD:

> I never could use birth control. I tried the pill for a while but I kept forgetting to take it. And I always figured I wouldn't feel comfortable using a diaphragm because I'd always have to carry it with me. But with the IUD, it's just in there and I don't have to do anything about it. I feel much safer with the IUD than I ever did before. (Bell, 1980, p. 186)

The IUD is almost as effective as the pill. It gives a woman complete control over her own fertility. Since the IUD is always in place, it does not depend on memory (as the pill does), and it does not interfere with spontaneous sexual activity.

## The diaphragm

**diaphragm** a birth control device in the shape of a domed rubber cap that covers the cervix

The **diaphragm**, a dome-shaped rubber cap designed to cover the cervix (see Figure 19.2), was developed by Wilhelm Mensinga, a German professor of anatomy, in the 1880s. The device was soon adopted in Holland, where the first family planning clinic opened in 1882, and the diaphragm became known as the "Dutch cap." Margaret Sanger saw the diaphragm as the birth control technique that would finally free women from unwanted pregnancy and encouraged its use.

For generations, women in the United States used this method with considerable success. In the 1960s, when the pill and the IUD became available, there was a sharp decrease in the popularity of the diaphragm, and it began to receive a bad press. Women heard that it was messy, difficult to use, and ineffective. In recent years, however, the well-publicized side effects of the pill and the IUD seem to be sending a growing number of women back to the safety of the diaphragm. At family planning clinics, it is now almost three times as popular as the IUD (*Family Planning Perspectives*, 1982).

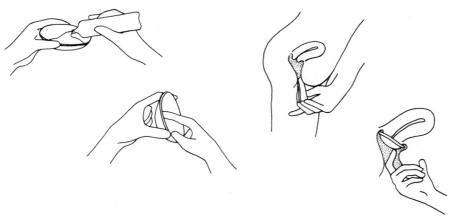

***Figure 19.2***

The diaphragm is gaining in popularity among women who are unwilling to risk the side effects of the pill or IUD. (left) The application of spermicidal jelly to the diaphragm. The jelly must be used every time the diaphragm is inserted. (right) The insertion of the diaphragm into the vagina.

Diaphragms come in a variety of sizes (from 50 to 105 mm) and types, depending on the construction of the spring that maintains the diaphragm's shape. The main function of the diaphragm is not to act as a physical barrier against sperm, but to hold a spermicidal (sperm-killing) cream or jelly over the cervix.

There is some disagreement as to when the diaphragm should be inserted and how much spermicide is necessary. The conservative view, presented by most authorities, is that a diaphragm should be inserted no more than two hours before intercourse and should remain in place at least eight hours afterward. If intercourse is repeated within those eight hours, additional cream or jelly is added for each sexual act. Some researchers have suggested that spermicides are more powerful than most people suppose and that a single application may prevent pregnancy for up to twenty-four hours. Until research verifies this proposal, the standard instructions are probably safest. In addition, other researchers have reported that wearing a diaphragm for such a long period may cause a woman to risk toxic shock syndrome (discussed in Chapter 3). Several cases of toxic shock have occurred among women who wore a diaphragm for at least thirty-six hours (Baehler et al., 1982).

Since the diaphragm must be fitted individually, it can be obtained only by medical prescription. Generally, the health professional prescribes the largest size that can be used comfortably. Too large, and the diaphragm becomes painful; too small, and it will not protect against conception. Once a properly fitted diaphragm is in place, a woman cannot feel it. A woman should be refitted after she bears a child or has an abortion, if the tone of her vaginal muscles changes, or if she loses or gains more than twenty pounds, for her size may change in any of these situations.

Most diaphragms are inserted by hand, although some types come with a notched inserter that may make it easier to position them. After the diaphragm is in place, the woman checks its position, making certain that the front rim is tucked behind the ridge of the pubic bone and the cervix felt through the dome. If a diaphragm is cared for properly it lasts about two years, but its fit should be checked on a yearly basis.

One reason for the diaphragm's decline in popularity is esthetic. A generation that has grown up with the pill may see the diaphragm as messy and intrusive. (Actually, many diaphragm users have discovered that the diaphragm holds back the menstrual flow, making intercourse during menstruation *less* messy.) It's true that if women do not plan their sexual activity in advance, stopping to insert the diaphragm can interrupt the flow of sexual activity. But insertion does not have to destroy the sexual mood, as one man discovered:

> Most of the women I've been with in the last five years used a diaphragm, and
> I've bought the cream. Several have showed me how to put it in but, even
> though I've tried a number of times, I'm not very good at it. But we laugh at
> my bumbling attempts and that becomes part of our being together.
> (Zilbergeld, 1978, p. 201)

Although sex manuals suggest that the male partner become involved in the process of insertion, checking the position, and removal, when a man does not cooperate the responsibility falls on the woman. Some men report they can feel the diaphragm during intercourse, but this usually presents no problem. Men may object to the taste of the spermicidal jelly or cream during oral sex, and it may be necessary to try several brands of spermicide until a type is found that both partners find nonirritating and acceptable.

While the diaphragm has some obvious drawbacks, it also has several clear advantages over other contraceptive methods. Most important, it has virtually no physical side effects. Other than the rare allergy to a particular brand of spermicide, the diaphragm is a completely safe and easily reversible birth control technique. It can be used by all women except those who have a severely displaced uterus or some structural problem in the vaginal area.

The diaphragm's effectiveness is extremely high when used correctly and consistently. But unless the method suits a person's needs and attitudes, it may fail. Perhaps the most important factor in predicting the diaphragm's effectiveness is the couple's motivation. Highly motivated couples generally find it an extremely effective method, but couples who are ambivalent about using it may find that carelessness can lead to an unplanned pregnancy.

## The cervical cap

**cervical cap** a birth control device shaped like a rubber thimble that fits snugly over the tip of the cervix

The small, thimble-shaped **cervical cap** operates on the same principle as the diaphragm. However, instead of extending across the vagina, it fits snugly over the tip of the cervix, blocking the cervical opening while providing a spermicidal barrier. The cap is held in place by suction rather than by the presence of the rim against the vaginal wall that secures the diaphragm.

The cervical cap has been in use longer than the diaphragm; a rubber cervical cap was developed in 1838 by Friedrich Wilde, a German physician, who made a wax impression of each patient's cervix and designed a cap to fit it exactly. Nearly a century before, however, the famous European lover Casanova provided some of his partners with a squeezed lemon half, which covered the cervix and provided an acid barrier against sperm (Fairbanks and Scharfman, 1980).

The cervical cap was used in the United States until the 1950s and is still popular in Europe. Its use is limited in the United States because there have been no widespread trials to provide the Food and Drug Administration with a statistical basis for approval. Physicians and clinics that prescribe it do so on an "investigational" basis (Littman, 1980). Preliminary studies indicate 8.4 pregnancies for every hundred woman-years of use (Koch, 1982b).

Like the diaphragm, the cap is fitted by a health professional. The Prentif cap, which is manufactured in England, comes in only four sizes, but a majority of women can be fitted with one of the sizes. Although spermicidal agents are recommended with the cervical cap, its snug fit may provide protection without any cream or jelly. However, the spermicide certainly provides added security.

Some women prefer the cap to the diaphragm because the cervical cap can be left in place for several days, and fresh spermicide does not have to be added for each act of intercourse. There may be some risk of toxic shock syndrome if the cap is left in too long, although no cases have yet been reported.

The cap is somewhat more difficult to insert and remove than the diaphragm (see Figure 19.3), and women tend to complain about an offensive odor, especially when removing the cap. Among nearly 400 women, about a third stopped using the cap within a year. By the end of the second year, less than half were still using it (Koch, 1982a). Odor, discomfort, and the dislodgement of the cap by their partner's penis were among the reasons given for stopping its use. Those who kept using it said they liked the cap's convenience, effectiveness, and safety, and the fact that it did not interfere with spontaneous sexual activity.

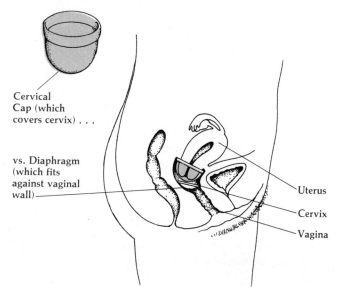

Cervical Cap (which covers cervix) . . .

vs. Diaphragm (which fits against vaginal wall)

Uterus

Cervix

Vagina

**Figure 19.3 The Cervical Cap**

This illustration shows the placement of the cervical cap over the cervix as compared to the diaphragm, which is positioned (in the vagina) as it should be for use during intercourse.

## Condoms

The condom has a long and varied history, perhaps dating back to ancient Egypt. However, it has not always been used as a contraceptive. In the sixteenth century, Gabrielle Fallopius, who first described the Fallopian tubes, urged European men to use a linen condom as protection against STDs. But Casanova, who was also in favor of the cervical cap, used condoms made of sheep's intestine for contraception. By the nineteenth century, the condom was recognized by the general population as an effective way to regulate fertility. At that time, animal-intestine condoms were bulky and expensive. Once the process of vulcanization of rubber was discovered in 1843, the mass production of thin, cheap condoms became possible, and their popularity increased. In this century, technological advances have improved the condom's reliability, comfort, and availability.

Like the diaphragm, the condom has become less popular in the era of the pill. However, people in many countries with low birth rates—such as Japan and Sweden—rely on the condom. In fact, among the Japanese, the condom and rhythm methods account for 90 percent of all contraceptive use (Giele and Smock, 1977). Part of the reason for the condom's success in Japan seems to be that the Japanese design condoms with pleasure in mind—their condoms are thinner than American condoms and come in a variety of sizes, colors, and textures. In Sweden, condoms are promoted for their ability to prevent a number of STDs. In the United States, the advertisement of condoms as either "sensuous" or "health-protecting" is a relatively recent development, but most newspapers, magazines, and television stations refuse to carry such advertising.

In an age when most contraceptives are designed for women, the condom is one of the few methods that allow the man direct responsibility for birth control. The condom has many advantages. When used properly, it is extremely effective, particularly if the female partner also uses a spermicide. It has the added bonus of providing protection for some STDs, it is a reversible method of contraception, and it has no side effects on health. Since the condom does not require a medical prescription, it is available to the sexually active adolescent. The condom is especially attractive to couples who have sex only occasionally, although condoms that have been carried around in a wallet often deteriorate from heat and are no longer effective. One man summed up his feelings:

> I can't say that I like using it, but at least it's there when we need it. I think a
> lot depends on your attitude, and we don't have any problems with the idea
> of a rubber. For us it's just a matter of convenience. (Authors' files)

There are objections to the condom. Some people feel that stopping to put on a condom disrupts sexual activity and mood, and some men say that it decreases sensitivity. Perhaps emphasizing the pleasurable aspects of the condom, as the Japanese do, would lessen these objections to the device. One problem is that standards set up by the Food and Drug Administration require American manufacturers to produce the thickest condoms made anywhere in the world (Djerassi, 1979). There is, nevertheless, a large variety to choose from, and condoms once again appear to be gaining in popularity.

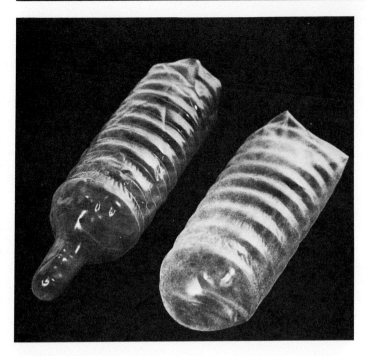

Condoms come in a variety of shapes and colors, and do more
than prevent conception; they also protect against many STDs.
(© Leonard Speier)

## Spermicides

**Spermicides** are contraceptives that provide a chemical barrier meant to kill sperm
before they can enter the cervix. Spermicides come in the form of foams, jellies,
creams, suppositories, and sponges. Creams and jellies are generally used with diaphragms or cervical caps, and foam is often used with condoms. In these cases,
they provide extremely effective protection. When used alone, spermicides provide
some protection, but not as much as other methods.

Researchers have worried that spermicides may cause miscarriages or birth defects in babies accidentally conceived when a spermicide was being used. A study
of more than 1,500 unplanned pregnancies among English women indicates that
miscarriages are no higher among women using spermicides than among women
who had planned their pregnancies. However, the study seemed to find a slight
increase in birth defects among women who were using spermicides at the time of
conception (Huggins et al., 1982).

Foam is a spermicidal agent in aerosol foam. It is used by shaking the aerosol
can, transferring the foam into an applicator, then depositing the foam in the vagina. Foam works well because it disperses throughout the vagina, spreading over

**spermicide** creams,
jellies, or foams that
prevent conception by
killing sperm

the cervical opening and working into vaginal folds and creases. Creams, jellies, and spermicidal suppositories are used in a similar manner, but disperse less efficiently and so provide less protection.

Foam seems to be nearly as effective as the diaphragm, but it has additional drawbacks. It remains effective for a shorter span of time and so must be applied almost immediately before intercourse and reapplied each time intercourse is repeated. It should not be washed out until about eight hours after the last act of intercourse. Some men and women report allergic reactions to foam, and there are wide variations in the effectiveness and appropriate dosages of different brands. What's more, a good many people dislike foam for esthethic reasons—it may leak from the vagina or have an unpleasant taste.

Foam does have major advantages. It is easily available, it is reversible, and it requires no medical intervention. The adolescent whose sexual activity is infrequent may find foam a good fit to her contraceptive needs, as did this young woman:

> Foam and rubbers are just about the only kind of birth control you can use
> when you need it and forget when you don't need it. I carry those little tubes
> of foam in my purse when I go out with my boyfriend and it's just like
> carrying Tampax, which everybody does. (Bell, 1980, pp. 170–171)

In addition, foam seems to decrease the likelihood of some STDs and vaginal infections.

The spermicide-saturated sponge is a new contraceptive, available since mid-1983. The spermicide kills sperm while the inserted sponge seems to block the cervix as it traps and absorbs semen (Pear, 1983b). The disposable sponge is about as effective as the diaphragm and once inserted it protects for at least 24 hours. Like foam, it is easily available, reversible, and requires no medical intervention.

## Rhythm

**rhythm method** birth control achieved by temporary abstinence during a woman's fertile period

Contraception can also be achieved by temporary abstinence during a woman's fertile period, a method known as **rhythm**. For thousands of years, there has been an awareness that the fertility of women varies during the month, but only during the past fifty years have we known that the fertile period occurs roughly in the middle of the menstrual cycle.

Although the approximate fertile period has been established, individual differences in ovulation make it extremely difficult to be certain just when a couple can safely have unprotected intercourse. The establishment of a "safe" period when a woman cannot become pregnant has taken three different forms: the calendar method, the temperature method, and the cervical mucus method.

The *calendar method* is based on two assumptions: that ovulation occurs about 14 days before the onset of the next menstrual period, and that sperm can fertilize an egg for only about 48 hours. Before using the calendar method, a woman first records the length of her menstrual cycles for at least six months. She then subtracts 14 from the longest and shortest cycles. For instance, if the shortest cycle was 26 days and the longest cycle 32 days, her fertile period would be from 12 to 18 days after the onset of menstruation. However, since sperm can survive in the vagina for 48 hours, a safety margin of several days is added to each end of the fertile period. This woman would abstain on days 8 to 21 of her cycle.

Even under the best of conditions, calendar calculations of fertility are risky. The calculations are easily thrown off because few women have completely regular cycles, and because emotional or physical stress can alter the pattern at any time, making information from past cycles misleading. Some women attempt to use this technique without having a clear idea of just when their fertile period occurs, further increasing the risks involved.

Somewhat more reliable than the calendar method is *temperature rhythm,* which is based on the fact that basal temperature (the lowest body temperature reached during waking hours) follows a monthly pattern related to ovarian hormone levels. Body temperature changes are very small, and the measurement of basal temperature requires a special thermometer that is marked in tenths of a degree. Basal temperature is taken immediately upon waking each morning, since getting out of bed and moving around, taking a drink, or smoking a cigarette changes the temperature. If a woman records her temperature every morning at about the same time, she will probably notice a drop around the middle of her cycle, followed by a sharp rise which signals that she has ovulated (see Figure 19.4). About three days after a sustained temperature rise, the egg can no longer be fertilized and intercourse is safe.

## Figure 19.4

Basal body temperature graph showing variations during a model menstrual cycle.

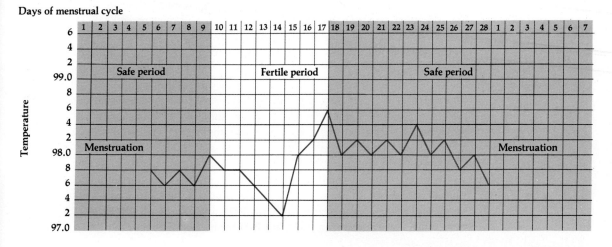

Although this technique is more precise than the calendar rhythm method, it has several disadvantages. Not every woman shows the clear patterns of temperature changes that are needed to pinpoint the day of ovulation. Such factors as emotional upset or a common cold may make it difficult to interpret temperature changes. In addition, the technique accurately determines the safe period *after* ovulation, but does not predict when ovulation will occur. This means that a couple relying on the temperature method will practice abstinence for about half of every menstrual cycle—a span they may find unacceptably long.

Some couples have met this problem by combining calendar rhythm with temperature rhythm. The calendar method predicts the earliest onset of ovulation, allowing them to have intercourse in the early part of the menstrual cycle, and the temperature method indicates when ovulation is over, allowing them to resume intercourse.

Finally, the *cervical mucus* method is based on changes in cervical mucus during the menstrual cycle. Just after ovulation, the cervix is rather dry and mucus is scanty. Then it becomes white and sticky until, at about the time of ovulation, it tends to become thin and perhaps transparent, indicating that it is now a hospitable environment for sperm. After ovulation, it returns to the sticky, white consistency. By learning to recognize these changes, a woman might be able to predict when ovulation is about to occur. However, not every woman has a clear pattern of mucus changes, and as we've seen, such factors as illness or diet may alter the pattern.

Researchers are working on a home method of predicting the onset of ovulation by detecting the presence of guaiacol peroxidase (G-Px), an enzyme in the mucus that apparently decreases sharply just before ovulation (Tsibris et al., 1982). If the method is successful, a woman would be able to have intercourse as long as G-Px could be detected in a sample of her mucus. When G-Px levels dropped too low to register, the woman would know that she was due to ovulate in about four days and that she had entered her fertile period.

In order to practice "natural birth control," a woman becomes a devoted student of her own body. She learns to identify the physical changes that are part of her menstrual cycle: temperature, mucosal secretions, cervical size and shape, mood, sexual arousal, water retention and swelling, the cramping some women feel at ovulation, and so on. Since each woman has a different pattern of signs and symptoms, personal experience is the only reliable guide. Ideally, this method leads to birth control that requires no external contraceptives and only a short period of abstinence. Actually, it requires self-control and an understanding sex partner. Some couples make it work by combining rhythm methods with the temporary use of a diaphragm during the fertile period. In any case, rhythm methods require sharp attention to bodily changes and the ability to tolerate the risk of unwanted pregnancy.

Although rhythm methods are the only contraceptive technique accepted by the Roman Catholic Church, they have been just as unpopular with Catholic women as with the rest of the population. In 1975, the National Fertility Study indicated that only 5.9 percent of married Catholic women were using rhythm. However, recent dissatisfaction with pills, IUDs, condoms, and spermicides has led a small but growing number of people to advocate a return to contraceptive methods that work in harmony with the body.

## Withdrawal

Removing the penis from the vagina before ejaculation, called **withdrawal**, or coitus interruptus, is perhaps the oldest method of birth control. It remains popular in parts of the world to this day. Its obvious advantage is that it requires no preparation, planning, or devices.

    Theoretically, if a man withdraws his penis before ejaculating, there should be no chance of impregnation. In reality, the failure rate of withdrawal is relatively high. In order to have any hope of success, the man has to predict his ejaculation accurately and maintain enough self-control to remove his penis. But if he ejaculates near the vagina, he may impregnate his partner. Besides, a small amount of "preejaculate," containing sperm cells, is released before the actual ejaculation. Although some men may become comfortable with their ability to withdraw soon enough, others may find that this method of birth control is tense and distracting. Since the woman has no control over the process, she may find herself so tense and worried that she can't enjoy sexual activity.

    Withdrawal has the advantage of being free, reversible, and without physical side effects. It requires no medical intervention. It has the disadvantage of being unreliable as compared with other techniques. In fact, withdrawal is so unreliable that many authorities do not regard it as an acceptable form of birth control.

**withdrawal** an unreliable method of birth control in which the penis is removed from the vagina before ejaculation

## STERILIZATION

Not all couples who do not wish to have children use contraception. Voluntary sterilization, which makes a person incapable of reproducing but does not interfere with sexual function, is fast becoming the most prevalent method of birth control in the world. In the United States, either the husband or wife has been sterilized in about one out of every three married couples between the ages of 15 and 44 (Kessel and Mumford, 1982). In the early 1970s, the procedure for sterilizing women was complex and fairly dangerous, so most sterilizations were performed on men. With the development of simpler procedures for female sterilization, about half the operations are now performed on women.

    The obvious advantages of sterilization are that it is completely effective and requires no further action to ensure birth control. Its major disadvantage is that sterilization is considered irreversible. Although it is sometimes possible to reverse the procedure, people who contemplate this form of birth control are encouraged to think of it as permanent.

    Both male and female sterilizations are almost always safe and effective, but their lack of reversibility means that it is unwise to undertake them lightly. The United States government has instituted a waiting period for all individuals requesting sterilization, so that they may consider their decision. During this period, both partners are advised to ask themselves several questions: Are we positive that we will never want another child under any circumstances? Will the operation be completely voluntary? Do we think we will feel the same about each other after the operation? Do we think this procedure will solve our marital difficulties?

The most controversial aspect of sterilization is its potential for coercion or abuse. A marital partner or physician may put pressure on an individual who is considering sterilization. In several instances, the procedure has been performed on women who did not understand its consequences and would not have consented to it if they had. In India, the government's sterilization program was halted when it was discovered that gifts and money were being used to persuade men to undergo sterilization. Responsible sterilization requires fully informed consent.

## Male sterilization

**vasectomy** male sterilization by cutting or blocking the vas deferens

Vasectomy, the sterilization procedure for men, is relatively uncomplicated. It is almost always performed in a physician's office and usually takes no more than thirty minutes. After a local anesthetic has been applied, the surgeon makes two incisions in the scrotum and cuts or blocks the vas deferens, the duct that carries sperm from the testes to the penis (Figure 19.5). Vasectomy causes no physical changes other

### Figure 19.5

Male reproductive organs showing stage one (left) and stage two (right) of the vasectomy procedure.

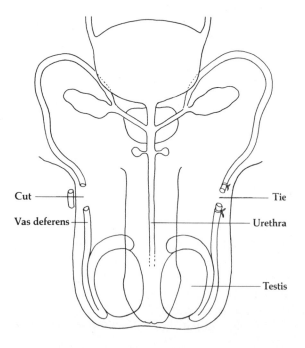

Cut

Vas deferens

Tie

Urethra

Testis

than the absence of sperm in the ejaculate, and the procedure is considered both safe and reliable.

The emotional effects of vasectomy vary and are apparently influenced by a man's prior commitment to the procedure and attitude toward it. Men who are certain they want a vasectomy and who are well informed about its effects tend to be the most satisfied with the outcome. In fact, the overwhelming majority of men who have had vasectomies report that they are completely satisified.

Vasectomy has been reported to have a failure rate of about .15 pregnancies per 100 men. Two types of failure are possible. First, in rare cases the vas deferens reconnects, and sperm are again carried through the penis during ejaculation. Second, after the surgery sperm may still inhabit the reproductive tract. For this reason, a man is usually advised to use some form of contraception until the reproductive tract is completely cleared, a process that may take several months.

Occasionally, a man changes his mind and asks a surgeon to reverse the vasectomy, reconnecting the vas deferens. Although a specialist can reconnect the tubes, the operation is generally not successful. In some cases, although sperm reappear in the semen, conception does not occur. When this happens, inability to conceive seems due to lack of sperm motility—that is, the sperm aren't active after ejaculation—or else the sperm have developed abnormal tails (Pelfrey, Overstreet, and Lewis, 1982).

## Female sterilization

At one time the most common technique for female sterilizaton was hysterectomy, or removal of the uterus. Hysterectomy effectively prevents pregnancy, but in the absence of other health problems, few physicians advise it. Hysterectomy is more risky than other sterilization techniques and can have many more side effects on health (Johnson, 1982). Removing the ovaries also provides permanent contraception, but is not advisable because it deprives the body of hormones.

Today the preferred technique for female sterilization is **tubal ligation**, in which the Fallopian tubes are either cut and tied or cauterized. Since eggs can no longer be fertilized or reach the uterus, they simply dissolve within the tube. The ovaries and uterus remain intact, and the menstrual cycle and hormone levels are unchanged.

**tubal ligation** female sterilization by cauterizing or cutting and tying the Fallopian tubes

Tubal ligation can be performed in several different ways. The Fallopian tubes can be approached through the vagina, a technique that is generally performed under general anesthetic in the hospital. The major disadvantage of the vaginal approach seems to be an increased incidence of complications, such as infection and hemorrhage. The most popular method in the United States is an abdominal approach, in which one or two small incisions are made in the abdomen and an instrument called a laparoscope is inserted. This permits the surgeon to see the Fallopian tubes, which he cuts and ties (see Figure 19.6). Although this procedure is sometimes performed under general anesthesia, it can also be done in a physician's office and does not require hospitalization. Laparoscopic sterilization has

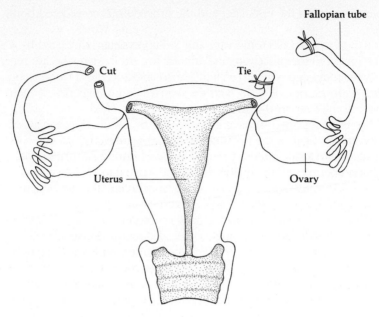

### *Figure 19.6*

Female reproductive organs showing stage one (left) and stage two (right) in a typical tubal ligation procedure.

been called a "Band-Aid" operation because the abdominal incisions are small enough to be covered with adhesive strips. As a result, the scars are small and do not disfigure the abdomen.

The effectiveness and safety of tubal ligation depend on the skill of the physician. In rare cases, the severed tubes grow back together and the woman becomes pregnant. Since there is a risk of ectopic pregnancy, the situation can become serious. Although serious complications of tubal ligation are rare, they include damage to other organs, infection, and hemorrhage.

New methods of sterilization without surgery are being developed. In one technique, now being tested in the United States, the physician inserts silicone plugs into the tubes. This technique is called bilateral tubal occlusion, and it can be performed in a physician's office under a local anesthetic. The physician inserts an instrument through the vagina into the uterus and pumps silicone rubber into the tubes. The silicone hardens, forming a plug. So far, no side effects have been detected from this method of sterilization (Brozan, 1982).

A different nonsurgical method uses the drug quinicrine, which is a common treatment for malaria. With an IUD inserter, the physician places several pellets of quinicrine inside the uterus. The drug, which has no harmful effects on the body, sets up an inflammation that closes the Fallopian tubes. Once this method has been thoroughly tested, authorities (Kessel and Mumford, 1982) expect it to become the preferred method of sterilization in the developing world, because it does not require a high degree of skill on the part of the physician.

# ABORTION

Most birth control techniques prevent conception—the meeting of egg and sperm—from taking place. A few, such as the IUD or the "morning-after" pill, permit conception but keep the fertilized egg from implanting itself in the uterine wall. Abortion disrupts fertility *after* the developing egg is implanted. This basic difference makes abortion an extremely controversial procedure.

Most people accept the desirability of preventing unwanted conceptions, but ending an established pregnancy often presents a moral dilemma. Some people believe every fetus has the "right to life" and oppose all abortion on moral or ethical grounds. Others find abortion personally offensive, but believe the decision is a personal matter to be settled by a woman and her physician. Still others believe abortion involves no more moral concern than any other means of birth control.

## Techniques of induced abortion

There are many medical techniques for abortion, and the procedure selected depends largely on how long the woman has been pregnant. Basically, the shorter the duration of the pregnancy, the quicker, the simpler, and the safer an abortion is.

**Early abortion** Although most physicians prefer to wait for a positive diagnosis of pregnancy before performing an abortion, a technique called **menstrual extraction** can be used even before pregnancy has been established for certain. This technique is generally used within six weeks after the last menstrual period, and it involves inserting a thin, flexible plastic tube through the cervix into the uterus. Through some form of suction—either a small pump or a syringe—the lining of the uterus, together with a small amount of fetal material, is removed through the tube. This procedure is considered very safe and usually takes only a few minutes. However, it has one disadvantage: Since the fetus is so small, it is hard to be sure the pregnancy has actually been ended. Women who are aborted by this method are advised to take a pregnancy test a week later to make certain the abortion was successful.

If the pregnancy continues more than 6 weeks after the last menstrual period, a technique called **vacuum suction** or **uterine aspiration** can be used. Abortion can be performed in this manner any time within the first 12 weeks of pregnancy, and the procedure is based on the same principle as menstrual extraction. Since a nonflexible tube has to be inserted into the uterus, it is usually necessary to dilate—or

**menstrual extraction** an abortion technique, using suction to extract the uterine lining, that is appropriate only very early in pregnancy—within six weeks of the last menstrual period

**vacuum suction** an abortion technique using suction to extract the uterine lining that is appropriate through the twelfth week of pregnancy; also called uterine aspiration

*Focus*

THE STATUS
OF ABORTION

Although induced abortion has been for centuries the world's most widely used method of birth control (Tietze, 1977), its legal and moral status has varied. As of 1976, more than half of the world's people lived in countries that allow abortion on demand or grant it under certain conditions. Only one person in every twelve lived in a country that forbade abortion for any reason. Among the countries with high rates of legal abortion are China, Japan, and the USSR. Abortions are most likely to be restricted in countries with strong Catholic traditions. However, these countries generally have extremely high rates of illegal abortion.

Although abortion is hotly debated in the United States, it was once widely tolerated. In both the United States and Europe, Abortion was permitted any time before "quickening"—the mother's first perception of fetal movement, usually between sixteen and twenty weeks after the last menstrual period. Early abortion was acceptable to the Catholic Church until 1868, when Pope Pius IX made all

abortions punishable by excommunication.

By this time abortion had been prohibited in England for more than half a century, and the United States was gradually following suit. In 1829, New York became the first state to restrict abortion, and over the next century each state adopted its own laws, with the majority forbidding abortion unless it was necessary to save the mother's life. These early laws may not have been concerned with the life of the fetus. The conditions surrounding surgery in the nineteenth century often meant dangerous infection or death to the patient, and the first abortion laws were seen as protecting the life of the pregnant woman (David, 1973).

Laws against abortion did little to prevent the procedure, however. In the 1960s, when about 8,000 legal abortions were performed in the United States each year, it is estimated that from fifty to eighty times that number were performed illegally. Affluent women had their abortions certified as legal, traveled to countries where abortion was per-

mitted, or obtained an illegal abortion from a competent physician. Poor women generally resorted to unsafe illegal abortions—often self-induced with coat hangers, knitting needles, or corrosive material packed into the uterus. Needless to say, many women died from such procedures.

In the early 1960s, restrictive abortion laws were challenged. The American Law Institute suggested that abortion be made legal if the physical or mental health of the mother was threatened, if the child might be born with a serious physical or mental defect, or if pregnancy was the result of rape or incest.

The public's attention was caught by the abortion issue when Sherry Finkbine, an Arizona mother of four who had taken thalidomide during early pregnancy, sought an abortion. The drug had been linked to serious birth defects, and she had been granted the right to a therapeutic abortion at a local hospital. But when the case was publicized, the hostile reaction caused the hospital to withdraw its permission. In

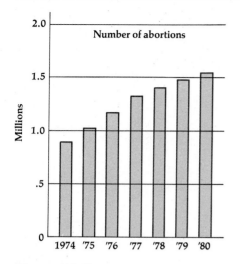
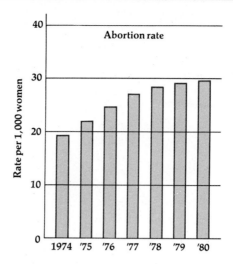

## Figure 19.7

Legal Abortions—Number and Rate per 1,000 Women Ages 15–44: 1974–1980.
(Statistical Abstract of the United States, 1982–1983. U.S. Bureau of the Census,
1982)

order to obtain a legal abortion, Finkbine had to go to Sweden. The publicity surrounding this and similar cases led to the gradual liberalization of abortion laws in a few states, with most following the guidelines set forth by the American Law Institute.

Abortion became available in all states in 1973, when the Supreme Court ruled that abortion during the first 12 weeks of pregnancy was a private matter between a mother and her physician and that from 12 to 24 weeks the state could not forbid an abortion but could regulate the conditions under which it was performed.

This landmark decision did not end the abortion controversy. Although surveys (Granberg and Granberg, 1980) consistently show that the majority of American people view abortion as essentially a private decision, a well-organized minority has continued to press for laws restricting the right to abortion and for a constitutional amendment that would once more outlaw it. Few people accept the use of abortion as a routine method of birth control, but an increasing number have come to regard it as a valid backup for contraceptive failure.

Sine 1975, the number of abortions has increased (see Figure 19.7), a rise generally attributed to a decline in the use of the pill and the IUD, coupled with an increase in the proportion of sexually active unmarried women (Henshaw et al., 1982). By the 1980s, about a million and a half legal abortions were performed in the United States each year, and the rate is expected to stabilize at that level.

During the first 12 weeks of pregnancy, the preferred method of abortion involves vacuum suction, which removes the uterine contents in about ten minutes. (© Erich Hartmann/Magnum Photos, Inc.)

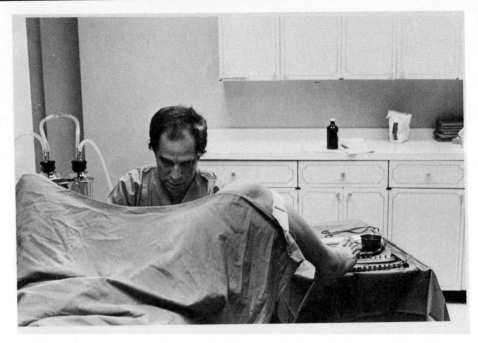

**dilation and evacuation (D&E)** an abortion technique used between the twelfth and sixteenth weeks of pregnancy in which the physician performs a vacuum suction abortion and then scrapes the inside of the uterus with a curette

**saline abortion** an abortion technique used after the sixteenth week of pregnancy in which amniotic fluid is replaced by saline solution, triggering labor

**prostaglandin abortion** an abortion technique used after the sixteenth week of pregnancy in which prostaglandins are injected into the amniotic fluid or the bloodstream, triggering labor

stretch—the cervical opening. The tube is attached to a mechanical or electrical suction pump, and when the uterine contents have been removed, they can be examined to be sure all fetal material is included. A local anesthetic is usually given with this procedure, and the abortion may be completed within ten minutes.

After the twelfth week of pregnancy but before the sixteenth week, most physicians use a procedure called **D&E (dilation and evacuation)**. After performing a vacuum suction abortion, the physician scrapes the inside of the uterus with a sharp metal curette to remove any tissue left behind by the suction pump. This procedure may be more painful than a simple vacuum suction and usually requires extensive local, or even a general, anesthetic.

**Late abortion** After sixteen weeks, abortion becomes a more serious procedure. Changes in the size and structure of the uterus, as well as the growth of the fetus, make it impossible to end a pregnancy with vaginal evacuation methods. In most late abortions, labor is induced so that the fetus can be removed through a "natural" delivery. There are two ways of doing this.

In **saline abortion,** a part of the fluid surrounding the fetus is withdrawn through a needle inserted into the woman's abdomen and replaced with a saline solution. This procedure usually starts labor within 12 to 36 hours. In **prostaglandin abortion,** prostaglandins may be administered into the fluid surrounding the fetus or through the bloodstream. These hormonelike substances occur naturally when a woman is giving birth, and they induce labor much more quickly than a saline solution. The disadvantage of prostaglandin abortion is that it has an increased number of side effects.

Surgical procedures are rarely used in abortions. They are usually reserved for very late abortions when other attempts to induce labor have failed or the woman is hemorrhaging. In a hysterotomy, the fetus is removed through a small incision in the abdomen, in a procedure similar to a birth by Caesarean section. The hysterotomy is a major surgical procedure requiring general anesthesia and a prolonged recovery. In a few cases, hysterectomy, or the surgical removal of the uterus, is used to abort a woman who is certain she wants no more children. Neither of these techniques is likely to be used merely to abort a fetus, for both have a high rate of complications.

## Physical risks of abortion

The physical risks of abortion are directly related to the length of time a woman has been pregnant. When legal abortions are performed before eight weeks of pregnancy, the death rate is 0.4 deaths pers 100,000 abortions. After 16 weeks of pregnancy, this rate increases to 17 deaths per 100,000 abortions (Tietze, 1977). Since most legal abortions are performed early in pregnancy, it's been estimated that there are two deaths per 100,000 legal abortions in the United States (Binkin, Gold, and Cates, 1982).

Since the mortality rate for women who carry their infants to delivery is estimated at sixteen deaths per 100,000 live births, it's safer to have a legal abortion than to have a baby. However, when abortion is illegal—performed in unsterile conditions by untrained people, or self-induced—the risk of death or complications rises sharply. An analysis of the abortion deaths between 1975 and 1979 indicates that illegal abortions are still sought by women who cannot afford a legal abortion, who are trying to keep the abortion a secret, who think an abortion requires consent of a husband or parent, or who live in areas where no abortion services are available (Binkin, Gold, and Cates, 1982).

The physical complications of abortion can be immediate, delayed, or late. Immediate complications are very rare with legal abortions. They include uterine perforation from the instruments used in vacuum and D&E abortions, damage to the cervix, hemorrhage, and negative reactions to anesthesia. Delayed complications generally involve a retention of tissue that results in bleeding and infection. Little is known about late complications of abortion, but there is some concern that repeated abortions may increase the risk of miscarriage or premature birth in later pregnancies. Some researchers have found fertility problems in women who have had abortions, but others have found no such problems.

## Psychological factors

Unlike other methods of birth control, abortion is often a highly emotional experience. Some authorities believe abortion presents a major risk to mental well-being. However, there is little evidence that abortion need present long-term psychological problems. For many women, it has the positive effect of eliminating the stress of an unwanted pregnancy (David, 1973). It would seem that the emotional stress of abortion may be far less damaging than the stress of bearing and rearing an unwanted child.

Several factors influence a woman's response to abortion. Early abortions seem to cause less emotional stress than abortions late in pregnancy. The surroundings in which an abortion takes place are also important. A legal abortion in a specialized clinic is likely to be much less traumatic than an illegal abortion performed in a clandestine location. Finally, a great many personal factors affect a woman's reaction to abortion: whether she has the support of friends and family; whether she is pressured into the abortion; the quality of her relationship to the man who impregnated her; her own views about abortion.

Most women feel tremendous relief after an abortion, as did this twenty-eight-year-old single photographer:

> The day after he left, I had the abortion. The pregnancy was a nuisance. It was very inconvenient. You have all the little frustrations in your day-to-day life and some big ones, but then something like this comes along, and you think, no way. . . . The abortion was nothing. We drove back into the city afterwards, and I felt just incredible. I have never felt so in control of my life. I could really make that decision. It felt fantastic. I never had a bad moment. (Francke, 1978, p. 52)

Many women are filled with negative feelings: sadness, regret, anger, or guilt. A twenty-three-year-old single receptionist reported such feelings:

> Emotionally I felt terrible. I just didn't know how I'd gotten myself into this situation. I hated myself. I felt abandoned and lost. There was no one's shoulder to cry on, and I wanted to cry like hell. And I felt guilty about killing something. I couldn't get it out of my head that I'd just killed a baby. (Francke, 1978, p. 61)

Cultural values tend to shape the personal experience of abortion, and American culture views abortion negatively. In some ways, however, single women, who have two-thirds of the abortions, face less censure than do the married (Francke, 1978). For a single woman, the lingering stigma of being an unwed mother and the financial obligations of caring for a child alone can make the decision to abort a simple one. Because a married woman is under more pressure to have the baby, she may find the decision to abort more complicated.

## THE BIRTH CONTROL DECISION

Those of us who are sexually active can choose from an array of sophisticated, inexpensive contraceptives. The use of these devices is legal, and the idea of limiting family size and spacing childbearing is supported by the culture (Figure 19.8). In addition, society disapproves of births that take place out of wedlock. Why, then, are there still so many unwanted and unplanned pregnancies?

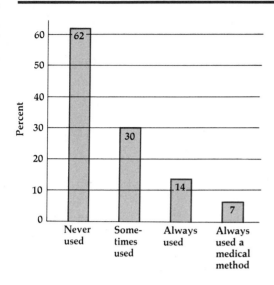

**Figure 19.8**

It can be seen in this figure that most teenagers who become pregnant have never used a contraceptive at any time.
(The Alan Suttmacher Institute, 1981)

The failure to use contraceptives—or to use them correctly and consistently— is most obvious among unmarried teenage women. As we saw in Chapter 12, at least a million adolescent women become pregnant each year in the United States. Older women also have unwanted pregnancies. For every adolescent who unintentionally became pregnant in 1978, nearly three women between the ages of twenty and forty-four found themselves involved in unplanned pregnancies (Dryfoos, 1982).

At each stage in a woman's fertility career, she is likely to have different concerns and desires regarding pregnancy (McCormick et al., 1977). The financial costs of childbearing vary, and so do the emotional, social, and physical consequences of motherhood. For instance, the unmarried adolescent who becomes pregnant pays a higher price for contraceptive failure than does the married woman whose pregnancy is unplanned but not unwanted. At the same time, the emotional and social barriers to effective birth control are often severe for the unmarried adolescent. Such factors mean that women's contraceptive needs also differ as they pass through their fertility careers. It makes sense, then, to separate the discussion of birth control decisions into the three stages of the fertility career: adolescence, young adulthood, and older adulthood.

## The adolescent

We hear most concern voiced about contraceptive failure in the young and unmarried, but as a society we can't seem to decide just how to deal with the contraceptive needs of sexually active adolescents. This conflict is probably due to the gap between attitudes toward premarital sexuality and its actual frequency.

Data gathered over the past few decades show a clear trend toward greater adolescent sexual activity. Despite substantial social disapproval, premarital intercourse has been rising steadily among adolescents, as we saw in Chapter 12.

Since both teenage sexual activity and out-of-wedlock pregnancies have been increasing, it might seem that adolescents are not making use of the contraceptive devices available to them. Studies have supported this conclusion, indicating that 31 percent of sexually active adolescent women never use contraceptives and only 27 percent always use them (Zelnick, Kantner and Ford, 1981). However, there has been a dramatic shift toward greater contraceptive use. Between 1971 and 1976, the proportion of young women who said they had used contraception during their most recent intercourse rose from 47 to 64 percent.

During the same period there was a trend toward increasing use of effective methods of birth control. Use of the pill, the IUD, and the diaphragm had increased from 38 to 57 percent. However, by 1979 use of the pill had declined, and more adolescent women were relying on withdrawal, probably because of the negative publicity given the pill in recent years (Zelnick, Kantner, and Ford, 1981). As a result, although more young women were using some method of birth control and using it consistently, the rate of unwanted pregnancies was continuing to climb.

A substantial number of young women still use contraception inconsistently, incorrectly, or not at all. Although adolescents sometimes find their access to contraceptives blocked by disapproving adults, the major barriers to effective contraception appear to be informational or emotional.

**Lack of information**   In an age of increasing sexual freedom, there still seems to be considerable ignorance about how the body works and how contraceptives should be used. In general, the younger a woman, the less she knows about the contraceptive facts of life. And because young women are becoming sexually active at earlier ages, the number who are uninformed has also increased.

Only six states and the District of Columbia require or encourage schools to provide adolescents with information about birth control, and only one state (Illinois) and the District of Columbia encourage the discussion of abortion (Alan Guttmacher Institute, 1981). Perhaps as a result, many adolescents severely underestimate their chances of pregnancy, and only about half of these women can identify the period during the menstrual cycle when they run the greatest risk. The lack of explicit information about how to use contraceptives may also increase pregnancies. A young woman may *think* she is protected if she takes one of her mother's birth control pills before a date, if she has intercourse only in certain positions, or if she uses a spermicidal foam after intercourse.

**Emotional obstacles**   The sexual "double standard," though in modified form, may also play a major role in the contraceptive decisions of many young women. On the one hand, they are told that premarital sex is improper, which may make some young women feel that planning for it is a sign of shame. On the other hand, they are the ones who bear the unpleasant consequences when an unplanned sexual encounter leads to pregnancy. They are blamed for using contra-

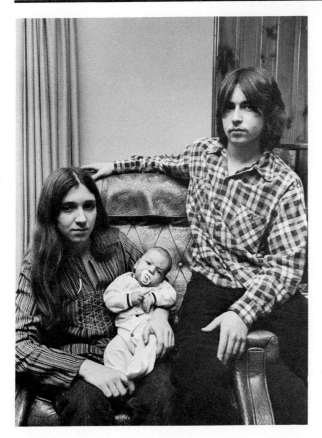

Because many adolescents either use ineffective contraceptives or none at all, teenage pregnancy rates continue to increase. (© Sepp Sertz 1978/Woodfin Camp & Assoc.)

ceptives and for not using them. A young woman who carries a diaphragm in her purse or takes birth control pills every day is admitting that her sexual behavior is intentional.

Since planned contraception requires assuming personal and sexual responsibility, it's not surprising that women who use effective contraception differ from those who use ineffective methods—or none at all. Interviews with adolescent women between the ages of fourteen and eighteen at a family planning clinic found several striking differences between the two groups (Spain, 1980). Those who used contraceptives effectively planned for the future and understood that their actions in the present had consequences in the years ahead. They also felt in control of their own lives. Teenagers who used contraceptives ineffectively either never thought about the future or had unrealistic goals for themselves.

Feelings about sex also played a role. Women in the group who were comfortable with their sexuality and who were able to deal with any guilt or discomfort they felt tended to be effective contraceptive users. But women who continued sexual activity despite continued guilt or ambivalence tended to use contraceptives carelessly or sporadically.

A relationship between guilt and contraceptive methods also appeared among a group of college women (Keller and Sack, 1982). Those who showed a high degree of guilt over sex tended to rely on withdrawal or rhythm—or else used no contraceptives at all. Those who accepted their own sexuality used the pill, an IUD, or a diaphragm—or else insisted that their partner use a condom.

Some young women who use no contraceptives at all believe that they destroy the pleasure of sexuality or reduce the romantic atmosphere. And some are simply opposed to contraception on moral grounds (Zelnick, Kantner, and Ford, 1981).

We've stressed the young woman's role in contraception because, by and large, it is the woman who suffers the consequences of premarital pregnancies. However, the relationship between sexual partners can also play a major role in contraceptive choice. Even in a close, romantic relationship, communication about contraception may be difficult or embarrassing. If the young man refuses to use a condom, the woman may not feel able to assert her own contraceptive needs. Sometimes a man might assume that since his partner has no objections to intercourse, she must be using the pill or an IUD. Such miscommunication is probably most typical of young, sexually inexperienced men and women, but it can also occur when older adults have sexual contact with an unfamiliar partner.

## *The young adult*

During young adulthood, a woman's contraceptive concerns often change substantially. As the single woman becomes more confident and self-assured about her sexual and social life style, she finds that obtaining contraceptives is much simpler than it was during adolescence.

Although some women delay childbearing until their thirties or decide not to have any children at all, the majority of women complete their families while in their twenties. The ideal family size is usually reported as two children. Couples use contraceptives in attaining this ideal, both to limit the number of children and to space them so that one birth does not quickly follow another. Within this group, contraceptive failure takes the form of too many children or too short a time between births.

About 70 percent of young married women practice some form of birth control, and the first birth occurs an average of twenty-seven months after marriage (Rindfuss and Westoff, 1974). Two factors seem to play a role in the births of subsequent children: effective contraceptives and frequency of intercourse. There has been a trend toward the use of the pill, IUD, and vasectomy, and a decrease in the use of such unreliable methods as withdrawal. In addition, couples who want to end childbearing tend to have intercourse less frequently than couples who are simply delaying the birth of their next child (Westoff, 1974).

Despite the growing use of effective contraception, one-third of the births to married women in 1978 were unplanned pregnancies (Dryfoos, 1982). However, most of the contraceptive failures occurred among women using less effective methods. Although 64 percent of couples used the pill, IUD, or sterilization, they had only 16 percent of the unwanted pregnancies.

Large-scale studies have found a clear relationship between a couple's choice of contraceptive and frequency of intercourse. Couples using the pill, IUD, vasectomy, or diaphragm tend to have intercourse more often than do couples who use less reliable means of birth control, such as withdrawal or foam (Westoff, 1974). Although these data show a relationship between effective contraception and sexual activity, there's no way to tell whether the availability of effective contraceptives leads to a more active sex life, or whether sexually active women tend to select more effective contraceptives. Perhaps both factors are at work.

## The older adult

Most women have completed their families by the time they reach their mid-thirties. Since menopause usually takes place at about the age of fifty, this leaves a woman fifteen fertile years during which she wants no more children. The contraceptive task of the older adult becomes bridging this time span without becoming pregnant.

Increasingly, the solution has involved surgical sterilization. When a couple's family is complete, sterilization removes the need for all future contraceptive decisions or actions.

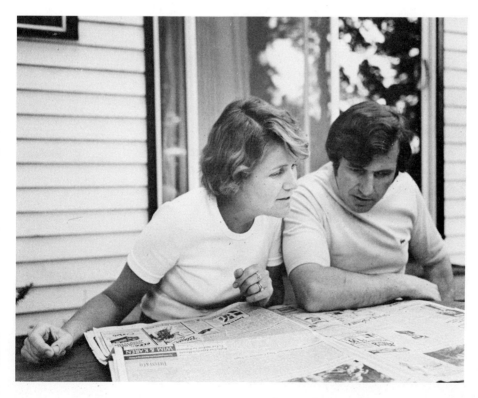

After couples have completed their families, the need for contraception continues. Among couples in their late thirties and forties, surgical sterilization has become increasingly popular. (© Richard Kalvar/ Magnum Photo)

Among older couples who do not choose sterilization, several factors tend to reduce fertility. Older women are usually less fertile than women in their twenties and are also more likely to have a spontaneous abortion. In addition, the frequency of sexual relations usually declines among older couples. Finally, the older woman has probably had many years of experience with contraceptives, knows how to use them, and has easy access to family planning resources (McCormick et al., 1977).

## Contraceptive fit

Since contraceptive needs and behavior change considerably with age, successful methods of contraception will suit these changes over the life span. When there is a poor fit between the individual's needs and a chosen contraceptive, it may be discarded—perhaps leaving the person with no protection from pregnancy. The concept of "contraceptive fit" may help to explain the prevalence of unwanted and unplanned pregnancies. When women fail in contraceptive use, it may be that they have selected—or been given—a method of birth control that does not suit their needs.

Every contraceptive technique has both advantages and disadvantages. Although the pill offers virtually complete protection, it is often associated with unpleasant side effects. Since the risks are lower for young women—especially for nonsmokers—those who do not suffer from side effects may find the pill a very acceptable means of birth control. The pill's particular advantage for the young is its independence from coitus, so the young woman who is not skilled at asserting her contraceptive needs is relieved of that burden at the time of intercourse. Yet the pill may not fit well with the needs of the older woman, who is at greater risk of side effects and may be more adept at suggesting such techniques as the diaphragm.

A contraceptive that fits a woman's life style is simply that contraceptive she is most likely to use both correctly and consistently. Women who dislike touching their own genitals probably will not do well with a diaphragm. Women who are disturbed by a heavy menstrual flow will probably dislike an IUD. A man who believes that condoms interfere with his sexual pleasure will probably object to using them. The married woman who uses contraceptives to delay pregnancy is likely to tolerate a method that carries a small risk of pregnancy, but a woman whose health or age prohibits further childbearing needs a method that guarantees complete protection.

A contraceptive that fits well into one phase of life may be unacceptable at another phase. And even the most effective contraceptive will not work if it does not match the individual's needs and preferences.

# Summary

**1** Effective, widespread, and socially approved **contraception**, or the intentional prevention of conception, is a relatively recent development. Because contraceptives sometimes fail, **sterilization** (the use of medical techniques to make a person incapable of conceiving a child) and **induced abortion** (the intentional termination of pregnancy) have also been used to prevent births.

**2** A society's attitude toward contraception is linked with population levels, and contraception has been encouraged as concern about overpopulation has grown. Contraceptives were once illegal; the work of people like Margaret Sanger, urbanization, industrialization, and the changing role of women have combined to make contraceptives freely available.

**3** The ideal contraceptive is effective, has no negative effects on users, is easily reversible, and fits their personal and sexual needs. The **pill**, which controls fertility with synthetic hormones, provides the most effective reversible contraception. Some women who take the pill for long periods experience the **oversuppression syndrome**, and the menstrual cycle does not return as soon as they stop taking the pill. The pill can have both pleasant and unpleasant side effects, but it may cause dangerous complications in some women, especially older women who smoke. The **intrauterine device (IUD)**, a small piece of plastic or metal that is inserted in the uterus, appears to keep the fertilized egg from implanting itself in the uterine wall. IUDs are highly effective; however, they may have unpleasant side effects or serious complications, such as pelvic inflammatory disease, ectopic pregnancy, or perforation of the uterus.

**4** The **diaphragm**, a dome-shaped rubber cap that holds a spermicide over the cervix, must be individually fitted. It has almost no side effects, but requires a highly motivated couple for greatest success. The **cervical cap**, which fits snugly over the tip of the uterus, is available in the United States on an "investigational" basis. Although it seems quite effective, it is more difficult to use than the diaphragm, and some women complain of odor. Condoms are extremely effective, especially if the female partner uses a **spermicide**. Spermicides and condoms require no prescription, but tend to interfere with sexual spontaneity. Among spermicides, foam and sponges are the most effective. They are easily available, decreasing the likelihood of vaginal infection and some STDs, but not as effective as medical methods.

**5** **Rhythm**, which requires abstinence during a woman's fertile period, has three major forms: The calendar method, the temperature method, and the cervical mucus method. To be successful, the rhythm method requires a woman to pay close attention to her bodily changes, to have self-control, and to have an understanding sex partner. **Withdrawal**, or coitus interruptus, is extremely unreliable and not recommended.

**6** Sterilization is a completely effective method of birth control, suitable for people who are sure they want no more children. It is virtually irreversible. **Vasectomy**, the sterilization procedure for men, involves cutting or blocking the vas deferens. It is both safe and reliable. **Tubal ligation**, in which the Fallopian tubes are cut and tied or cauterized, is the preferred technique for female sterilization. Laparoscopic sterilization, which can be performed in a physician's office, is a simple operation that leaves no disfiguring scars.

**7** Abortion is controversial because it disrupts fertilization after the developing egg is implanted in the uterine wall. Early in pregnancy, physicians can perform safe, quick abortions with one of the methods that use suction to remove the uterine lining. After the sixteenth week of pregnancy, abortion becomes a more risky procedure. Labor must be induced, using a **saline** solution or **prostaglandins**. Abortion is a highly emotional experience, and a woman's response depends on the length of time she has been pregnant, the surroundings in which the abortion takes place, and such personal factors as family support and the woman's own views on abortion.

**8** Although more adolescents are using contraceptives, informational or emotional barriers may keep them from using contraceptives correctly or consistently. Adolescent women who use contraceptives effectively tend to plan for the future, feel in control of their own lives, and be comfortable with their sexuality. Among younger women, the contraceptive concern is often limiting family size and spacing children. Among older women, the concern is usually to prevent pregnancy completely. A contraceptive fit exists when a contraceptive meets a person's life style and needs. For most people, contraceptive concerns will change over the life span, and the successful method of contraception will change as well.

## a mother's view.

Despite the childbirth classes and the books and the exercises, I was apprehensive when I went into the hospital. But afterward I felt so good I wanted to shout. I felt triumphant—and so sorry for men because they could never have the experience of giving birth. (Authors' files)

## a father's view

I remember when I first became a father, I was standing on a street corner, experiencing the most remarkable feeling I ever knew, as if I were being blown up like a balloon and expanded in all directions. From then on I think I had moved in a new world. I did not just go downtown anymore, but when I went to work I went bouncing, knowing that I had left part of me sitting back there at home. (C. Romalis, 1981, p. 106)

# 20 Pregnancy and Childbirth

*Chapter* 20

In each normal pregnancy, two tiny cells unite deep within a woman's body and thirty-eight weeks later a new human being emerges, ready for independent life. The miracle of birth can reduce a bystander to awestruck silence and is often a profound emotional experience for both parents.

Birth takes place within a social context, and the attitudes of society have a powerful influence on most people's decisions to reproduce and their feelings about the experience. Societies can encourage or discourage reproduction; they can make the experience of childbirth a fearful or a natural—even joyous—occasion.

Whether or not pregnancy is inevitable can also affect attitudes toward the process. Safe, inexpensive ways to eliminate the reproductive consequences of sexual activity have revolutionized attitudes, behavior, and the course of people's lives. For the first time in human history, childbirth is truly a choice. As a result, for most people most of the time and for some people all of the time, pregnancy and childbirth are separated from sexuality. Yet at least once in the lives of most people, pregnancy and the birth of a child become a matter of hope, happiness, concern, or despair. Few joys exceed the birth of a wanted child, and few sorrows are deeper than the inability to conceive such a child (Menning, 1980).

In this chapter, we begin our exploration of pregnancy and childbirth with the mechanics of conception. After following the course of pregnancy, we examine methods of childbirth and the period just after birth. Since pregnancies don't always progress smoothly, we'll investigate some of the possible complications. Finally, we take up the problem of infertility from both the male and female perspectives and suggest some solutions.

# Pregnancy and Childbirth

## CONCEPTION

Considering all the obstacles that stand in their way, it's a wonder that an ovum and a sperm ever manage to meet. By tracing their journey toward each other, we can see how the deck is stacked against conception.

The single ovum released at ovulation is about 50,000 times larger than the sperm. The mature ovum contains genetic material and a mass of nutrient substances surrounded by a gelatinous capsule. The egg's journey along the Fallopian tube to the uterus usually takes between three and five days, but it can probably be fertilized during only eight hours of that journey. Since the egg is released into the abdominal cavity, as we saw in Chapter 3, its first task is to get into the tube. Once within the tube, it begins the passage toward the uterus.

A single ejaculation may contain as many as 400 million sperm, but only a few will ever reach the ovum while it can still be fertilized. Millions of sperm are lost if the woman changes her position after intercourse and spills ejaculate out of the vagina. Millions more are killed by the acid environment of the uterus or lost in the folds of its surfaces.

Sperm swim toward the uterus by lashing their tails. Once they reach the cervix, they face a formidable barrier. Most of the time the cervical mucus is opaque and thick, arranged in a dense net that sperm cannot pierce. Just before ovulation, the mucus becomes thin and transparent, and its structure changes so that sperm can pass through. Within forty-eight hours, the mucous barrier will again become impenetrable (Silver, 1980).

Even if the mucus is open, less than 200,000 of those 400 million sperm deposited in the vagina will ever make their way into the uterus. Sperm that do not penetrate the cervical mucus within half an hour of ejaculation are too weak to get through at all. Those that do get into the uterus have forty-eight hours to reach the egg; after that time, they are no longer capable of fertilization. Some of the successful sperm become lost in the uterus, and half of those that continue the trip travel up the "wrong" Fallopian tube. Sperm that get into the tube must swim upstream against the strong current created by the tiny hairs within the tube that move the egg toward the uterus. Among the sperm still in the race, many get lost within the tube or miss the egg by as little as a millionth of an inch.

A few sperm do make it to the outer surface of the egg, where they face a final set of barriers. The genetic material in the egg is protected by several walls, and sperm cannot get through them without resorting to chemical aids. Enzymes released from the head of the sperm dissolve the first barrier, then cut a slit in the inner barrier just large enough for a single sperm to get through (Silber, 1980). Once this happens, the outer layer of the egg hardens so that other sperm cannot enter. The tail of the sperm drops off, and its twenty-three chromosomes combine with the twenty-three chromosomes in the egg to form the first cell of a new human being.

**zygote** a fertilized ovum, formed by the union of two cells

During the next few days, the fertilized egg, now called a **zygote**, divides into two cells, then four, then eight, and so on (Figure 20.1). At this phase, it is passed from the Fallopian tube into the uterus, where it floats freely for another four or five days. Then, about a week after conception, the egg becomes implanted in the uterine wall. If the egg's passage through the tube has been too fast, it will enter the uterus too soon and will die before it is ready to implant itself. Once successfully implanted, however, the egg develops rapidly.

Some of the obstacles to fertilization can be lessened by couples who are trying to conceive a child. According to Sherman Silber (1980), attention to position, timing, and frequency of intercourse can increase the chances of conception. If the traditional missionary position is used and the woman remains on her back for half an hour (preferably with her hips raised), the sperm's chances of entering the cervix multiply.

More frequent sexual activity is usually helpful. A man who has intercourse infrequently—say, once a month—will deposit more sperm with each ejaculation, but a high percentage of them will be too old to fertilize an egg. Unless a man's sperm count is low, a good rule is the more sex, the better. Fertile couples who have intercourse less than once a week have a 16 percent chance of conceiving within six months. Intercourse once a week improves the chances to 32 percent, but intercourse four times a week ups the chances to 80 percent. However, it may be possible to have sex too frequently: ejaculating once a day or more can lead to a decrease in sperm count.

Finally, although a rise in the woman's temperature indicates ovulation, the process has already occurred when her temperature goes up. Once the couple have charted a few cycles, they probably should stop worrying about hitting the woman's brief fertile period exactly. This kind of anxiety sometimes causes a woman to stop ovulating altogether, destroying any chance of conception.

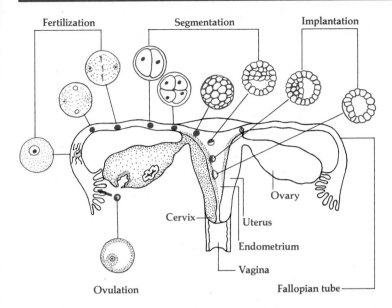

Fertilization  Segmentation  Implantation

Ovary

Cervix  Uterus

Endometrium

Vagina

Ovulation  Fallopian tube

**Figure 20.1**

Schematic Representation of the Passage of the Egg from Ovulation (1)
to Implantation (10).
Note that the size of the ovum and the blastosphere have been
exaggerated for the purpose of illustration.

## PREGNANCY

During the thirty-eight weeks of pregnancy, what was once a single fertilized cell
develops into a baby. This process has far-reaching effects on the mother's body,
which must provide the growing organism with nourishment and remove its
wastes. In addition, her hormone levels alter sharply in order to maintain the pregnancy. But pregnancy is not simply a biological event; its psychological effects can
be equally profound. Within her body the mother carries another being, and from
the moment of her awareness a close relationship begins to form. The birth will
make enormous changes in her life and in the life of her sexual partner. They will
have to shift their roles, living patterns, and needs in order to accommodate a child
(Grossman, Eichler, and Winickoff, 1980).

The thirty-eight weeks of pregnancy (or forty weeks from the time of the
mother's last menstrual period) are commonly divided into three periods, or **trimesters**, each lasting three calendar months. By the time a woman is certain she is
pregnant she may be well along into the first trimester.

### Signs of pregnancy

Anyone who has ever missed a menstrual period knows it is an emotional event. A
sexually active woman and her partner invariably react with emotion—with excite-

ment or joy if they are trying to conceive, with apprehension or fear if they are trying not to conceive.

Although the missing period is usually the first sign of pregnancy, it is not an infallible guide. Menstrual periods can be delayed or skipped for other reasons—emotional stress, illness, a radical change in diet or climate. As we saw in Chapter 3, women joggers sometimes menstruate erratically. Yet bleeding does not always signal the absence of pregnancy. Some women have short, scanty periods when they are pregnant.

Since the missing period may be due to other causes, a woman can end the suspense by having a pregnancy test. The most commonly used tests check the urine for the presence of human chorionic gonadotropin (HCG), a hormone secreted only by pregnant women. Chemicals are added to a sample of urine, and if the woman is at least two weeks pregnant, the HCG in her urine prevents the liquid from coagulating. If she is not pregnant, the urine thickens within a few minutes. A more expensive blood test can detect an HCG-like substance as early as four to six

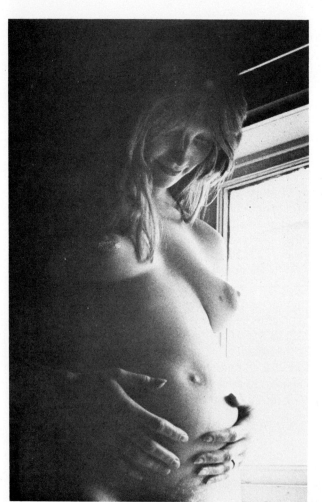

By the time a woman has reached the third trimester of pregnancy, her condition is obvious to the world and her attention is often absorbed by the growing fetus within her. (© Joel Gordon 1980)

days after conception, even before the fertilized egg has become implanted in the uterus.

It is possible to perform a urine test for HCG at home. Test kits available at any drugstore can detect the hormone about two weeks after a missed period—or four weeks after conception. A woman takes a sample of her urine when she first gets up in the morning, puts a few drops into a test tube containing chemicals, adds a little water, shakes it up, and forgets it for a few hours. If she is pregnant, the HCG will cause a dark-brown, doughnut-shaped ring to form in the bottom of the tube.

All these tests are highly accurate, but they are not perfect. They occasionally indicate that a woman is not pregnant when she is indeed carrying a zygote. For that reason, a woman with a negative test who does not begin to menstruate within a week or so should repeat the test. If the test is still negative she should see a physician immediately, because an ectopic pregnancy, in which the zygote embeds itself into the wall of the Fallopian tube, will produce a negative test.

If a woman is willing to be patient, the HCG test is not necessary. She can wait until she thinks she is about eight weeks pregnant and then consult a physician, for by that time a manual examination will confirm a pregnancy. As hormone levels increase during early pregnancy, the uterus and cervix begin to soften. By eight weeks, the cervix, when prodded, no longer feels much like the tip of a nose; instead it feels more like a chin. In addition, the color of the vagina and cervix may have changed from their normal pink to a bluish shade, the result of blood congestion in the pelvic area.

## *The first trimester*

During the first trimester, most women experience some or all the signs of early pregnancy. The breasts may swell and become tender, and the nipples and aerolae may enlarge and darken in color. Some women are nauseated and may vomit, but not all women become sick. In one study, about two-thirds of the women said they had been nauseated, but less than half of them ever vomited (Newton and Modahl, 1978). Most women find that they need to urinate frequently, or that they are often tired. Many women are excessively sleepy and complain that they could sleep all day.

**trimester** a period of approximately three months, often used when discussing pregnancy

As old wives' tales remind us, pregnant women often crave unusual foods, although the craving is rarely severe. No one is certain whether the urge for strawberries in winter, ice cream, pickles, or even cornstarch reflects dietary deficiencies, anxiety, or cultural expectations (Newton and Modahl, 1978).

A woman's personal feelings about her pregnancy are important. The positive emotions of feeling special, fertile, and womanly, excited and impatient are common. Negative emotions, such as fear, exhaustion, worry about the health of the child, and concern about the ability to cope with motherhood are also natural. Most women who are healthy and comfortable with their lives adapt fairly easily to pregnancy and feel good about the experience. However, women who are accustomed to severe bouts of premenstrual tension often have trouble adapting (Grossman, Eichler, and Winickoff, 1980).

Another factor in the experience of pregnancy is the reaction of those around the woman. The response of a male partner to the pregnancy can be vital. To some

*Focus*

PRENATAL
HEALTH
CARE

**fetal alcohol syndrome** a condition affecting many babies born to alcoholic mothers, marked by small size at birth, conical head, and physical defects or mental retardation

Most prenatal health care is a matter of following the usual health rules. A nutritious diet is essential. Proteins, vitamins, and minerals are needed to build the body of the fetus, and a woman's energy requirements increase about 300 calories a day. Because protein requirements also increase, the addition of three cups of skim milk a day, or cottage cheese, yogurt, lean meat, fish, or chicken are good places to pick up the extra calories.

Today physicians feel that the average woman should gain at least twenty-five pounds during a pregnancy. That may seem like too much weight, but it has places to go. When the weight of fetus, amniotic fluid, placenta, uterus, breast expansion, added maternal blood, and fluid are added up, the total comes to more than twenty pounds (Newton and Modahl, 1978). Extra vitamins as insurance are a good idea, and some authorities urge pregnant women to take additional iron and folic acid.

As for taking anything else into the body, the best advice is *don't*. Don't smoke, don't drink, don't take drugs—either recreational or over-the-counter preparations. Many such substances, as well as some antibiotics and other prescription drugs, have been connected with birth complications, extra-small babies, high rates of miscarriage or stillbirths, or fetal malformations. For example, babies born to alcoholic mothers often have **fetal alcohol syndrome.** They are extra-small, they may have an odd, conical-shaped head, and they may be mentally retarded. Some babies with fetal alcohol syndrome have cleft palates, heart murmurs, hernias, damaged kidneys, and eye or skeletal defects (Streissguth et al., 1980).

The roll call of substances that can harm the fetus is a long one and seems to grow almost daily. One obstetrician (Schulman, 1982) has suggested that a pregnant woman ask her doctor four questions before taking any medication: Is this medication necessary? Does taking the medication endanger my baby? What risks might I face if I do *not* take this medication? Is the medication in question the best one for a pregnant woman to take? Table 20.1 indicates what substances are relatively safe to take for the discomforts of pregnancy and which should be avoided.

Exercise is important, and walking or swimming is probably the best way to get it. In most cases, exercises a woman customarily does can be continued as long as they are comfortable, but pregnancy is not the time to take up a new sport. In fact, some authorities (Holt and Weber, 1981) recommend that joggers switch to walking, cycling, or swimming because of the strain jogging places on abdominal muscles, hips, knees, and ankles.

## Table 20.1   *Medication in pregnancy*

| COMMON DISCOMFORTS | REMEDIES | DRUGS TO AVOID | ACCEPTABLE ALTERNATIVES |
|---|---|---|---|
| Morning sickness (nausea) | Eat a few dry crackers before arising and frequent, small, low-fat meals during the day. Drink liquids between meals. | Antinausea drugs, such as cyclizine, meclizine (Antivert), trimethobenzamide. | *Avoid all medication during first trimester except that prescribed by a physician for a specific condition.* |
| Fatigue | Exercise regularly. Get plenty of sleep, with frequent naps during the day. | Stimulants, such as amphetamines, excessive caffeine. | |
| Sleeplessness | A glass of warm milk before bedtime. | Tranquilizers, narcotics, barbiturates, antihistamines, alcohol. | *Avoid X rays.* |
| Faintness or dizziness | Sit with feet up when possible; rise slowly and with support. | Tranquilizers, alcohol. | Smelling salts, aromatic spirit of ammonia. |
| Skin changes | | Antibiotics: tetracycline. | If nipples or abdomen itch, use a lanolin-based cream or baby oil. |
| Headaches | Change body position slowly; rest with damp cloth on forehead; drink milk and/ or eat a small snack. | Analgesics: aspirin, phenacetin/caffeine, Darvon, Indocin; tranquilizers. | Acetaminophen (Tylenol). |
| Leg and muscle cramps | Exercise regularly. Elevate legs and flex toes while resting. Increase milk consumption. | Aspirin, tranquilizers. | Calcium supplements with little or no phosphorus. |
| Heartburn | Drink milk between small, frequent meals. | Antacids: calcium carbonate, Gaviscon; sodium bicarbonate, Tagamet. | Antacids: Maalox, Mylanta. |
| Swollen ankles | Elevate legs for an hour or so each day. Sleep on left side. | Most diuretics. | |
| Constipation | Eat foods containing roughage. Drink liquids. Exercise often. | Laxatives: mineral oil, castor oil. | Laxatives: Metamucil, Senokot, milk of magnesia. |
| Backaches | Back exercises to strengthen muscles. Wear low-heeled shoes or flats. Avoid heavy lifting. | Analgesics: aspirin, Darvon, phenacetin/caffeine, codeine. | Acetaminophen (Tylenol). |

*Source:* H. Schulman, "Common Discomforts of Pregnancy," *Childbirth Educator* 1 (Spring 1982): 11–12.

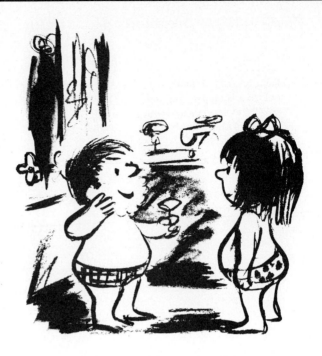

*"Let's play pregnant. I'll shave and you'll throw up."*

**placenta** a pliable
structure of tissue and
blood vessels that
transmits nourishment
and wastes between
mother and fetus

**fetus** the developing
organism from eight
weeks after conception
to birth

women, pregnancy is a time of vulnerability, when male support is necessary. However, men are susceptible to the same anxieties as women and are not always able to meet the emotional needs of the mother-to-be.

While the mother is adapting to pregnancy, rapid physical development is taking place within her. Before she has missed a menstrual period, the zygote has implanted itself in the uterine wall, where a tiny network of roots anchors it securely. This network grows into the **placenta**, a flexible structure of tissue and blood vessels that transmits nourishment and wastes.

By four weeks (two weeks after the missed period), there is already a rudimentary brain, heart, kidney, liver, and digestive tract. At seven weeks gonads appear, but they have not yet differentiated into testes or ovaries. By the eighth week the developing zygote, now known as a **fetus**, is almost an inch long. It floats in a sac filled with amniotic fluid, which protects it from the outside world. The umbilical cord, which connects the abdomen of the fetus to the placenta, has developed.

As the first trimester ends, the fetus is about four inches long and is clearly male or female. The tiny brain is beginning to coordinate the action of other organs, but it will be several months before the organs are truly functional (Pritchard and McDonald, 1976).

Because a developing organ is most vulnerable to harmful influences, drugs, disease, environmental chemicals, or radiation are most likely to affect the fetus during the first trimester. The mother's health is important all during pregnancy, but special care is essential during the early weeks.

## The second trimester

During the second trimester many women first feel truly pregnant, for it is now that they can detect the fetus moving within them, a sensation called "quickening." This perception often causes whatever doubts a woman has about her potential mother-hood to disappear. A woman who has firmly rejected the idea of becoming a moth-er may now embrace it.

Quickening is felt by the mother-to-be; her changing appearance toward the end of the second trimester is obvious to the world. Some women enjoy the visible signs of pregnancy; others, adhering to the social standard that "slim is beautiful," may try to hide their condition as long as possible.

A woman's breasts may become fuller and heavier, and begin to secrete a yel-lowish substance called colostrum. The skin around the nipples may deepen in col-or, as may the line between the navel and the pubic hair, and the skin on the face. This faint skin pigmentation usually disappears from the face after delivery, but tends to remain around the nipples.

Physically, most women feel well during the second trimester. Their nausea has vanished, they no longer feel tired and sleepy, and the need to urinate fre-quently has disappeared. As one woman described this period:

Development within the uterus progresses rapidly; at just over five weeks, the zygote (A) has rudimentary internal organs but no gonads. By the beginning of the eighth week, the fetus (B) is about an inch long, has asexual gonads, and an umbilical cord. When the first trimester ends (C), the fetus is four inches long and clearly male or female. (© Landrum B. Shettles)

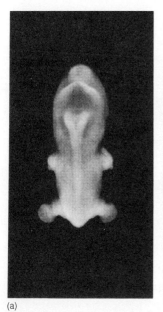
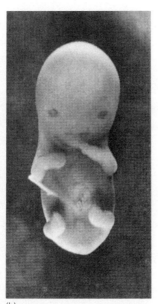
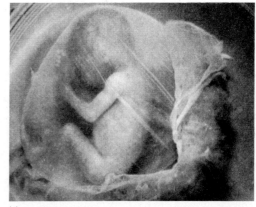

(a)          (b)          (c)

I felt on top of the world. I was full of energy and almost euphoric. I seemed capable of doing almost anything. (Author's files)

Not all women respond this way. Some play the "sick role," a role that exempts them from normal responsibilities and a sense of personal responsibility for their "illness" (Laws and Schwartz, 1977). Women who treat pregnancy as an illness tend to be surrounded by people who regard the pregnant woman as "not normal" or "unusual." Physicians may unwittingly pressure the pregnant woman into acting as though she had a medical condition. Some pregnant women learn to play a sick role even though the physical changes of pregnancy rarely require it.

During the second trimester, fetal development continues. Arms and legs develop, and the face now looks human. By the end of the second trimester, the fetus can open and close its eyes. It sleeps, wakes, and tends to nap in the same general posture. It now weighs about a pound and a half. A few infants born toward the end of the second trimester have survived, but only with intensive care, including intravenous feeding and oxygen.

## The third trimester

During the last trimester, a woman's size and weight may restrict her movements and activity. She certainly feels clumsy, and if she lives in a society that encourages strict birth control, the unmistakable bulge of her uterus may make her feel out of place (Newton and Modahl, 1978).

Physical symptoms often return during this period. Indigestion, heartburn, and constipation are common, as are swollen hands, feet, and face caused by the body's retention of water. The large uterus may exert pressure on other pelvic organs, and it may tighten in what are called "Braxton-Hicks" contractions, which may strengthen uterine muscles. A woman's back may ache, and feelings of tiredness return. Sharp kicks and punches from the fetus, especially in the middle of the night, may be uncomfortable or annoying.

As delivery draws near, the nine months of waiting can seem endless. Most women want to have the whole thing over and wish that **labor**, or the birth process, would start. At the same time, however, they may become somewhat anxious about the delivery process or the health of the baby.

**labor** the birth process, from the first contractions until the placenta emerges

During the last trimester, the fetus responds to loud noises outside the mother's body. Within the uterus it hears the whooshing of its mother's heart and the rumbling of gas in her intestines (Newton and Modahl, 1978). All through this period, the fetus is putting on weight. By the close of pregnancy it probably weighs about seven pounds, although a full-term baby can range from less than five pounds to more than twelve.

## Sex during pregnancy

Human attitudes and rules concerning sexual activity during pregnancy vary widely in tribal cultures around the world. Members of the African Masai tribe demand abstinence as soon as a woman misses one or two menstrual periods. Women of the Crow Indian tribe are expected to give up coitus as soon as the fetus quickens. Other tribes permit intercourse almost until time of delivery or as long as the woman can comfortably participate. In most tribes the limits are placed only on women, and a culture often provides some other sexual outlet for their partners (Ford and Beach, 1951). In cultures that prohibit intercourse, it is usually feared that coitus will in some way harm the unborn child.

American physicians often warn against intercourse during the last six or eight weeks of pregnancy, but definite harm to the fetus has never been established. These prohibitions are usually based on fears that intense uterine contractions accompanying orgasm may prematurely start labor, that membranes may rupture, or that bacteria in the semen may harm the fetus.

Whether orgasm does trigger the delivery process is uncertain. Some studies show more frequent orgasms late in pregnancy among women who have premature births, but other studies show no such relationship. For example, among one group of women, whether or not they abstained from sex or continued to have orgasms throughout pregnancy, the prematurity rate was the same: about 6 percent (Solberg et al., 1978). Researchers have also been unable to find any difference in the rate of premature rupture of the membranes or infant death between women who have intercourse in the last month of pregnancy and those who abstain (Mills, Harlap, and Harley, 1981). It seems likely that the vast majority of women can have sexual activity with no danger to the fetus. But if coitus or orgasm is followed by pain or bleeding, it may be wise to avoid sexual contact.

Another concern among researchers is that sexual activity during pregnancy causes amniotic fluid infections. Such infections account for about 17 percent of fetal and newborn deaths, usually because the infection leads to premature deliv-

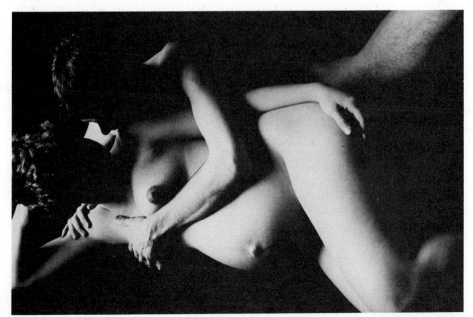

As pregnancy progresses, rear-entry or side-by-side positions are generally the most comfortable and they allow couples to continue intercourse until delivery if they wish. (© Flip & Debra Schulke)

ery. In an analysis of more than 26,000 pregnancies, one researcher (Naeye, 1979) discovered that coitus increased both the frequency and severity of amniotic fluid infections. What's more, coitus during the second trimester was more strongly associated with infection than coitus in the third trimester. However, these cases were all pregnancies that occurred between 1959 and 1966, when the risk of mortality from such infections was greater than it is today. So this study remains controversial, and we have no final word on the hazards of intercourse during pregnancy.

Couples who are concerned about amniotic infections can switch to other forms of sexual activity. In any case, as pregnancy progresses, couples may find the man-above position uncomfortable. The rear-entry and side-by-side positions are likely to be more satisfactory and to allow couples to continue intercourse until delivery, if they wish.

Whether intercourse is "permitted" or not, women show a wide range of sexual response during pregnancy (White and Reamy, 1982). They may show a decrease in interest during the first trimester or no change at all; during the second trimester, sexual interest and activity may increase or decrease. During the last trimester, most women report a decrease in interest, and many give up sexual activity.

A few pregnant women were taken into the laboratory and their sexual response measured all during pregnancy (Masters and Johnson, 1966). Among these women, vaginal lubrication and vasocongestion intensified as pregnancy progressed. Perhaps increased blood flow to the pelvic area accounts for the strong sexual interest, multiple orgasms during the second trimester, and awareness of sexual tension reported by these women. By the third trimester, the vagina was so engorged with blood during arousal that its orgasmic contractions were barely observable. Yet the women said they could feel them. Orgasm during this third trimester produced intense uterine response, sometimes lasting thirty minutes.

Not all women report this pattern of increased sexual tension. Among a large group of American women, there was a steady decrease in frequency of intercourse during pregnancy. Only 5 percent of the women abstained during the first two trimesters. During the third trimester more and more couples gave up sexual activity, until in the ninth month 60 percent were abstaining. Individual differences in response were clear. Many women reported that orgasm was less intense during the third trimester or that they were less likely to reach orgasm. Others reported a steady increase in the intensity of their orgasms all during pregnancy (Solberg et al., 1978).

Women give various reasons for abstaining from sexual activity during pregnancy: physical discomfort, fear of harming the baby, a loss of sexual interest, and a physician's advice. No matter what their reason, many women tend to feel confused, anxious, or guilty about sexual activity. The feelings of a woman's sexual partner may also vary; he may fear harming the fetus, believe that sex during pregnancy is "immoral," find himself turned off by his partner's visible pregnancy, or respond to it with an increase in sexual desire (White and Reamy, 1982). However, few physicians discuss sex with pregnant women unless it is to establish an arbitrary period of abstention. Since such apparently unnecessary restrictions can place the marital relationship under severe stress, an individual approach that considers each woman's physical condition would seem preferable.

# CHILDBIRTH

The last trimester ends and a child is born. The exact changes that begin labor are not known, but a variety of hormones secreted by mother and fetus appear to be involved. Any of several signs can indicate the beginning of labor.

The clearest sign is strong and regular uterine contractions. However, in some women other indications precede contractions of the uterus. One such sign is the "bloody show"—the expulsion of the mucus plug that has sealed the cervix during pregnancy, accompanied by a small amount of bleeding. Another sign is rupture of the amniotic membrane, so that the fluid surrounding the fetus leaks from the vagina. Some women have diarrhea for a few days preceding delivery, perhaps nature's way of emptying the bowels to provide more room for passage of the fetus through the birth canal (the term applied to the vagina during delivery).

During the last month of pregnancy, the fetal head usually drops down into the pelvis. Although most babies are born in this head-down position, some try to emerge in a way that complicates birth. A few babies are in the breech position, lying so that the buttocks emerge first. Less common is the transverse position, in which the fetus lies crosswise and an arm or leg enters the birth canal first. When a fetus is in a difficult position, a physician may try to rotate it before it can leave the uterus. If this attempt fails, a Caesarean section is usually performed, and the baby is removed surgically through the wall of the abdomen.

The duration of labor varies greatly from one woman to another and often for the same woman in different pregnancies. A woman having her first child can expect to labor between twelve and fourteen hours, on the average. For a second or subsequent child, the average labor lasts about seven hours. In rare cases, birth can occur in a matter of minutes or take as long as thirty hours. With very short labors, the mother's tissues may not have stretched enough to allow passage of the baby, and the physician sometimes tries to slow the process. Long labors can also be risky because of the great physical stress they place on mother and child. If labor seems unduly prolonged, the physician may intervene surgically.

## *The stages of labor*

Labor is usually divided into three stages. During the first, and longest, stage, the cervix, which has remained tightly closed throughout pregnancy, opens to accommodate the baby's head. During the second stage, the baby passes down the birth canal and is born. During the final stage, the placenta is expelled.

The dilation of the cervix in the first stage is caused by muscular contractions of the uterus. These contractions start from the top of the uterus and move downward toward the cervix, causing it to open up. Each wavelike contraction starts slowly, builds to a peak, and then slowly declines.

As first-stage labor begins, contractions are usually between ten and twenty minutes apart, with each contraction lasting about thirty seconds. At first the contractions are often faint, and only their rhythmic nature tells some women that labor has begun. Although they get stronger, they are not too uncomfortable, and the woman has time between them to rest and relax. In fact, the more relaxed a woman is, the more quickly this phase passes.

However, if a woman lies flat in bed during this period, the contractions are likely to be less efficient and more painful. Studies (Roberts, 1982) have shown that women who are encouraged to walk during the first stage have shorter labors and need less medication than women who lie down.

Now first-stage labor enters its active phase; contractions become even stronger and are close together. Discomfort increases, and in a short time the woman passes out of this phase into the most difficult part of childbirth. The cervix reaches full dilation in about a dozen enormously powerful contractions, with only a minute's pause between them. Women may report nausea, intense irritability, trembling, or chills.

Up to this point, the mother's role has been to relax as much as possible. Once she enters the second stage of labor, she can take an active role in pushing the baby out. At the beginning of this stage, the baby's head begins to move from the uterus down into the birth canal (see Figure 20.2). It moves forward with each contraction, then slides back slightly between contractions. As the baby inches down the birth canal, the mother bears down with each contraction, shoving the baby farther ahead. Bearing down seems to relieve much of the pain, and some women feel as if they were having an orgasm (Cooke and Dworkin, 1981).

Toward the end of this stage, the baby's head "crowns"—that is, it can be seen at the vaginal opening. The moment when the baby is born is often highly emotional. Some women describe it as an intense "high" or as a religious experience. Once the baby is born, the umbilical cord is cut. The second stage of labor normally lasts between one and two hours for women having their first child.

In the final stage of labor, the uterus continues to contract, detaching the placenta from the uterine wall and passing it down the birth canal. Normally, the placenta emerges within five to twenty minutes of the baby's arrival. Some physicians administer hormones to stimulate contractions during this stage, speeding the process. However, if the mother is allowed to breastfeed her baby immediately, the sucking triggers the release of **oxytocin** within the mother's body. This hormone stimulates the uterus to contract and expel the placenta.

**oxytocin** a hormone involved with coitus, labor, and the production of milk

## *The experience of childbirth*

Cultural attitudes toward childbirth vary around the world. In some societies it is a fearful and secret process, and women have lengthy, painful labors. In other societies childbirth is expected to be a simple, natural process, with short, uncomplicated labors (Mead and Newton, 1967). Many women in Western societies have long and painful labors, perhaps because religious traditions demand it.

The Bible tells us that because Eve tempted Adam to eat from the forbidden apple, all women were punished with the pain of childbirth. Since Eve's curse dictated a painful childbirth, few attempts were made to alleviate that pain until the nineteenth century. Then a Scottish physician named James Simpson found that the new anesthetics, ether and chloroform, could relieve the pains of labor. Religious authorities opposed his work on the ground that pain was necessary, even

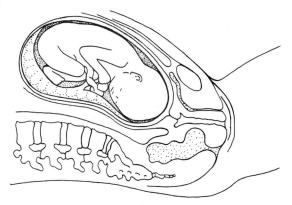

1. Fetus ready to be born

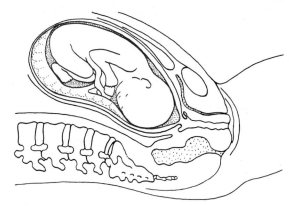

2. Cervix dilating

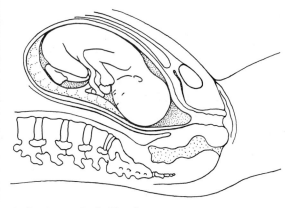

3. Cervix completely dilated

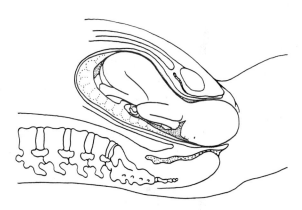

4. Head appearing

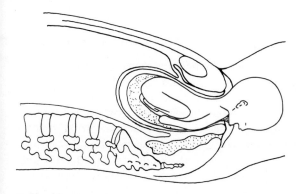

5. Shoulders appearing

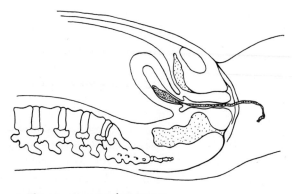

6. Placenta separating from uterus

### *Figure 20.2 The Birth of a Baby.*

Schematic representation of the birth process, from before the beginning of labor to the delivery and afterbirth.

desirable, for the laboring woman. This opposition collapsed when England's conservative Queen Victoria accepted anesthetics for the birth of her seventh child. She made painkillers an integral part of the childbirth process for most women, and the principle that attempts should be made to minimize the pain of childbirth is generally accepted today.

Until recently, however, few women regarded childbirth as anything but a painful experience that was unbearable without medical intervention. Most pregnant women had little information about what actually happened during labor except that they should expect pain. Birth was a mysterious process surrounded by fear: fear of the unknown, fear of suffering, fear generated by countless tales of agonizing labor. It was only natural that women feared childbirth—to the extent of calling the normal muscular contractions of labor "pains."

Two general approaches have evolved to deal with the pain of childbirth. In keeping with cultural traditions, one approach is to administer drugs to lessen pain. This method is used in most hospitals. A second approach is to view childbirth as a natural process that has been made excessively painful and alienating by society. In this view, fear and anxiety pour adrenalin into a woman's bloodstream, counteracting the hormones that control the labor process. Anxiety translates into muscular tension and converts simple contractions into painful cramps. This position has been supported by studies indicating that women who are highly anxious during pregnancy tend to have complicated deliveries, and those who regard pregnancy as an illness tend to have long labors (Grossman, Eichler, and Winickoff, 1980).

Both approaches are used in American society. In the past few years, however, some hospitals have begun to incorporate methods used in "natural" childbirth into their obstetric routines.

## The traditional hospital birth

The elements of the traditional hospital birth arise in part from the view that the birthing woman is a patient suffering from the disease of pregnancy. A variety of medical inventions (such as shaving pubic hair, enemas, the denial of food and drink) have been adopted to streamline or hasten the resolution of what is seen as a medical problem.

Many hospitals have begun to use fetal monitors, electronic devices that record the fetal heart rate and trace uterine contractions during labor. When used in problem pregnancies this equipment is valuable, for it alerts physicians to fetal distress and allows some mothers who would have been routinely delivered by Caesarean section to go through a normal delivery. Some hospitals use it with all laboring women, a procedure that has been criticized on several grounds. It may lead to unnecessary fetal and maternal injury, and false signals of fetal distress may lead to needless Caesarean sections (Hurst and Summey, 1982). In addition, it keeps the woman on her back, slowing labor.

Most hospitals make painkilling drugs freely available to the woman and may even encourage her to use them. Two kinds of drugs are commonly used: analgesics, which are given during labor; and anesthetics, which are given during delivery. Analgesics reduce the sensations of pain and relax the mother. Anesthetics remove the sensation of pain entirely. General anesthesia, which causes unconsciousness, is most often used when there are serious complications. Partial anesthesia, which numbs a specific part of the body, is fairly common. Either the entire body below the waist is numbed or only the external genital area.

Drugs certainly minimize pain during labor and delivery, and for this reason their use is likely to continue. They also play an important role when there are complications, such as forceps delivery, Caesarean section, or maternal illness. In the past decade, however, a trend has developed toward using the mildest types of drugs and in the smallest possible doses.

Researchers have found that all drugs can cross the placenta and affect the baby. They often produce a sluggish and unresponsive infant. As long as a year after birth, babies born to drugged mothers do not do as well on some tests as babies of undrugged mothers, with some drugs having more severe effects than others (Brackbill, 1979).

Drugs can also have a negative effect on the mother, giving her the feeling she has lost control of the labor process. They may even affect the relationship between mother and baby, for in those first days after delivery a drugged mother and a drugged baby have a hard time relating to each other (Newton and Modahl, 1978).

A procedure so common in traditional hospital births as to be almost standard is the episiotomy, an incision made just before the baby's head emerges in order to enlarge the vaginal opening. It has been estimated that more than 80 percent of women in American hospitals have this incision. The practice is far less prevalent in other countries; only about 15 percent of women in England have episiotomies, and the rate is even lower in Holland and Denmark.

Why are rates so high in the United States? In part, episiotomies are performed as preventive medicine—as a way of keeping tissues from tearing. However, in the majority of women in Europe, tissues do not tear. The American need for episiotomies may be due to the position in which most hospitals place women for delivery. In this position, the woman lies flat on her back, and great stress is placed on the tissues surrounding the vaginal opening. When women are allowed to give birth in a semi-upright position, the force of gravity may eliminate any need for episiotomy.

Episiotomies do speed delivery; once the head is in the birth canal, the enlarged opening hastens the baby's expulsion, making the physician's task simpler. In cases of fetal distress, this hastening of delivery is necessary and valuable. However, the medical description of the procedure as a "tiny cut" ignores the discomfort that generally follows it. Although the incision heals within a couple of weeks, it can make walking and sitting extremely uncomfortable and severely restrict the new mother's mobility.

The exclusion of family and friends and the early separation of mother and newborn, together with the medical aspects of hospital delivery already described, can make hospital births into a procedure called "alienated labor" (Rich, 1977). Alienated labor promotes the feeling that the woman is having an abnormal experience, one that is beyond her control, rather than a normal event in which her active participation is required. This alienation shows in some women's responses to birth:

The doctor had my husband leave, and I remember being wheeled into the delivery room. The doctor just gave me a shot, and the next thing he held up the baby, and put her on my stomach. And I remember yelling, "Take her away!" (Tanzer, 1968, p. 69)

## Natural childbirth

The term **natural childbirth** encompasses a wide variety of techniques, procedures, and attitudes aimed at making birth a rewarding and less painful experience. All methods of natural childbirth tend to emphasize three factors: the importance of educating parents about the birth process; the value of a trusted companion or "coach" during labor; and the use of techniques that minimize pain as they encourage the woman to participate actively in the birth.

The modern era of natural childbirth began with the work of British obstetrician Grantly Dick-Read. His books—*Natural Childbirth* (1932) and *Childbirth Without Fear* (1944)—challenged the popular notion that birth must be accompanied by anxiety and pain. Dick-Read, who had been trained in traditional methods, said he "discovered" natural childbirth when one of his patients in a home delivery refused chloroform. As he was about to leave, he asked her why she had not accepted the anesthetic. Her reply was, "It didn't hurt. It wasn't meant to, was it, Doctor?" (1944, p. 18).

**natural childbirth** any method of childbirth that stresses educating parents about the process, the use of a "coach," and the minimization of pain without drugs

In his travels through Africa and in his practice in Britain, Dick-Read saw many births which confirmed the belief that childbirth "wasn't meant to hurt." He also saw births in which women experienced a great deal of pain. Dick-Read concluded that fear and the anticipation of pain were the causes of painful childbirth and offered suggestions to deal with the "fear-tension-pain" syndrome.

All people, he advised, should learn that childbirth is strenuous but not painful. Pregnant women could be made aware of the physiology of pregnancy and delivery. Doctors and other birth attendants could work with the woman to reduce her fear and tension. Dick-Read also stressed the importance of exercise and breathing techniques to promote relaxation, both before and during delivery. Although he believed anesthesia was justified in some births, Dick-Read emphasized that uncomplicated birth and delivery should be a spiritual and not a medical experience.

The second major figure in the acceptance of natural childbirth was Fernand Lamaze (1972), a French obstetrician. Lamaze based his method on a Russian technique in which pain was prevented through psychological means. In the Lamaze method, a woman learns to substitute new responses for learned responses of pain and to focus her attention during labor on breathing, using a set of specific breathing techniques. A coach—usually the husband—encourages her to use the pain-inhibiting techniques and provides emotional support.

Many methods of natural childbirth have been developed and popularized in the past two decades. Each stresses the importance of education, preparatory exercises, minimal medical intervention, and the absence of painkilling drugs. There is no doubt that the natural childbirth movement has expanded a woman's options, and some women describe such births in almost ecstatic terms:

Like an orgasm . . . a different kind . . . the wonderful free feeling. Joy, a wild joy. I had known it, but it was very special. . . . Seeing a real, honest-to-good-ness baby. He looked like a porcelain eskimo, and all kinds of colors—blue, green, red, and shiny. And having Bill there . . . great! (Tanzer, 1968, p. 17)

However, natural childbirth does not work for every woman. Pain thresholds vary, as do physical and emotional needs. Women who have been trained in natu-ral childbirth and expect a painless delivery are often disappointed with themselves when they find they want medication. They mistakenly feel their need for drugs makes them a "failure." In addition, most natural childbirth training does little to prepare a woman for an unusual birth experience, such as Caesarean section.

Although the promise of a painless birth is inviting, it is not always fulfilled. For many women, three months of education and training cannot overcome a life-time of fear and anxiety about birth. For that reason, women who attempt natural childbirth need to understand that asking for drugs is not a sign of failure and that some deliveries are so complicated or painful that drugs are needed.

As the female sex role becomes less traditional, the popularity of natural child-birth may increase. After examining the research, sociologist Alice Rossi (1973) concluded that assertive, independent women tended to choose natural childbirth. The traditional hospital birth, she believes, places women in a submissive position and establishes the male physician as a dominant "deliverer" instead of as someone who assists her in giving birth.

## The Leboyer method

One method of childbirth concentrates not on the mother, but on the needs of the infant. Frederick Leboyer (1975), a French physician, looks at birth from the new-born's point of view and finds it a traumatic and agonizing experience. He regards traditional childbirth as a violent experience for the baby, who is rudely pushed out of the warm, comfortable uterus into a cold, hard, brightly lit, and noisy world.

An advocate of "birth without violence," Leboyer offers many suggestions to humanize birth for the child. He urges dim lights in the delivery room, a delay in severing the umbilical cord in order to give the infant extra oxygen, immediate con-tact between infant and mother, a massage, and a bath in warm water heated to body temperature. Finally, the infant is wrapped in warm, soft materials and left alone for a short while to discover its own stillness and immobility. Since the birth has been designed to minimize pain, fear, and shock, the baby is calm enough to enjoy this moment of tranquility. In traditional childbirth, the baby comes into the world screaming with shock and pain; in the Leboyer method, the baby is born peacefully and enters the world with a smile.

Leboyer's method of birth without violence is not always possible. If a serious problem arises—if, for example, the umbilical cord is wrapped tightly around the child's neck, then every technique must be used to start the child's breathing as soon as possible. However, in an uncomplicated and undrugged birth, Leboyer's method is an alternative to the traditional birth. In fact, some of its aspects—the dim lights, the delay in cutting the umbilical cord, the peace and quiet, and some-times the warm bath—are part of the obstetric routine in Holland (Newton, 1975).

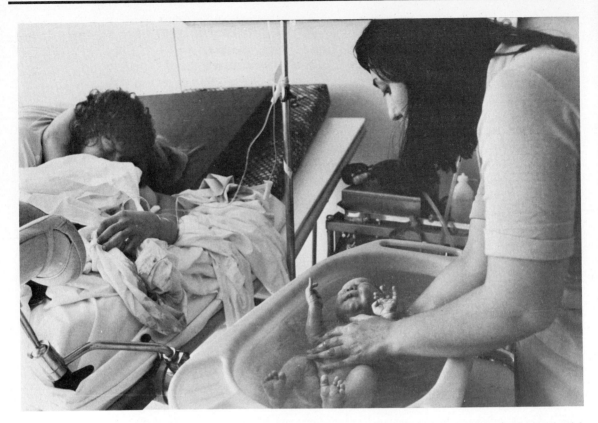

This infant has just been born by the Leboyer method, which stresses a calm, peaceful atmosphere, dim lights, and immersion in a bath heated to body temperature. (© Irene Barhi 1979/Woodfin Camp & Assoc.)

## *Male roles in childbearing*

Until recently, most literate societies denied fathers any role in childbearing. Pregnancy and birth were almost exclusively "women's business," and fathers were expected to remain apart and uninvolved until after the birth.

**couvade** childbirth rituals in which the male partner mimics the birth process

In contrast, men in some nonliterate societies take an important role in childbearing. In childbirth rituals called **couvade** (from the French word *couver,* meaning "to brood or hatch"), the husband may take a starring role. Before the birth he may be expected to rest, observe dietary restrictions, and remain in seclusion. When labor starts, the pregnant woman may go off quietly with a female companion to deliver the baby while her husband lies in bed and mimics the pains and stresses of birth. He may take a considerable amount of time to recover, and remain in bed and eat special foods while receiving visitors.

Several explanations for couvade customs have been proposed. One proposal is that the couvade ritual enables a man to demonstrate his paternity and to claim the newborn child as his offspring (Paige and Paige, 1973). Another explanation involves a belief in sympathetic magic. By mimicking the activities of pregnancy and birth, the father fools the evil spirits, diverting them away from the mother and protecting the unborn child.

It is possible that couvade fills a psychological need and enables the husband to feel he is an important part of the mystery of birth. This explanation is strengthened by research indicating that American fathers tend to be jealous of the attention received by pregnant women and new mothers and to resent being displaced as the center of their wives' attention (C. Romalis, 1981).

In a traditional hospital birth, the physician takes complete control and the father is pushed to the side. By bringing the husband back into pregnancy and childbirth as an active participant, natural childbirth methods may serve a couvade-like purpose in helping him adjust to the birth of the child. Most fathers who acted as coaches in Lamaze deliveries say they felt they had an important role to play only *after* they had taken part in the delivery (C. Romalis, 1981). Among a group of women, those who had a natural childbirth with their husbands present described them as strong, positive, and competent. But women who had a traditional hospital birth tended to see their husbands as more weak, impatient, and childlike (Tanzer, 1976).

## The new hospital birth

The popularity of natural methods of childbirth, together with the burgeoning home birth movement, has forced medical professionals to reevaluate the traditional hospital birth. They have concluded that childbearing should be a family experience and have endorsed family-centered childbirth procedures under the direction of a hospital.

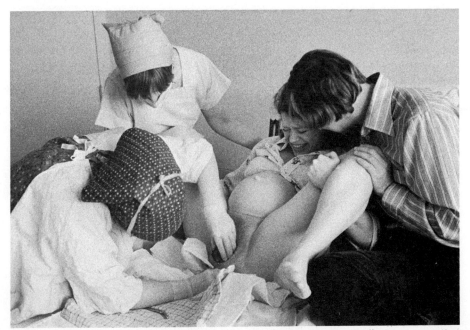

New methods of childbirth allow both parents to take an active role in the birth process. The mother is awake and alert, and the father is at her side, providing support and encouragement. (© Abigail Heyman/ Archive)

## *Focus*

### THE HOME BIRTH MOVEMENT

A small but growing number of couples have become disenchanted with childbirth procedures in the typical American hospital on the grounds that they interfere with the natural rhythms of delivery. As an alternative, these couples choose home birth—delivery of the child in the home, attended by a physician or trained nurse-midwife. Compared with a century ago few births take place at home, but compared with ten years ago the number of home births has shown a dramatic increase. Between 1972 and 1975, for example, reported out-of-hospital births increased by 60 percent (Parfitt, 1977). The home birth movement seems most popular in the western states, particularly California, and among members of the middle class.

The movement has been severely criticized by the medical profession. Physicians, who are trained to view birth as an event that may require medical attention, believe home birth represents an unnecessary risk to the health of mother and child. They stress the importance of hospital technology to deal with last-minute complications. Even physicians who approve of home births have difficulty participating in them, since they may lose hospital privileges or insurance coverage by becoming involved in a home delivery.

Yet routine hospitalization of women has its own problems. In addition to all the alienating medical procedures that sometimes induce their own complications, there are high medical costs, separation of family members and of mother and child after birth, and long isolation of mother and infant from other siblings (Arms, 1975). In contrast, the woman who gives birth at home goes through labor in familiar surroundings with attendants of her own choice, following whatever procedures soothe and encourage her. The annoying and sometimes dangerous hospital routines are eliminated, and birth becomes a family event (Boston

Although the official statement is silent about such procedures as shaving, intravenous solutions, fetal monitoring, medication, and episiotomies, it does urge a homelike atmosphere for births (Interprofessional Task Force in Health Care of Women and Children, 1978). Until labor becomes active, a woman is allowed to have her husband and children with her and to move about in a family lounge. Once labor becomes active, the woman and her husband move into an attractively furnished "birthing room," which serves as a combination labor and delivery room. The woman's bed permits her to labor and deliver in a semi-sitting position. Immediately after delivery, she is urged to breastfeed her baby, and both parents are encouraged to handle the child. Physicians believe that such an arrangement combines the best features of each approach to childbirth: Natural procedures are used, but medical assistance is immediately available.

Birthing rooms are not available in all hospitals, and hospitals that provide them generally have only one such room. If the birthing room is in use when a woman enters the hospital, she must use separate labor and delivery rooms. However, in this case delivery tables that allow a semi-sitting position are urged and the participation of her husband or "supporting other" is encouraged, as is breastfeeding and handling of the newborn.

Women's Health Collective, 1976).

Home birth is certainly a more pleasant experience than hospital delivery in cases of uncomplicated childbirth. But just how safe are home births? The answer is not clear. In Holland and England, where home birth is relatively common, infant mortality rates are lower than in the United States. Medical personnel trained in home birth are available, and backup emergency procedures are well established. Such assistance is not generally available in the United States.

The safety of home birth can be greatly increased by screening expectant mothers. Women who face any risk of complica-

tion should not try home delivery. The National Association of Parents and Professionals for Safe Alternatives in Childbirth (NAPSAC) provides a set of standards for home birth. To ensure safety, the mother should be less than ten miles from a hospital and willing to go there immediately in case of complications. She should locate a pediatrician who will see the infant soon after birth, be well informed about birth, learn to identify the complications that may occur during labor, and agree to prepare her home for delivery.

As far as medical standards go, NAPSAC recommends against home birth if the mother is not in

good health, if she has a history of complications in previous births, or if there is any chance of prematurity, breech or transverse delivery, multiple birth, blood incompatibility between mother and baby, or disproportion between the baby's head and the mother's pelvis.

Active prenatal care and screening can discover the vast majority of high-risk mothers and discourage them from home birth. Even with the most satisfactory screening procedures, however, there is always a slight risk of last-minute complications. The couple contemplating home delivery must weigh this risk against the expected benefits.

In some areas, birthing centers that are separate from hospitals have been established. These centers, run by nurse-midwives, are a sort of "half-way house" between the complete naturalness of the home birth and the medical atmosphere of the hospital. In case of emergency, the woman is transported to a nearby hospital.

## Caesarean section

Childbirth does not always progress smoothly, and sometimes a baby cannot safely be born through the birth canal. In such cases, a **Caesarean section**, in which a surgical incision is made in the mother's abdomen and uterus, may be necessary. The incision is usually made horizontally, just above the pubic hair line, so that the scar—called "the bikini scar"—will not be noticeable. The operation can be performed under either general or local anesthetic. Since a Caesarean section is major surgery, recovery time—typically one to two weeks—is considerably longer than recovery from a vaginal delivery.

In some cases, a physician can predict the need for a Caesarean section well in advance. For example, the infant's head may clearly be too large to pass through

**Caesarean section** the delivery of a child through a surgical incision in the abdomen and uterus

the mother's birth canal, the mother may suffer from high blood pressure or diabetes, or she may have had a Caesarean section in the past. (A previous Caesarean does not always mean that a woman can never deliver vaginally, but it dramatically increases the likelihood of future Caesareans.) In other cases, the decision to perform a Caesarean section is made after labor has started. The operation may become necessary if the placenta becomes detached; if the umbilical cord prolapses, preceding the infant down the birth canal; if the baby is in a breech position; or if mother or baby shows signs of distress. Some physicians perform a Caesarean section if labor seems unduly prolonged.

Caesarean section often saves the lives of both mother and child. Although Caesareans are much safer than they once were, they present some risks: jaundice and respiratory problems for the baby, and infection or dangerous bleeding for the mother (S. Romalis, 1981).

Concern has developed over the rising rate of Caesarean section in the United States, where it is higher than in other Western countries. According to a national survey, about one child in eight is delivered by Caesarean section—a rate three times as high as in 1967 (Brody, 1978). Rates are even higher in many teaching hospitals, where one child in four may be delivered through the abdomen. These rates have caused medical authorities to reassess the need for so many Caesareans.

When the parents know in advance that a Caesarean will be necessary, they have time to learn about the procedure and to adjust to it. Last-minute Caesareans are often a serious shock and disappointment to expectant parents. The mother may feel inadequate because she could not deliver vaginally, and both parents may feel "cheated." To lessen such disappointment, childbirth classes have begun to educate expectant parents about Caesarean procedures and about the possible last-minute need for such surgery. Afterward, to help women reconcile their need for a Caesarean with their plans for a natural birth, some health facilities provide support groups for women who have had such deliveries.

## AFTER BIRTH: THE POSTPARTUM PERIOD

**postpartum period** the period following the birth of a child

The time after the birth of a child, called the **postpartum period**, is both exhilarating and stressful. The mother's body undergoes enormous changes while she faces the stress of assuming responsibility for the well-being of a newborn. If caregiving chores fall primarily to the mother, the father's task is to adjust to the presence of a newcomer for whom he has financial responsibility. In families where caregiving is shared, mother and father may have to develop complex schedules to balance the needs of their child with the needs of the work world—and with their own emotional and sexual needs.

### Recovery and adjustment

The postpartum period consists of two major stages: the days immediately following the birth, and the first few months of caring for the infant at home.

Not too many years ago, women spent the first stage in the hospital, staying

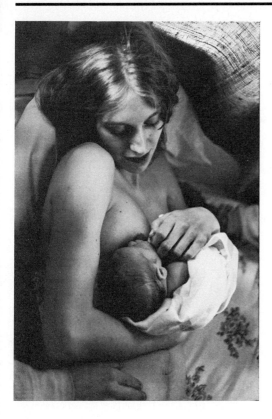

This family is still in the delivery room, sharing the first few moments of their child's life. (© Jim Harrison/Stock, Boston)

about ten days in order to recover from the stress of childbirth. Today, the average hospital stay is about three days, and the mother is often out of bed within a day of delivery. There is some evidence that women who get on their feet quickly are less likely to suffer from bladder and bowel problems and more likely to recover quickly than those who are kept in bed.

During this early stage, major physical changes take place within a woman's body. The uterus contracts to its normal size, and the contractions—stimulated by the secretion of oxytocin—may be felt by the new mother as "afterpains." Since sucking stimulates the release of oxytocin, for a few weeks a woman may experience afterpains each time she begins breastfeeding her baby.

As the uterus heals, it discharges **lochia**, a flow that begins as bleeding and gradually changes to first a pink, then a tan or whitish discharge. The flow gradually diminishes, ending within three or four weeks to indicate that healing is complete. The episiotomy also must heal, and the stitches either fall out or become absorbed.

**lochia** the vaginal discharge during the postpartum period

On the second or third day, the breasts become full and tender as they fill with milk. Until the milk comes in the breasts secrete colostrum, a fluid that is extremely valuable to the new baby because it contains antibodies that protect the infant against infection. If a mother decides not to breastfeed her infant, she can easily suppress milk production by taking estrogen.

During the second postpartum stage, a mother continues to undergo physical and emotional stress. Her body must adjust to a decreased volume of blood and changes in metabolism. Hormone balance shifts as levels of estrogen and progesterone decline. Some women hardly notice these physical changes, but others experience such unpleasant side effects as sweating, constipation, or loss of appetite. Perhaps the most common physical side effect is fatigue—the demands of caring for a newborn baby, combined with the stresses of childbirth and physical recovery, can produce a tired feeling that lasts for months.

Accompanying these physical stresses are emotional or psychological changes. For many women, the euphoria of delivery is often followed by an emotional letdown known as **postpartum depression.** This emotional reaction, sometimes called the "baby blues," may include crying, nightmares, and fears or worries about the baby. It is usually shortlived, but some women may experience mild or even severe depression that lasts for several months. One woman described her feelings during the period:

**postpartum depression** an emotional letdown that often follows the birth of a child

> I can't say that it's been a joyful experience. Everyone says it's wonderful and that the child brings so much joy but it's hard to see that joy in the first few months. . . . I was really in bad shape for about three or four weeks. I really didn't believe in postpartum depression. I thought you could avoid if it you're smart and you know enough about it. And that was hard for him [her husband] because he's used to seeing me cope, and I wasn't coping. (Grossman, Eichler, and Winickoff, 1980, pp. 92–93)

For a very few women, the postpartum period can precipitate a psychotic reaction. But in such cases, pregnancy and delivery are probably only one of several stresses reponsible for the disturbance.

The most common explanation for postpartum depression is the dramatic drop in hormone levels after delivery. Yet all women experience this drop, but not all become depressed. Perhaps the strain of adapting to the role of mother is actually the primary cause of depression (Laws and Schwartz, 1977).

Although motherhood is considered both natural and rewarding, there are negative aspects of the mother's role. Many women report feeling trapped after the birth of a first child, a response that could easily arise from being the only and the constant caregiver. Postpartum depression seems to be particularly common among women who have a strong commitment to work or career, perhaps because society views the role of mother as incompatible with the role of worker (Laws and Schwartz, 1977). The most predictable consequence of motherhood—and one that is often overlooked—is loss of sleep. Researchers have shown that sleep deprivation can lead to psychological distress, and almost every new mother goes through a considerable period when an uninterrupted night's sleep seems like an impossible dream.

## Sexual function in the postpartum period

Since sexual activity in most species depends on hormonal influence, intercourse is not resumed until breastfeeding has been completed. Although breastfeeding also tends to suppress the menstrual cycle in women, human sexual behavior is relatively free of hormonal influence. Most women are ready to resume sexual intercourse long before they are ready for a second pregnancy.

Breastfeeding is not, however, a reliable contraceptive technique. In societies where breast milk is a baby's only nourishment, breastfeeding seems a relatively reliable—although not foolproof—method of contraception. In Botswana and Namibia, for example, where women resume intercourse soon after birth but rely on breastfeeding as their only form of contraception, births are generally spaced about three years apart (Konner and Worthman, 1980). But in societies where infants have supplemental food, the stimulation from breastfeeding seems to be too weak to prevent ovulation for long. A mother is likely to be fertile long before she weans her baby. Since ovulation precedes menstruation, the appearance of the first menstrual period is not a reliable signal for resuming contraception.

Most cultures have developed rules concerning the resumption of sexual activity after birth. In some tribal societies, sexual intercourse is resumed as early as one week after delivery; others insist on abstinence for several years. Some societies forbid intercourse until a child can sit up or walk (Ford and Beach, 1951).

Only a decade or so ago, American physicians advised that intercourse be postponed until six weeks after delivery. By this time the episiotomy is fully healed and lochia has stopped. Yet many women heal long before the six weeks have passed, and if the discharge has stopped and there is no vaginal discomfort, there is little risk of infection. The six-week prohibition is an arbitrary rule, probably chosen because most physicians schedule the first postpartum checkup at this time and can ascertain that healing is complete.

It would seem that many women can safely resume intercourse within two or three weeks—if the episiotomy has healed and intercourse is not uncomfortable. However, as long as lochia continues the cervix is open, so a condom is essential to prevent infection.

A woman may be physically healed but not psychologically ready to resume intercourse. Among women studied by Masters and Johnson (1966), about half reported little or no interest in sexual activity three months after their babies' birth. Many of these women believed that intercourse might cause them physical harm; others were too tired or suffering from vaginal pain or discharge. Psychological factors are also important in this lack of sexual interest. The influences implicated in postpartum depression can also cause a woman to lose interest in sexual activity.

However, fully half the women showed intense interest in sexual activity during the first few months after delivery. Within three weeks, the sexual interest of some had returned to prepregnancy levels, and others found that their interest was considerably higher than it had been before they became pregnant. High levels of sexual tension were most evident among women who were breastfeeding their babies. Nursing mothers were the most eager to resume intercourse with their husbands, and some noted high levels of arousal, even orgasm, while breastfeeding their infants.

Since oxytocin is released during orgasm, labor, and breastfeeding, the link between sexual arousal and breastfeeding is not surprising. In fact, studies (Newton, 1978) have found that women who say they enjoy coitus are much more likely to breastfeed their babies than are women who have only mildly positive attitudes toward coitus, tolerate it, or dislike it.

# PROBLEM PREGNANCIES

Although most pregnancies are normal, from time to time the process goes awry. Among the hazards that can face a pregnant woman are ectopic pregnancy, miscarriage, Rh incompatibility, and toxemia.

If the fertilized egg implants itself in the Fallopian tubes, or more rarely in the ovary, the cervix, or the abdominal cavity, it cannot develop into a normal baby. This misplacement of the zygote, known as an **ectopic pregnancy**, is most likely to occur in women whose Fallopian tubes have been damaged by disease or surgery, or who have used an IUD for contraception.

**ectopic pregnancy** a pregnancy in which the fertilized egg implants itself outside the uterus, generally in the Fallopian tubes

A woman may not realize that she has an ectopic pregnancy until the growing zygote ruptures the tube and blood fills the abdominal cavity. Pains in the abdomen are often the first sign of ectopic pregnancy, which is a gynecological emergency that requires immediate medical attention.

**Miscarriage**, which is a spontaneous abortion, ends about 15 percent of confirmed pregnancies. An even greater proportion of conceptions end in miscarriage before the pregnancy has been confirmed. A woman may believe that her menstrual period is simply late or note that it is quite heavy and never realize that she has been pregnant and miscarried. About 75 percent of miscarriages take place during the first trimester, and the rest in the second trimester. After the second trimester, an early birth is called a premature delivery.

**miscarriage** a spontaneous abortion; the expulsion of the fetus from the uterus during the first two trimesters

Miscarriage is usually an emotionally distressing experience. It may also be physically stressful for the woman, depending on the stage of her pregnancy. The more advanced the pregnancy, the more severe the experience, which can range from a heavy menstrual period or several days of cramps and bleeding to a process resembling labor, with uterine contractions and cervical dilation.

Several factors can induce spontaneous abortion, but in most cases the aborted fetus is defective. A genetic defect or an accident in the early division of chromosomes often produces a fetus that is eliminated by the body through miscarriage. If the women becomes pregnant again, she is likely to have a normal pregnancy and produce a normal baby.

In other cases, a normal fetus is aborted because it has not been securely implanted in the uterine wall, because the cervix dilates prematurely, or because of abnormal hormone levels. If the corpus luteum does not secrete enough progesterone to maintain the pregnancy, the zygote will miscarry. Women who are prone to miscarry because of low hormone levels can be given natural progesterone to maintain the pregnancy. (Synthetic hormones are not recommended by most authorities because they may produce a malformed infant.)

Bleeding or cramping—or both—during pregnancy often signals a miscarriage. However, these symptoms may have some other cause and may disappear on their own. In the past, women who threatened to miscarry were put to bed until the bleeding stopped, but research has indicated that bed rest has no effect on the outcome of most pregnancies. Many physicians recommend sexual abstinence, but there is no conclusive evidence that sexual activity can cause a miscarriage (White and Reamy, 1982). Once the process of miscarriage has begun—particularly if the fetus is defective—there is little that can be done to halt it.

About one in two hundred births involves an incompatibility in blood type between mother and infant. This incompatibility is a crucial difference in the Rh factor—the antigens that stimulate production of antibodies. When an Rh-negative mother carries an Rh-positive fetus, there may be a slight mixing of blood cells across the placenta. If this is the mother's first child, there is unlikely to be a problem. But if the mother carries another Rh-positive baby, her immune system may produce antibodies that cross the placenta and enter the baby's circulatory system, destroying the developing red blood cells. Such a baby, if untreated, may be mentally retarded, have cerebral palsy, or even be stillborn.

This complication can be prevented by a relatively simple procedure. After each delivery, the Rh-negative mother is given an injection of RhoGAM, a substance that stops the formation of antibodies in her blood, making her body safe for the development of an Rh-positive baby (Freda et al., 1975).

Should the Rh-negative mother already have developed antibodies against Rh-positive blood, their presence can be detected during the sixth month of pregnancy by a process known as **amniocentesis**. A hollow needle is inserted through the abdomen into the amniotic fluid and a sample withdrawn for testing (Figure 20.3).

**amniocentesis** a method of detecting fetal abnormalities by drawing out a sample of amniotic fluid for analysis

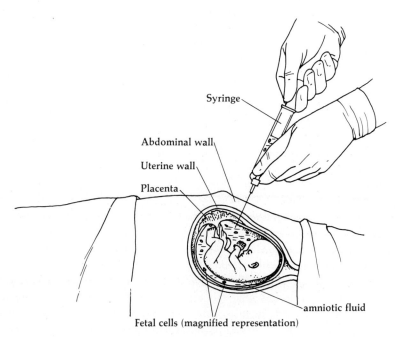

Syringe

Abdominal wall

Uterine wall

Placenta

amniotic fluid

Fetal cells (magnified representation)

### Figure 20.3

An amniocentesis involves removing a small quantity of amniotic fluid for analysis of fetal cells found in the fluid. This procedure is recommended for determining the presence of chromosomal abnormalities in women over 35.

If it contains the substance produced by a fetus in response to antibodies, a transfusion of Rh-negative blood into the umbilical vein of the fetus will protect it from the effects of antibodies.

**toxemia** a disorder of pregnancy characterized by high blood pressure, swollen legs and feet, high levels of protein in the urine, and—sometimes—convulsions

No one knows exactly why some pregnant women develop **toxemia**, a disorder that involves high levels of protein in the urine, high blood pressure, swollen legs and feet, and—in severe cases—convulsions. It is most likely to be found during pregnancy among adolescents, women who are having their first child, and women who already have high blood pressure. One reason a physician tests a woman's urine and takes her blood pressure at each visit is to detect early signs of the toxemia disorder.

If the condition is discovered early enough, the woman simply goes to bed. But if the condition is allowed to progress, she may have to be hospitalized. As soon as the baby is delivered, the toxemia disappears.

The best way to avoid the dangerous complications of pregnancy is to have regular prenatal care. By preventing some problems from starting and catching other problems before they become serious, prenatal care can help to ensure a healthy baby and a healthy mother.

## FERTILITY PROBLEMS

About 15 percent of American couples find it difficult to conceive children. Some fertility problems are mild and respond to simple treatment; others are severe and untreatable. Although most couples who attempt to conceive a child expect it may take them some time, the discovery that they are unable to conceive can lead to overwhelming disappointment and doubts about their function as males and females. As one man said:

> To find out that you're sterile makes you realize that every time you had sex with somebody there was always a grain of thought that you could have a child. . . . A man takes it for granted that he's going to be able to father a child any time he wants in his life. Picasso had a child when he was 67. It's a fantasy no one really expects to fulfill, but it's jolting to lose it. (Bouton, 1982, p. 100)

Women often express similar feelings, and the couple who cannot conceive may first experience surprise or shock, then become angry or guilty. When they abandon all hope of having a child, they often grieve as if they had experienced a death in the family (Menning, 1980).

Although recent articles in the media have indicated that women who postpone pregnancy until their thirties tend to become infertile, the worry has been greatly exaggerated. Early reports were based on studies of women who were trying to conceive through artificial insemination, a technique we'll examine later. Women in their thirties who attempt conception using natural intercourse have much higher rates of success, although not as high as women in their twenties (Bongaarts, 1982).

Among people who can conceive, some are more fertile than others. Fertility lies along a continuum: some couples are so fertile that pregnancy occurs despite the careful use of contraceptives; others may try for several years before they are successful. Among couples who are trying to conceive, about 25 percent of the women will be pregnant after one month, about 60 percent within six months, and about 80 percent within twelve months. Most specialists recommend that a couple try for at least a year before seeking medical advice.

In the past, fertility was viewed as a female problem, so much so that some cultures allowed a man to divorce his wife on grounds of "barrenness." To this day, some men refuse to undergo tests of their own fertility. However, it is estimated that about 40 percent of infertility is due to factors in the man, and about 40 percent to factors in the woman. The rest are due to some problem of the couple as a unit. In about 5 percent of the cases, emotional factors may be responsible (Seibel and Taymor, 1982). In the rest, it is the interaction of the two reproductive systems so that—although both are fertile—the woman's body rejects her husband's sperm.

Fertility problems are much easier to diagnose in a man; it is a simple matter to examine a sample of semen, and the male genitals are relatively accessible. Testing for female fertility may require extensive examination of hormone levels, and even exploratory surgery. However, medical intervention tends to be more successful with problems of female fertility.

Regardless of which partner is low in fertility, both are generally involved in treatment, for sometimes increasing the fertility of the more fertile member can counterbalance the low fertility of the partner. Medical testing and intervention begin only after the physician is sure that the couple's infertility is not the result of sexual dysfunciton, sexual misinformation, or low rates of sexual activity. As noted earlier, some of the obstacles to fertility can be surmounted by paying attention to the timing, frequency, and position of intercourse.

## Male fertility problems

In Chapter 4, the male genitals were described as a "sperm delivery system." In order to conceive through this system, the male must produce an adequate number of healthy sperm and deposit them near the female partner's cervix.

Simply producing an adequate number of sperm does not guarantee fertility. Sperm that are to be successful in fertilizing an egg must show adequate motility— that is, between 60 and 85 percent of them should still be active an hour after ejaculation. They must also be capable of swimming straight ahead; sperm that swim in circles will never make their way through the cervix. What's more, between 60 and 85 percent should be of normal shape and structure, because an abnormally shaped sperm cannot penetrate the ovum. Finally, the sperm must have vitality— some proportion should be motile at least 24 hours after ejaculation.

Sperm quality and quantity can be evaluated by microscopic examination of semen provided through masturbation. A low sperm count may be caused by several temporary factors. Since sperm production is most efficient at temperatures slightly lower than the normal body temperature, exposure to heat temporarily lowers fertility. A man who works in a hot environment—say, a bakery—or who wears tight underwear or a jock strap, who soaks in hot baths or hot tubs, or jogs in a rubber sweatsuit can temporarily impair his fertility. Sperm production can also be depressed by drugs, an illness that is accompanied by a high fever, or poor general health. Sometimes the cause is as simple as an abscessed tooth (Silber, 1980). In any of these cases, sperm counts may return to normal within three months after the cause is eliminated.

When low sperm count persists without an obvious cause, there may be a hormonal disturbance, an impairment in sperm production, or a problem in the sperm delivery system. The mechanisms of sperm production are not completely understood, so the use of hormones to treat low fertility is still in an experimental stage. When the problem is a blockage in one of the delivery tubes, surgery may be able to repair the problem. For example, sometimes an old infection has scarred the tube so that sperm cannot pass through. In other cases, variocele, varicose veins in the scrotal sac, are responsible for infertility, perhaps by increasing the temperature of the scrotum. Once again, surgical repair can often increase sperm counts.

## Female fertility problems

So many problems can interfere with female fertility that determining just which factor is responsible is often a complex and lengthy process. Once the factor is isolated, however, the problem can often be treated successfully.

Perhaps the most common cause of female infertility is the failure to ovulate. This condition may be caused by temporary factors that reverse themselves with time. In some cases, emotional stress or physical illness has interfered with ovulation. Sometimes women who have just stopped using birth control pills do not ovulate for several months. In other women, the hormones that induce ovulation are not present in large enough quantities.

The simplest method of testing for ovulation is the basal temperature chart used in the temperature rhythm method of birth control. When the chart fails to show a temperature rise at midcycle, it's likely that the woman is not ovulating. Additional tests can be used to evaluate the hormone level in the bloodstream. When it becomes apparent that a woman is not ovulating, fertility drugs are often successful in reestablishing ovulation. Sometimes these drugs cause more than one ovum to mature during a cycle, resulting in multiple births. But for a couple who have nearly given up hope of conceiving, the birth of twins could be a welcome event.

Another common cause of infertility in women is blockage or disturbance of the Fallopian tubes. If a tube is blocked, or if it does not contain essential nutrients, or if the mechanisms that transport the egg toward the uterus are disturbed, the woman may become infertile. Tubal problems can be due to a number of causes. Sometimes the problem is due to a pelvic infection—untreated gonorrhea, general pelvic inflammation, or appendicitis. Eight out of ten women with such conditions conceive after surgery opens the tubes (Silber, 1980).

Another condition often involved in tubal problems is **endometriosis**, in

**endometriosis** a condition in which cells from the uterine lining become attached to the ovaries or Fallopian tubes

which cells from the lining of the uterus become displaced to other parts of the body. Although the uterus sheds its lining every month, the cells attached to the ovaries or tubes cannot be shed, but instead bleed into the body cavity. This may cause scarring and adhesions that block fertility. Once this condition is discovered, it can often be cleared up by the administration of hormones over a period of months.

Another relatively common fertility problem is known as "hostile" cervical mucus; that is, the mucus that keeps sperm from entering the uterus for most of the month continues to bar the entrance during a woman's fertile period. Cervical mucus can be evaluated through the "postcoital test," in which the couple has intercourse at midcycle, and four to twelve hours later a sample of mucus is taken from the cervix. If the sperm within the sample are dead or show little activity, the cervical mucus is considered "hostile."

Since cervical mucus is normally made receptive to sperm by the high estrogen levels of midcycle, inadequate levels of estrogen are one possible cause of hostile mucus. The mucus may also become hostile from a cervical infection. A third form occurs when a woman develops antibodies to her partner's sperm. Sometimes a woman develops immunity to sperm, and her body treats her partner's sperm as an infectious agent, developing antibodies in the cervical mucus that destroy the sperm. Since antibody levels drop when a foreign agent is no longer present in the body, treatment for sperm immunity often consists of simply using a condom during intercourse. After several months, the level of sperm antibodies may drop far enough to permit conception.

## The new technology of fertilization

Although many couples who have difficulty conceiving can be helped by surgery, hormones, or other treatment that allows them to conceive through sexual intercourse, the best efforts sometimes fail. Within the past few years, a number of these couples have at last become parents through either artificial insemination or test-tube fertilization.

**Artificial insemination,** in which sperm is deposited on the cervix without any sexual contact, may be the answer for couples when the woman seems able to conceive but the man's problems cannot be treated. In this procedure, a woman's ovulatory cycle is determined, and during her fertile period sperm are deposited onto the cervix through a glass tube. The sperm used in such conceptions are anonymously donated, usually by a medical student intern, who is not aware of the couple's identity. When insemination occurs within two hours after the sperm is obtained through masturbation, from 60 to 80 percent of women treated will conceive after several attempts (Aiman, 1982). The success rate with frozen sperm appears to be much lower, perhaps because freezing seems to reduce sperm motility by 30 to 40 percent.

It is believed that each year about 10,000 babies are conceived by artificial insemination in the United States. Couples who consider the technique need to resolve their feelings about certain issues connected with it. For some couples, the

**artificial insemination** a method of fertilization in which sperm is deposited on the cervix without sexual contact

This sonogram was produced by bouncing sound off the fetus and converting the echoes into a picture. Sonograms can find visible abnormalities, detect multiple births, and guide physicians as they perform amniocentesis. (© James Holland/ Stock, Boston)

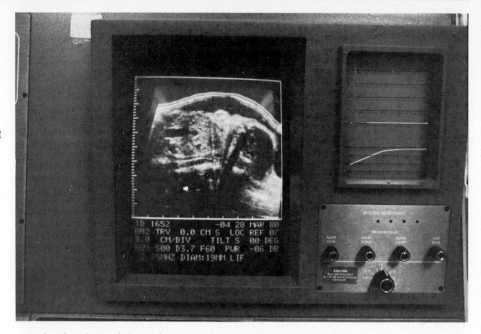

moral, ethical, or philosophical aspects may be troubling. For example, the Roman Catholic Church views artificial insemination as "adultery" and regards any child born from this procedure as "illegitimate." For other couples, the husband's lack of genetic contribution to the infant may create problems. The wife may feel "selfish" or the husband grieve over his inability to have a physical part in the conception. Once the issue is resolved, it is often possible for the husband to regain a sense of participation by becoming an active partner in childbirth education classes and by acting as a coach in labor and delivery (Menning, 1980).

**test-tube fertilization** a method of fertilization in which sperm and ovum are joined in a laboratory dish, and the fertilized ovum is then returned to the uterus

In **test-tube fertilization**, the egg and sperm meet in a laboratory container instead of in the Fallopian tubes. The first successful birth from test-tube fertilization occurred in England on July 25, 1978, when a healthy five-pound, twelve-ounce girl was born. This procedure can be used when a woman's tubes are so heavily scarred and blocked that she cannot conceive.

At the time a woman is due to ovulate, the physician uses a surgical technique to remove her own egg from the ovary just as it is ready to burst free. The egg is mixed with her partner's sperm in a laboratory dish containing a nutrient substance. In two days, when the fertilized egg consists of about eight cells, it is returned to her uterus. From there, the pregnancy proceeds in the usual fashion.

Since 1978, a number of test-tube babies have been born. By the end of 1981, two babies conceived in this manner had been born, and five more women were pregnant in a program at Norfolk, Virginia (Jones et al., 1982). The researchers who conduct this program first give women a fertility drug to stimulate ovulation. In this way, they are sometimes able to obtain more than one mature egg, which they believe greatly increases the chances of conception.

Although some people have expressed the fear that such techniques might lead to the birth of deformed children, a number of researchers believe that the chances of producing an infant with some birth defect may even drop when test-tube fertilization is used. They propose that only perfect zygotes will survive to implant themselves in the uterine wall and point to animal studies, in which all test-tube offspring have been healthy, to support their position (Silber, 1980).

Only a few years ago, couples who could not conceive naturally were advised to stop fretting and adopt a child. Today at least half of these couples can have children. Although some couples who want their own children cannot as yet have them, we seem to be moving closer to that ideal state in which birth control guarantees that unwanted children are not conceived and fertility techniques allow all couples who want a child to have one.

## Summary

**1** There are many physical obstacles to conception: the brief period in which the ovum can be fertilized, the loss of ejaculate from the vagina, the mucous barrier that shields the cervix, the sperm's inability to find the ovum, and the resistant walls of the ovum. Attention to position, timing, and frequency of intercourse can increase the chances of conception. Once fertilized, the egg is called a **zygote**, and about a week after conception it implants itself in the uterus.

**2** The thirty-eight weeks of pregnancy are divided into three **trimesters**, each lasting three calendar months. The first sign of pregnancy is usually a missed menstrual period. Pregnancy tests, which check the urine for human chorionic gonadotropins (HCG), a hormone secreted only by pregnant women, can detect pregnancy after the second week. A woman in the first trimester of pregnancy may be nauseated, sleepy, tired, and have to urinate frequently; her breasts may be swollen and tender. From eight weeks, the zygote is known as a **fetus**, and it is most vulnerable to harmful influences during the first trimester, when organ systems are forming. A woman in the second trimester of pregnancy usually feels well. By the end of the second trimester, a fetus that is born prematurely may survive if given intensive care. Unpleasant physical symptoms may plague a woman in the third trimester. American physicians often warn against intercourse during the last six to eight weeks of pregnancy, fearing premature labor, rupture of membranes, or amniotic fluid infections. However, definite harm to the fetus has never been established.

**3** Signs of **labor** include strong and regular uterine contractions, the expulsion of the mucous plug from the cervix, or the rupture of the amniotic membranes. Labor is divided into three stages: in the first stage, the cervix dilates; in the second stage, the fetus leaves the uterus, passes down the birth canal, and is born; in the third stage, the **placenta** is expelled. In American society, the pain of childbirth is handled by drugs or through attempts to reduce the fear and anxiety that surround the birth process. The traditional medical view is that the woman is a patient suffering from the disease of pregnancy. Physicians intervene with medical techniques to hasten or streamline delivery. Natural childbirth emphasizes education, coaching, and exercises to minimize pain and to enable the woman to participate in the process. Many couples, dissatisfied with hospital procedures, have taken part in the home birth movement. Recently, the medical establishment has incorporated some of the features of **natural childbirth** into the medical management of labor and delivery in hospitals. When the infant cannot be safely born through the birth canal, a **Caesarean section**, in which the baby is delivered through an abdominal incision, is performed.

**4** The **postpartum period** consists of two major stages: the days immediately following the birth and the first few months of caring for the infant at home. During the early stage a woman's uterus contracts to normal size, discharging **lochia** as it heals, and her breasts begin to produce milk. During the second stage, the woman faces physical and emotional stress. Many women have **postpartum depression,** a usually brief period of depression that may include tears, nightmares, and worry about the baby. The causes of postpartum depression are unknown, but hormones, the strain of adapting to the role of motherhood, and loss of sleep may be involved. Many women can safely resume intercourse within two or three weeks of delivery if the episiotomy is healed and intercourse is not comfortable. As long as lochia persists, a condom should be used to prevent infection. Interest in sexual activity among new mothers varies from a total absence of interest to a high degree of sexual tension.

**5** Among the major hazards of pregnancy are **ectopic pregnancy, miscarriage,** incompatibility of blood types, and **toxemia.** In an ectopic pregnancy, the zygote generally implants itself in the Fallopian tubes. If undetected, the growing zygote ruptures the tube, causing a gynecological emergency. Miscarriage, or spontaneous abortion, ends about 15 percent of confirmed pregnancies. The aborted fetus is usually defective, although insecure implantation, dilation of the cervix, or abnormal hormone levels can also cause miscarriage. When the blood type of mother and fetus is incompatible, the cause is a difference in Rh factor, with the mother's blood being Rh negative and that of the fetus Rh positive. Once the mother's system is sensitized to Rh-positive blood, her immune system produces antibodies that cross the placenta, damaging or destroying the Rh-positive fetus. Injections of RhoGAM after each Rh-positive birth can prevent the problem. The cause of toxemia is unclear, but the disorder is most often found during pregnancy among adolescents, women who have never before borne children, and women with high blood pressure. Toxemia disappears after delivery.

**6** When fertility problems exist, 40 percent can be traced to the male, 40 percent to the female, and the rest to some problem of the couple as a unit. Male fertility problems are due to sperm quality or quantity. Low sperm count can be a temporary condition (caused by exposure to heat, drugs, illness, or poor health), or a permanent condition (caused by hormonal disturbance, impaired sperm production, or a problem in sperm delivery). Female fertility problems may be due to a failure to ovulate (caused by stress, illness, recent use of birth control pills, or low hormone levels), to tubal problems (caused by blocked Fallopian tubes, a lack of essential nutrients, or a disturbance in the mechanism that transports the egg), or to **endometriosis.** Hostile cervical mucus, which keeps sperm from entering the uterus, may be due to low estrogen levels or to the development of antibodies against sperm.

**7** Couples who cannot conceive through intercourse may be able to have a child through **artificial insemination** or **test-tube fertilization.** Artificial insemination is used when male fertility problems cannot be treated; sperm from an anonymous donor is deposited onto the woman's cervix without sexual contact. Test-tube fertilization is used when the woman's tubes are so heavily scarred or blocked that she cannot conceive; an ovum is surgically removed, mixed with her partner's sperm in a laboratory dish, and two days later returned to her uterus.

# Glossary

**acception** the phase of pair bonding that consists of genital sexual activity, including vaginal, anal, and oral sex

**acquired immune deficiency syndrome (AIDS)** a disease that involves a breakdown of the body's natural immune system

**acrotomophilia** dependence on having an amputee as a partner for sexual arousal or gratification

**adolescence** transitional phase of life between puberty and adulthood

**afterplay** touching and kissing that follow sexual activity

**ambisexual** a bisexual with no interest in a continuing relationship with one person

**amenorrhea** absence of menstruation

**amniocentesis** a method of detecting fetal abnormalities by drawing out a sample of amniotic fluid for analysis

**anal stage** the second of Freud's psychosexual stages of development, occupying the second and third years of life; the rectum is the focus of sensual pleasure

**androgen insensitivity syndrome** a condition in which a genetic male cannot use the androgen secreted by his testes; his external genitals are female but his internal genitals are male

**androgenital syndrome** a condition in which a genetic female's adrenal cortex produces an improper form of cortisone, which masculinizes the appearance of her external genitals

**androgens** male hormones

**androgyny** the presence of both traditional male and traditional female characteristics in the same person

**aphrodisiac** a drug that heightens sexual desire, pleasure, or performance

**apotemnophilia** dependence on fantasies about becoming an amputee for sexual arousal or gratification

**areola** the dark, circular area surrounding the nipple

**artificial insemination** a method of fertilization in which sperm is deposited on the cervix without sexual contact

**assertive** able to act in one's personal interest, expressing honest feelings and exercising personal rights without denying the rights of others

**asynchrony** the maturation of different body parts at different rates, a growth characteristic typical of adolescence

**autonomic nervous system** that part of the PNS connecting the CNS with organs involved in functions that operate without conscious control

**aversion therapy** elimination of unwanted responses by punishing them with electric shock or other painful stimuli

**Bartholin's glands** glands on either side of the vaginal opening that secrete fluid

**behavioral rehearsal** imaginative practice of a planned interaction, saying aloud statements you propose making

**behavior shaping** a procedure which encourages behavior that comes closer and closer to an ultimate goal, a step at a time

**bisexuality** sexual activity with both men and women

**brain dimorphism** sex differences in brain structure and function, believed to be caused by prenatal exposure to hormones

**Caesarean section** delivery of a child through surgical incision in the abdomen and uterus

**castration** removal or destruction of the testes or their function

**celibacy** abstention from sexual activity

**central nervous system (CNS)** the brain and spinal cord

**cervical cap** birth-control device shaped like a thimble that fits snugly over the tip of the cervix

**cervix** the neck of the uterus, which is the passageway between the uterus and the vagina

**chancre** a hard, painless sore that is the first visible sign of syphilis

**chancroid** a sexually transmitted disease that is caused by a bacterium and characterized by a soft, painful sore resembling the syphilis chancre

**child molestation** sexual contact between an adult and a child

**chromosomes** beadlike structures made up of many genes carrying the information required to turn a single cell into a human being

**circumcision** an operation in which the foreskin is pulled forward over the penis and cut away, leaving the glans permanently exposed

**clitoral glans** the small, rounded portion of the clitoris that is visible on the body surface

**clitoral hood**   upper part of the labia minora, which meet, partially covering the clitoris

**clitoridectomy**   surgical removal of the clitoris

**clitoridotomy**   surgical removal of the clitoral hood

**clitoris**   the female erectile organ, which is highly responsive to sexual stimulation; part of the vulva

**cohabitation**   the sharing of living quarters by unmarried heterosexual couples

**coitus**   genital intercourse, in which the penis is inserted into the vagina

**comarital relationship**   an extramarital relationship that is allowed under the marriage rules established by both partners

**conception**   the phase of pair bonding that consists of conception, pregnancy, and parent-hood; also, the fertilization of an ovum

**condom**   a thin rubber sheath that covers the penis, worn to prevent conception or the transmission of disease

**contraception**   the intentional prevention of conception

**coprophilia**   dependence on the smell, taste, or sight of feces for sexual arousal or gratification

**corona**   the ridge of tissue separating the head of the penis from the shaft

**corpora cavernosa**   hollow, spongelike cylinders found in both the clitoris and the penis

**corpus luteum**   "yellow body"; the ovarian follicle after the eruption of the ovum

**corpus spongiosum**   the hollow cylinder within the penis through which the urethra runs

**couvade**   childbirth rituals in which the male partner mimics the birth process

**covert sensitization**   elimination of unwanted responses by imagining unpleasant consequences following them

**Cowper's gland**   a gland located on either side of the urethra whose alkaline secretion neutralizes the normally acid urethra

**crura**   leglike structures that join to form the clitoral body in women and to anchor the penis to the pubic bone in men

**cryptorchidism**   a condition in which the testes do not descend from the abdomen into the scrotum

**cunnilingus**   oral stimulation of the female genitals

**delayed ejaculation**   the inability to ejaculate

**desire discrepancy**   a difference in the general level of sexual interest between sexual partners

**detumescence**   loss of penile erection caused by the flow of blood out of the pelvic area after orgasm

**diaphragm**   a birth-control device in the shape of a domed rubber cap that covers the cervix

**diethylstilbestrol (DES)**   a synthetic hormone that seems to be associated with cervical cancer in the daughters of women who took the hormone while they were pregnant

**dilation and evacuation (D and E)**   an abortion technique used between the twelfth and sixteenth weeks of pregnancy in which the physician performs a vacuum suction abortion and then scrapes the inside of the uterus with a curette

**dysmenorrhea** painful menstruation

**dyspareunia** pain or discomfort during intercourse

**ectopic pregnancy** a pregnancy in which the fertilized egg implants itself outside the uterus, generally in the Fallopian tube

**editing** leaving out complaints and rude, offensive, or snide comments in favor of specific requests and honest statements

**ejaculation** expulsion of semen during orgasm

**ejaculatory duct** continuation of the vas deferens through the prostate to the urethra

**ejaculatory dysfunction** a condition in which a man either cannot ejaculate or ejaculates prematurely

**endometriosis** a condition in which cells from the uterine lining become attached to the ovaries or Fallopian tubes

**endometrium** inner lining of the uterus

**epididymis** a system of ducts within the testes where sperm mature

**erectile dysfunction** a condition in which a man cannot achieve or maintain an erection

**erogenous zone** a body area that is especially responsive to touch and involved in sexual arousal

**erotica** literature or art dealing with sexual love

**estrogens** female hormones

**eunuch** a man who was castrated before puberty

**excitement stage** first stage of Masters and Johnson model of the sexual response cycle

**exhibitionism** the deliberate exposure of the genitals in a public place with the intent of obtaining sexual stimulation; also called "flashing"

**Fallopian tubes** the tubes that transport ova from the ovaries to the uterus

**fellatio** oral stimulation of the penis

**fetal alcohol syndrome** a condition affecting many babies born to alcoholic mothers, marked by small size at birth, a conical head, and often by physical defects or mental retardation

**fetishism** dependence on some inanimate object or particular part of a partner's body for sexual arousal or gratification

**fetus** the developing organism from eight weeks after conception to birth

**fibroadenoma** multiplication of cells enclosed in a fibrous capsule that forms a harmless lump within the breast

**fibrinogenase** substance in the prostatic secretion that causes semen to coagulate temporarily when deposited in the vagina

**follicle** one of the many compartments within the ovary where ova mature

**foreplay** kissing, hugging, stroking, and oral stimulation that may precede intercourse or may make up the entire sexual encounter

**foreskin** the fold of skin that covers the glans

**frenulum** a thin strip of skin attached to the glans on the underside of the penis

**frotteurism**   dependence on rubbing against a stranger, especially in a crowd, for sexual arousal or gratification

**gay**   male homosexual, although the term is sometimes applied to female homosexuals

**gender**   all differences between males and females, including biological, social, and psychological

**gender identity**   a person's inner sense of being male or female

**glans**   the head of the penis

**gonadotropins**   sex hormones produced by the pituitary gland

**gonads**   sex organs, called testes in the male and ovaries in the female

**gonorrhea**   sexually transmitted disease caused by the bacterium gonococcus

**Graafian follicle**   the ovarian follicle that is in the process of maturing an egg

**Grafenberg spot (G spot)**   a small area within the vagina that supposedly is highly responsive to sexual stimulation

**granuloma inguinale**   sexually transmitted disease that is caused by a bacterium and characterized by continual growth of scar tissue in the genital area

**group marriage**   marriage of three or more partners, in which each considers him- or herself married to more than one of the other partners

**gynecomastia**   enlargement of the male breasts

**hebephilia**   sexual contact between an adult and a young adolescent

**hepatitis B**   inflammation of the liver caused by a virus that can be passed by sexual contact

**herpes**   infection of the mucous membranes or skin surface, caused by herpes type 1 or herpes type 2 virus, and often transmitted by sexual contact

**homologues**   organs or structures with the same embryonic origin, such as the clitoris and the penis

**homophobia**   an irrational fear of homosexuality

**homosexuality**   sexual activity with a partner of the same sex

**hymen**   a thin membrane that separates the vagina from the external genitals

**hypospadia**   a condition in which the urethra opens on the underside of the penis instead of at the tip

**imperative elements of gender**   the physical differences between males and females that are necessary in order to carry out reproductive functions

**incest**   intimate, sexually arousing physical contact between members of a family who are not married to each other

**induced abortion**   the intentional termination of pregnancy

**intimacy**   an emotional state marked by acceptance, self-disclosure, and feelings of trust and closeness

**intrauterine device (IUD)**   a small piece of plastic or metal that—when inserted into the uterus—sets up an inflammation that prevents implantation of a fertilized egg

**intromission**   insertion of the penis into the vagina

**Klinefelter's syndrome**   a condition in which boys are born with an extra X chromosome in each body cell, resulting in small external genitals, sterility, and a diminished sex drive

**klismaphilia**   dependence on receiving an enema for sexual arousal or gratification

**labia majora**   outer lips surrounding the vaginal opening; part of the vulva

**labia minora**   inner lips surrounding the vaginal opening; part of the vulva

**labor**   the birth process, from the first contractions until the placenta emerges

**latency period**   the fourth of Freud's psychosexual stages of development, lasting from age six until puberty; the sex drive is supposedly repressed during this period

**lesbian**   female homosexual

**leveling**   expressing feelings in clear, simple language in order to clarify expectations, likes, and dislikes

**libido**   the basic sexual instinct, or life force

**limerence**   passionate love

**lochia**   vaginal discharge during the postpartum period

**lymphogranuloma venereum (LGV)**   a sexually transmitted disease caused by chlamydia, which is characterized by swollen, tender lymph nodes and grotesque swelling of the genitals

**mammary lobes**   milk glands within the breast

**masochism**   dependence on submission or the reception of pain for sexual arousal or gratification

**mastectomy**   the surgical removal of a breast

**mastodynia**   tender, swollen, lumpy condition of the breasts that is common just before menstruation

**masturbation**   deliberate self-stimulation that produces a sexual response

**meatus**   the slit-shaped opening in the head of the penis

**menarche**   the first menstruation

**menopause**   the time of the last menstrual cycle, which usually comes at about age 51

**menstrual extraction**   an abortion technique, using suction to extract the uterine lining, that is appropriate only very early in pregnancy—within six weeks of the last menstrual period

**miscarriage**   a spontaneous abortion; the expulsion of the fetus from the uterus during the first two trimesters

**monilia**   a yeast fungus, usually transmitted by sexual activity, that can cause vaginal infection

**monogamy**   sexual pair bond between one male and one female

**Mullerian ducts**   primitive sexual structures that develop into female internal reproductive organs

**multiple orgasm**   a succession of orgasms in which the person drops back to the plateau phase, then with further stimulation has a second, third, or more orgasms; also called sequential orgasms

**myotonia**   increase in muscle tension

**natural childbirth**  any method of childbirth that stresses educating parents about the birth process, the use of a "coach," and the minimization of pain without drugs

**necrophilia**  dependence on seeing, fondling, or having intercourse with the dead for sexual arousal or gratification

**nipple**  the conical structure in the center of each breast containing the outlet of the milk ducts

**nocturnal emission**  ejaculation during sleep; also known as a "wet dream"

**nongonococcal urethritis (NGU)**  any urethral infection that is not caused by gonococcal bacteria

**obscene**  an object that causes sexual excitement or lust, but is offensive, disgusting, or repulsive

**open marriage**  a marriage in which husband and wife agree that each is free to form outside sexual liaisons, so that fidelity shifts from faithfulness to placing the partner first

**optional elements of gender**  the social and psychological aspects of gender

**oral stage**  the first stage in Freud's scheme of psychosexual development, which lasts through the first year of life; the lips and mouth are the focus of sensual pleasure

**orgasm**  an intense physiological reflex that releases sexual tension

**orgasmic platform**  narrowing of the vagina during the plateau stage of the sexual response cycle

**orgasmic reconditioning**  the transfer of sexual responses from unacceptable objects or acts to acceptable objects or acts by masturbating to thoughts or representations of the acceptable stimuli

**orgasm stage**  third stage of the Masters and Johnson model of the sexual response cycle

**ovary**  female sex organ, which secretes sex hormones and produces ova

**oversuppression syndrome**  temporary infertility in women who take the pill for so long that ovulation does not resume when they stop taking it

**ovum**  the egg cell produced by the female ovary

**oxytocin**  a hormone involved with coitus, labor, and the production of milk

**pair bond**  an intimate, committed relationship between two human beings or animals, usually between an adult male and female and generally involving a sexual component

**paraphilia**  preference for or dependence on unusual or bizarre objects, partners, or acts for sexual arousal and gratification

**parasympathetic system**  the division of the autonomic nervous system that dominates during periods of relaxation

**pedophilia**  dependence on sexual activity with pre-pubertal children as a primary source of sexual arousal or gratification

**penile plethysmograph**  a device that measures penile arousal through changes in the flow of electrical current

**penile prosthesis**  an inflatable or semi-rigid device surgically implanted inside the penis to provide an erection

**penis**  the male erectile organ, which is highly responsive to sexual stimulation

**penis envy** Freudian belief that envy of the male penis overshadows the life of girls and women

**performance anxiety** the fear of failing at sexual performance

**peripheral nervous system (PNS)** nerve fibers that link muscles, glands, and sense organs with the central nervous system

**petting** tactile stimulation of any part of the body that stops short of intercourse

**phallic stage** the third of Freud's psychosexual stages of development, occupying the years from three to six; the genitals are the focus of sensual pleasure

**pheromone** any chemical messenger produced by one individual that influences the behavior of another individual of the same species

**phimosis** a condition in which the penile foreskin is so tight that it cannot be pulled back

**pill** a synthetic hormone preparation that prevents conception

**placenta** a pliable structure of tissue and blood vessels that transmits nourishment and wastes between mother and fetus

**plateau stage** second stage of the Masters and Johnson model of the sexual response cycle

**polyandry** sexual pair bond between one female and several males

**polygyny** sexual pair bond between one male and several females

**pornography** obscene literature, art, or photography, especially that having no artistic merit

**postpartum depression** emotional letdown that often follows the birth of a child

**postpartum period** the period following the birth of a child

**precocious puberty** puberty that appears before the age of eight in girls or the age of nine in boys

**premature ejaculation** lack of control over the ejaculatory reflex so that a man ejaculates rapidly and involuntarily

**premenstrual syndrome (PMS)** an uncomfortable condition, with both physiological and emotional symptoms, that can develop just before menstruation

**preorgasmic** a woman with primary orgasmic dysfunction

**priapism** prolonged erection in the absence of sexual stimulation

**primary erectile dysfunction** a condition in which a man has never been able to keep an erection long enough to have intercourse

**primary orgasmic dysfunction** a condition in which a woman has never experienced orgasm from any kind of stimulation

**proception** the courtship phase of pair bonding, which includes the solicitation and attraction of the partner

**prostaglandin abortion** an abortion technique used after the sixteenth week of pregnancy in which prostaglandins are injected into the amniotic fluid or the bloodstream, triggering labor

**prostate** a gland that secretes the portion of the seminal fluid that gives semen its characteristic color and odor

**prostatectomy** surgical removal of the prostate gland

**prostatitis** inflammation of the prostate

**prostitution**   the emotionally indifferent but voluntary sale of sexual services

**psychogenic**   arising from the mind; processed by higher brain centers

**psychophysiology**   study of the connection between mental processes and bodily responses

**puberty**   period of early adolescence when biological changes are transforming children into sexually mature adults

**pubic lice**   parasites that infest human hair, primarily in the genital areas, and are often transmitted by sexual activity

**rape**   sexual relations with another person obtained by using force, threat, or intimidation

**reflexogenic**   involuntary physiological response; processed in the spinal cord

**refractory period**   period after ejaculation when a man's penis will not respond to stimulation

**resolution stage**   fourth stage of the Masters and Johnson model of the sexual response cycle

**retrograde ejaculation**   "backward" ejaculation into the bladder instead of out through the urethra

**rhythm method**   birth control achieved by temporary abstinence during a woman's fertile period

**sadism**   dependence on dominance or the inflicting of physical or psychological pain for sexual arousal or gratification

**saline abortion**   an abortion technique used after the sixteenth week of pregnancy in which amniotic fluid is replaced by saline solution, triggering labor

**scabies**   parasites that burrow into human skin, causing intense itching; they are often transmitted by sexual activity

**scrotal sac**   pouch behind the penis that holds the testes; also called scrotum

**scrotum**   scrotal sac; pouch of skin that holds the testes

**secondary erectile dysfunction**   a condition in which a man fails to keep an erection in at least 25 percent of his attempts at intercourse

**Semans technique**   a method of treating premature ejaculation in which a man masturbates until he is about to ejaculate, stops, then resumes stimulation, repeating the process until he can experience intense arousal without ejaculating

**semen**   the fluid produced by the prostate, seminal vesicles, and Cowper's glands in which sperm are carried from the body

**seminal vesicle**   a coiled and bulging tube that secretes part of the seminal fluid

**seminiferous tubules**   the tightly coiled tubes within the testes where sperm develop

**sensate focus**   exercises in which couples experiment by gently stroking and caressing each other's bodies free from the performance demands of intercourse

**serial polygamy**   a series of legal monogamous relationships

**sex**   the anatomical and physiological differences between males and females

**sex flush**   a measlelike rash that spreads over the skin of some people as orgasm approaches

**sexology** the science of human sexual behavior

**sex role** the pattern of attitudes, behavior, and beliefs dictated by society for members of each sex

**sex-role stereotype** exaggerated concepts of the traits and behavior of each gender

**sex-typed** possessing only the characteristics of a single gender

**sexual differentiation** the process of becoming male or female

**sexual dysfunction** an incapacity that interferes with sexual functioning

**sexual harassment** unwelcome sexual advances that are a condition of employment, that affect personnel decisions, that interfere with job performance, or that make the work environment offensive

**sexually transmitted disease** any disease that can be passed by sexual contact

**sexual orientation** a person's choice of sex partner, which may be heterosexual, homosexual, or bisexual; also called sexual preference

**sexual response cycle** the orderly sequence of physiological responses identified with sexual arousal

**sexual script** the mental plan that guides a person's sexual activity

**simultaneous orgasm** an orgasm in which both partners climax at the same time

**situational orgasmic dysfunction** a condition in which a woman is unable to have an orgasm from certain kinds of stimulation

**smegma** secretion that accumulates beneath the foreskin

**socialization** the process of absorbing a culture's behavior, attitudes, values, and sex roles

**sociobiology** the study of the biological basis of all social behavior

**somatic nervous system** that part of the PNS connecting the CNS with muscles used in motor activity

**spermache** the first ejaculation, a sign of puberty in boys

**spermicide** creams, jellies, or foams that prevent conception by killing sperm

**spermatogenesis** the process of sperm development

**squeeze technique** a variation of the Semans technique for treating premature ejaculation, in which a woman stimulates her partner, then squeezes the frenulum of his penis each time he feels the urge to ejaculate

**sterilization** the use of medical techniques to make a person incapable of conceiving a child

**swinger** person who engages in group sex

**sympathetic system** the division of the automatic nervous system that dominates during periods of stress

**synergism** interaction of psychogenic and reflexogenic stimuli to achieve a single goal or response

**syphilis** a chronic disease caused by a spirochete, which is transmitted by sexual activity

**telephone scatophilia** dependence on making obscene telephone calls for sexual arousal or gratification

**testosterone** male hormone

**test-tube fertilization**   a method of fertilization in which sperm and ovum are joined in a laboratory dish and the fertilized ovum is then returned to the uterus

**toxemia**   a disorder of pregnancy characterized by high blood pressure, swollen legs and feet, high levels of protein in the urine, and—sometimes—convulsions

**toxic shock syndrome**   a violent pathological reaction to the growth of a bacterium, Staphylococcus aureus, which has been connected with tampon use

**transsexual**   a person whose gender identity conflicts with his or her biological sex and prescribed sex role

**transvestism**   a compulsion to dress in the clothing of the opposite sex in order to obtain sexual arousal or gratification

**trichomoniasis**   a protozoan, usually transmitted by sexual activity, that can cause vaginal infection

**trimester**   a period of approximately three months, often used when discussing pregnancy

**tubal ligation**   female sterilization by cauterizing or cutting and tying the Fallopian tubes

**tumescence**   the condition arising when blood flows into the pelvic area during sexual arousal

**Turner's syndrome**   a condition in which girls are born with only one X chromosome in each body cell, no ovaries, but apparently normal external genitals

**urophilia**   dependence on the sight, smell, or taste of urine for sexual arousal or gratification

**uterine aspiration**   see vacuum suction

**uterus**   the womb

**vacuum suction**   an abortion technique, using suction to extract the uterine lining, that is appropriate through the twelfth week of pregnancy; also called uterine aspiration

**vagina**   the canal extending from the vulva to the cervix

**vaginal photocell plethysmograph**   a device that measures vaginal arousal through changes in the reflection of light

**vaginismus**   a condition in which intercourse is difficult or impossible because muscles around the vagina involuntarily contract

**vas deferens**   a long duct that transports sperm from the epididymis to the urethra

**vasectomy**   male sterilization by cutting or blocking the vas deferens

**vasocongestion**   increased blood flow due to the dilation of small blood vessels

**venereal disease**   any disease that is primarily passed by sexual conduct

**venereal warts**   soft, pink, fleshy growths on the genitals, which are caused by a virus and transmitted by sexual activity

**vestibular bulbs**   two masses of tissue on either side of the vaginal opening that swell when sexually stimulated

**vestibule**   area between the labia minora containing small mucous glands

**viability**   ability of the fetus to survive outside the uterus; any expulsion of the fetus from the uterus before viability is considered abortion

**voyeurism** preference for or dependence on the illicit observation of a woman or couple undressing or engaging in sexual activity for sexual arousal and gratification

**vulva** the external female genitals

**withdrawal** an unreliable method of birth control in which the penis is removed from the vagina before ejaculation

**Wolffian ducts** primitive sexual structures that develop into male internal reproductive organs

**zoophilia** dependence on sexual activity with an animal for sexual arousal or gratification

**zygote** fertilized ovum, formed by the union of two cells

# References

The number(s) in brackets after each entry refers to the chapter(s) in the book in which that work is cited.

Abel, G. G., and E. B. Blanchard. "The Measurement and Generation of Sexual Arousal in Male Sexual Deviates," *Progress in Behavior Modification.* Vol. 2. New York: Academic Press, 1976, pp. 99–136. [15]

Abel, G. G., W. D. Murphy, J. V. Becker, and A. Bitar. "Women's Vaginal Responses During REM Sleep," *Journal of Sex and Marital Therapy,* 5 (1979), 5–14. [7]

Abelson, H., R. Cohen, F. Heaton, and C. Suder. "Public Attitudes Toward and Experience with Erotic Materials," *Technical Reports of the Commission on Obscenity and Pornography.* Vol. 6. Washington, D.C.: U.S. Government Printing Office, 1971. [17]

Abernathy, T. J. "Adolescent Cohabitation: A Form of Courtship or Marriage?" *Adolescence,* 16 (1981), 791–797. [12]

Addegio, F., E. G. Belzer, Jr., J. Comolli, W. Moger, J. D. Perry, and B. Whipple, "Female Ejaculation: A Case Study," *Journal of Sex Research,* 17 (1981), 13–21. [5]

Aiman, J. "Factors Affecting the Success of Donor Insemination," *Fertility and Sterility,* 37 (1982), 94–99. [20]

Alan Guttmacher Institute. *Teenage Pregnancy: The Problem That Hasn't Gone Away.* New York: Alan Guttmacher Institute, 1981. [19]

Alberti, R. E., and M. L. Emmons. *Your Perfect Right: A Guide to Assertive Behavior.* 3rd ed. San Luis Obispo, Calif.: Impact Publishers, 1978. [10]

Alcott, W. B. *The Physiology of Marriage.* New York: Arno Press and New York Times, 1972 (orig. pub. 1866). [13]

Altschuler, M. "Capaya Personality and Sexual Motivation." In D. S. Marshall and R. C. Suggs (eds.), *Human Sexual Behavior.* New York: Basic Books, 1971, pp. 38–58 [8]

American Cancer Society. *Teaching Breast Self-Examination.* No date. [6]

Amir, M. *Patterns of Forcible Rape.* Chicago: University of Chicago Press, 1971. [16]

Anonymous. *A Man with a Maid.* New York: Grove Press, 1968. [5]

Antonovsky, H. F., I. Shoham, S. Kavenocki, B. Modan, and M. Lancet. "Sexual Attitude-Behavior Discrepancy Among Israeli Adolescent Girls," *Journal of Sex Research,* 14 (1978), 260–272. [12]

Apfelbaum, B. "The Diagnosis and Treatment of Retarded Ejaculation." In S. R. Leiblum and L. A. Pervin (eds.), *Principles and Practice of Sex Therapy.* New York: Guilford Press, 1980, pp. 263–298. [14]

Arms, S. *Immaculate Deception: A New Look at Women and Childbirth in America.* Boston: Houghton Mifflin, 1975. [20]

Athanasiou, R., P. Shaver, and C. A. Tavris. "Sex," *Psychology Today,* 4 (July 1970), 39–52. [7]

Avellan, L. "Morphology of Hypospadias," *Scandinavian Journal of Plastic and Reconstructive Surgery,* 14 (1980), 239–247. [4]


Babson, S. G., M. L. Pernoll, G. I. Benda, and K. Simpson. *Diagnosis and Management of the Fetus and Neonate at Risk.* 4th ed. St. Louis: C. V. Mosby, 1980. [17]

Bach, G. R., and L. Torbet. *A Time for Caring.* New York: Delacorte, 1982. [2, 10]

Bach, G. R., and P. Wyden. *The Intimate Enemy.* New York: Avon, 1968. [10]

Baehler, E. Z., W. P. Dillon, T. J. Cumbo, and R. V. Lee. "Prolonged Use of a Diaphragm and Toxic Shock Syndrome," *Fertility and Sterility,* 38 (1982), 248–250. [19]

Bancroft, J. *Deviant Sexual Behavior.* London: Oxford University Press, 1974. [15]

Bancroft, J. "Psychophysiology of Sexual Dysfunction." In Van Praag (ed.), *Handbook of Biological Psychiatry.* New York: Marcel Dekker, 1980, pp. 359–392. [16]

Bancroft, J. "Hormones and Human Sexual Behavior," *British Medical Bulletin,* 37 (1981), 153–158. [4, 9]

Bandura, A. *Aggression: A Social Learning Analysis.* Englewood Cliffs, N.J.: Prentice-Hall, 1973. [16]

Bandura, A. *Social Learning Theory.* Englewood Cliffs, N.J.: Prentice-Hall, 1977. [11]

Barash, D. P. *Sociobiology and Behavior.* New York: Elsevier Press, 1977. [2]

Barbach, L. G. *For Yourself: The Fulfillment of Female Sexuality.* Garden City, N.Y.: Doubleday, 1975. [6–7, 14]

Barbach, L. G. *For Each Other: Sharing Sexual Intimacy.* Garden City, N.Y.: Doubleday, 1982. [13, 14]

Barbach, L. G., and L. Levine. *Shared Intimacies: Women's Sexual Experiences.* New York: Bantam, 1981. [2, 10]

Barlow, D. H., G. G. Abel, and E. B. Blanchard. "Gender Identity Change in Transsexuals," *Archives of General Psychiatry,* 36, (1979), 1001–1007. [15]

Bartel, G. B. "Group Sex Among the Mid-Americans." In L. G. Smith and J. R. Smith (eds.), *Beyond Monogamy.* Baltimore: Johns Hopkins University Press, 1974, pp. 185–201. [13]

Beach, F. "It's All in Your Mind," *Psychology Today,* 3 (July 1969), 33–35+. [5]

Beach, F. A. *Human Sexuality in Four Perspectives.* Baltimore: Johns Hopkins University Press, 1976. [2, 8]

Becker, E. F. "Sexuality and the Spinal Cord-Injured Woman." In D. G. Bullard and S. E. Knight (eds.), *Sexuality and Physical Disability: Personal Perspectives.* St. Louis: C. V. Mosby, 1981, pp. 18–24. [18]

Becker, J. V., L. J. Skinner, G. G. Abel, and E. C. Treacy. "Incidence and Types of Sexual Dysfunction in Rape and Incest Victims," *Journal of Sex and Marital Therapy,* 8 (1982), 65–74. [16]

Bell, A. P., and M. S. Weinberg. *Homosexualities: A Study of Diversity Among Men and Women.* New York: Simon and Schuster, 1978. [9]

Bell, A. P., M. S. Weinberg, and S. K. Hammersmith. *Sexual Preference: Its Development in Men and Women.* Bloomington: Indiana University Press, 1981. [9, 12]

Bell, D. H. *Being a Man: The Paradox of Masculinity.* Lexington, Mass.: Lewis Publishing, 1982. [1, 2]

Bell, R. *Changing Bodies, Changing Lives.* New York: Random House, 1980. [1, 4, 6–7, 9, 11–12, 17, 19]

Belsky, J. "Early Human Experience: A Family Perspective," *Developmental Psychology,* 17 (1981), 3–23. [13]

Belzer, E. G., Jr. "Orgasmic Expulsions of Women: A Review and Heuristic Inquiry," *Journal of Sex Research,* 17 (1981), 1–12. [5]

Bem, S. L. "The Measurement of Psychological Androgyny," *Journal of Consulting and Clinical Psychology,* 42 (1974), 155–162. [1]

Bem, S. L. "Gender Schema Theory: A Cognitive Account of Sex Typing," *Psychological Review,* 88 (1981), 354–364. [1]

Bennetts, L. "Tootsie Taught Dustin Hoffman About the Sexes," *New York Times,* December 21, 1982, p. C11. [1]

Bernard, J. "How to Make Marital Sex More Exciting." In L. Gross (ed.), *Sexual Issues in Marriage.* New York: Spectrum, 1975, pp. 17–18. [13]

Berne, E. *Sex in Human Loving.* New York: Simon and Schuster, 1970. [6, 8]

Bernstein, A. C. *The Flight of the Stork.* New York: Delacorte, 1978. [11]

Berry, C. "Doing Your Own Vaginal Self-Exam," *Medical Self-Care,* 2 (Winter 1977–1978), 24–26. [6]

Berscheid, E., E. Walster, and G. Bohrnstedt. "Body Image," *Psychology Today,* 7 (November 1973), 119–131. [6]

Bieber, I. "A Discussion of 'Homosexuality: The Ethical Challenge,'" *Journal of Consulting and Clinical Psychology,* 44 (1976), 163–166. [9]

Bieber, I., et al. *Homosexuality: A Psychoanalytic Study of Male Homosexuals.* New York: Basic Books, 1962. [9]

Binkin, N., J. Gold, and W. Cates, Jr. "Illegal-Abortion Deaths in the United States: Why Are They Still Occurring?" *Family Planning Perspectives,* 14 (1982), 163–167. [19]

Bird, D. "Defense Linked to Menstruation Dropped in Case," *New York Times,* November 4, 1982, p. B4. [3]

Black, S. L., and C. Biron. "Androstenol as a Human Pheromone: No Effect on Perceived Physical Attractiveness," *Behavioral and Neural Biology,* 34 (1982), 326–330. [6]

Blank, A. M., S. E. Goldstein, and N. Chatterjee. "Pre-Menstrual Tension and Mood Change," *Canadian Journal of Psychiatry,* 25 (1980), 577–585. [3]

Blumstein, P. W., and P. Schwartz. "Bisexuality in Women," *Archives of Sexual Behavior,* 5 (1976), 171–181. [9]

Blumstein, P. W., and P. Schwartz. "Bisexuality in Men." In C. Warren (ed.), *Sexuality: Encounters, Identities, and Relationships.* Beverly Hills, Calif.: Sage, 1977, pp. 79–98. [9]

Boffey, P. M. "Injected Contraceptive: Hazard or a Boon?" *New York Times,* January 11, 1983, p. 13. [19]

Bohlen, J. G., J. P. Held, and M. O. Sanderson. "The Male Orgasm: Pelvic Contractions Measured by Anal Probe," *Archives of Sexual Behavior,* 9 (1980), 503–521. [5]

Bolton, F. G., Jr. *The Pregnant Adolescent: Problem or Premature Parenthood.* Beverly Hills, Calif.: Sage, 1980. [12]

Bongaarts, J. "Infertility After Age 30: A False Alarm," *Family Planning Perspectives,* 14 (March–April 1982), 75–78. [20]

Bootzin, R. R., and J. R. Acocella. *Abnormal Psychology: Current Perspectives.* 3rd ed. New York: Random House, 1980. [18]

Boston Women's Health Book Collective. *Our Bodies, Ourselves.* 2nd ed. New York: Simon and Schuster, 1976. [20]

Boston Women's Health Book Collective. "Menopause." In S. H. Zarit (ed.), *Readings in Aging and Death: Contemporary Perspectives.* New York: Harper & Row, 1977, pp. 156–164. [13]

Boston Women's Health Book Collective. *Ourselves and Our Children.* New York: Random House, 1978. [20]

Boswell, J. *Christianity, Social Tolerance, and Homosexuality.* Chicago: University of Chicago Press, 1980. [9]

Bouton, K. "Fighting Male Infertility," *New York Times Magazine,* June 13, 1982, 86–100. [20]

Boyd, M. *Take Off the Masks.* New York: Doubleday, 1978. [9]

Brackbill, Y. "Obstetrical Medication and Infant Behavior." In J. D. Osofsky (ed.), *Handbook of Infant Development.* New York: Wiley-Interscience, 1979, pp. 76–125. [20]

Bralove, M. "A Cold Shoulder: Career Women Decry Sexual Harassment by Bosses and Clients," *Wall Street Journal,* January 1, 1976, p. 15. [16]

Brannon, R. "The Male Sex Role: Our Culture's Blueprint of Manhood and What It's Done for Us Lately." In D. David and R. Brannon (eds.), *The Forty-Nine Percent Majority: The Male Sex Role.* Reading, Mass.: Addison-Wesley, 1976. [1]

Brecher, E. *The Sex Researchers.* Boston: Little, Brown, 1969. [7]

Bremer, J. *Asexualization: A Follow-Up Study of 244 Cases.* New York: Macmillan, 1959. [4]

Briddell, D. W., and G. T. Wilson. "The Effects of Alcohol and Expectancy Set on Male Sexual Arousal," *Journal of Abnormal Psychology,* 85 (1976), 225–234. [18]

Brody, J. E. "Personal Health," *New York Times,* March 8, 1978, p. C10. [20]

Brody, J. E. "Effects of Exercise on Menstruation," *New York Times,* September 1, 1982, p. C1+. [3]

Brooks, M. B., and S. W. Brooks. *Lifelong Sexual Vigor: How to Avoid and Overcome Impotence.* New York: Doubleday, 1981. [4]

Brooks-Gunn, J., and D. N. Ruble. "Menarche: The Interaction of Physiological, Cultural, and Social Factors." In A. J. Dan and E. M. Srahawn (eds.), *The Menstrual Cycle: Synthesis of Interdisciplinary Research.* New York: Springer, 1981. [12]

Brooks-Gunn, J., and D. N. Ruble. "The Development of Menstrual-Related Beliefs and Behavior During Early Adolescence," *Child Development,* 53 (1982a), 1567–1577. [12]

Brooks-Gunn, J., and D. N. Ruble. "Psychological Correlates of Tampon Use in Adolescents," *Annals of Internal Medicine,* 96 (Part 2) (1982b), 962–965. [12]

Brooks-Gunn, J., and W. S. Matthews. *He & She: How Children Develop Their Sex-Role Identity.* Englewood Cliffs, N.J.: Prentice-Hall, 1979. [12]

Brown, C. *The New Celibacy: Why More Men and Women are Abstaining from Sex—And Enjoying It.* New York: McGraw-Hill, 1980. [13]

Brownmiller, S. *Against Our Will: Men, Women, and Rape.* New York: Simon and Schuster, 1975. [16]

Brozan, N. "Sterilization Without Surgery Has Promise," *New York Times,* September 6, 1982, p. C38. [19]

Budoff, P. W. "Zompirac Sodium in the Treatment of Primary Dysmenorrhea Syndrome," *New England Journal of Medicine,* 307 (1982), 714–719. [3]

Bullard, D. G. "Sexual Enhancement in Physical Disability and Disorders," *International Journal of Mental Health,* 10 (1981), 169–180. [18]

Bullough, V. L. *Sexual Variance in Society and History.* New York: Wiley, 1976. [2, 4, 6, 8–9, 15–16]

Bullough, V. L. *Homosexuality: A History.* New York: New American Library, 1979. [9]

Bullough, V. L. "Technology and Female Sexuality and Physiology: Some Implications," *Journal of Sex Research,* 16 (1980), 59–71. [1]

Bullough, V. L. "Age of Menarche: A Misunderstanding," *Science,* 213 (1981), 365–366. [12]

Bullough, V. L., and B. Bullough. *The Subordinate Sex: A History of Attitudes Toward Women.* Urbana, Ill.: University of Illinois Press, 1973. [1, 2]

Burger, E. "Radical Hysterectomy and Vaginectomy for Cancer." In D. G. Bullard and S. E. Knight (eds.), *Sexuality and Physical Disability: Personal Perspectives.* St. Louis: C. V. Mosby, 1981, pp. 44–58. [18]

Burgess, A. W., and L. L. Holmstrom. "Rape Trauma Syndrome," *American Journal of Psychiatry,* 131 (1974), 981–986. [16]

Burgess, A. W., and L. L. Holstrom. "Rape: Sexual Disruption and Recovery," *American Journal of Orthopsychiatry,* 49 (1979), 648–657. [16]

Burt, M. R. "Cultural Myths and Supports for Rape," *Journal of Personality and Social Psychology,* 38 (1980), 217–230. [16]

Buscaglia, L. F. *Personhood: The Art of Being Fully Human.* New York: Fawcett Columbine, 1978. [10]

Byrne, D., and L. Byrne. *Exploring Human Sexuality.* New York: Crowell, 1977. [7]

Calderone, M. S., and E. W. Johnson. *The Family Book About Sexuality.* New York: Harper & Row, 1981. [13, 14]

Cargan, L., and M. Melko. *Singles: Myths and Realities.* Beverly Hills, Calif.: Sage, 1982. [13]

Castleman, M. "A Field Guide to Men's Reproductive Health," *Medical Self-Care,* 3 (1978), 27–32. [6]

Chambless, D. L., T. Stern, F. E. Sultan, A. J. Williams, A. J. Goldstein, M. H. Lineberger, J. L. Lifschitz, and L. Kelly. "The Pubococcygens and Female Orgasm: A Correlation Study with Normal Subjects," *Archives of Sexual Behavior,* 11 (1982), 479–490. [6]

Chang, J. *The Tao of Love and Sex.* New York: Dutton, 1977. [8]

Chesser, E. *Human Aspects of Sexual Deviation.* London: Jerrolds, 1971. [15]

Chilman, C. *Adolescent Sexuality in a Changing American Society: Social and Psychological Perspectives.* Bethesda, Md.: DHEW Public Health Service, National Institutes of Health, No (NIH) 79-1426, 1979. [12]

Cicone, M. V., and D. N. Ruble. "Beliefs About Males," *Journal of Social Issues,* 34 (1978), 5–15. [1]

Clarke-Stewart, K. A., and C. M. Hevey. "Longitudinal Relations in Repeated Observations of Mother-Child Interaction from 1 to 2½ Years," *Developmental Psychology,* 17 (1981), 127–145. [11]

Clayton, R. R., and J. L. Bokemeier. "Premarital Sex in the Seventies," *Journal of Marriage and the Family,* 42 (1980), 759–774. [12]

Cohen, H., R. C. Rosen, and L. Goldstein. "Elecroencephalographic Laterality Changes During Human Sexual Orgasm," *Archives of Sexual Behavior,* 5 (1976), 189–199. [5, 7]

Cohen, Y. "The Disappearance of the Incest Taboo," *Human Nature,* 1 (July 1978), 72–78. [16]

Cole, T. M. "Sexuality and the Spinal Cord Injured." In R. Green (ed.), *Human Sexuality: A Health Practitioner's Text.* Baltimore: Williams & Wilkins, 1975, pp. 181–196. [18]

Coleman, J. C. *Abnormal Psychology and Modern Life.* Glenview, Ill.: Scott, Foresman, 1972. [15]

Collins, E. G., C., and T. B. Blodgett. "Sexual Harassment: Some See It . . . Some Won't," *Harvard Business Review,* 59 (March–April 1981), 76–95. [16]

Comfort, A. *The Joy of Sex.* New York: Simon and Schuster, 1972. [8, 15]

Comfort, A. *A Good Age.* New York: Simon and Schuster, 1976. [13]

Comfort, A. (ed.), *Sexual Consequences of Disability.* Philadelphia: George F. Stickley, 1978. [18]

Constantine, L. L., and J. M. Constantine. "Sexual Aspects of Group Marriage." In R. W. Libby and R. N. Whitehurst (eds.), *Marriage and Alternatives: Exploring Intimate Relationships.* Glenview, Ill.: Scott, Foresman, 1977, pp. 186–195. [13]

Cook, M., and R. McHenry. *Sexual Attraction.* New York: Pergamon, 1978. [10]

Cooke, C. W., and S. Dworkin. *The Ms. Guide to a Woman's Health.* Rev. ed. New York: Berkeley Books, 1981. [17, 19–20]

Cope, O. *The Breast: A Health Guide for Women of All Ages.* Boston: Houghton Mifflin, 1978. [3, 18]

Cox, C., and R. G. Smart. "Social and Psychological Aspects of Speed Use," *International Journal of the Addictions,* 7 (1972), 201–217. [18]

Crepault, C., and M. Couture. "Men's Erotic Fantasies," *Archives of Sexual Behavior,* 9 (1980), 565–581. [7]

Croughan, J. L., M. Saghir, R. Cohen, and E. Robins. "A Comparison of Treated and Untreated Male Cross-Dressers," *Archives of Sexual Behavior,* 10 (1981), 515–528. [15]

Crovitz, E., and A. Steinmann. "A Decade Later: Black-White Attitudes Toward Women's Familial Role," *Psychology of Women Quarterly,* 5 (1980), 170–176. [2]

Cuber, J. F., and P. B. Harroff. *Sex and the Significant Americans.* Baltimore: Penguin Books, 1965. [1]

Cushman, P. "Sexual Behavior in Heroin Addiction and Methadone Maintenance," *New York State Journal of Medicine,* 48 (1972), 1261–1265. [18]

Dalton, K. *The Pre-Menstrual Syndrome.* Springfield, Ill.: Charles C Thomas, 1964. [3]

David, H. P. "Psychological Studies in Abortion." In J. T. Fawcett (ed.), *Psychological Perspectives on Population.* New York: Basic Books, 1973, pp. 241–273. [19]

Davidson, J. M. "Hormones and Sexual Behavior in the Male," *Hospital Practice,* September 1975, pp. 126–132. [4]

Davis, A. J. "Sexual Assaults in the Philadelphia Prison System." In J. H. Gagnon and W. Simon (eds.), *The Sexual Scene.* Chicago: Aldine, 1970, pp. 107–124. [16]

Davis, S. K., and P. W. Davis. "Meanings and Process in Erotic Offensiveness." In C. Warren (ed.) *Sexuality: Encounters, Identities, and Relationships.* Beverly Hills, Calif.: Sage, 1977, pp. 117–136. [15]

Davis, S. M., and M. B. Harris. "Sexual Knowledge, Sexual Interests, and Sources of Sexual Information of Rural and Urban Adolescents from Three Cultures," *Adolescence,* 17 (1982), 471–491. [12]

Davison, G. C. "Homosexuality: The Ethical Challenge," *Journal of Consulting and Clinical Psychology,* 44 (1976), 157–162. [9]

Davison, G. C. "Not Can But Ought: The Treatment of Homosexuality," *Journal of Consulting and Clinical Psychology,* 46 (1978), 170–172. [9]

de Bruijn, G. "From Masturbation to Orgasm with a Partner: How Some Women Bridge the

Gap—and Why Others Don't," *Journal of Sex and Marital Therapy,* 8 (1982), 151–167. [14]

Delaney, J., M. J. Lupton, and E. Toth. *The Curse: A Cultural History of Menstruation.* New York: Dutton, 1976. [3]

DeLeon, G., and H. K. Wexler. "Heroin Addiction: Its Relation to Sexual Behavior and Sexual Experience," *Journal of Abnormal Psychology,* 81 (1973), 36–38. [18]

DeLora, J. S., and C. A. Warren. *Understanding Sexual Interaction.* Boston: Houghton Mifflin, 1977. [13]

Deutsch, H. *The Psychology of Women.* New York: Grune and Stratton, 1944. [16]

Diamond, M. "Human Sexual Development: Biological Foundations for Social Development." In F. Beach (ed.), *Human Sexuality in Four Perspectives.* Baltimore: Johns Hopkins University Press, 1976, pp. 22–61. [1]

Diamond, M. "Sexual Identity, Monozygotic Twins Reared in Discordant Sex Roles and a BBC Follow-Up," *Archives of Sexual Behavior,* 11 (1982), 181–186. [11]

Diaz, S., M. Pavez, P. Miranda, D. N. Robertson, I. Sivin, and H. B. Croxatto. "A Five-Year Clinical Trial of Levonorgestrel Silastic Implants (Norplant)," *Contraception,* 25 (1982), 447–456. [19]

Dickinson, R. L. *Human Sex Anatomy.* Baltimore: Williams & Wilkins, 1933. [3–4, 7]

Dickinson, R. L., and L. Beam. *A Thousand Marriages: A Medical Study of Sex Adjustment.* Baltimore: Williams & Wilkins, 1931. [8]

Dick-Read, G. *Childbirth Without Fear.* New York: Harper & Row, 1944. [20]

Dingfelder, J. R. "Prostaglandin Inhibitors: New Treatment for an Old Nemesis," *New England Journal of Medicine,* 307 (1982), 746–747. [3]

Djerassi, C. *The Politics of Contraception.* New York: Norton, 1979. [19]

Dodson, B. *Liberating Masturbation.* New York: Bodysex Designs, 1974. [6, 7]

Dodson, B. *Self Love and Orgasm.* New York: B. Dodson, 1983. [6, 7]

Donnerstein, E., and L. Berkowitz. "Victim Reactions in Aggressive Erotic Films as a Factor in Violence Against Women," *Journal of Personality and Social Psychology,* 41 (1981), 710–724. [16]

Dornbusch, S. M., J. M. Carlsmith, R. T. Gross, J. A. Martin, D. Jennings, A. Rosenberg, and P. Drake. "Sexual Development, Age, and Dating: A Comparison of Biological and Social Influences upon One Set of Behaviors," *Child Development,* 52 (1981), 179–185. [12]

Dosey, M. F., and M. A. Dosey. "The Climacteric Woman," *Patient Counselling and Health Education,* 4 (1980), 14–21. [13]

Downey, L. "Intergenerational Change in Sexual Behavior: A Belated Look at Kinsey's Males," *Archives of Sexual Behavior,* 9 (1980), 267–317. [9, 13]

Downing, G. *The Massage Book.* New York: Random House, 1972. [10]

Dryfoos, J. G. "Contraceptive Use, Pregnancy Intentions and Pregnancy Outcomes Among U.S. Women," *Family Planning Perspectives,* 14 (1982), 81–94. [19]

Dunn, M., E. E. Lloyd, and G. H. Phelps. "Sexual Assertiveness in Spinal Cord Injury." In D. G. Bullard and S. E. Knight (eds.), *Sexuality and Physical Disability: Personal Perspectives.* St. Louis: C. V. Mosby, 1981, pp. 249–255. [18]


Edwardes, A., and R. E. L. Masters. *The Cradle of Erotica.* New York: Bantam Books, 1962. [8]

Ehrhardt, A. A., G. Grisanti, and E. A. McCauley. "Female-to-Male Transsexuals Compared to Lesbians: Behavioral Patterns of Childhood and Adolescent Development," *Archives of Sexual Behavior,* 8 (1979), 481–490. [15]

Ehrhardt, A. A., and H. F. L. Meyer-Bahlburg. "Psychological Correlates of Abnormal Pubertal Development," *Clinics in Endocrinology and Metabolism,* 4 (1975), 207–222. [12]

Ehrhardt, A. A., and H. F. L. Meyer-Bahlburg. "Effects of Prenatal Hormones on Gender-Related Behavior," *Science,* 211 (1981), 1312–1318. [11]

Ellenstein, N. S., and J. W. Cavanaugh. "Sexual Abuse of Boys," *American Journal of Disabled Children,* 134 (1980), 255–257. [16]

Ellis, A. "What Is Normal Sexual Behavior?" In A. Ellis and R. Brancale (eds.), *The Psychology of Sex Offenders.* Springfield, Ill.: Charles C Thomas, 1956, pp. 120–132. [15]

Ellis, E. M., K. S. Calhoun, and B. M. Atheson. "Sexual Dysfunction in Victims of Rape," *Women and Health,* 5 (Winter 1980), 39–47. [16]

Ellis, H. *Studies in the Psychology of Sex.* New York: Random House, 1906. [5]

Engels, F. *The Origin of the Family, Private Property, and the State.* 4th ed. New York: International Publishers, 1942 (orig. pub. 1884). [1]

Equal Employment Opportunity Commission. *Guidelines on Discrimination on the Basis of Sex.* Washington, D.C.: EEOC, November 10, 1980. [16]

Erikson, E. H. *Childhood and Society.* 2nd ed. New York: Norton, 1963. [11]

Erikson, E. H. *Identity and the Life Cycle.* New ed. New York: Norton, 1980. [13]

Evans, L. J. "Sexual Harassment: Women's Hidden Occupational Hazard." In J. R. Chapman and M. Gates (eds.), *The Victimization of Women.* Beverly Hills, Calif.: Sage, 1978, pp. 203–223. [16]

Fagot, B. I. "Sex Differences in Toddlers' Behavior and Parental Reaction," *Developmental Psychology,* 10 (1974), 554–558. [11]

Fagot, B. I. "The Influence of Sex of Child on Parental Reactions to Toddler Children," *Child Development,* 49 (1978), 459–465. [11]

Fairbanks, B., and B. Scharfman. "The Cervical Cap: Past and Current Experience," *Women and Health,* 5 (Fall 1980), 61–77. [19]

Falicov, C. J. "Mexican Families." In M. McGoldrick, J. K. Pearce, and Joseph Giordana (eds.), *Ethnicity and Family Therapy.* New York: Guilford Press, 1982, pp. 134–141. [2]

*Family Planning Perspectives.* "Digest: Pill and IUD Use at PPFA Clinics Decline; Diaphragm Use Rises," *Family Planning Perspectives,* 14 (1982), 152. [19]

Farkas, G., and R. C. Rosen. "Effects of Alcohol on Elicited Male Sexual Response," *Quarterly Journal of Studies on Alcohol,* 37 (1976), 265–272. [18]

Farrell, W. *The Liberated Man.* New York: Random House, 1975. [1]

Federal Bureau of Investigation. *Uniform Crime Reports for the United States.* Washington, D.C.: U.S. Government Printing Office, 1980. [16]

Feinbloom, D. H. *Transvestites and Transsexuals: Mixed Views.* New York: Delacorte, 1976. [1, 15]

Feldman, M. P., and M. J. McCullough. *Homosexual Behavior: Therapy and Assessment.* Oxford: Pergamon, 1978. [9]

Feldman-Summers, S., and C. D. Ashworth. "Factors Related to Intentions to Report a Rape," *Journal of Social Issues,* 37 (1981), 53–70. [16]

Feldman-Summers, S., P. E. Gordon, and J. R. Meagher. "The Impact of Rape on Sexual Satisfaction," *Journal of Abnormal Psychology,* 88 (1979), 101–105. [16]

Feldman-Summers, S., and G. C. Palmer. "Rape as Viewed by Judges, Prosecutors, and Police Officers," *Criminal Justice and Behavior,* 7 (1980), 19–40. [16]

Feldman, Y. M., and J. A. Nikitas. "Nongonococcal Urethritis: A Clinical Review," *Journal of the American Medical Association,* 245 (1981), 381–386. [17]

Fenichel, O. *The Psychoanalytic Theory of Neurosis.* New York: Norton, 1945. [15]

Fensterheim, H., and J. Baer. *Don't Say Yes When You Want to Say No.* New York: Dell, 1975. [10]

Field, T. M., S. M. Widmayer, S. Stringer, and E. Ignatoff. "Teenage, Lower-Class, Black Mothers and Their Preterm Infants: An Intervention and Developmental Follow-up," *Child Development,* 51 (1980), 426–436. [12]

Finkelhor, D. "Sex Among Siblings: A Survey on Prevalence, Variety, and Effects," *Archives of Sexual Behavior,* 9 (1980), 171–194. [16]

Finn, J. D. "Sex Differences in Educational Outcomes: A Cross-National Study," *Sex Roles,* 6 (1980), 9–26. [1]

Finney, J. C. "Maternal Influences on Anal or Compulsive Character in Children," *Journal of Genetic Psychology,* 103 (1963), 351–367. [11]

Fischer, J. L., and L. R. Narus, Jr. "Sex Roles and Intimacy in Same Sex and Other Sex Relationships," *Psychology of Women Quarterly,* 5 (1981), 444–455. [2]

Fisher, C., J. Gross, and J. Zuch. "Cycle of Penile Erection Synchronous with Dreaming (REM) Sleep," *Archives of General Psychiatry,* 12 (1965), 29–45. [7]

Fisher, S. *The Female Orgasm.* New York: Basic Books, 1973. [14]

Fisher, S. and R. P. Greenberg. *The Scientific Credibility of Freud's Theories and Therapy.* New York: Basic Books, 1977. [11]

Fleming, M., C. Steinman, and G. Bocknek. "Methodological Problems in Assessing Sex-Reassignment Surgery: A Reply to Meyer and Reter," *Archives of Sexual Behavior,* 9 (1980), 451–456. [15]

Ford, C. S., and F. A. Beach. *Patterns of Sexual Behavior.* New York: Harper & Row, 1951. [1, 3, 4, 7, 8, 9, 10, 11, 13, 20]

Forgac, G. E., and E. J. Michaels. "Personality Characteristics of Two Types of Male Exhibitionists," *Journal of Abnormal Psychology,* 91 (1982), 287–293. [15]

Fotherby, K., G. Benagiano, H. K. Topozada, A. Abdel-Rahman, F. Navaroli, B. Arce, R. Ramos-Cordero, C. Gual, B. M. Landgren, and E. Johannisson. "A Preliminary Pharmacological Trial of the Monthly Injectable Contraceptive Cycloprovera," *Contraception,* 25 (1982), 261–272. [19]

Fox, C. A., and B. Fox. "Blood Pressure and Respiratory Patterns During Human Coitus," *Journal of Reproductive Fertility,* 19 (1969), 405–415. [5]

Fracher, J. C., S. R. Leiblum, and R. C. Rosen. "Recent Advances in the Comprehensive Evaluation of Erectile Dysfunction," *International Journal of Mental Health,* 10 (1981), 110–121. [14]

Francis, D. P., et al. "The Prevention of Hepatitis B with Vaccine," *Annals of Internal Medicine,* 97 (1982), 362–366. [17]

Francke, L. B. *The Ambivalence of Abortion.* New York: Random House, 1978. [19]

Francoeur, R. T., and A. K. Francoeur, "Hot and Cool Sex: Fidelity in Marriage." In R. W. Libby and R. N. Whitehurst (eds.), *Marriage and Alternatives: Exploring Intimate Relationships.* Glenview, Ill.: Scott, Foresman, 1977, pp. 302–319. [13]

Frank, E., C. Anderson and D. Rubinstein. "Frequency of Sexual Dysfunction in 'Normal' Couples," *New England Journal of Medicine,* 299 (1978), 111–115. [13, 14]

Freda, V. J., J. G. Gorman, W. Pollack, and E. Howe. "Prevention of Rh Hemolytic Disease—Ten Years' Clinical Experience with Rh Immune Globulin," *New England Journal of Medicine,* 282 (1975), 19. [20]

Freimuth, M. J., and G. A. Hornstein. "A Critical Examination of the Concept of Gender," *Sex Roles,* 8 (1982), 515–532. [1]

Freud, S. "Femininity." In J. Strouse (ed.), *Women and Analysis: Dialogues on Psychoanalytic Views of Femininity.* New York: Dell, 1974. [4]

Freud, S. *Ueber Coca.* Reprinted by Dunequin Press, 1963 (orig. pub. 1884). [18]

Friedman-Kien, A. E., et al. "Disseminated Kaposi's Sarcoma in Homosexual Men," *Annals of Internal Medicine,* 96 (1982), 693–700. [17]

Frieze, I. H., J. E. Parsons, P. B. Johnson, D. N. Ruble, and G. L. Zellman. *Women and Sex Roles: A Social Psychological Perspective.* New York: Norton, 1978. [1]

Fryer, J. G., and J. R. Ashford. "Trends in Perinatal and Neo-natal Mortality in England and Wales 1960–1969," *British Journal of Preventive and Social Medicine,* 26 (1972), 1–9. [11]

Furstenberg, F. F., Jr. *Unplanned Parenthood: The Social Consequences of Teenage Childbearing.* New York: Free Press, 1976. [12]

Furstenberg, F. F., Jr. "Burdens and Benefits: The Impact of Early Childbearing on the Family," *Journal of Social Issues,* 36 (1980), 64–87. [12]

Gadpaille, W. J. *The Cycles of Sex.* New York: Scribner, 1975. [11, 12]

Gadpaille, W. J. "Homosexuality." In R. C. Simons and H. Pardes (eds.), *Understanding Human Behavior in Health and Illness.* 2nd ed. Baltimore: Williams & Wilkins, 1981, pp. 362–371. [9]

Gagnon, J. H. "Sex Research and Social Change," *Archives of Sexual Behavior,* 4 (1975), 111–141. [1, 2]

Gagnon, J. H. *Human Sexualities.* Glenview, Ill.: Scott, Foresman, 1977. [8–9, 11]

Gagnon, J. H. "Books: *Greek Homosexuality* and *Homosexualities: A Study of Diversity Among Men and Women,*" *Human Nature,* 2 (March 1979), 20–24. [9]

Gagnon, J. H., and C. S. Greenblatt. *Life Designs: Individuals, Marriages, and Families.* Glenview, Ill.: Scott, Foresman, 1978. [13]

Gagnon, J. H., and E. J. Roberts "Parents' Messages to Pre-Adolescent Children About Sexuality." In J. M. Samson (ed.), *Childhood and Sexuality.* Montreal: Editions Etudes Vivantes, 1980, pp. 275–285. [11, 12]

Gagnon, J. H., R. C. Rosen, and S. R. Leiblum. "Cognitive and Social Aspects of Sexual Dysfunction: Sexual Scripts in Sex Therapy," *Journal of Sex and Marital Therapy,* 8 (1982), 44–56. [1, 8, 13–14]

Gagnon, J. H., and W. E. Simon. "They're Going to Learn It in the Street Anyway," *Psychology Today,* 3 (July 1969), 46–47+. [11]

Gagnon, J. H., and W. E. Simon. *Sexual Conduct: The Social Sources of Human Sexuality.* Chicago: Aldine, 1973. [1, 8–9, 12, 15–16]

Galin, D., and R. Ornstein. "Lateral Specialization of Cognitive Mode: An EEG Study," *Psychophysiology,* 9 (1972), 412. [5]

Gannon, L. "Evidence for a Psychological Etiology of Menstrual Disorders," *Psychological Reports,* 48 (1981), 287–294. [3]

Garcia-Preto, N. "Puerto-Rican Families." In M. McGoldrick, J. K. Pearce, and J. Giordano (eds.), *Ethnicity and Family Therapy.* New York: Guilford Press, 1982, p. 164. [2]

Gardiner, S., and J. Torge. *A Book About Sexual Assault.* Montreal: Montreal Health Press, 1979. [16]

Gates, M. "Introduction." In J. R. Chapman and M. Gates (eds.). *The Victimization of Women.* Beverly Hills, Calif.: Sage, 1978, pp. 9–27. [16]

Gay, G. R., and C. W. Sheppard. "Sex-Crazed Dope Fiends—Myths or Reality?" *Drug Forum,* 2 (1973), 125–140. [18]

Gebhard, P. H., "Sexuality in Cross-Cultural Perspective." In W. H. Masters, V. E. Johnson, and R. C. Kolodny, *Human Sexuality.* Boston: Little, Brown, 1982, pp. 484–499.[6]

Gebhard, P. H., J. H. Gagnon, W. B. Pomeroy, and C. V. Christenson. *Sex Offenders: An Analysis of Types.* New York: Harper & Row, 1965 [15, 16]

Geer, J. H. "The Relationship Between Sexual Arousal Experience and Genital Response." *Psychophysiology,* 20 (1983), 121–127. [6]

Geer, J. H., and R. Fuhr. "Cognitive Factors in Sexual Arousal: The Role of Distraction," *Journal of Consulting and Clinical Psychology,* 44 (1976), 238–243. [5]

Gelman, D., et al. "Just How the Sexes Differ," *Newsweek,* May 18, 1981, pp. 72–83. [1]

Gelman, E. "In Sports, 'Lions vs. Tigers.' " *Newsweek,* May 18, 1981, p. 75. [1]

Giele, J. Z., and A. C. Smock. *Women: Roles and Status in Eight Countries.* New York: Wiley, 1977. [19]

Gilbert, F. S., and K. L. Bailis "Sex Education in the Home: An Empirical Task Analysis," *Journal of Sex Research,* 16 (1980), 148–161. [12]

Gilmartin, B. G. "Swinging: Who Gets Involved and How?" In R. W. Libby and R. N. Whitehurst (eds.), *Marriage and Alternatives: Exploring Intimate Relationships.* Glenview, Ill.: Scott, Foresman, 1977, pp. 161–186. [13]

Glick, P. C. "Remarriage: Some Recent Changes and Variations," *Journal of Family Issues,* 1 (1980), 455–478. [13]

Gochros, H. L., and J. Fischer. *Treat Yourself to a Better Sex Life.* Englewood Cliffs, N.J.: Prentice-Hall, 1980. [6, 10]

Goldberg, A. S., and S. Shiflett. "Goals of Male and Female College Students: Do Traditional Sex Differences Still Exist?" *Sex Roles,* 7 (1981), 1213–1222. [1]

Goldberg, H. *The New Male: From Self-Destruction to Self-Care.* New York: William Morrow, 1979. [1]

Goldman, R. J., and J. D. G. Goldman. "How Children Perceive the Origin of Babies and the Roles of Mothers and Fathers in Procreation: A Cross-National Study," *Child Development,* 53 (1982), 491–504. [11]

Goldstein, M. J., and H. S. Kant. *Pornography and Sexual Deviance.* Berkeley: University of California, 1973. [7]

Goldstein, M. J., H. Kant, L. Judd, C. Rice, and R. Green. "Experience with Pornography: Rapists, Pedophiles, Homosexuals, Transsexuals, and Controls," *Archives of Sexual Behavior,* 1 (1971), 1–15. [16]

Goode, E. *Drugs in American Society.* New York: Knopf, 1972. [18]

Goode, R. S., and M. A. Capone. "Emotional Considerations in the Care of the Gynecologic Cancer Patient." In D. D. Youngs and A. A. Ehrhardt (eds.), *Psychosomatic Obstetrics and Gynecology.* New York: Appleton-Century-Crofts, 1980. [18]

Gordis, R. "Designated Discussion." In W. H. Masters, V. E. Johnson, and R. C. Kolodny (eds.), *Ethical Issues in Sex Therapy and Research.* Boston: Little, Brown, 1977, pp. 32–38. [2]

Gordon, L. *Women's Body, Women's Right: A Social History of Birth Control in America.* New York: Grossman, 1976. [19]

Gordon, S. *The Sexual Adolescent: Communicating with Teenagers About Sex.* Belmont, Calif.: Duxbury Press, 1973. [12]

Gottman, J., C. Notarius, J. Gonso, and H. Markman. *A Couple's Guide to Communication.* Champaign, Ill.: Research Press, 1976. [10]

Granberg, D., and B. W. Granberg. "Abortion Attitudes, 1965–1980: Trends and Determinants," *Family Planning Perspectives,* 12 (1980), 250–261. [19]

Green, C., and J. E. Mantell. "The Need for Management of the Psychosexual Aspects of Mastectomy." In A. Comfort (ed.), *Sexual Consequences of Disability.* Philadelphia: George F. Stickney, 1978, pp. 193–205. [18]

Green, R. *Sexual Identity Conflict in Children and Adults.* New York: Basic Books, 1974. [1, 11]

Green, R. "Sexual Identity of 37 Children Raised by Homosexual or Transsexual Parents," *American Journal of Psychiatry,* 135 (1978), 692–697. [15]

Green, R. "Patterns of Sexual Identity in Childhood: Relationship to Subsequent Sexual Partner Preference." In J. Marmor (ed.), *Homosexual Behavior: A Modern Reappraisal.* New York: Basic Books, 1980, pp. 255–266. [15]

Gross, A. E. "The Male Role and Heterosexual Behavior," *Journal of Social Issues,* 34 (1978), 87–107. [1]

Grossman, F. K., L. S. Eichler, and S. A. Winickoff. *Pregnancy, Birth, and Parenthood.* San Francisco: Jossey-Bass, 1980. [20]

Groth, A. N. "Patterns of Sexual Assault Against Children and Adolescents." In A. W. Burgess, A. N. Groth, L. L. Holmstrom, and S. M. Serdi (eds.), *Sexual Assault of Children and Adolescents.* Lexington, Mass.: Lexington Books, 1978, pp. 3–24. [16]

Groth, A. N., and H. J. Birnbaum. *Men Who Rape: The Psychology of the Offender.* New York: Plenum, 1979. [16]

Guttman, D. "Parenthood: A Key to the Comparative Study of the Life Cycle." In N. Datan and L. H. Ginsberg (eds.), *Life-Span Developmental Psychology: Normative Life Crises.* New York: Academic Press, 1975, pp. 167–184. [1]


Hacker, H. M. "Blabbermouths and Clams: Sex Differences in Self-Disclosure in Same-Sex and Cross-Sex Friendship Dyads," *Psychology of Women Quarterly,* 5 (1981), 385–401. [2]

Hackett, T. P. "The Psychotherapy of Exhibitionists in a Court Clinic Setting," *Seminars in Psychiatry,* 3 (1971), 297–306. [15]

Haeberle, E. J. *The Sex Atlas.* New York: Seabury Press, 1978. [6–9]

Hall, E., M. E. Lamb, and M. Perlmutter. *Child Psychology Today.* New York: Random House, 1982. [11]

Hall, J. E. "Sexuality and the Mentally Retarded." In R. Green (ed.), *Human Sexuality: A Health Practitioner's Text.* Baltimore: Williams & Wilkins, 1975, pp. 181–196. [18]

Halleck, S. L. "Another Response to 'Homosexuality: The Ethical Challenge," *Journal of Consulting and Clinical Psychology,* 44 (1976), 167–170. [9]

Hamburg, D. A., and D. T. Lunde. "Sex Hormones in the Development of Sex Differences in Human Behavior." In E. E. Maccoby (ed.), *The Development of Sex Differences.* Stanford, Calif.: Stanford University Press, 1966, pp. 1–24. [11]

Hamilton, R. *The Herpes Book.* Los Angeles: J. P. Tarcher, 1980. [17]

Hammond, C. B., and W. S. Maxon. "Current Status of Estrogen Therapy for the Menopause," *Fertility and Sterility,* 37 (1982), 5–25. [13]

Harlow, H. F., and M. K. Harlow. "Learning to Love," *American Scientist,* 54 (1966), 244–272. [11]

Harlow, H. F., and M. K. Harlow. "Effects of Various Mother-Infant Relationships on Rhesus Monkey Behavior." In B. M. Foss (ed.), *Determinants of Infant Behavior.* Vol. 4. London: Methuen, 1969, pp. 15–36. [11]

Harris, R., R. S. Good, and L. Pollack. "Sexual Behavior of Gynecologic Cancer Patients," *Archives of Sexual Behavior,* 11 (1982), 503–510. [18]

Hartman, W. E., and M. A. Fithian. *Treatment of Sexual Dysfunction.* 2nd ed. New York: Jason Aronson, 1974. [14]

Hass, A. *Teenage Sexuality.* New York: Macmillan, 1979. [12]

Hatcher, R. A., G. K. Stewart, F. Guest, D. W. Schwartz, and S. A. Jones. *Contraceptive Technology, 1980–1981.* New York: Irvington, 1980. [19]

Hedblom, J. H., and J. J. Hartman. "Research on Lesbianism: Selected Effects of Time, Geographic Location, and Data Collection Technique," *Archives of Sexual Behavior,* 9 (1980), 217–234. [9]

Heim, N. "Sexual Behavior of Castrated Sex Offenders," *Archives of Sexual Behavior,* 10 (1981), 11–19. [4]

Heiman, J. "The Physiology of Erotica," *Psychology Today,* 8 (April 1975), 90–94. [7]

Heiman, J., L. LoPiccolo, and J. LoPiccolo. *Becoming Orgasmic: A Sexual Growth Program for Women.* Englewood Cliffs, N.J.: Prentice-Hall, 1976. [6–7, 10]

Heinrichs, W. L., and G. D. Adamson. "A Practical Approach to the Patient with Dysmenorrhea," *Journal of Reproductive Medicine,* 25 (1980), 236–242. [3]

Hellerstein, H. K., and E. H. Friedman. "Sexual Activity and the Post-Coronary Patient," *Archives of Internal Medicine,* 125 (1970), 987–999. [18]

Hellerstein, H. K., T. P. Hackett, A. A. Kattus, R. Stein, C. L. Witten, and L. Zohman. *Sex and the Heart Patient: Truths and Myths.* New York: Synthesis Communications, 1977. [18]

Henshaw, S. K., J. D. Forrest, E. Sullivan, and C. Tietze. "Abortion Services in the United States, 1979 and 1980," *Family Planning Perspectives,* 14 (1982), 5–15. [19]

Herman, J. L., and L. Hirschman. *Father-Daughter Incest.* Cambridge, Mass.: Harvard University Press, 1981. [16]

Hetherington, E. M., M. Cox, and R. Cox. "Stress and Coping in Divorce: A Focus on Women." In J. E. Gullahorn (ed.), *Psychology and Women: In Transition.* New York: Wiley, 1979, pp. 95–128. [13]

Hiltner, S. "Theological Perspectives on the Ethics of Scientific Investigation and Treatment of Human Sexuality." In W. H. Masters, V. E. Johnson, and R. C. Kolodny (eds.), *Ethical Issues in Sex Therapy and Research.* Boston: Little, Brown, 1977, pp. 20–32. [2]

Hite, S. *The Hite Report.* New York: Macmillan, 1976. [5, 7–8, 14]

Hite, S. *The Hite Report on Male Sexuality.* New York: Knopf, 1981. [2, 4, 8–9, 13–14]

Hoffman, M. "The Male Prostitute." In M. P. Levine (ed.), *Gay Men: The Sociology of Male Homosexuality.* New York: Harper & Row, 1979, pp. 275–284. [16]

Holstrom, L. L., and A. W. Burgess. "Sexual Behavior of Assailants During Reported Rapes," *Archives of Sexual Behavior,* 9 (1980), 427–439. [16]

Holt, L. H., and M. Weber. *The American Medical Association Book of Woman Care.* New York: Random House, 1981. [19, 20]

Hooker, E., interviewed by P. Chance. "Facts That Liberated the Gay Community," *Psychology Today,* 9 (December 1975), 52–55+. [9]

Hoon, P. W., K. Bruce, and B. Kinchloe. "Does the Menstrual Cycle Play a Role in Sexual Arousal?" *Psychophysiology,* 19 (1982), 21–26. [3]

Horvath, T. "Physical Attractiveness: The Influence of Selected Torso Parameters," *Archives of Sexual Behavior,* 10 (1981), 21–24. [6]

Houser, B. B. "An Investigation of the Correlation Between Hormonal Levels in Males and Mood, Behavior, and Physical Discomfort," *Hormones and Behavior,* 12 (1979), 185–197. [4]

Hoyt, M. F. "Primal-Scene Experiences: Quantitative Assessment of an Interview Study," *Archives of Sexual Behavior,* 8 (1979), 225–245. [11]

Hrdy, S. B. *The Woman That Never Evolved.* Cambridge, Mass: Harvard University Press, 1981. [8]

Huelsman, B. R. "An Anthropological View of Clitoral and Other Female Genital Mutilations." In T. R. Lowry and T. S. Lowry (eds.), *The Clitoris.* St. Louis: Warren H. Green, 1976, pp. 111–161. [3]

Huggins, G., M. Vessey, R. Flavel, D. Yeates, and K. McPherson. "Vaginal Spermicides and Outcome of Pregnancy: Findings in a Large Cohort Study," *Contraception,* 25 (1982), 219–230. [19]

Humphreys, L. *Tearoom Trade: Impersonal Sex in Public Restrooms.* Chicago: Aldine, 1970. [9]

Hunt, M. *Sexual Behavior in the 1970's.* New York: Dell, 1974. [7–9, 12–15]

Hunt, M. *Gay: What You Should Know About Homosexuality.* New York: Farrar, Straus & Giroux, 1977. [9]

Hurst, M., and P. S. Summey. "Who Needs Electronic Fetal Monitoring?" *Childbirth Educator,* 1 (Spring 1982), 35–42. [20]

Interprofessional Task Force on Health Care of Women and Children. *The Development of Family-Centered Maternity/Newborn Care in Hospitals.* Chicago: Interprofessional Task Force Secretariat, 1978. [20]

Irving, J. *The World According to Garp.* New York: Dutton, 1978. [15]

James, J. "The Prostitute as Victim." In J. R. Chapman and M. Gates (eds.), *The Victimization of Women.* Beverly Hills, Calif.: Sage, 1978, pp. 175–201. [16]

Johnson, A. G. "On the Prevalence of Rape in the United States," *Signs,* 6 (1980), 136–146. [16]

Johnson, J. H. "Tubal Sterilization and Hysterectomy," *Family Planning Perspectives,* 14 (1982), 28–30. [19]

Johnson, W. R. "The Handicapped: Recreational Sex and Procreational Responsibility." In J. Money and H. Musaph (eds.), *Handbook of Sexology.* Amsterdam: Elsevier/North Holland Biomedical Press, 1977, pp. 933–937. [18]

Jones, H. W., G. S. Jones, M. C. Andrews, A. Acosta, C. Bundren, J. Garcia, B. Sandow, L. Veeck, C. Wilkes, J. Witmyer, J. E. Wortham, and G. Wright. "The Program for In Vitro Fertilization at Norfolk," *Fertility and Sterility,* 38 (July 1982), 14–21. [20]

Justice, B., and R. Justice. *The Broken Taboo: Sex in the Family.* New York: Human Sciences Press, 1979. [16]

Kagan, J. *The Growth of the Child.* New York: Norton, 1978. [11]

Kaplan, H. S. *The New Sex Therapy.* New York: Brunner/Mazel, 1974. [4, 7, 14]

Kaplan, H. S. "Hypoactive Sexual Desire," *Journal of Sex and Marital Therapy,* 3 (1977), 3–9. [14]

Kaplan, H. S. *Disorders of Sexual Desire.* New York: Simon and Schuster, 1979. [5]

Karacan, I., C. J. Hursch, R. L. Williams, and J. I. Thornby. "Some Characteristics of Nocturnal Penile Tumescence in Young Adults," *Archives of General Psychiatry,* 26 (1972), 351–356. [7]

Katz, J. *Gay American History: Lesbians and Gay Men in the U.S.A.* New York: Crowell, 1976. [9]

Katz, S., and M. A. Mazur. *Understanding the Rape Victim: A Synthesis of Research Findings.* New York: Wiley, 1979. [16]

Kay, B., and J. N. Neelley. "Sexuality and the Aging: A Review of Current Literature," *Sexuality and Disability,* 5 (1982), 38–46. [13]

Kaye, H. E., et al. "Homosexuality in Women," *Archives of General Psychiatry,* 17 (1967), 626. [9]

Kedia, K. R., C. Markland, and E. F. Fraley. "Sexual Function After High Retroperitoneal Lymphadenectomy," *Urologic Clinics of North America,* 4 (1977), 523–528. [18]

Kegel, A. H. "Sexual Functions of the Pubococcygeus Muscle," *Western Journal of Surgery,* 60 (1952), 521–524. [6]

Keith, L., and J. Brittain. *Sexually Transmitted Diseases.* Aspen, Colo.: Creative Infomatics, 1978. [17]

Keller, J. F., and A. R. Sack. "Sex Guilt and the Use of Contraception Among Unmarried Women," *Contraception,* 25 (1982), 387–393. [19]

Kelly, J. "The Aging Male Homosexual: Myth and Reality." In M. P. Levine (ed.), *Gay Men: The Sociology of Male Homosexuality.* New York: Harper & Row, 1979, pp. 253–262. [9]

Kelly, J. A., G. G. O'Brien, and R. Hosford. "Sex Roles and Social Skills: Considerations for Interpersonal Adjustment," *Psychology of Women Quarterly,* 5 (1981), 758–766. [1]

Kenney, A. M., J. D. Forrest, and A. Torres. "Storm over Washington: The Parental Notification Proposal," *Family Planning Perspectives,* 14 (1982), 185–197. [19]

Kessel, E., and S. D. Mumford. "Potential Demand for Voluntary Female Sterilization in the 1980s: The Compelling Need for a Nonsurgical Method," *Fertility and Sterility,* 37 (1982), 725–733. [19]

Kesselman, S. "Circumcision Reconsidered," *Childbirth Educator,* 1 (Spring 1982), 43–48. [4]

Kessler, S. J., and W. McKenna. *Gender: An Ethnomethodological Approach.* New York: Wiley, 1978. [1]

Keverne, E. B. "Pheromones and Sexual Behavior." In J. Money and H. Musaph (eds.), *Handbook of Sexology.* Amsterdam: Elsevier/North Holland Biomedical Press, 1977, pp. 413–428. [6]

Kilpatrick, D. G., P. A. Resick, and L. J. Veronen. "Effects of a Rape Experience: A Longitudinal Study," *Journal of Social Issues,* 37 (1981), 105–123. [16]

Kimmel, D. C. "Adult Development and Aging: A Gay Perspective," *Journal of Social Issues,* 34 (1978), 113–130. [1]

King, M., and D. Sobel. "Sex on the College Campus: Current Attitudes and Behavior," *Journal of College Student Personnel,* 16 (1975), 48–65. [12]

Kiniery, G. L. "Technical Virgins: What and Who Are They? A Scientific Investigation." Honors thesis. Rutgers University, 1982. [12]

Kinsey, A. C., W. B. Pomeroy, and C. E. Martin. *Sexual Behavior in the Human Male.* Philadelphia: Saunders, 1948. [1–2, 5, 7–8, 9, 11–14, 16]

Kinsey, A. C., W. B. Pomeroy, C. E. Martin, and P. H. Gebhard. *Sexual Behavior in the Human Female.* Philadelphia: Saunders, 1953. [1–2, 5, 7–9, 11–14]

Klein, F. *The Bisexual Option.* New York: Arbor House, 1978. [9]

Knox, D. H., Jr., and M. J. Sporakowski. "Attitudes of College Students Toward Love," *Journal of Marriage and the Family,* 30 (1968), 638–642. [2]

Koch, J. P. "The Prentif Contraceptive Cervical Cap: Acceptability Aspects and Their Implications for Future Cap Design," *Contraception,* 25 (1982a), 161–173. [19]

Koch, J. P. "The Prentif Contraceptive Cervical Cap: A Contemporary Study of Its Clinical Safety and Effectiveness," *Contraception,* 25 (1982b), 135–159. [19]

Koff, W. C. "Marihuana and Sexual Activity," *Journal of Sex Research,* 10 (1974), 194–204. [18]

Kohlberg, L. "A Cognitive-Developmental Analysis of Children's Sex Role Concepts and Attitudes." In E. E. Maccoby (ed.), *The Development of Sex Differences.* Stanford, Calif.: Stanford University Press, 1966, pp. 82–173. [11]

Kolodny, R. C. "Evaluating Sex Therapy: Process and Outcome at the Masters and Johnson Institute," *Journal of Sex Research,* 17 (1981), 301–318. [14]

Kolodny, R. C., W. H. Masters, J. Hendryx, and G. Toro. "Plasma Testosterone Levels and Semen Analysis in Male Homosexuals," *New England Journal of Medicine,* 285 (1971), 1170–1174. [9]

Kolodny, R. C., W. H. Masters, and V. E. Johnson. *Textbook of Sexual Medicine.* Boston: Little, Brown, 1979, [4, 18]

Konner, M., and C. Worthman. "Nursing Frequency, Gonadal Function, and Birth Spacing Among !Kung Hunter-Gatherers," *Science,* 207 (1980), 788–791. [20]

Koss, M., and C. Oros. "Hidden Rape: A Survey of the Incidence of Sexual Aggression

Among University Males." Paper presented at the annual meeting of the Midwestern Psychological Association. St. Louis, 1980. [16]

Kradjian, R. M. *Breast Lumps: A Guide to Understanding Breast Problems and Breast Surgery.* Daly City, Calif.: Physicians Art Service, 1980. [6]

Kraemer, H. C., H. B. Becker, H. K. Brodie, C. H. Doering, R. H. Moos, and D. A. Hamburg. "Orgasmic Frequency and Plasma Testosterone Levels in Normal Human Males," *Archives of Sexual Behavior,* 5 (1976), 125–132. [4]

Kriss, R. "Self-Image and Sexuality After Mastectomy." In D. G. Bullard and S. E. Knight (eds.), *Sexuality and Physical Disability: Personal Perspectives.* St. Louis: C. V. Mosby, 1981, pp. 185–192. [18]

Kuhn, M. E. "Sexual Myths Surrounding the Aging." In W. W. Oaks, G. A. Melchiode, and I. Ficher (eds.), *Sex and the Life Cycle.* New York: Grune and Stratton, 1976, pp. 117–134. [13]


Ladas, A. K., B. Whipple, and J. D. Perry. *The G Spot and Other Recent Discoveries About Human Sexuality.* New York: Holt, Rinehart and Winston, 1982. [3, 5]

Ladner, J. A. *Tomorrow's Tomorrow: The Black Woman.* New York: Doubleday, 1971. [2]

Lamaze, F. *Painless Childbirth: The Lamaze Method.* New York: Simon and Schuster, 1972. [20]

Lamb, M. E., and J. J. Campos. *Development in Infancy.* New York: Random House, 1982. [11]

Langevin, R., D. Paitich, G. Ramsay, C. Anderson, J. Kamrad, S. Pope, G. Geller, L. Pearl, and S. Newman. "Experimental Studies of the Etiology of Genital Exhibitionism," *Archives of Sexual Behavior,* 8 (1979), 307–331. [15]

Lanson, L. T. *Woman to Woman.* New York: Knopf, 1975. [3]

LaPlante, M. N., N. McCormick, and G. G. Brannigan. "Living the Sexual Script: College Students' Views of Influences in Sexual Encounters," *Journal of Sex Research,* 16 (1980), 338–355. [12]

LaRocco, S. A., and D. F. Polit. "Women's Knowledge About the Menopause," *Nursing Research,* 29 (1980), 10–13. [13]

Lasagna, L. *The VD Epidemic.* Philadelphia: Temple University Presss, 1975. [17]

Lawrence, D. H. *Lady Chatterley's Lover.* New York: Grove Press, 1959 (orig. pub. 1928), [5, 6]

Laws, D. R., J. Meyer, and M. L. Holmen. "Reduction of Sadistic Sexual Arousal by Olfactory Aversion: A Case Study," *Behavior Research and Therapy,* 16 (1978), 281–285. [15]

Laws, J. L., and P. Schwartz. *Sexual Scripts: The Social Construction of Female Sexuality.* Washington, D.C.: University Press of America, 1977. [2, 13, 20]

Layde, P. M., H. W. Ory, and J. J. Schlesselman. "The Risk of Myocardial Infarction in Former Users of Oral Contraceptives." *Family Planning Perspectives,* 14 (1982), 78–80. [19]

Leary, W. E. "Drug Can Stop Infant Herpes," *Reporter-Dispatch,* November 9, 1980. [17]

Leboyer, F. *Birth Without Violence,* New York: Knopf, 1975. [20]

Leiber, L., M. M. Plumb, M. O. Gerstenzang, and J. Holland. "The Communication of Affection Between Cancer Patients and Their Spouses," *Psychosomatic Medicine,* 38 (1976), 376–389. [18]

Leiblum, S. R., G. Bachmann, E. Kenmann, D. Colburn, and L. Swartzman. "Vaginal Atrophy in the Post-Menopausal Woman: The Importance of Sexual Activity and Hormones," *Journal of the American Medical Association* 249 (1983), 2195–2198. [13]

Leiblum, S. R., and L. A. Pervin. "Introduction: The Development of Sex Therapy from a Sociocultural Perspective." In S. R. Leiblum and L. A. Pervin (eds.), *Principles and Practices of Sex Therapy.* New York: Guilford Press, 1980, pp. 1–24. [14]

Leiblum, S. R., L. A. Pervin, and E. H. Campbell. "The Treatment of Vaginismus: Success and Failure." In S. R. Leiblum and L. A. Pervin (eds.), *Principles and Practices of Sex Therapy*. New York: Guilford Press, 1980, pp. 167–194. [14]

Lenz, R., and B. Chaves. "Becoming Active Partners." In D. G. Bullard and S. E. Knight (eds.), *Sexuality and Physical Disability: Personal Perspectives*. St. Louis: C. V. Mosby, 1981, pp. 65–71. [18]

Lerner, R. M., and G. B. Spanier. *Adolescent Development: A Life-Span Perspective*. New York: McGraw–Hill, 1980. [12]

Levine, A. S. "The Epidemic of Acquired Immune Dysfunction in Homosexual Men and Its Sequelae—Opportunistic Infections, Kaposi's Sarcoma, and Other Malignancies: An Update and Interpretation," *Cancer Treatment Reports, 66* (1982), 1391–1395. [17]

Levine, S. B., and D. P. Agle. "The Effectiveness of Sex Therapy for Chronic Secondary Psychological Impotence," *Journal of Sex and Marital Therapy, 4* (1978), 235–258. [14]

Levine, S. B., and L. M. Lothstein. "Transsexualism or the Gender Dysphoria Syndromes," *Journal of Sex and Marital Therapy, 7* (1981), 85–113. [1, 15]

Levitt, E. E., and R. E. Duffy. "Objective Estimates of the Duration of Sexual Behaviors: A Laboratory Analog Study." Paper presented at the International Academy of Sex Research. Bloomington, Indiana, August 1977. [8]

Lewis, M. L. "The History of Female Sexuality in the United States." In M. Kirkpatrick (ed.), *Women's Sexual Development: Explorations of Inner Space*. New York: Plenum, 1980, pp. 19–38. [1]

Lewis, R. A. "Emotional Intimacy Among Men," *Journal of Social Issues, 34* (1978), 108–121. [2]

Lilius, H. G., E. J. Valtonen, and J. Wikström. "Sexual Problems in Patients Suffering from Multiple Sclerosis," *Journal of Chronic Diseases, 29* (1976), 643–647. [18]

Littman, K. J. "Contraception: The Cervical Cap—Back to Basics," *Ms.,* (October 1980), 91–93. [19]

Loftus, E. *Memory*. Reading, Mass.: Addison-Wesley, 1980. [9]

Loh, W. D. "Q: What Has Reform of Rape Legislation Wrought? A.: Truth in Criminal Labeling," *Journal of Social Issues, 37* (1981), 28–52. [16]

LoPiccolo, J. "Direct Treatment of Sexual Dysfunction in the Couple." In J. Money and J. Musaph (ed.), *Handbook of Sexology*. Amsterdam: Elsevier/North Holland Press, 1977, pp. 1227–1244. [14]

LoPiccolo, J., and W. C. Lobitz. "The Role of Masturbation in the Treatment of Orgasmic Dysfunction," *Archives of Sexual Behavior, 2* (1973), 153–164. [14]

LoPiccolo, L. "Low Sexual Desire." In S. R. Leiblum and L. A. Pervin (eds.), *Principles and Practices of Sex Therapy*. New York: Guilford Press, 1980, pp. 29–64. [14]

Lothstein, L. M. "The Postsurgical Transsexual: Empirical and Theoretical Considerations," *Archives of Sexual Behavior, 9* (1980), 547–564. [15]


Maccoby, E. E., and C. N. Jacklin. *The Psychology of Sex Differences*. Stanford, Calif.: Stanford University Press, 1974. [1]

MacFarlane, K. "Sexual Abuse of Children." In J. R. Chapman and M. Gates (eds.), *The Victimization of Women*. Beverly Hills, Calif.: Sage, 1978, pp. 81–109. [16]

Mackey, F. G., "Sexuality and Heart Disease." In A. Comfort (ed.), *Sexual Consequences of Disability*. Philadelphia: George F. Stickley, 1978, pp. 107–120. [18]

MacKinnon, C. A. *Sexual Harassment of Working Women*. New Haven, Conn.: Yale University Press, 1979. [16]

Macklin, E. D. "Nontraditional Family Forms: A Decade of Research," *Journal of Marriage and the Family, 42* (1980), 905–922. [13]

Magee, M. "Psychogenic Impotence: A Critical Review," *Journal of Urology,* 15 (1980), 5–14. [14]

Mahoney, E. R. "Religiosity and Sexual Behavior Among Heterosexual College Students," *Journal of Sex Research,* 16 (1980), 97–113. [12]

Malamuth, N. M. "Rape Proclivity Among Males," *Journal of Social Issues,* 37 (1981), 138–157. [16]

Malatesta, V. J., R. H. Pollack, and T. D. Crotty. "Alcohol Effects on the Orgasmic Response in Human Females." Paper presented at the annual meeting of the Psychonomic Society. Phoenix, Arizona, November 1979a. [18]

Malatesta, V. J., R. H. Pollack, W. A. Wilbanks, and H. E. Adams. "Alcohol Effects on the Orgasmic-Ejaculatory Response in Human Males," *Journal of Sex Research,* 15 (1979b), 101–197. [18]

Mamay, P. D., and R. L. Simpson. "Three Female Roles in Television Commercials," *Sex Roles,* 7 (1981), 1223–1232. [1]

Manaster, G. J. *Adolescent Development and the Life Tasks.* Boston: Allyn & Bacon, 1977. [12]

Mann, J. "Retarded Ejaculation and Treatment." Paper presented at the International Congress of Medical Sexology. Rome, October 1976. [14]

Marks, C. "Positions of Intercourse in Three Cultures." Paper presented at the International Congress of Medical Sexology. Rome, October 1978. [8]

Marmor, J. "Homosexuality and Sexual Orientation Disturbances." In B. J. Sadock, H. I. Kaplan, and A. M. Freedman (eds.), *The Sexual Experience.* Baltimore: Williams & Wilkins, 1976, pp. 374–391. [9]

Marshall, D. S. "Sexual Behavior on Mangaia." In D. S. Marshall and R. C. Suggs (eds.), *Human Sexual Behavior.* New York: Basic Books, 1971, pp. 103–162. [2, 8]

Martin, C. E. "Sexual Activity in the Aging Male." In J. Money and H. Musaph (eds.), *Handbook of Sexology.* Amsterdam: Elsevier/North Holland Biomedical Press, 1977, pp. 813–824. [13]

Mastalli, G. L. "Appendix: The Legal Context," *Harvard Business Review,* 59 (March–April 1981), 94. [16]

Masters, R. E. L. *Sexual Self-Stimulation.* Los Angeles: Sherbourne Press, 1967. [7]

Masters, W. H., and V. E. Johnson. *Human Sexual Response.* Boston: Little, Brown, 1966. [2–5, 13, 20]

Masters, W. H., and V. E. Johnson, interviewed by M. H. Hall. "A Conversation with Masters and Johnson," *Psychology Today,* 3 (July 1969), 50–54+. [11]

Masters, W. H., and V. E. Johnson. *Human Sexual Inadequacy.* Boston: Little, Brown, 1970. [7–8, 10, 13, 14]

Masters, W. H., and V. E. Johnson. *The Pleasure Bond.* Boston: Little, Brown, 1975. [10]

Masters, W. H., and V. E. Johnson. *Homosexuality in Perspective.* Boston: Little, Brown, 1979. [9]

May, R. A. *Freedom and Destiny.* New York: Norton, 1981. [2]

McCauley, E., and A. A. Ehrhardt. "Female Sexual Response: Hormonal and Behavioral Interactions," *Primary Care,* 3 (1976), 455–476. [3]

McCormick, E. P., R. L. Johnson, H. L. Friedman, and H. P. David. "Psychosocial Aspects of Fertility Regulation." In J. Money and H. Musaph (eds.), *Handbook of Sexology.* Amsterdam: Elsevier/North Holland Biomedical Press, 1977, pp. 621–653. [19]

McFarland, L. Z. "Comparative Anatomy of the Clitoris," In T. R. Lowry and T. S. Lowry (eds.), *The Clitoris.* St. Louis: Warren H. Green, 1976, pp. 22–34. [3]

McGregor, I. A. "Skin Grafts to the Vulva." In C. E. Horton (ed.), *Plastic and Reconstructive Surgery of the Genital Area.* Boston: Little, Brown, 1973, pp. 605–612. [18]

McKoewn, T. *The Modern Rise of Population.* New York: Academic Press, 1977. [1]

McMullen, S., and R. C. Rosen. "The Use of Self-Administered Masturbation Training in the Treatment of Primary Orgasmic Dysfunction," *Journal of Consulting and Clinical Psychology,* 47 (1979), 912–918. [7, 14]

McWhirter, D. P., and A. M. Mattison. "Treatment of Sexual Dysfunction in Homosexual Male Couples." In S. L. Leiblum and L. A. Pervin (eds.), *Principles and Practice of Sex Therapy.* New York: Guilford Press, 1980. [9]

Mead, M., and N. Newton. "Cultural Patterning of Perinatal Behavior." In S. A. Richardson and A. F. Guttmacher (eds.), *Childbearing: Its Social and Psychological Factors.* Baltimore: Williams & Wilkins, 1967. [20]

Meiselman, K. C. *Incest.* San Francisco: Jossey-Bass, 1978. [16]

Menning, B. E. "Psychological Issues in Infertility." In B. L. Blum (ed.), *Psychological Aspects of Pregnancy, Birthing, and Bonding.* New York: Human Sciences Press, 1980, pp. 33–55. [20]

Messenger, J. C. "Sex and Repression in an Irish Folk Community." In D. S. Marshall and R. D. Suggs (ed.), *Human Sexual Behavior.* New York: Basic Books, 1971, pp. 3–37. [6]

Meyer, J. K., and D. J. Reter. "Sex Reassignment: Follow-up," *Archives of General Psychiatry,* 36 (1979), 1010–1015. [15]

Meyer-Bahlburg, H. F. L. "Sex Hormones and Male Homosexuality in Comparative Perspective," *Archives of Sexual Behavior,* 6 (1977), 297–325. [9]

Meyer-Bahlburg, H. F. L. "Sex Hormones and Female Sexuality: A Critical Examination," *Archives of Sexual Behavior,* 8 (1979), 101–119. [9]

Miller, N. E., and J. Dollard. *Social Learning and Imitation.* New Haven, Conn.: Yale University Press, 1941. [11]

Miller, P. Y., and W. E. Simon. "The Development of Sexuality in Adolescence." In J. Adelson (ed.), *Handbook of Adolescent Psychology.* New York: Wiley-Interscience, 1980, pp. 383–407. [12]

Mills, J. L., S. Harlap, and E. E. Harley. "Should Coitus Late in Pregnancy Be Discouraged?" *The Lancet,* 2 (1981), 136–138. [20]

Mohr, J. W., R. E. Turner, and M. B. Jerry. *Pedophilia and Exhibitionism.* Toronto: University of Toronto Press, 1964. [16]

Money, J. "The American Heritage of Three Traditions of Pair-Bonding: Mediterranean, Nordic, and Slave." In J. Money and H. Musaph (eds.), *Handbook of Sexology.* Amsterdam: Elsevier/North Holland Biomedical Press, 1977a, pp. 497–504. [2]

Money, J. "Determinants of Human Gender Identity/Role." In J. Money and H. Musaph (eds.), *Handbook of Sexology.* Amsterdam: Elsevier/North Holland Biomedical Press, 1977b, pp. 57–79. [11]

Money, J. *Love and Love Sickness: The Science of Sex, Gender Difference, and Pair-Bonding.* Baltimore: Johns Hopkins University Press, 1980. [2, 6, 15]

Money, J. "Paraphilias: Phyletic Origins of Erotosexual Dysfunction," *International Journal of Mental Health,* 10 (1981), 75–109. [15]

Money, J., and R. G. Bennett. "Postadolescent Paraphiliac Sex Offenders: Antiandrogenic and Counseling Therapy Follow-Up," *International Journal of Mental Health,* 10 (1981), 122–133. [15]

Money, J., and C. Bohmer. "Prison Sexology: Two Personal Accounts of Masturbation, Homosexuality, and Rape," *Journal of Sex Research,* 16 (1980), 258–266. [16]

Money, J., and A. A. Ehrhardt. *Man and Woman, Boy and Girl.* Baltimore: Johns Hopkins University Press, 1972. [1, 9, 11–12]

Montagu, A. *The Humanization of Man.* New York: Grove Press, 1962. [2]

Montagu, A. *Touching: The Human Significance of the Skin.* New York: Columbia University Press, 1971. [8, 11]

Moos, R. H. "A Typology of Menstrual Cycle Symptoms," *American Journal of Obstetrics and Gynecology,* 103 (1969), 390–402. [3]

Moreland, J. "Age and Change in the Adult Male Sex Role," *Sex Roles,* 6 (1980), 807–818. [1]

Morin, S. F. "Heterosexual Bias in Psychological Research on Lesbianism and Male Homosexuality," *American Psychologist,* 32 (1977), 629–639. [9]

Morin, S. F., and E. M. Garfinkle. "Male Homophobia," *Journal of Social Issues,* 34 (1978), 29–47. [1]

Morneau, R. H., Jr., and R. R. Rockwell. *Sex, Motivation, and the Criminal Offender.* Springfield, Ill.: Charles C Thomas, 1980. [15]

Morokoff, P. "Determinants of Female Orgasm." In J. LoPiccolo and L. LoPiccolo (eds.), *Handbook of Sex Therapy.* New York: Plenum, 1978, pp. 147–166. [14]

Morris, N. M., and J. R. Udry. "Pheromonal Influences on Human Sexual Behavior: An Experimental Search," *Journal of Biosocial Science,* 1978. [13]

Mosher, D. L. "Sex Guilt and Sex Myths in College Men and Women," *Journal of Sex Research,* 15 (1979), 224–234. [12]

Mosher, D. L., and H. J. Cross "Sex Guilt and Premarital Sexual Experiences of College Students," *Journal of Consulting and Clinical Psychology,* 36 (1971), 27–32. [12]

Mosher, D. L., and B. B. White. "Effects of Committed or Casual Erotic Guided Imagery on Females' Subjective Sexual Arousal and Emotional Response," *Journal of Sex Research,* 16 (1980), 273–299. [7]

Moss, H. A. "Early Sex Differences and Mother-Infant Interaction." In R. C. Friedman, R. M. Richcart, and R. L. Van de Wiele (eds.), *Sex Differences in Behavior.* New York: Wiley, 1974, pp. 149–164. [11]

Murdock, G. P. *Social Structure.* New York: Macmillan, 1949. [16]

Murstein, B. I. "Swinging, or Comarital Sex." In B. I. Murstein (ed.), *Exploring Intimate Life Styles.* New York: Springer, 1978, pp. 109–130. [13]

Murstein, B. I. "Mate Selection in the 1970s," *Journal of Marriage and the Family,* 42 (1980), 777–792. [13]

Naeye, R. L. "Coitus and Associated Amniotic-Fluid Infections," *New England Journal of Medicine,* 22 (1979), 22–27. [20]

Napoli, M. "Breast Self-Examination: The Promises and Premises—As Handed Down by the Cancer Establishment." Paper presented at the annual meeting of the American Public Health Association. Detroit, October 21, 1980. [6]

Narus, L. R., Jr., and J. L. Fischer. "Strong but Not Silent: A Reexamination of Expressivity in the Relationships of Men," *Sex Roles,* 8 (1982), 159–168. [1]

National Academy of Sciences, Institute of Medicine. *Marijuana and Health.* Washington, D.C.: National Academy Press, 1982. [18]

National Commission on the Causes and Prevention of Violence. *Crimes of Violence.* Vol. 2. Washington, D.C.: U.S. Government Printing Office, 1969. [16]

Nawy, H. "The San Francisco Erotic Marketplace," *Technical Reports of the Commission on Obscenity and Pornography.* Vol. 4. Washington, D.C.: U.S. Government Printing Office, 1970. [16]

Neubeck, G. *Extramarital Relations.* Englewood Cliffs, N.J.: Prentice-Hall, 1969. [13]

Neugarten, B. L., interviewed by E. Hall. "Acting One's Age: New Rules for Old," *Psychology Today,* 13 (April 1980). 66–80. [1]

Neugarten, B. L., V. Wood, R. J. Kraines, and B. Loomis. "Women's Attitude Toward the Menopause," *Vita Humana,* 6 (1963), 140–151. [13]

Newton, N. "Putting the Child Back in Childbirth," *Psychology Today,* 9 (August 1975), 24–25. [20]

Newton, N. "The Role of the Oxytocin Reflexes in Three Interpersonal Reproductive Acts: Coitus, Birth, and Breastfeeding." In L. Carenz, P. Pancheri, and L. Zichella (eds.), *Clinical Psychoneuroendocrinology in Reproduction: Proceedings of the Serono Symposia.* Vol. 22. London: Academic Press, 1978, pp. 411–418. [20]

Newton, N., and C. Modahl. "Pregnancy: The Closest Human Relationship," *Human Nature,* 1 (March 1978), 40–49. [20]

*New York Times.* "Judge Reduces Award in Case of Sexual Harassment on Job," August 30, 1982, p. A15. [16]

*New York Times.* "Death Benefit Voted for Homosexual's Lover," November 11, 1982, p. A26. [9]

Nichols, M., and S. R. Leiblum. "Lesbianism as Personal Identity and Social Role: Conceptual and Clinical Issues," *Journal of Sex and Marital Therapy* (in press). [9]

Nowinski, J. *Becoming Satisfied: A Man's Guide to Sexual Fulfillment.* Englwood Cliffs, N.J.: Prentice-Hall, 1980. [6, 10]

O'Connor, J. F. "Sexual Problems, Therapy, and Prognostic Factors." In J. K. Meyer (ed.), *Clinical Management of Sexual Disorders.* Baltimore: Williams & Wilkins, 1976, pp. 74–98. [14]

Offer, D., E. Ostrov, and K. I. Howard. *The Adolescent: A Psychological Self-Portrait.* New York: Basic Books, 1981. [12]

Ory, H. W. "The Noncontraceptive Health Benefits from Oral Contraceptive Use," *Family Planning Perspectives,* 14 (1982), 182–184. [19]

Ostrow, D. G., et al. "Preliminary Report on the Task Force on Vaccination Strategies for Sexually Transmitted Hepatitis B Infection," *Sexually Transmitted Diseases,* 9 (1982), 151–153. [17]

Paige, K. E. "Women Learn to Sing the Menstrual Blues." In J. L. McCary and D. R. Copeland (eds.), *Modern Views of Human Sexual Behavior.* Chicago: Science Research Associates, 1976, pp. 109–115. [3]

Paige, K. E., and J. M. Paige. "The Politics of Birth Practices: A Strategic Analysis," *American Sociological Review,* 38 (1973), 663–676. [20]

Parfitt, R. R. *The Birth Primer.* Philadelphia: Runnin Press, 1977. [20]

Parlee, M. B. "The Premenstrual Syndrome." In S. Cox (ed.), *Female Psychology: The Emerging Self.* Chicago: Science Research Associates, 1976. [3]

Pear, R. "Another Judge Bars Birth-Control Rule for Minors," *New York Times,* February 19, 1983a. [19]

Pear, R. "F.D.A. Approves New Sponge Contraceptive," *New York Times,* April 7, 1983b. [19]

Pelfrey, R. J., J. W. Overstreet, and E. L. Lewis. "Abnormalities of Sperm Morphology in Cases of Persistent Infertility After Vasectomy Reversal," *Fertility and Sterility,* 38 (1982), 112–114. [19]

Peplau, L. A., Z. Rubin, and C. T. Hill. "Sexual Intimacy in Dating Relationships," *Journal of Social Issues,* 33 (1977), 86–109. [2]

Perlmutter, L. H., T. Engel, and C. J. Sager. "The Incest Taboo: Loosened Sexual Boundaries in Remarried Families," *Journal of Sex and Marital Therapy,* 8 (1982), 83–95. [16]

Perry, J. D., and B. Whipple. "Pelvic Muscle Strength of Female Ejaculators: Evidence in Suport of a New Theory of Orgasm," *Journal of Sex Research,* 17 (1981), 22–39. [5]

Peterman, D. J., C. A. Ridley, and S. M. Anderson. "A Comparison of Cohabiting and Noncohabiting College Students," *Journal of Marriage and the Family,* 36 (May 1974), 344–354. [12]

Petersen, A. C., and B. Taylor. "The Biological Approach to Adolescence: Biological Change and Psychological Adaptation." In J. Adelson (ed.), *Handbook of Adolescent Psychology.* New York: Wiley-Interscience, 1980, pp. 117–155. [12]

Petersen, J. R., A. Kretchmer, B. Nellis, J. Lever, and R. Hertz. "The *Playboy* Readers' Sex Survey," Part One, *Playboy,* 30 (January 1983), 108, 241–250. [13]

Phillips, D., and R. Judd. *Sexual Confidence.* New York: Bantam, 1982. [10]

Phillips, S., S. King, and L. DuBois. "Spontaneous Activities of Female Versus Male Newborns," *Child Development,* 49 (1978), 590–597. [11]

Phipps, W. E. *The Sexuality of Jesus.* New York: Harper & Row, 1973. [2]

Pirke, K. M., G. Kockott, and F. Dittmen. "Psychosexual Stimulation and Plasma Testosterone in Men," *Archives of Sexual Behavior,* 3 (1974), 577–584. [4]

Plummer, K. *Sexual Stigma: An Interactionist Account.* London: Routledge & Kegan Paul, 1975. [15]

Prial, F. J. "More Women Work at Traditional Male Jobs," *New York Times,* November 15, 1982, pp. Al, C20. [1]

Pritchard, J. A., and P. C. MacDonald. *Obstetrics.* 15th ed. New York: Appleton-Century-Crofts, 1976. [20]

Purvis, K., B. M. Landgren, Z. Cekan, and E. Diczfalusy. "Endocrine Effects of Masturbation in Men," *Journal of Endocrinology,* 70, (1976), 439–444. [4]


Rachman, S. "Sexual Fetishism: An Experimental Analogue," *Psychological Record,* 16 (1966), 293–296. [15]

Rada, R. T. "Psychological Factors in Rapist Behavior." In R. T. Rada (ed.), *Clinical Aspects of the Rapist.* New York: Grune and Stratton, 1978, pp. 21–58. [16]

Rada, R. T., D. R. Laws, and R. Kellner, "Plasma Testosterone Levels in the Rapist," *Psychosomatic Medicine,* 38 (1976), 257–268. [16]

Rasmussen, P. K., and L. L. Kuhn. "The New Masseuse: Play for Pay." In C. Warren (ed.), *Sexuality: Encounters, Identities, and Relationships.* Beverly Hills, Calif.: Sage, 1977, pp. 11–32. [16]

Reedy, M. N., J. E. Birren, and K. W. Schaie. "Age and Sex Differences in Satisfying Love Relationships Across the Adult Life Span," *Human Development,* 24 (1981), 52–66. [13]

Reid, R. L., and S. S. C. Yen. "Premenstrual Syndrome," *American Journal of Obstetrics and Gynecology,* 139 (1981), 85–104. [3]

Reik, T. *Sex in Men and Women: Its Emotional Variations.* New York: Noonday Press, 1960. [1]

Reinisch, J. M. "Prenatal Exposure to Synthetic Progestins Increases Potential for Aggression in Humans," *Science,* 211 (1981), 1171–1173. [1, 11]

Reinisch, J. M., R. Gandelman, and F. S. Speigel. "Prenatal Influences on Cognitive Abilities: Human Genetic and Endocrine Syndromes." In M. A. Wittig and A. C. Peterson (eds.), *Sex-Related Differences in Cognitive Functioning.* New York: Academic Press, 1979, pp. 215–239. [1]

Reiss, A. J. "The Social Integration of Queers and Peers," *Social Problems,* 9 (1961), 102–120. [12]

Reiss, I. L. "Changing Sociosexual Mores." In J. Money and H. Musaph (eds.), *Handbook of Sexology.* Amsterdam: Elsevier/North Holland Biomedical Press, 1977, pp. 311–324. [12]

Renshaw, D. C. "Impotence in Diabetics," *Diseases of the Nervous System,* 36 (1975), 369–371. [18]

Renshaw, D. C. "Stroke and Sex." In A. Comfort (ed.), *Sexual Consequences of Disability.* Philadelphia: George F. Stickley, 1978, pp. 121–131. [18]

Resick, P. A., K. S. Calhoun, B. M. Atkeson, and E. M. Ellis. "Social Adjustment in Victims of Sexual Assault," *Journal of Consulting and Clinical Psychology,* 49 (1981), 705–712. [16]

Reynolds , B. S. "Psychological Treatment Models and Outcome Results for Erectile Dysfunction: A Critical Review," *Psychological Bulletin,* 84 (1977), 1218–1238. [14]

Rich, A. *Of Woman Born.* New York: Bantam Books, 1977. [20]

Rindfuss, R., and C. F. Westoff. "The Initiation of Contraception," *Demography,* 11 (1974), 75–87. [19]

Robbins, M., and G. D. Jensen. "Multiple Orgasm in Males," *Journal of Sex Research,* 14 (1978), 21–26. [5]

Roberts, E. J. "Sex Education Versus Sexual Learning." In M. Kirkpatrick (ed.), *Women's Sexual Development: Explorations of Inner Space.* New York: Plenum, 1980, pp. 239–250. [1]

Roberts, E. J. "Children's Sexual Learning: A Report on the Project on Human Sexual Development, 1974–1980." Doctoral dissertation. Harvard University, 1982. [11, 12]

Roberts, E. J., D. Kline, and J. H. Gagnon. *Family Life and Sexual Learning.* Vol. 1. Cambridge, Mass.: Population Education, Inc., 1978. [12]

Roberts, J. "Which Position for the First Stage?" *Childbirth Educator,* 1 (Summer 1982), 35–41. [20]

Robertson, N. "Toxic Shock," *New York Times Magazine,* September 12, 1982, pp. 30–33+. [3]

Robinson, P. *The Modernization of Sex.* New York: Harper & Row, 1976. [5]

Romalis, C. "Taking Care of the Little Woman: Father-Physician Relations During Pregnancy and Childbirth." In S. Romalis (ed.) *Childbirth: Alternatives to Medical Control.* Austin: University of Texas Press, 1981, pp. 92–121. [20]

Romalis, S. "Overview." In S. Romalis (ed.), *Childbirth: Alternatives to Medical Control.* Austin: University of Texas Press, 1981, pp. 3–32. [20]

Rose, R. M. "Plasma Testosterone Levels in the Male Rhesus: Influences of Sexual and Social Stimuli," *Science,* 178 (1972), 643–645. [4]

Rosebury, T. *Microbes and Morals.* New York: Viking, 1971. [17]

Rosen, L. J., and R. C. Rosen. "How Long Should a Man Last?" *Forum,* July 1977 [8]

Rosen, R. C. "Suppression of Penile Tumescence by Instrumental Conditioning," *Psychosomatic Medicine,* 35 (1973), 509–514. [5]

Rosen, R. C. "Current Research on the Psychophysiology of Sexual Response." Paper presented at the Society for the Scientific Study of Sex. New York, November 1981. [5]

Rosen, R. C. "Clinical Issues in the Assessment and Treatment of Impotence: A New Look at an Old Problem," *The Behavior Therapist* 6 (1983), 81–85. [14]

Rosen, R. C., and E. S. Gendel. "Sexual Problems: Current Approaches in Primary Care Practice," *Postgraduate Medicine,* 69 (1981) 127–134. [14]

Rosen, R. C., and F. J. Keefe. "The Measurement of Human Penile Tumescence," *Psychophysiology,* 45 (1978), 366–376. [15]

Rosen, R. C., and S. Kopel. "The Use of Plethysmography and Biofeedback in the Treatment of a Transvestite-Exhibitionist," *Journal of Consulting and Clinical Psychology,* 45 (1977), 908–916. [15]

Rosen, R. C., and S. R. Leiblum. "Unequal Sex Drives—Helping Mates Match Up," *Sexology,* 42 (1976), 11–16. [10, 14]

Rosen, R. C., and S. R. Leiblum. "Current Perspectives on Sexual Desire." Paper presented at the Society for Scientific Study of Sex. San Francisco, November 1982. [11]

Rosen, R. C., D. Shapiro, and G. E. Schwartz. "Voluntary Control of Penile Tumescence," *Psychosomatic Medicine,* 37 (1975), 479–483. [5]

Rossi, A. S. "Maternalism, Sexuality, and the New Feminism." In J. Zubin and J. Money (eds.), *Contemporary Sexual Behavior: Critical Issue in the 1970s*. Baltimore: Johns Hopkins University Press, 1973, pp. 145–173. [20]

Roth, P. *Portnoy's Complaint*. New York: Random House, 1967. [7]

Rothman, S. M. *Woman's Proper Place*. New York: Basic Books, 1978. [1]

Rubin, L. *Worlds of Pain: Life in the Working Class Family*. New York: Basic Books, 1976. [1]

Rubin, R. T., J. M. Reinisch, and R. F. Haskett. "Postnatal Gonadal Steroid Effects on Human Behavior," *Science,* 211 (1981), 1318–1324. [4, 11]

Rubin, Z., L. A. Peplau, and C. T. Hill. "Loving and Leaving: Sex Differences in Romantic Attachments," *Sex Roles,* 7 (1981), 821–835. [2]

Rubinstein, C. "Wellness Is All," *Psychology Today,* 16 (October 1982), 28–37. [Part VI Intro]

Rubinstein, C., P. Shaver, and L. A. Peplau. "Loneliness," *Human Nature,* 2 (February 1979), 58–65. [13]

Ruble, D. N., T. Balaban, and J. Cooper. "Gender Constancy and the Effects of Sex-Typed Televised Toy Commercials," *Child Development,* 52 (1981), 667–673. [11]

Ruble, D. N., and J. Brooks-Gunn. "The Experience of Menarche," *Child Development,* 53 (1982), 1557–1566. [12]

Russell, D. E. H. *Rape in Marriage*. New York: Macmillan, 1982. [16]

Rytting, M. B. "Sex or Intimacy: Male and Female Versions of Heterosexual Relationships." Paper presented at the meeting of the Midwestern Psychological Association. Chicago, May 1976. [1]


Sagarin, E. "Power to the Peephole." In L. Gross (ed.), *Sexual Behavior: Current Issues*. Flushing, N.Y.: Spectrum Publications, 1974, p. 205–214. [15]

Sage, W. "Inside the Colossal Closet." In M. P. Levine (ed.), *Gay Men: The Sociology of Male Homosexuality*. New York: Harper & Row, 1979, pp. 148–163. [9]

Sanday, P. R. "The Socio-Cultural Context of Rape: A Cross-Cultural Study," *Journal of Social Issues,* 37 (1981), 705–712. [16]

Sanford, L. T. *The Silent Children*. Garden City, N.Y.: Doubleday, 1980. [16]

Saral, R., W. H. Burns, O. L. Laskin, G. W. Santos, and P. S. Lietman. "Acyclovir Prophylaxis of Herpes-Simplex-Virus Infection," *New England Journal of Medicine,* 305 (1981), 63–67. [17]

Sarrel, P. M., and W. H. Masters. "Sexual Molestation of Men by Women," *Archives of Sexual Behavior,* 11 (1982), 117–131. [16]

Sarrel, P., and L. Sarrel. "The *Redbook* Report on Sexual Relationships," *Redbook,* 150 (October 1980), 73–80. [13]

Scanzoni, J., and G. L. Fox. "Sex Roles, Family, and Society: The Seventies and Beyond," *Journal of Marriage and the Family,* 42 (1980), 743–756. [1]

Scanzoni, J., and M. Szinovacz. *Family Decision-Making: A Developmental Sex Role Model*. Beverly Hills, Calif.: Sage, 1980. [13]

Schell, R. E., and E. Hall. *Developmental Psychology Today*. 4th ed. New York: Random House, 1983. [1, 13]

Schiavi, R. C., C. Fisher, D. White, P. Beers, M. Fogel, and R. Szechter. "Hormonal Variations During Sleep in Men with Erectile Dysfunction and Normal Controls," *Archives of Sexual Behavior,* 11 (1982), 189–200. [4, 7]

Schiavi, R. C., and D. White. "Androgen and Male Sexual Function: A Review of Human Studies," *Journal of Sex and Marital Therapy,* 2 (1976), 214–228. [4]

Schiller, P. *Creative Approach to Sex Education and Counseling*. 2nd ed. Chicago: Follett, 1977. [11]

Schonbuch, S. S., and R. E. Schell. "Judgments of Body Appearance by Fat and Skinny Male College Students," *Perceptual and Motor Skills,* 24 (1967), 999–1002. [6]

Schram, D. D. "Rape." In J. R. Chapman and M. Gates (eds.), *The Victimization of Women.* Beverly Hills, Calif.: Sage, 1978, pp. 53–79. [16]

Schreeder, M. T. "Hepatitis B in Homosexual Men: Prevalence of Infection and Factors Related to Transmission," *Journal of Infectious Diseases,* 146 (1982), 7–15. [17]

Schulman, H. "Common Discomforts of Pregnancy," *Childbirth Educator,* 1 (Spring 1982), 11–12. [20]

Schumacher, S., and C. W. Lloyd. "Physiological and Psychological Factors in Impotence," *Journal of Sex Research,* 17 (1981), 40–53. [14]

Schwartz, M. F., J. Money, and K. Robinson. "Biosocial Perspectives on the Development of the Proceptive, Acceptive, and Conceptive Phases of Eroticism," *Journal of Sex and Marital Therapy,* 7 (1981), 243–255. [2]

Sears, R. R., E. E. Maccoby, and H. Levin. *Patterns of Child-Rearing.* Evanston, Ill.: Row, Peterson, 1957. [11]

Secondi, J. J. *For People Who Make Love: A Doctor's Guide to Sexual Health.* New York: Taplinger, 1975. [17]

Seemanova, E. "A Study of Children of Incestuous Matings," *Human Heredity,* 21 (1971), 108–128. [16]

Seibel, M. M., and M. L. Taymor. "Emotional Aspects of Infertility," *Fertility and Sterility,* 37 (February 1982), 137–145. [20]

Selkin, J. "Rape: When to Fight Back," *Psychology Today,* 8 (January 1975), 71–76. [16]

Semans, J. H. "Premature Ejaculation: A New Approach," *Southern Medical Journal,* 49 (1956), 353–357. [14]

Sevely, J. L., and J. W. Bennett. "Concerning Female Ejaculation and the Female Prostate," *Journal of Sex Research,* 14 (1978), 1–20. [5]

Shanor, K. *The Shanor Study: The Sexual Sensitivity of the American Male.* New York: Dial Press, 1978. [5, 7, 8]

Sherfey, M. J. *The Nature and Evolution of Female Sexuality.* New York: Vintage Books, 1973. [3, 8]

Shiono, P. H., S. Harlap, and S. Ramcharan. "Sex of Offspring of Women Using Oral Contraceptives, Rhythm, and Other Methods of Birth Control Around the Time of Conception." *Fertility and Sterility,* 37 (1982), 367–372. [19]

Shipman, A. "The Psychodynamics of Sex Education." In R. E. Muuss (ed.), *Adolescent Behavior and Society: A Book of Readings.* New York: Random House, 1971. [12]

Silber, S. J. *How to Get Pregnant.* New York: Scribner, 1980. [20]

Silber, S. J. *The Male: From Infancy to Old Age.* New York: Scribner, 1981. [4, 18]

Simpson, G. M., J. H. Blair, and D. Amuso. "Effects of Antidepressants on Genito-Urinary Function," *Diseases of the Nervous System,* 26 (1965), 787–789. [18]

Singer, M. I. "Comparison of Indicators of Homosexuality on the MMPI," *Journal of Consulting and Clinical Psychology,* 34 (1970), 15–18. [9]

Sintchak, G., and J. Geer. "A Vaginal Plethysmograph System," *Psychophysiology,* 12 (1975), 113–115. [5]

Slater, P. *Footholds.* New York: Dutton, 1977. [1]

Sloane, E. *Biology of Women.* New York: Wiley, 1980. [6]

Smith, D. "Spinal Cord Injury." In D. G. Bullard and S. E. Knight (eds.), *Sexuality and Physical Disability: Personal Perspectives.* St. Louis: C. V. Mosby, 1981, pp. 12–16. [18]

Smith, T. M. "Sexual Psychosocial Approaches to the AIDS Epidemic Among Gay Men," *Official Newsletter of the National Coalition of Gay STDS Services,* 4 (October 1982), 14–17. [17]

Socarides, C. W. *Beyond Sexual Freedom*. New York: Quadrangle Books, 1975. [17]

Solberg, D. A., J. Butler, and N. A. Wagner. "Sexual Behavior in Pregnancy." In J. LoPiccolo and L. LoPiccolo (eds.), *Handbook of Sex Therapy*. New York: Plenum, 1978. [20]

Sorenson, R. C. *Adolescent Sexuality in Contemporary America*. New York: World Books, 1973. [7, 12]

Spain, J. "Psychological Aspects of Contraceptive Use in Teenage Girls." In B. L. Blum (ed.), *Psychological Aspects of Pregnancy, Birthing, and Bonding*. New York: Human Sciences Press, 1980, pp. 67–83. [19]

Spanier, G. B., and R. A. Lewis. "Marital Quality: A Review of the Seventies," *Journal of Marriage and the Family*, 42 (1980), 825–839. [13]

Spark, R. F., R. A. White, and P. B. Connolly. "Impotence Is Not Always Psychogenic: Newer Insights into Hypothalamic-Pituitary-Gonadal Dysfunction," *Journal of the American Medical Association*, 243 (1980), 750–755. [14]

Spence, J. T. "Traits, Roles, and the Concept of Androgyny." In J. E. Gullahorn (ed.), *Psychology and Women: In Transition*. Washington, D.C.: Winston, 1979, pp. 167–188. [1]

Spence, J. T., and R. L. Helmreich. "Masculine Instrumentality and Feminine Expressiveness: Their Relationship with Sex Role Attitudes and Behavior," *Psychology of Women Quarterly*, 5 (1980), 147–163. [1]

Spence, J. T., and R. L. Helmreich. "Theoretical Notes: Androgyny Versus Gender Schema: A Comment on Bem's Gender Schema Theory," *Psychological Review*, 88 (1981), 365–368. [1]

Sprenkle, D. H., and D. L. Weis. "Extramarital Sexuality: Implications for Marital Therapy," *Journal of Sex and Marital Therapy*, 3 (1978), 279–291. [13]

Staples, R. "A Study of the Influence of Liberal Conservative Attitudes on the Premarital Sexual Standards of Different Racial, Sex Role, and Social Class Groupings." Doctoral dissertation. University of Minnesota, 1971. [2]

Staples, R. "Research on Black Sexuality: Its Implications for Family Life, Sex Education, and Public Policy," *Family Coordinator*, 21 (April 1972), 183–188. [2]

Starr, B. D., and M. B. Weiner. *The Starr-Weiner Report on Sex and Sexuality in the Mature Years*. New York: Stein and Day, 1981. [13]

Stein, M. L. "Prostitution." In J. Money and H. Musaph (eds.), *Handbook of Sexology*. Amsterdam: Elsevier/North Holland Biomedical Press, 1977, pp. 1069–1085. [16]

Stein, P. "Singlehood: An Alternative to Marriage," *Family Coordinator*, 24 (1975), 489–505. [13]

Stein, R. A. "The Effect of Exercise Training on Heart Rate During Coitus in the Postmyocardial Infarction Patient," *Circulation*, May 1977. [18]

Steinman, D. L., J. P. Wincze, B. Sakheim, D. H. Barlow, and M. Mavissakalian. "A Comparison of Male and Female Patterns of Sexual Arousal," *Archives of Sexual Behavior*, 10 (1981), 529–547. [6]

Stock, W. E., and J. H. Geer. "A Study of Fantasy-Based Sexual Arousal in Women," *Archives of Sexual Behavior*, 11 (1982), 33–47. [7]

Stoller, R. J. *Sex and Gender: On the Development of Masculinity and Femininity*. New York: Science House, 1968. [1]

Storaska, F. *How to Say No to a Rapist . . . and Survive*. New York: Random House, 1975. [16]

Storms, M. D. "Theories of Sexual Orientation," *Journal of Personality and Social Psychology*, 38 (1980), 783–792. [9]

Streissguth, A. P., S. Landesman-Dwyer, J. C. Martin, and D. W. Smith. "Teratogenic Effects of Alcohol in Humans and Laboratory Animals," *Science*, 209 (1980), 353–361. [20]

Sue, D. "Erotic Fantasies of College Students During Coitus," *Journal of Sex Research,* 15 (1979), 299–305. [7]

Suomi, S. J., and H. F. Harlow. "The Role and Reason of Peer Relationships in Rhesus Monkeys." In M. Lewis and L. A. Rosenblum (eds.), *Friendship and Peer Relations.* New York: Wiley, 1975, pp. 153–185. [11]

Sussman, L., and E. Bordwell. *The Rapist File.* New York: Chelsea House, 1981. [16]

Sussman, N. "Sex and Sexuality in History." In B. J. Sadock, H. I. Kaplan, and A. M. Freedman (eds.), *The Sexual Experience.* Baltimore: Williams & Wilkins, 1976, pp. 7–70. [6, 7]

Symons, D. *The Evolution of Human Sexuality.* New York: Oxford University Press, 1979. [6]

Szasz, T. S. "Legal and Moral Aspects of Homosexuality." In J. Marmor (ed.), *Sexual Inversion.* New York: Basic Books, 1965, pp. 124–139. [9]

Szasz, T. S. *Sex by Prescription.* New York: Anchor Press, 1980. [14]


Tannahill, R. *Sex In History,* New York: Stein and Day, 1980. [1]

Tanner, J. M. *Fetus into Man.* Cambridge, Mass.: Harvard University Press, 1978. [12]

Tanzer, D. "Natural Childbirth: Pain or Peak Experience?" *Psychology Today,* 2 (October 1968), 17–21+. [20]

Tanzer, D. (with J. L. Block). *Why Natural Childbirth? A Psychologist's Report on the Benefits to Mothers, Fathers, and Babies.* New York: Schocken, 1976. [20]

Tart, C. T. *On Being Stoned: A Psychological Study of Intoxication.* Palo Alto, Calif.: Science and Behavior Books, 1971. [18]

Tavris, C. A. "Women in China: The Speak Bitterness Revolution," *Psychology Today,* 7 (May 1974), 43–49+. [2]

Tavris, C. A. "Men and Women Report Their Views on Masculinity," *Psychology Today,* 10 (January 1977), 34–42+. [1, 6]

Tavris, C. A., and C. W. Offir. *The Longest War: Sex Differences in Perspective.* New York: Harcourt Brace Jovanovich, 1977. [1]

Tavris, C. A., and S. Sadd. *The Redbook Report on Female Sexuality.* New York: Delacorte, 1977. [2, 8, 13]

Tennov, D. *Love and Limerence: The Experience of Being in Love.* New York: Stein and Day, 1979. [2]

Terkel, S. *Working.* New York: Avon Books, 1976. [16]

Thompson, S. K. "Gender Labels and Early Sex Role Development," *Child Development,* 46 (1975), 339–347. [11]

Thorburg, H. *Teenage Pregnancies: Have They Reached Epidemic Proportions?.* Phoenix: Arizona Governor's Council on Children, Youth and Families, 1979. [12]

Thornton, V. "Growing Up with Cerebral Palsy." In D. B. Bullard and S. E. Knight (eds.), *Sexuality and Physical Disability: Personal Perspectives.* St. Louis: C. V. Mosby, 1981, pp. 26–30. [18]

Tiefer, L. "The Kiss," *Human Nature,* 1 (July 1978), 28–37. [8]

Tiefer, L. "A Survey of College Women's Experiences with and Attitudes Toward Pelvic Examinations," *Women and Health,* 4 (1979), 385–395. [6]

Tietze, C. "Induced Abortion." In J. Money and H. Musaph (eds.), *Handbook of Sexology.* Amsterdam: Elsevier/North Holland Biomedical Press, 1977, pp. 605–620. [19]

Tollison, C. D., and H. E. Adams. *Sexual Disorders: Treatment, Theory, and Research.* New York: Gardner Press, 1979. [15]

Tripp, C. A. *The Homosexual Matrix.* New York: McGraw-Hill, 1975. [9]

Tsai, M., S. Feldman-Summers, and M. Edgar. "Childhood Molestation: Variables Related to Differential Impacts on Psychosexual Functioning in Adult Women," *Journal of Abnormal Psychology,* 88 (1979), 407–417. [16]

Tsibris, J. C. M., J. L. Thomason, A. Kunigk, R. S. Khan-Dawood, C. V. Kirschner, and W. N. Spellacy. "Guiacol Peroxidase Levels in Human Cervical Mucus: A Possible Predictor of Ovulation," *Contraception,* 25 (1982), 59–67. [19]

Udry, J. R. "Changes in the Frequency of Marital Intercourse from Panel Data," *Archives of Sexual Behavior,* 9 (1980), 319–325. [13]

U.S. Bureau of the Census. *Marital Status and Living Arrangements:* March 1980 (Current Population Reports, Series P-20, No. 365). Washington, D.C.: U.S. Government Printing Office, 1981. [13]

U.S. Public Health Service. "Nonreported Sexually Transmitted Disease—United States," *MMWR: Morbidity and Mortality Weekly Report,* 28 (February 16, 1979), 61–63. [17]

U.S. Public Health Service. *STD Fact Sheet.* Edition 35. HHS Publication No. (CDC) 8–8195. Atlanta, 1980. [17]

U.S. Public Health Service. "Follow-up on Toxic Shock Syndrome: United States," *MMWR: Morbidity and Mortality Weekly Report,* 29 (1980), 297–299. [3]

U.S. Public Health Service. "Genital Herpes Infection—United States, 1966–1979," *MMWR: Morbidity and Mortality Weekly Report,* 31 (March 26, 1982a), 137–139. [17]

U.S. Public Health Service. "Sexually Transmitted Diseases: Treatment Guidelines," *MMWR: Morbidity and Mortality Weekly Report,* 31 (August 20, 1982b), 35S-62S. [17]

U.S. Public Health Service. "Oral Contraceptives and Cancer Risk," *MMWR: Morbidity and Mortality Weekly Report,* 31 (1982), 393. [19]

U.S. Public Health Service: "Update on Acquired Immune Deficiency Syndrome (AIDS)—United States," *MMWR: Morbidity and Mortality Weekly Report,* 31 (1982), 507–514. [9, 17]

Vance, E. B., and N. W. Wagner. "Written Descriptions of Orgasm: A Study of Sex Difference," *Archives of Sexual Behavior,* 5 (1976), 87–98. [5]

Van de Velde, T. H. *Ideal Marriage: Its Physiology and Technique.* New York: Random House, 1957 (orig. pub. 1926). [5, 8]

Wabrek, A. J., and C. J. Wabrek. "Mastectomy: Sexual Implications," *Primary Care,* 3 (1976), 803. [18]

Wagner, G., J. Hilsted, and S. B. Jensen. "Diabetes Mellitus and Erectile Failure." In G. Wagner and R. Green (eds.), *Impotence: Physiological, Psychological, Surgical Diagnosis and Treatment.* New York: Plenum, 1981. [18]

Wagner, N. M. "Sexual Activity and the Cardiac Patient." In R. Green (ed.), *Human Sexuality: A Health Practitioner's Text.* Baltimore: Williams & Wilkins, 1975, pp. 173–180. [18]

Wahl, P., C. Walden, R. Knopp, J. Hoover, R. Wallace, G. Heiss, and B. Rifkind. "Effect of Estrogen/Progestin Potency on Lipid/Lipoprotein Cholesterol," *New England Journal of Medicine,* 308 (1983), 862–867. [19]

Walfish, S., and M. Myerson. "Sex Role Identity and Attitudes Toward Sexuality," *Archives of Sexual Behavior,* 9 (1980), 199–203. [1]

Walinder, J., and I. Thuwe. *A Social-Psychiatric Follow-up Study of 24 Sex Reassigned Transsexuals.* Copenhagen: Scandinavian University Books, 1975. [15]

Wallerstein, E. *Circumcision: An American Health Fallacy.* New York: Springer, 1980. [4]

Walster, E., and G. W. Walster. *A New Look at Love.* Reading, Mass.: Addison-Wesley, 1978. [2]

Watson, J. S., L. A. Hayes, L. Dorman, and P. Vietze. "Infant Sex Differences in Operant Fixation with Visual and Auditory Reinforcement," *Infant Behavior and Development,* 3 (1980), 107–114. [11]

Webb, L. J., C. C. DiClemente, E. E. Johnstone, J. L. Sanders, and R. A. Perley (eds.). *DSM-III Training Guide.* New York: Brunner/Mazel, 1981. [15]

Weinberg, M. S., and C. J. Williams. *Male Homosexuals.* New York: Oxford University Press, 1974. [9]

Weiss, H. D. "The Physiology of Human Penile Erection," *Annals of Internal Medicine,* 76 (1972), 793–799. [5]

Wentworth, H., and S. B. Flexner. *Dictionary of American Slang.* 2nd ed. New York: Crowell, 1975. [6]

Westoff, C. F. "Coital Frequency and Contraception," *Family Planning Perspectives,* 6 (1974), 136–141. [19]

Whalen, R. E. "Cyclic Changes in Hormones and Behavior," *Archives of Sexual Behavior,* 4 (1975), 313–314. [3]

White, D. "Pursuit of the Ultimate Aphrodisiac," *Psychology Today,* 15 (September 1981), 9–12. [6]

White, S. E., and K. Reamy. "Sexuality and Pregnancy: A Review," *Archives of Sexual Behavior,* 11 (1982), 429–444. [20]

Wilsnack, S. C. "Alcohol, Sexuality, and Reproductive Dysfunction in Women." In E. L. Abel (ed.), *Fetal Alcohol Syndrome.* Vol. 2. *Human Studies.* Boca Raton, Fla.: CRC Press, 1982, pp. 21–46. [18]

Wilson, G. T. "The Effects of Alcohol on Human Sexual Behavior." In N. K. Mello (ed.), *Advances in Substance Abuse.* Vol. 2. Greenwich, Conn.: JAI Press, 1981, pp. 1–40. [18]

Winick, C. "Some Observations of Patrons of Adult Theaters and Bookstores," *Technical Reports of the Commission on Obscenity and Pornography.* Vol. 4. Washington, D.C.: U.S. Government Printing Office, 1970. [16]

Witzig, J. S. "The Group Treatment of Male Exhibitionists," *American Journal of Psychiatry,* 125 (1970), 179–185. [15]

Wolfe, L. *The Cosmo Report.* New York: Arbor House, 1981. [2, 5, 7–8, 13]

Wolfe, L. "The Good News," *New York,* December 28, 1981–January 4, 1982, pp. 33–35. [13]

Wong, H. "Typologies of Intimacy," *Psychology of Women Quarterly,* 5 (1981), 435–443. [2]

Woolsey, J. M. "Opinion A. 110-59," *United States v. One Book Called "Ulysses."* In James Joyce, *Ulysses.* New York: Random House, 1934. [16]

Working Women United Institute. *Sexual Harassment on the Job: Results of a Preliminary Survey.* Ithaca, N.Y.: Working Women United Institute, 1975. [16]


Yang, R. K., and H. A. Moss. "Neonatal Precursors of Infant Behavior," *Developmental Psychology,* 14 (1978), 607–613. [11]

Yankelovich, D. *New Rules.* New York: Random House, 1981. [13]

Yorburg, B. *Sexual Identity: Sex Roles and Social Change.* New York: Wiley, 1974. [1]

Young, M. "Attitudes and Behavior of College Students Relative to Oral-Genital Sexuality," *Archives of Sexual Behavior,* 9 (1980), 61–67. [8]


Zelnick, M., J. F. Kantner, and K. Ford. *Sex and Pregnancy in Adolescence.* Beverly Hills, Calif.: Sage, 1981. [12, 19]

Zelnick, M., and J. Y. Kim. "Sex Education and Its Association with Teenage Sexual Activity, Pregnancy, and Contraceptive Use," *Family Planning Perspectives,* 14 (1982), 117–126. [12]

Zilbergeld, B. *Male Sexuality: A Guide to Sexual Fulfillment*. Boston: Little, Brown, 1978. [1, 4, 6–8, 10, 14, 19]

Zilbergeld, B. "Pursuit of the Grafenberg Spot," *Psychology Today,* 16 (1982), 82–84. [3, 5]

Zilbergeld, B., and C. R. Ellison. "Desire Discrepancies and Arousal Problems in Sex Therapy." In S. R. Leiblum and L. A. Pervin (eds.), *Principles and Practices of Sex Therapy.* New York: Guilford Press, 1980, pp. 65–101. [14]

Zilbergeld, B., and M. Evans. "The Inadequacy of Masters and Johnson," *Psychology Today,* 14 (August 1980), 28–43. [14]

Zohar, J., D. Meiraz, B. Maoz, and N. Durst. "Factors Influencing Sexual Activity After Prostatectomy: A Prospective Study," *Journal of Urology,* 116 (1976), 332–334. [18]

Zuckerman, M. "Research on Pornography." In W. W. Oaks, G. A. Melchiode, and I. I. Ficher (eds.), *Sex and the Life Cycle.* New York: Grune and Stratton, 1976, pp. 147–161. [17]

Zuckerman, M., R. Tushup, and S. Finner. "Sexual Attitudes and Experience: Attitude and Personality Correlates and Changes Produced by a Course in Sexuality," *Journal of Consulting and Clinical Psychology,* 44 (1976), 7–19. [12]

# Index

## About the Authors

**Raymond Charles Rosen**, since receiving his Ph.D. in clinical psychology from SUNY at Stony Brook in 1972, has taught on the faculty at Rutgers Medical School and Rutgers University. In addition to his clinical position as co-director of the Sexual Counselling Service, he has taught courses in human sexuality and behavioral science. Dr. Rosen's major research interest has been in the psychophysiology of sexual response for which he has received a number of research grants; in addition, he has numerous professional publications in this field. In 1976, he was elected a member of the International Academy of Sex Research. In 1982 he was appointed chairman of the N.I.M.H. Review Committee on Sexual Assault.

**Elizabeth Hall** is the co-author of *Developmental Psychology Today* (3rd ed.) and *Child Psychology Today*. Before she turned to college textbooks, she was Editor-in-Chief of *Human Nature*, a magazine about the human sciences. From 1967 to 1976, she was with *Psychology Today*, and was Managing Editor of that magazine at the time she left to start *Human Nature*. As a science writer, Hall has interviewed many prominent psychologists, including Jean Piaget, Bärbel Inhelder, Jerome Bruner, B. F. Skinner, D. O. Hebb, George A. Miller, Bruno Bettelheim, Joseph Adelson, and Bernice Neugarten. She has also written a number of books for children; two of them, *Why Do We Do What We Do: A Look at Psychology* and *From Pigeons to People: A Look at Behavior Shaping*, received Honorable Mention in the American Psychological Foundation's National Media Awards. Hall was graduated with highest honors from California State University, Fresno, in 1962.